ATHEROGENESIS

VOLUME II

ATHEROGENESIS

VOLUME II

PROCEEDINGS OF THE SECOND INTERNATIONAL SYMPOSIUM ON ATHEROGENESIS, THROMBOGENESIS AND PYRIDINOLCARBAMATE TREATMENT

Tokyo, 18–20 May 1972

UNDER THE AUSPICES OF
THE JAPAN ARTERIOSCLEROSIS RESEARCH FOUNDATION

Edited by

T. SHIMAMOTO / F. NUMANO
Tokyo, Japan

and

G. M. ADDISON
Cardiff, United Kingdom

EXCERPTA MEDICA

International Congress Series No. 269

ISBN Excerpta Medica 90 219 0222 2
ISBN American Elsevier 0-444-15007-2
Library of Congress Catalog Card Number 72-96568

Publisher: Excerpta Medica
335 Jan van Galenstraat
Amsterdam
P.O. Box 1126

Sole Distributors for the USA and Canada:
American Elsevier Publishing Company, Inc.
52 Vanderbilt Avenue
New York, N.Y. 10017

Printed in The Netherlands by Reidel, Dordrecht

SECOND INTERNATIONAL SYMPOSIUM ON ATHEROGENESIS, THROMBOGENESIS AND PYRIDINOLCARBAMATE TREATMENT

ORGANIZING COMMITTEE

President: TAKIO SHIMAMOTO, M.D.
General Secretary: FUJIO NUMANO, M.D.

CONTENTS

II. Clinical Studies on the Treatment of Atherosclerosis and Thrombosis

PREFACE

This book is a record of the Proceedings of the Second International Symposium on Atherogenesis, Thrombogenesis and Pyridinolcarbamate Treatment held in Tokyo in 1972, in which atherogenesis was discussed mainly from a quite different point of view compared with other symposia of this kind.

Almost 20 years ago, Louis N. Katz destroyed the historical dogma that atherosclerosis is an incurable and inevitable aging process. He clearly demonstrated in his brilliant experiments, carried out in collaboration with Jeremiah Stamler, Ruth Pick and others, that atherosclerosis is a preventable and curable disease. With this as turning point, many risk factors involved in atherosclerosis have since been found and especially hyperlipemia or hypercholesterolemia has been extensivcly studied.

However, the mechanism involved in these risk factors has not yet been elucidated, so that, generally speaking, no specific treatment has been available – only desperate efforts to avoid or reduce risk factors in the treatment of atherosclerosis. As a result, the increasing incidence of premature death due to atherosclerosis is still a common problem in every civilized country.

In this Symposium the most essential problems in atherogenesis, namely how so-called 'risk factors' act on the arterial wall, how they promote the infiltration of cholesterol-bearing lipoproteins and various plasma proteins causing inflammation into the arterial wall, how this infiltration can be prevented, and how established atherosclerosis can be treated, were discussed and historically first answered to some extent.

In relation to these problems, contraction of endothelial cells was first highlighted at this Symposium and the efficacy of treatment of atherosclerotic disorders with the endothelial cell relaxant, pyridinolcarbamate, was reported and discussed.

From these papers and discussions some suggestions will be found on developing further research on the treatment of various atherosclerotic disorders and related severe conditions like diabetic angiopathy. This was our aim in publishing the Proceedings of this Symposium on 'Atherogenesis'.

February, 1973

TAKIO SHIMAMOTO

President of the Second International Symposium on Atherogenesis, Thrombogenesis and Pyridinolcarbamate Treatment

I

BASIC STUDIES ON ATHEROGENESIS AND THROMBOGENESIS

THE CONTRACTION AND BLEBBING OF ENDOTHELIAL CELLS ACCOMPANIED BY ACUTE INFILTRATION OF PLASMA SUBSTANCES INTO THE VESSEL WALL AND THEIR PREVENTION

TAKIO SHIMAMOTO and TOSHIAKI SUNAGA
Institute for Cardiovascular Diseases, Medical School, Tokyo Ika-Shika National University, Tokyo, Japan

The most important physiological functions of vascular endothelial cells, such as repelling function against the blood and blood corpuscles as well as active selective permeability, have been shown to be reduced or temporarily impaired by a single administration of atherogenic substances such as cholesterol, saturated fat and adrenaline (Shimamoto, 1960, 1963; Shimamoto et al., 1959). As a consequence, the large arteries exhibit an edematous change in their subendothelial space and often in the medial layers and the sticking of platelets to endothelial cells can be observed by histochemical techniques and transmission electron microscopy. The immediate response of animals to the challenge with atherogenic substances, such as cholesterol, saturated fat, adrenaline, angiotensin, etc. or to traumatic stress, has been called the 'edematous arterial reaction' by the author since 1958 (Shimamoto, 1963, 1969*a*). At the same time, the sticking and margination of platelets and leukocytes were also observed in the capillaries, arterioles and venules by a cinematographic technique in the mesentery or ear (Sandison-Clark's technique) (Shimamoto, 1960). These changes are always accompanied by enhancement of platelet aggregability and blood coagulability and all these alterations were prevented by pyridinolcarbamate (10 mg/kg) in the rabbit (Shimamoto, 1969*b*, 1972*a*, *b*; Shimamoto et al., 1971).

In previous experiments with rabbits and cockerels, the author (Shimamoto, 1969*b*) injected horseradish peroxidase intravenously as a marker to observe transendothelial transport of these large particles into the subendothelial space of the aorta and found that the infiltration of such large particles (40 Å) into the subendothelial space takes place mainly through the intercellular junction of endothelial cells of the aorta. The protein was also transported into the subendothelial space by a vesicle system of endothelial cells, but this was rather small in amount. Thus the plasma substance, infiltrated into the subendothelial and medial layers after a single-dose treatment of animals with adrenaline and cholesterol, was reasonably considered to be transported mainly through the intercellular junction of endothelial cells, producing the edematous arterial reaction (Shimamoto, 1963). Such evidence shows the importance of regulation by endothelial cells of the transendothelial transport of plasma substances into the blood vessel wall as well as the extravascular space.

In order to see the effect of single-dose treatment of animals with adrenaline and cholesterol on the endothelial cells, the author used a scanning and transmission electron microscope and the morphological changes of endothelial cells were re-examined in this experiment, because the combination of scanning and transmission electron-microscopic observation yields better information than independent observation with either of these methods. At the same time, the author utilized the immunofluorescent technique to watch the alteration in the regulatory activity of endothelial cells on the transendothelial transport of plasma proteins into the aortic wall which is induced by the above-mentioned challenges.

I. SCANNING AND TRANSMISSION ELECTRON-MICROSCOPIC OBSERVATION

A. Materials and methods

50 rabbits weighing 1.6 ~ 2.7 kg were divided into 5 groups of 10 animals each. Those of the first group received adrenaline (1 μg/kg i.v.) and were sacrificed 30 min thereafter. The same experiment was performed on the second group after pretreatment with pyridinolcarbamate (10 mg/kg p.o.) 1 hour before the challenge without anesthesia. The third group received cholesterol (1 g/kg p.o.) before anesthesia and they were sacrificed 2 hours after, under the anesthetic. The same experiment was performed on the fourth group except that pyridinolcarbamate (10 mg/kg p.o.) pretreatment was given 1 hour before the challenge without anesthesia. The fifth group received placebo (starch powder in 2 animals 2 hours before sacrifice without anesthesia and saline injection 30 min before sacrifice in 3 animals under anesthesia) as the control. The other 3 animals received angiotensin II (1 μg/kg i.v.) and were sacrificed 30 minutes thereafter. For the fixation of the arterial wall, all animals were anesthetized with 1.5 ml/kg of 60% urethane given intraperitoneally, the chest and abdomen were opened under anesthesia and a polyethylene tube (3 mm in diameter) was rapidly introduced into the ascending aorta through the left ventricle of the heart. Into the aorta was infused 500 ml of ice-cold 2.5% glutaraldehyde in isotonic phosphate buffer (pH 7.4) for 15 min under a pressure of 110 mm Hg; immediately after the start of perfusion with glutaraldehyde, the abdominal aorta was incised to allow the outflow of the perfusate. After the perfusion of the thoracic aorta, the aorta with heart was removed and the thoracic aorta was isolated. The lumen was rinsed with the ice-cold fixative and samples of aortic specimens were taken from the middle section of the dorsal part of the thoracic aorta at the level of the orifice of the second intercostal artery, and from the orifice of either the left or the right second intercostal artery. The specimens were cut into 5 blocks of 2 × 4 mm and the blocks were rinsed in the phosphate buffer with 0.25 M sucrose (pH 7.4) for 10 hours; then they were transferred into 1% osmium tetroxide in veronal buffer containing 0.25 M sucrose (pH 7.4) for 1–2 hours at 0°C. They were refrigerated for 1 hour, followed by dehydration in graded acetone solutions. After air drying, a coat of about 100 Å of gold was deposited. The specimens were studied with scanning electron microscopes (JSM-II and JSM-UIII) using a beam voltage of 5 ~ 25 kV. The focal distance was set at × 100 magnification, under which the details of endothelial surface, including crater-like structures (Nelson et al., 1972), were not recognizable. The center area of the field was automatically photographed at × 1,000 magnification. In this way, one photograph covering 1,000 μ^2 of endothelial surface from 2 different fields was obtained at random from each specimen. Thus, 10 photographs covering 10,000 μ^2 were obtained from each of the 2 parts of thoracic aorta for the present study.

In order to verify the results obtained by scanning electron-microscopic observation, the same area, i.e. the middle of the dorsal part of the thoracic area approximately at the level of the orifice of the second intercostal artery, was subjected to transmission electron-microscopic analysis using the same animals of all groups. In transmission electron micrography the same procedure of sampling and fixation was used, but after postfixation with osmium tetroxide, the blocks were washed with 50% ethanol and stained with saturated uranyl acetate for 30 min. Then the blocks were dehydrated in graded ethanol in the usual way and embedded in Epon by Luft's procedure. In order to make the horizontal or longitudinal section along the axis of the aorta the blocks were carefully trimmed to take the respective cutting plane. The blocks were cut with a diamond knife on a Sorvall Porter MT2-ultramicrotome. Sections were stained in lead citrate and examined in a Hitachi 11A electron microscope.

50 endothelial cells from 5 different blocks from each animal of all groups were photographed at random. After photography, blind observation was done, focussing attention on the morphological changes including those of individual endothelial cells, bleb formation, changes in protoplasm and nuclei, and subendothelial edema.

B. Results

1. Scanning electron-microscopic observation The results obtained were essentially the same as in the former observation. The endothelial surface in animals treated with either adrenaline or cholesterol seemed swollen, and sticking of platelets was observed at the same time. On the other hand, these changes were absent or minimal in the placebo control group and they were also markedly reduced in groups treated with either adrenaline or cholesterol after pyridinolcarbamate pretreatment.

The most important finding of the present observation was the appearance of areas of 800 to over 1,000 μ^2 with fine groove-like lines crossing the aortic lumen vertically on the surface of each endothelial cell in specimens from 9 of 10 animals given cholesterol ($p < 0.01$), from 8 of 10 animals given adrenaline ($p < 0.01$), and from all 3 animals given angiotensin. The distance between neighboring vertical groove-like lines was 0.6–1.8 μ, and the depth of the lines was 0.2–0.3 μ. There were also horizontally running groove-like lines, which were usually much smaller than vertical grooves; however, in certain areas, they dominated the vertical grooves, especially on the surface of some nuclear parts of endothelial cells of these areas. The distance between the groove-like lines was 0.4–1.5 μ, and the depth of the lines was 0.2–1 μ. The groove-like structures of each cell start from the cell boundaries and sometimes seem to connect with the same structure of the neighboring cells crossing the cell boundary, but there is usually no such direct connection and many groove-like structures are independent in each endothelial cell as shown in Figure 2. Lines were absent in 9 of all 10 animals given placebo and also in the 10 animals given cholesterol and in 8 of the 10 animals given adrenaline after pretreatment with pyridinolcarbamate, and the preventive effect of pyridinolcarbamate is statistically significant ($p < 0.01$ in both groups) as shown in Table I.

Crater-like structures were recognized in the scanning electron micrographs of the specimens obtained from all 5 groups, as shown in Tables I-III. They appeared relatively uniformly in all photographs of the specimens obtained from either the thoracic aorta or the orifices of the intercostal artery, and statistical evaluation was possible.

The crater-like structures appeared somewhat more numerous in the orifice of the intercostal artery, but there was no significant difference. On the other hand, the number of crater-like structures was larger to a statistically significant degree in animals given either

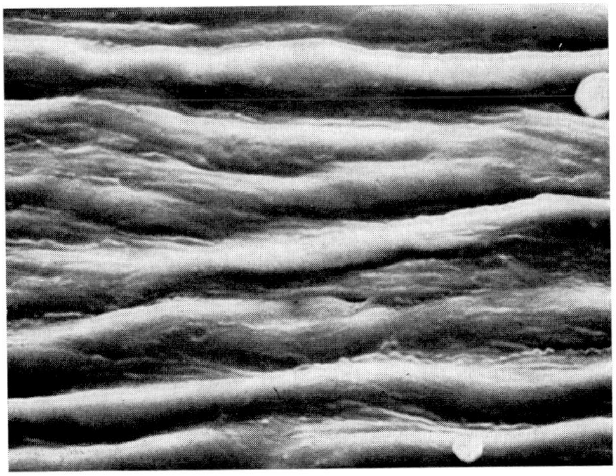

Fig. 1a

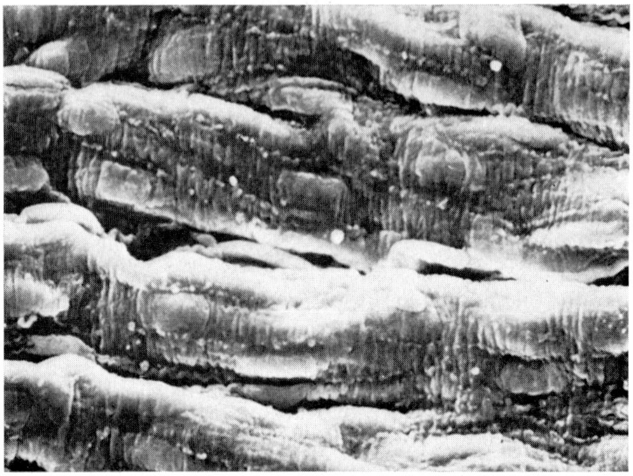

Fig. 1b

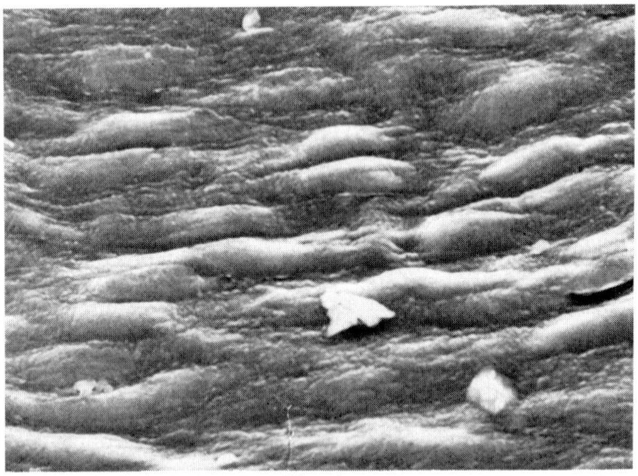

Fig. 1c

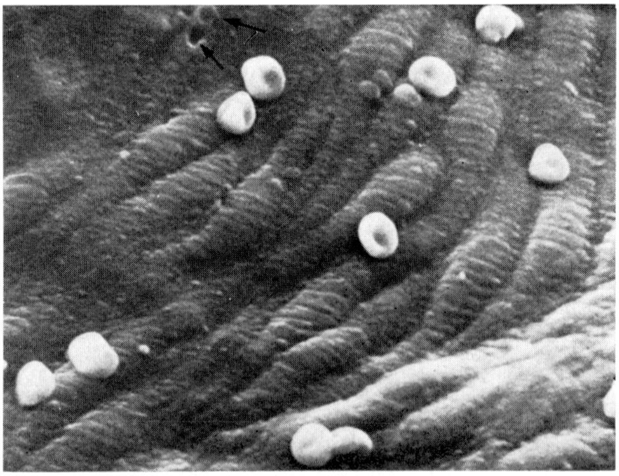

Fig. 1d

Fig. 1. Luminal surface of rabbit aorta (× 1,000). (*a*) Untreated. (*b*) Long-lasting contraction of endothelial cells induced by angiotensin II (1 μg/kg i.v.), (*c*) by adrenaline (1 μg/kg i.v.) and (*d*) cholesterol (1 g/kg p.o.). Crater-like structures (arrows) are seen in Fig. 1*d*.

cholesterol ($p < 0.01$) or adrenaline ($p < 0.01$) as compared with the placebo control group. In the case of cholesterol, relatively large crater-like structures with a diameter over 1 μ were more numerous ($p < 0.01$), while in the case of adrenaline, smaller crater-like structures with a diameter less than 0.5 μ were more numerous compared with the placebo control group ($p < 0.01$).

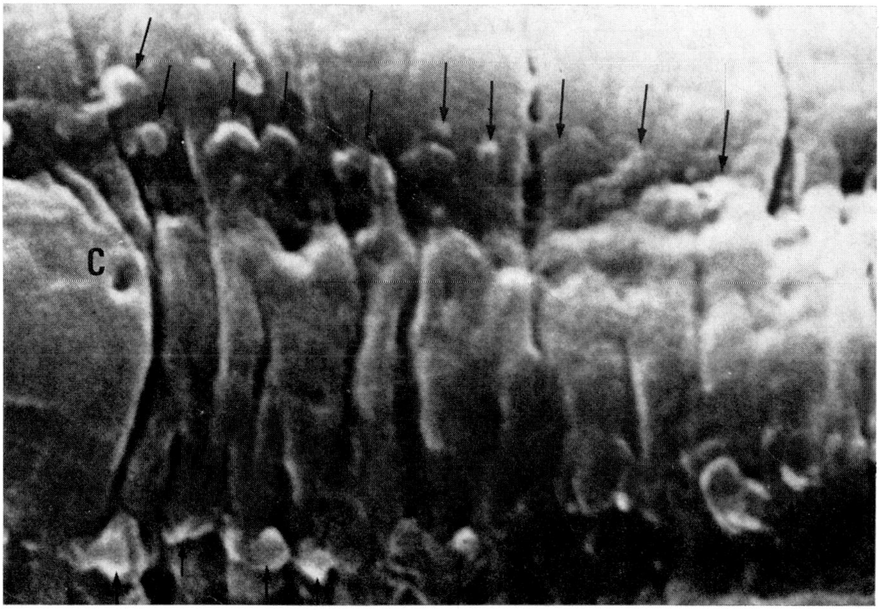

Fig. 2. Enlargement of Fig. 1*b* ($\times$ 21,000). Grooves and bulges are clearly shown in their relationship to the cell boundaries (arrows) and also between neighboring cells. One crater-like structure (C) is also seen.

TABLE I

Groove-like lines in the endothelial surface

Treatment	No. of animals		
	With grooves	Without grooves	Total
Placebo	1	9	10
Cholesterol	9**	1	10
Cholesterol after PDC	0	10††	10
Adrenaline	8*	2	10
Adrenaline after PDC	2	8†	10

PDC = pyridinolcarbamate pretreatment.
* $p < 0.05$, ** $p < 0.01$ Control vs challenged.
† $p < 0.05$, †† $p < 0.01$ Challenged vs challenged after PDC.

TABLE II

Number of crater-like structures with different diameters in scanning electron microscopy of aortic endothelial surface. Preventive effect of pyridinolcarbamate

	Challenge pretreatment \ Diameter of crater-like structures (μ)	<0.5	0.5	1	2	3	4	5	6	7	8	9	10
Thoracic aorta	Placebo control	43	24	15	7	2	2	0	0	0	0	0	0
	Cholesterol (1 g/kg p.o.)	**51**	**51**††	**48**††	**25**††	**12**†	**10**†	**4**†	**7**†	**0**	**0**	**0**	**0**
	Pyridinolcarbamate (10 mg/kg) +cholesterol (1 g/kg p.o.)	35	18**	21**	8**	2*	1*	0*	0*	0	0	0	0
Orifice to second intercostal artery	Placebo control	52	28	20	9	3	1	0	0	0	0	0	0
	Cholesterol (1 g/kg p.o.)	**41**	**62**††	**76**††	**32**††	**13**†	**9**†	**5**†	**8**†	**2**	**0**	**0**	**0**
	Pyridinolcarbamate (10 mg/kg) +cholesterol (1 g/kg p.o.)	43	30**	17**	13**	5*	2*	0*	1*	0	0	0	0

† p<0.05, †† p<0.01 Control vs challenged.
* p<0.05, ** p<0.01 Challenged vs challenged after pyridinolcarbamate.

TABLE III

Number of crater-like structures with different diameters in scanning electron microscopy of aortic endothelial surface. Preventive effect of pyridinolcarbamate

	Challenge pretreatment \ Diameter of crater-like structures (μ)	<0.5	0.5	1	2	3	4	5	6	7	8	9	10
Thoracic aorta	Placebo control	43	24	15	7	2	2	0	0	0	0	0	0
	Adrenaline (1 μg/kg i.v.)	**72**††	**48**††	**16**	**7**	**4**	**4**	**0**	**0**	**0**	**0**	**0**	**0**
	Pyridinolcarbamate (10 mg/kg) +adrenaline (1 μg/kg i.v.)	51	25**	9*	4*	1	2	0	0	0	0	0	0
Orifice to second intercostal artery	Placebo control	52	28	20	9	3	1	0	0	0	0	0	0
	Adrenaline (1 μg/kg i.v.)	**97**††	**77**††	**24**	**10**	**6**	**5**	**2**	0	**0**	**0**	**0**	**0**
	Pyridinolcarbamate (10 mg/kg) +adrenaline (1 μg/kg i.v.)	55	33**	14**	6*	4	3	1	0	0	0	0	0

† p<0.05, †† p<0.01 Control vs challenged.
* p<0.05, ** p<0.01 Challenged vs challenged after pyridinolcarbamate.

In animals pretreated with pyridinolcarbamate the number of crater-like structures showed a statistically significant decrease ($p < 0.01$). As shown in Figure 1, the crater-like structures appeared right on or close to the cell boundary, and this is one of their characteristic features.

2. Transmission electron-microscopic observation. 50 photographs were obtained from the same portions of the thoracic aorta of each animal in all groups and they were statistically analysed. In specimens cut along the long axis of the aorta, a marked unevenness of the surface of endothelial cells was clearly shown in animals of the group treated with adrenaline and angiotensin (Figs. 3 and 5) and in animals of the group treated with cholesterol. This unevenness corresponds quite closely with the fine groove-like lines seen in scanning electron microscopy; at the same time, they often correspond to the unevenness of nuclei as shown in Figure 4. A similar unevenness of cells and nuclei was found in endothelial cells in the sections in the aorta of animals treated with adrenaline, angiotensin and cholesterol. The most remarkable change in nuclei is the appearance of pinches (Majno et al., 1969) in which the opposing surfaces are pressed together so tightly that the opposing nuclear membranes come into contact along a part of the fold. The pinches appeared in $6.2 \pm 1.1\%$ of nuclei of the

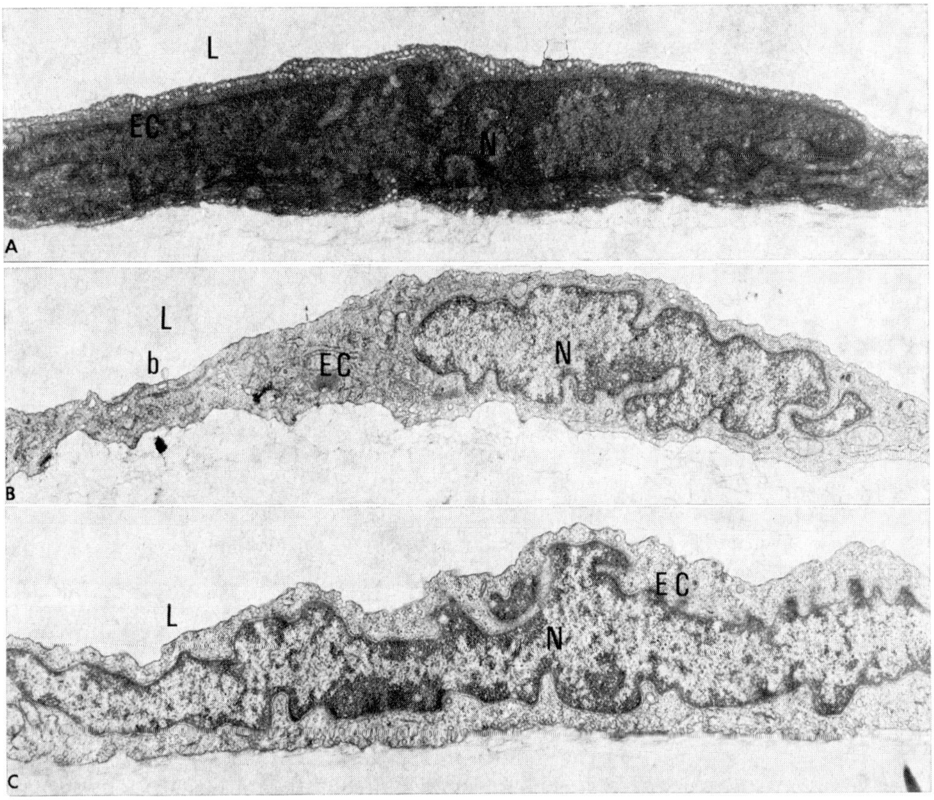

Fig. 3. Section of endothelial cells of aorta of rabbits treated with placebo (A), adrenaline (1 μg/kg i.v.) (B), and angiotensin (1 μg/kg i.v.) (C) showing unevenness of cells and nuclei in (B) and (C). L = vessel lumen, EC = endothelial cell, N = nucleus, b = bleb.

endothelial cells of animals which received cholesterol ($p < 0.001$) and in $2.4 \pm 2.1\%$ of nuclei of the endothelial cells of animals which received adrenaline ($p < 0.01$), while it was not seen in the placebo control group and the groups which received cholesterol or adrenaline after pyridinolcarbamate pretreatment. This unevenness of the surface of endothelial cells accompanied by such nuclear changes seems to represent, morphologically, the contraction of endothelial cells. Actually in the concave parts of the cytoplasm many filament-like structures appeared and the changes in the nuclei characterized by pinches were found only in animals

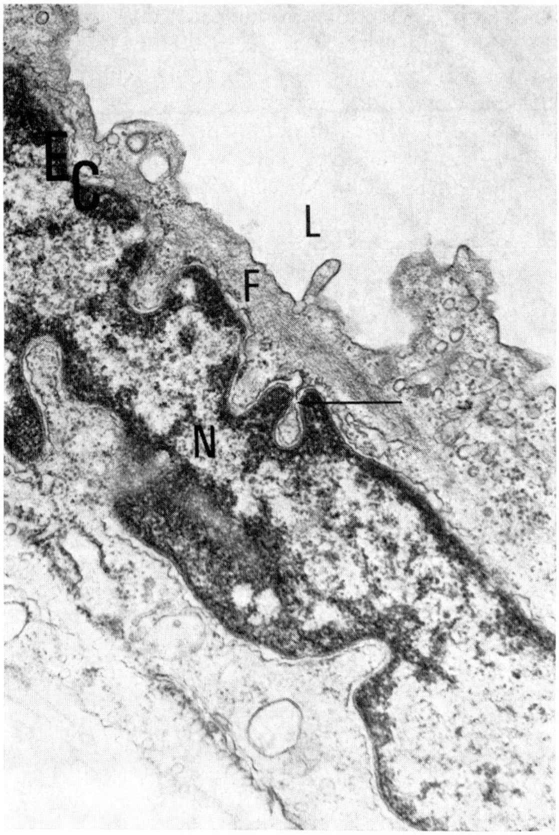

Fig. 4. Endothelial cell fixed in a contracted state, showing severe infolding of its nucleus following appearance of filament-like structures (F) running vertically in neighboring protoplasm. A pinch (arrow) is seen. EC = endothelial cell, L = vessel lumen, N = nucleus.

which received adrenaline, angiotensin and cholesterol. The mean percentage of endothelial cells, showing a certain degree of unevenness as seen in Figures 4 and 8(5) and calculated by a 'blind technique', amounted to 22.3% in the placebo control group, while it increased to 39.0% in the adrenaline group and to 34.5% in the cholesterol group. The mean percentage of endothelial cells showing unevenness of the same degree was reduced to 25.0% and 8.6% in the group given adrenaline or cholesterol respectively after pretreatment with pyridinolcarbamate. The milder forms of nuclear indentation such as notches, folds and closing folds (Majno et al., 1969) were also increased in animals receiving either cholesterol or adrenaline compared with animals receiving placebo and animals receiving adrenaline or cholesterol after pyridinolcarbamate pretreatment.

There was often a bleb characteristically located on the marginal fold or close to the fold. These blebs contain enlarged vesicles and vacuoles in a space with thinner electron density than the protoplasm, and sometimes contain relatively large granular structures. In some large blebs almost no fine structures were seen. The endothelial cells, especially those with blebs, exhibited certain changes characterized by enlargement of vesicles, cisternae of endoplasmic reticulum, Golgi apparatus and ribosomes, some edema of mitochondria and cytoplasm, deep indentations of nuclei, enlargement of the perinuclear space and condensation and margination of nuclear chromatin. It is important to note that blebs often had platelets sticking to them and the platelets often showed the formation of fibrin as seen in Figure 5.

The mean percentages of endothelial cells showing blebbing were 9.5% in the placebo control group, 18.9% in the adrenaline group, 12.8% in the adrenaline after pyridinolcarbamate group, 46.4% in the cholesterol group, and 23.7% in the cholesterol after pyridinolcarbamate

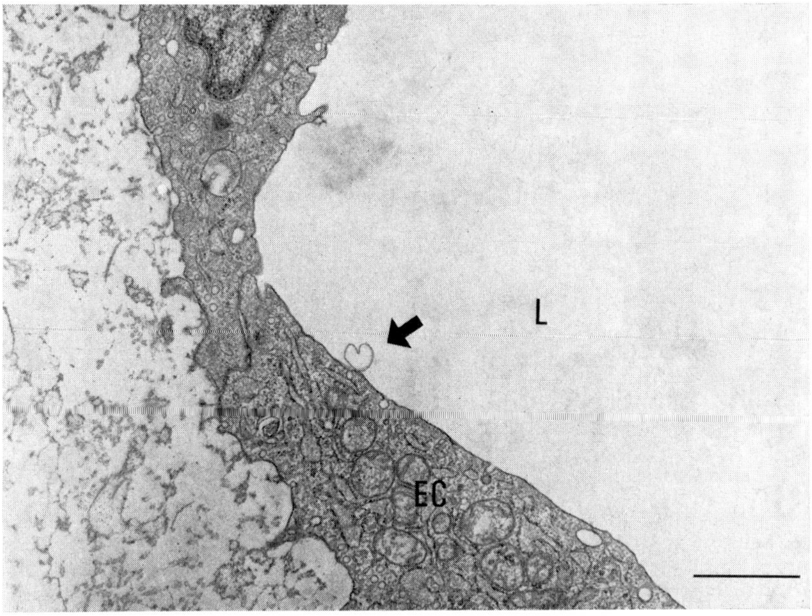

Fig. 5a. Endothelial cell of thoracic aorta of rabbit challenged with adrenaline showing a small bleb (arrow) and subendothelial edema. L = vessel lumen. EC = endothelial cell.

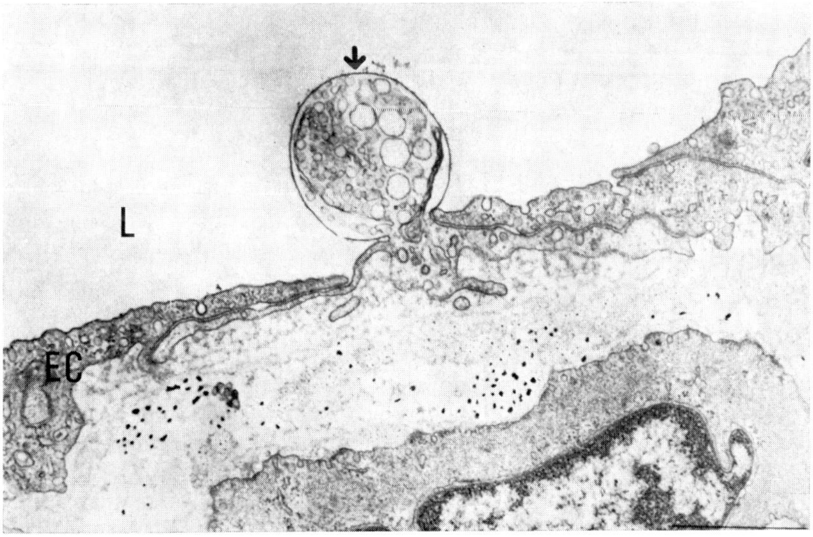

Fig. 5b. Large bleb (arrow) in endothelial cell (EC) of thoracic aorta of rabbit challenged with cholesterol. Note subendothelial edema. L = vessel lumen.

group (Fig. 6). These cells increased in the treated groups, and in the cholesterol group the increase is statistically significant ($p < 0.01$), while the p-value of the increase in the adrenaline group is less than 0.1. No statistically significant increase was seen in the group receiving cholesterol or adrenaline after pyridinolcarbamate pretreatment.

Large blebs with diameters of 1–4 μ appeared in 21.4% of the endothelial cells of animals given cholesterol ($p < 0.01$), but such large blebs were not found in the placebo control group. In animals given cholesterol after pyridinolcarbamate pretreatment, the number

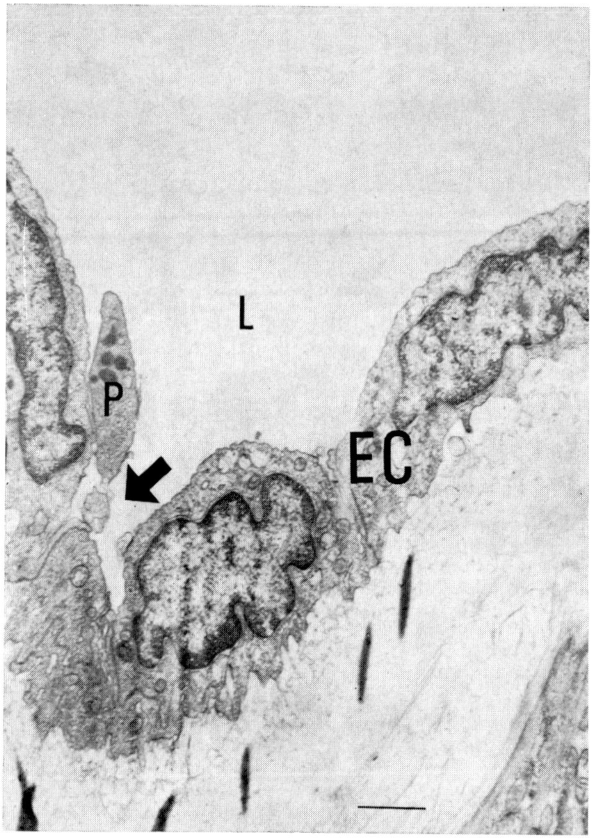

Fig. 5c. Bleb (arrow) with adherent platelet (P) in endothelial cell (EC) of thoracic aorta of rabbit challenged with cholesterol. L = vessel lumen.

of blebs, especially large ones, decreased. In animals given adrenaline, blebs of diameters of less than 1 μ increased compared with the placebo control group, but there was no statistical significance. Large blebs with a diameter over 1 μ, which were absent in the placebo control group, appeared in 2% of endothelial cells of the group receiving adrenaline only. In animals receiving adrenaline after pyridinolcarbamate pretreatment, the appearance of blebs was decreased compared to animals receiving adrenaline alone.

Edematous changes in the cytoplasm were marked in the group of animals given cholesterol ($p < 0.02$) but tended to decrease after pyridinolcarbamate pretreatment as shown in Group 5. Similar changes were seen in the adrenaline group, although much less than in the cholesterol group. On the other hand, the condensation and margination of chromatin particles of nuclei

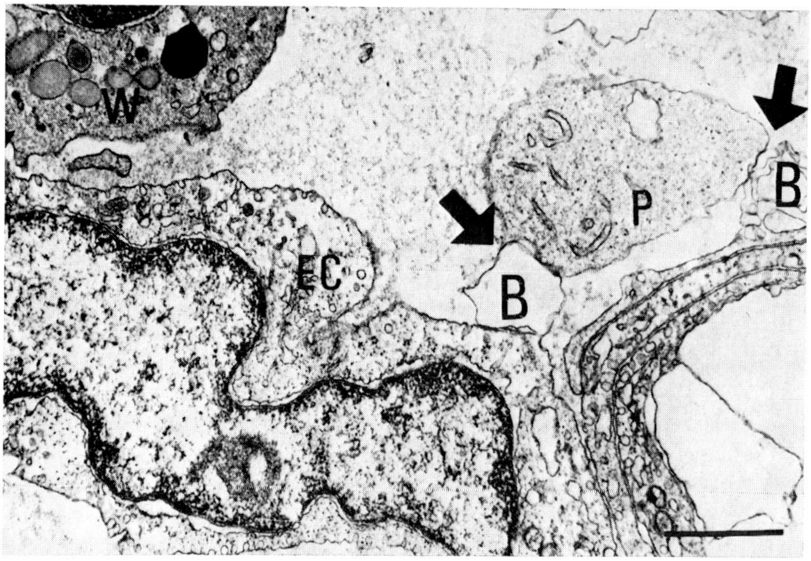

Fig. 5d. Large blebs (arrows) with adherent platelets (P) and fibrin in endothelial cell (EC) of thoracic aorta of rabbit challenged with cholesterol. B = bleb, W = leukocyte.

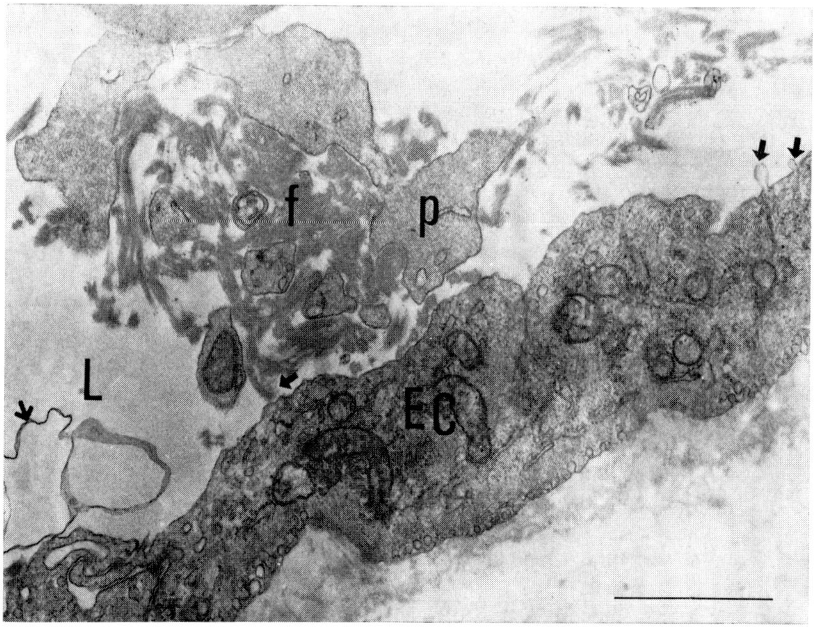

Fig. 5e. One large and 2 small blebs (arrows) on endothelial cells of thoracic aorta of rabbit challenged with cholesterol. Adherent platelets (p) and fibrin (f). The endothelial cell (EC) shows marked unevenness. L = vessel lumen.

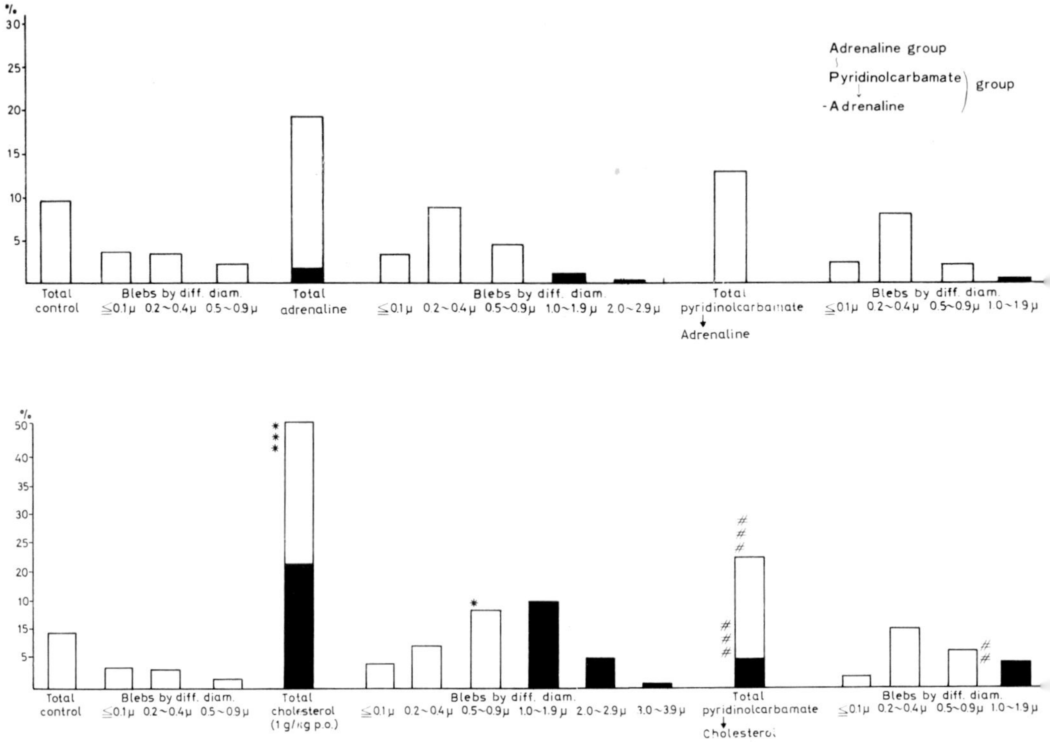

Fig. 6. Appearance of blebs in endothelial cells of thoracic aorta of rabbits of all 5 groups. Percentage of endothelial cells with blebs is shown.

* $p < 0.05$, *** $p < 0.001$	Placebo control group vs cholesterol group.
## $p < 0.01$, ### $p < 0.001$	Group with cholesterol after pyridinolcarbamate pretreatment vs cholesterol group.

and the widening of perinuclear spaces were marked in the adrenaline group ($p < 0.02$), but these changes tended to be reduced by pyridinolcarbamate pretreatment as seen in Group 3.

Subendothelial edema appeared to a statistically significant degree after administration of adrenaline or cholesterol as seen in Groups 2 and 4 ($p < 0.05$, in both cases) as shown in Figure 7, but in Groups 3 and 5 which were pretreated with pyridinolcarbamate, adrenaline or cholesterol administration did not induce subendothelial edema.

C. Discussion

Scanning electron-microscopic observation revealed two important phenomena, namely the groove-like lines and the crater-like holes on the luminal surface of the aorta. They are statistically significantly increased in animals receiving cholesterol and adrenaline, suggesting the biological significance of these structures. The vertical and horizontal groove-like lines especially appeared statistically significantly in animals receiving adrenaline and cholesterol compared with the placebo control group. Their appearance was also significantly prevented by pyridinolcarbamate pretreatment. In transmission electron-microscopic observation, the unevenness of endothelial cells, which corresponds well to the vertical and longitudinal lines respectively in the scanning electron-microscopic pictures, were seen on the luminal surface

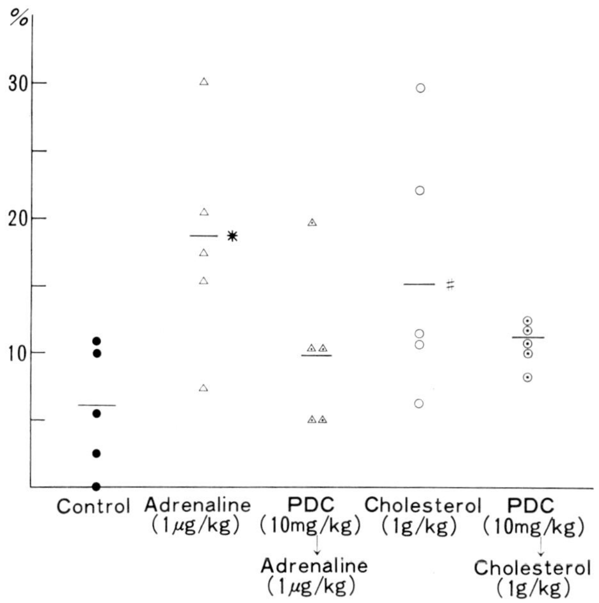

Fig. 7. Subendothelial edema, which was recognized in each electron-microscopic photograph obtained from each group of animals, is shown as a percentage. A statistically significant higher percentage of such changes was seen in photographs of animals challenged either with adrenaline or with cholesterol compared with those of the placebo control group. Such changes were not shown in groups pretreated with pyridinolcarbamate.

* $p < 0.05$ Control group vs adrenaline group.

\# $p < 0.05$ Control group vs cholesterol group.

of the longitudinal and vertical sections respectively of endothelial cells from animals receiving cholesterol or adrenaline. A similar unevenness was also found on the mural side.

In addition, marked indentations such as pinching of nuclei appeared in the endothelial cells of the aorta of animals receiving either cholesterol or adrenaline. Needless to say, the pinches appeared in the nuclei of striated muscle or endothelial cells of capillaries when they were fixed in their contracted state, as shown by Majno et al. (1969). These morphological changes undoubtedly represent the active contraction of the endothelial cells of the aorta which were fixed by glutaraldehyde. In these arterial specimens, the simultaneous appearance of subendothelial edema with infiltrated plasma proteins is a common finding. This evidence suggests that the above-mentioned morphological changes may show the contraction of endothelial cells which results in the widening of intercellular junctions for the transendothelial transport of plasma proteins. It is also clear that pyridinolcarbamate significantly inhibited this contraction of endothelial cells seen in the groups receiving either cholesterol or adrenaline. In the other experiment similar changes in endothelial cells of large arteries accompanied by edema of the arterial wall induced by noradrenaline and angiotensin were observed and these changes were also inhibited to a certain degree by pyridinolcarbamate and, at the same time, the subendothelial and medial edema with plasma proteins was inhibited by pyridinolcarbamate. These facts have suggested the possible relaxing effect of pyridinolcarbamate on the contractile protein of the endothelial cells.

In the present experiments, the morphological changes showing the contraction of endothelial cells induced by cholesterol are quite long-lasting (over 2 hours) and those induced by adrenaline are also a relatively long-lasting response lasting over half-an-hour. This differs from the hypertensive response of adrenaline, which ceases within 1 min after adrenaline injection. These long-lasting contractions, which are accompanied by the widening of intercellular spaces between neighboring endothelial cells and continue after the disappearance of the contraction of the vessel wall, undoubtedly contribute to the acute infiltration of plasma substances, including large particles such as plasma proteins, into the vessel wall as shown also in immunofluorescent observation (see below). This evidence undoubtedly shows that the contraction of endothelial cells is the most important trigger-mechanism in atherogenesis, and thus has not been appreciated enough until today.

The crater-like structures appearing in Groups 2 and 4 treated by adrenaline and cholesterol respectively are more numerous to a statistically significant degree compared with the placebo control group. In Group 2, receiving adrenaline, the number of small crater-like structures with a diameter less than 1 μ increased, while in Group 4, receiving cholesterol, the number of large crater-like structures with a diameter over 1 μ increased. These changes induced by adrenaline or cholesterol have been reduced by pyridinolcarbamate pretreatment to a significant degree as shown in Groups 3 and 5. In an experiment of Nelson et al. (1972) the crater-like structures were found to be produced by interruption of the blood flow, and to represent blebs mainly, although some of them seemed to be large vacuoles.

In observations with the transmission electron microscope, there was no vacuole formation, while blebs were increased significantly in the groups treated with adrenaline and cholesterol, appearing almost always on or close to the marginal fold. This characteristic localization was also confirmed by demonstrating the cell boundary by staining with silver nitrate (Garbarsch and Collatz Christensen, 1970) in another experiment. This fact also shows the biological significance of the crater-like structures, although blebs with a diameter of less than 1 μ appeared in the placebo control group and some of them, but not all, may possibly be artifacts. The large blebs with a diameter of over 1 μ were not found in untreated animals, but appeared in animals given cholesterol. Small blebs with a diameter of less than 1 μ were increased in animals given adrenaline, but appeared less frequently in animals pretreated with pyridinolcarbamate. This evidence corresponds to the appearance of crater-like structures in the scanning electron-microscopic pictures, and may indicate that the majority of crater-like structures seen in scanning electron microscopy may represent blebs destroyed by the dehydration procedures. Needless to say, bleb formation has been repeatedly produced by poor fixation procedures, so that it was quite essential to consider this possibility in our preparations. Therefore sampling and fixation were performed very carefully. Recently, Chiang et al. (1968) and Willms-Kretschmer and Majno (1969) observed bleb formation after the interruption of blood flow in the blood vessels of rat and rabbit brain and of rat skin. Their findings have been confirmed by Nelson et al. (1972) in the common carotid artery of rabbit and monkey. It is thus reasonable to suppose that single-dose treatment of animals with cholesterol or adrenaline produces blebbing in the endothelial cells. It is often observed that platelets stick to the blebs, and that some of these platelets have already produced fibrin around themselves. It is not unreasonable to assume that the blebs release ADP, which causes aggregation of platelets and release of their own ADP and clotting factors; this would explain the formation of fibrin on the surface of platelets. These observations also support the assumption that the apparent formation of blebs and the sticking of platelets to them are not artifacts due to poor fixation, because the fixative was given in situ in the living animals, and immediate fixation was performed. It seems clear that these findings show the thrombogenic significance of bleb formation.

The appearance of subendothelial edema after administration of adrenaline and cholesterol was also confirmed in this observation. As shown by immunofluorescent observation, the acute infiltration of plasma proteins such as β-lipoprotein, fibrinogen and γ-globulin was seen after the same challenges, and they appeared precisely in the same areas as the edematous features, so that the subendothelial edema indicates the increased infiltration of plasma fluid and plasma proteins through the endothelial lining, presumably through the enlarged intercellular spaces created by contraction of the contractile protein of endothelial cells, although the permeability of endothelium (French, 1966) has still not yet been fully clarified at the present moment.

The prevention of subendothelial edema by pyridinolcarbamate, confirmed in this experiment, may be reasonably considered to originate from its direct effect on the endothelial cells and to reflect the inhibitory effect on morphological changes brought about by the contraction of endothelial cells induced by adrenaline or cholesterol.

The contraction of the endothelial cell found in the present experiment seems to be the key mechanism in so-called 'episodic insudation', for which we have been looking. Recently we discovered that the effect of angiotensin and noradrenaline on the vascular endothelial cells is a powerful contraction similar to that seen in the case of cholesterol and adrenaline in the present experiment. These changes were shown to be significantly reduced by pyridinolcarbamate. As shown below, substances such as cholesterol, adrenaline, noradrenaline and angiotensin induce the acute infiltration of β-lipoprotein into the blood vessel wall in rabbit and monkey, thus showing their atherogenic property of initiating the key mechanism of so-called 'episodic insudation'. The results obtained in the present scanning and transmission electron-microscopic study suggest that the dynamic force opening the gate of the endothelial lining for plasma substances including β-lipoprotein in this mechanism may come mainly from the contraction of the contractile protein of endothelial cells in addition to the blood pressure, although the chemical and electrical changes on the surface of the endothelial cell membrane might play some limited role.

II. IMMUNOFLUORESCENT OBSERVATION

In the previous observation the author noted subendothelial and often medial edema after single-dose treatment of animals with cholesterol, adrenaline, noradrenaline or angiotensin, and it was assumed that the acute infiltration of plasma substances might be induced by such atherogenic stress. In the present observation, we tried to determine whether acute infiltration of large-sized plasma proteins such as β-lipoprotein, fibrinogen, IgG and γ-globulin is induced by single-dose treatment of animals with cholesterol (1 g/kg p.o.), saturated fat (1 ~ 2 g/kg p.o.), adrenaline or noradrenaline (1 μg/kg i.v.) into the arterial wall from the blood stream. For this purpose, immunofluorescent techniques (Kao and Wissler, 1965) were used with anti-rabbit β-lipoprotein antibody, anti-rabbit fibrinogen antibody, anti-rabbit IgG antibody and anti-rabbit γ-globulin antibody conjugated with fluorescein isothiocyanate.

A. Materials and methods

In this observation, 65 rabbits weighing 1.6–3.0 kg were used; 9 untreated animals served as controls and the remaining 57 animals were exposed to the following challenges and sacrificed at predetermined times from 5 min to 7 hours after the challenge. The challenges and modes of administration were: (1) adrenaline (Sankyo Co., Ltd.) given intravenously, 1 μg/kg in 15 animals; (2) noradrenaline (Sankyo Co., Ltd.) given intravenously, 1 μg/kg in 2 animals; (3) cholesterol given in a dose of 1 g/kg in 19 animals (in 10 of these cholesterol-fed animals an intravenous injection (1 μg/kg) of adrenaline was given 30 min before sacrifice which was performed 2 hours after cholesterol administration; in 5 of these animals 10 mg/kg of pyridinolcarbamate was given as pretreatment 2 hours before cholesterol administration; and in the remaining 5 animals, placebo was given 2 hours before the challenge); (4) lanolin, 1 g/kg given orally to 5 animals; (5) olive oil, 10 ml given orally to 5 animals; (6) 10% ethyl alcohol, 10 ml/kg given orally to 5 animals; (7) commercial rabbit pellets (Oriental Co., Ltd.), 50 g given to 5 animals; (8) butter, 1 and 2 g/kg to 2 animals; (9) linoleic acid, 2 g/kg to 2 animals.

The method used is principally the same as that described by Kao and Wissler (1965).

Unfixed cryostat-cut tissue sections of 1-2 and 4 μ were made from the wall of aorta, common carotid arteries, vena cava and the brain and heart. The sections underwent antigen-antibody reaction with goat anti-rabbit β-lipoprotein or fibrinogen (by courtesy of Prof. K. W. Walton, University of Birmingham) or γ-globulin (Behringwerke AG) or swine anti-IgG (Dakopatts AS) conjugated with fluorescein isothiocyanate by incubation for 30 min at room temperature. When the presence of fluorescence was demonstrated, evidence for each plasma protein antibody specificity was obtained by absorption techniques. Besides the classical immunofluorescent observation, a new method using Rygaard and Olsen's (1971) interference filter system was used in this experiment. In the classical observation the elastic fibers of the blood vessel wall exhibit non-specific fluorescence, but in the new method this non-specific fluorescence is eliminated.

B. Results

There was definite fluorescence due to the infiltration of β-lipoprotein, fibrinogen, IgG and γ-globulin into the subendothelial spaces of the aorta of all animals exposed to challenge with adrenaline, noradrenaline, cholesterol, butter or lanolin. This was marked at 30 min after the injection of adrenaline and noradrenaline, and at 1–3 hours after the administration of cholesterol, butter or lanolin, when the brilliant fluorescence occupied the entire subendothelial space.

In the early stage of infiltration, the fluorescence was mainly restricted to the subendothelial space and was fairly well limited by the internal elastic lamina, with some fluorescence found in or beyond the internal elastic lamina. Subendothelial stagnation of these plasma proteins, clearly dammed by the internal elastic lamina, was especially marked in animals receiving the combined administration of cholesterol and adrenaline. Examination of adjacent hematoxylin and eosin stained sections showed good correspondence between fluorescent areas and the previously described edematous change. Thus, β-lipoprotein, fibrinogen, IgG, and γ-globulin can be said to be present in the 'edematous arterial reaction' of the vessel wall (Shimamoto, 1960, 1963, 1969*a*; Shimamoto et al., 1959).

Later, fluorescence in the aorta penetrated into and through the internal elastic lamina, presumably at its fenestrations, since there was fine spotty or linear fluorescence at irregular intervals in the internal elastic lamina. In the aorta of animals sacrificed relatively late after the challenge, i.e. 3–5 hours after the administration of adrenaline or 3–6 hours after the challenge with cholesterol, the fluorescence was still present in the subendothelial spaces. However, it was also found here and there in the inner third muscle layer of the aorta. In the aorta of animals sacrificed 7 hours after the administration of adrenaline or 24 hours after cholesterol, β-lipoprotein, fibrinogen, IgG, and γ-globulin had already left the vessel wall. These 4 plasma proteins appeared concomitantly in the same area. However, among these 4 plasma proteins, the transportation through the internal elastic lamina of β-lipoprotein and fibrinogen seemed somewhat slower than that of IgG and γ-globulin.

In common carotid arteries a similar change was observed; however, the fluorescence did not always occupy the whole subendothelial space; it commonly appeared patchy and quite large areas remained free of infiltration. The fluorescence was more marked at the point of bifurcation, but generally it was relatively weak in these arteries compared with the aorta. In the larger coronary and cerebral arteries a definite subendothelial patchy fluorescence was often observed. In the vena cava there was a weak and diffuse fluorescence in the innermost layers.

In each section of the aorta from 4 of the 9 untreated animals and from one of the 5 animals treated with olive oil, there were a few small and faint patchy areas of subendothelial and medial fluorescence with anti-γ-globulin and anti-IgG antibody. In all other untreated animals and in all animals that received commercial pellets, olive oil or ethyl alcohol, there was sometimes a very faint and scattered fluorescence with anti-γ-globulin antibody and anti-IgG antibody, but there was almost no brilliant fluorescence to indicate definitely the presence of plasma

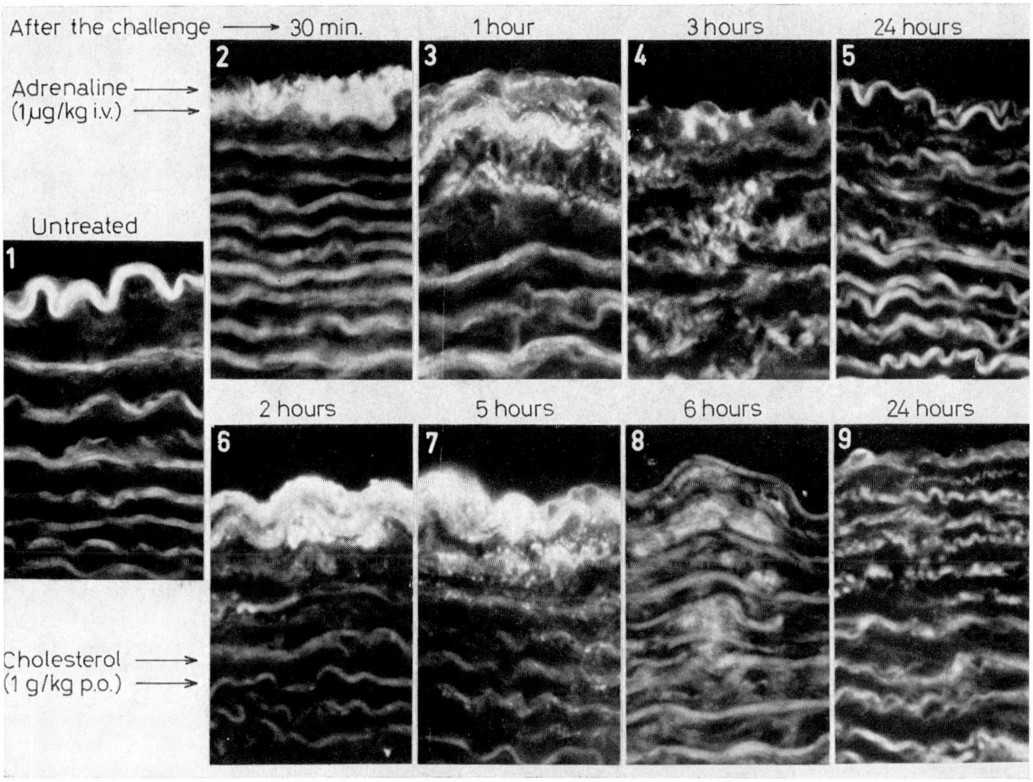

Fig. 8. Transportation of γ-globulin through aortic wall visualized by immunofluorescent method. Nos. 6–9 show effect of cholesterol which induces infiltration of γ-globulin into aortic wall.

1. Normal rabbit aorta. There is no fluorescence, except for normal autofluorescence of elastic tissues.
2. Definite fluorescence (γ-globulin) is seen in the subendothelial space 30 min after adrenaline injection.
3. Fluorescence (γ-globulin) is shown in subendothelial space and inner media in animals sacrificed 1 hour after injection.
4. Fluorescence is shown diffusely in media in animals sacrificed 3 hours after injection.
5. No fluorescence is seen 24 hours after injection.
6. Definite fluorescence (γ-globulin) is seen in the subendothelial space 2 hours after cholesterol administration.

7 and 8. Fluorescence (γ-globulin) is seen in medial layers in animals sacrificed 5 and 6 hours, respectively, after cholesterol administration.

9. No fluorescence is seen 24 hours after cholesterol administration.

proteins in the arterial or venous wall.

Among plasma proteins observed in this experiment, the infiltration of β-lipoprotein seemed sometimes to be delayed compared with the other proteins; however, all these plasma proteins were almost always demonstrated in the same place and in the same way.

C. Discussion

These experiments show the special effect of so-called 'atherogenic substances' (Shimamoto,

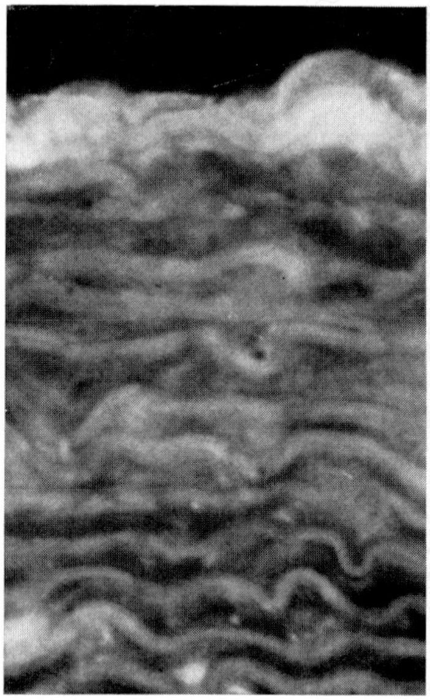

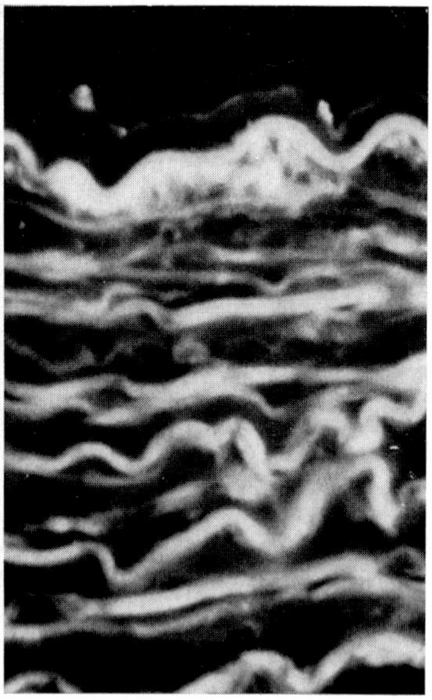

Fig. 9 *Fig. 10*

Fig. 9. Infiltration of fibrinogen is clearly shown in subendothelial and medial space of thoracic aorta in rabbit given an injection of adrenaline 30 min before sacrifice.

Fig. 10. Infiltration of β-lipoprotein is clearly shown in inner medial layer of thoracic aorta of rabbit treated with cholesterol 6 hours before sacrifice.

1969*a*; Shimamoto et al., 1959) such as cholesterol, saturated fat, adrenaline and noradrenaline in inducing an acute infiltration into the arterial wall, with temporary stagnation of plasma protein in subendothelial spaces dammed by the internal elastic lamina in large arteries. There is also infiltration of plasma protein into the venous wall, although to a much lesser extent and without subendothelial stagnation.

The acute and strong infiltration of cholesterol-bearing proteins such as β-lipoprotein has

→

Fig. 11. *a.* The clear-cut barrier function of the internal elastic lamina is shown in the aorta of animals challenged with adrenaline plus cholesterol. The stagnation of γ-globulin in the subendothelial space without any infiltration into the medial layer through the lamina is clearly shown at this stage, i.e. at 30 min after injection of adrenaline, which was given $1\frac{1}{2}$ hours after the administration of cholesterol. The contour of the internal elastic lamina is clearly shown.
b. Photo of the placebo control animal is shown for reference.

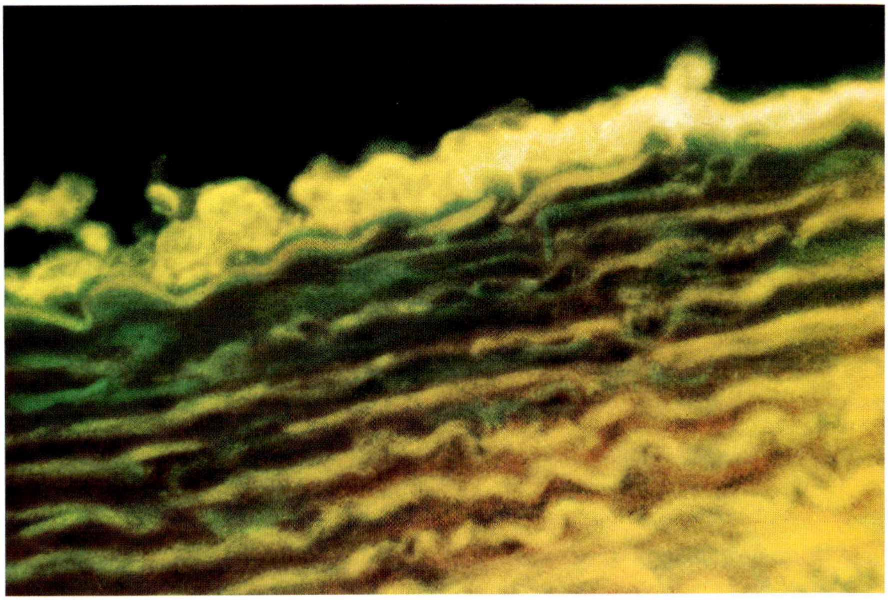

Fig. 11a

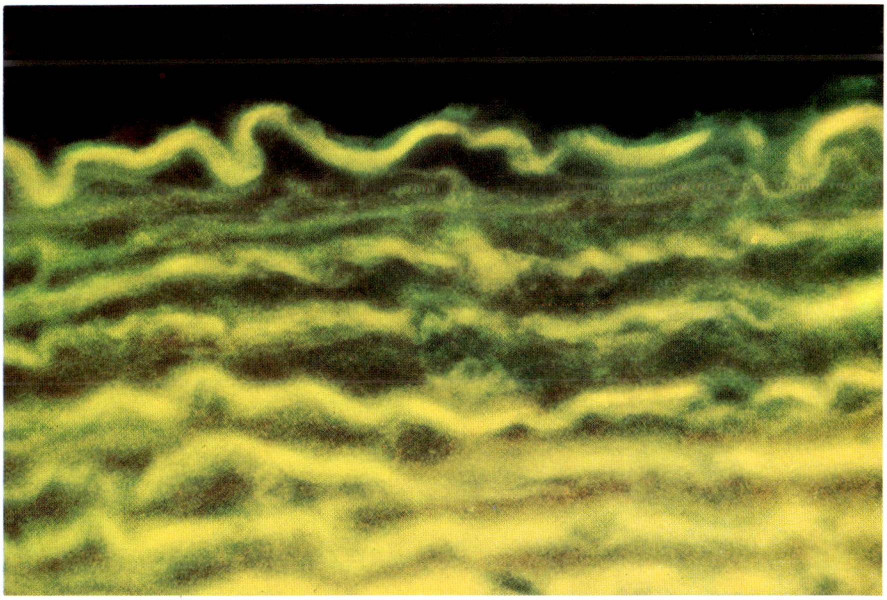

Fig. 11b

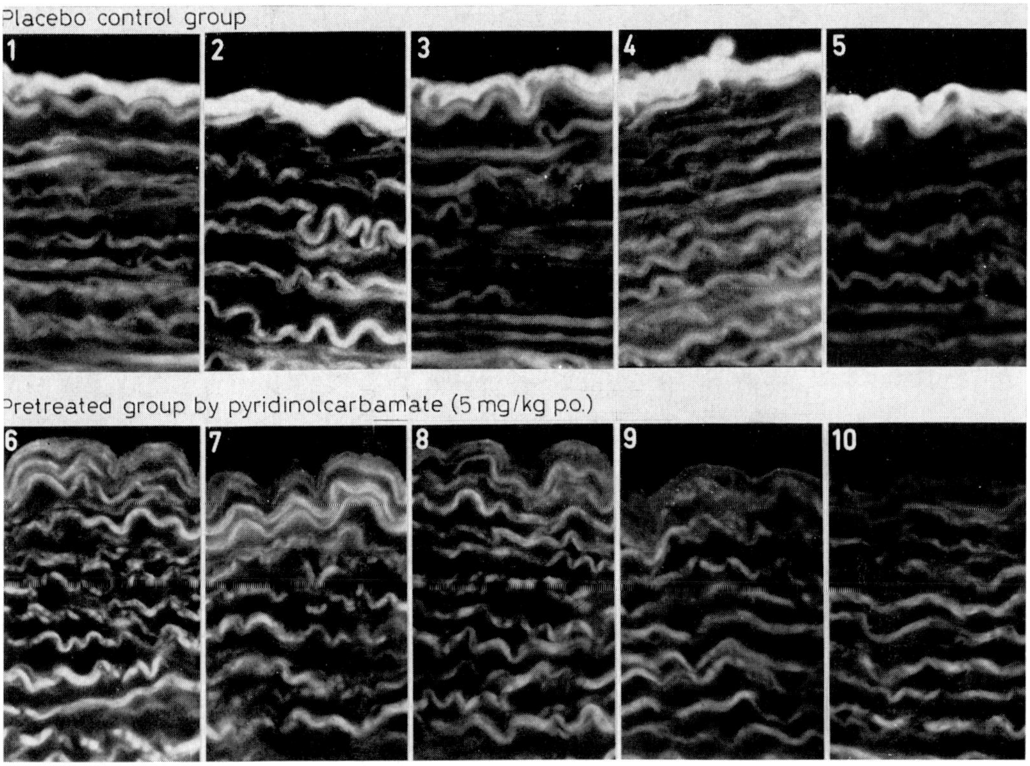

Fig. 12. Rabbit aorta sampled 2 hours after cholesterol (1 g/kg p.o.) and adrenaline (1 μg/kg i.v.) in 10 animals. Preventive effect of pyridinolcarbamate on infiltration of plasma proteins into the arterial wall induced by combined challenges of adrenaline plus cholesterol is shown in these photographs. Brilliant immunofluorescence shows presence of γ-globulin.
1–5: All 5 specimens from different animals of the placebo control group show definite infiltration and stagnation of γ-globulin in subendothelial space of aortae showing the relative barrier function of the internal elastic lamina.
6–10: All 5 specimens from different animals treated with adrenaline plus cholesterol after pretreatment with pyridinolcarbamate. Infiltration of γ-globulin is almost completely prevented.

thus been shown to be induced by the above-mentioned challenges in large arteries. This acute infiltration of plasma substances, with the barrier function of the internal elastic lamina causing stagnation of the infiltrate in the subendothelial spaces, may be the key-mechanism involved in the genesis and progress of atheromatous lesions. In the other experiment the author found a similar but stronger effect of angiotensin in inducing acute infiltration of β-lipoprotein into the blood vessel wall of rabbit and monkey.

Thus, the present immunofluorescent method has been shown to be extremely useful for visualizing 'episodic insudation' as well as for finding the atherogenic factors inducing it. Investigators have long been looking for such a method in order to find methods or drugs to prevent atherosclerosis or to halt its progress.

The atheromatous mass is characteristically localized in the subendothelial space, at least in the early stages. The absence of a well-developed internal elastic lamina that could act as a

TABLE IV

Presence and intensity of immunofluorescence of IgG

Treatment	No. of animal	Intima	Media: Internal	Media: Middle	Media: External
	320	± − − −	− − − −	− − − −	− − − −
		± − − −	− − − −	− − − −	− − − −
Untreated	321	± − − −	− − − −	− − − −	− − − −
		± − − −	− − − −	− − − −	− − − −
	336	± − − −	± − − −	± − − −	− − − −
		± − − −	− − − −	− − − −	− − − −
	337	+ ± − −	± − − −	± − − −	− − − −
		+ − − −	± − − −	− − − −	− − − −
	360	+ − − −	± − − −	± − − −	− − − −
		+ ± − −	± − − −	− − − −	− − − −
	367	± ± − −	± − − −	± − − −	− − − −
		± − − −	− − − −	− − − −	− − − −
	385	+ − − −	± − − −	− − − −	− − − −
		± − − −	− − − −	− − − −	− − − −
	403	+ ± − −	± − − −	± − − −	− − − −
		± ± − −	− − − −	− − − −	− − − −
	404	± ± − −	− − − −	− − − −	− − − −
		± − − −	− − − −	− − − −	− − − −
Olive oil	361	+ − − −	+ − − −	± − − −	± − − −
(2 g/kg)		+ ± − −	± − − −	− − − −	− − − −
Linoleic acid	362	+ ± ± −	+ ± − −	± − − −	± − − −
(2 g/kg)		+ ± − −	− − − −	− − − −	− − − −
Lanoline	363	+ ± − −	+ − − −	− − − −	− − − −
(2 g/kg)		+ ± − −	+ − − −	− − − −	− − − −
Alcohol (10 %	364	+ + − −	+ − − −	− − − −	− − − −
ethanol 50 ml)		+ ± − −	± − − −	− − − −	− − − −
Butter	365	+ + − −	± − − −	± − − −	− − − −
(2 g/kg)		+ ± − −	± − − −	− − − −	− − − −
Butter	366	+ ± ± −	+ − − −	± − − −	− − − −
(10 g/kg)		+ + ± −	+ ± − −	± − − −	− − − −
Noradrenaline	368	+ + + −	+ + ± −	+ ± − −	+ − − −
(0.5 hr)		+ + + −	+ + − −	+ − − −	± − − −
	433	+ + + −	+ + − −	+ − − −	− − − −
		+ + + −	± − − −	− − − −	− − − −
Adrenaline	332	+ + + ±	+ − − −	+ − − −	± − − −
(0.5 hr)		+ ± ± −	+ − − −	− − − −	− − − −
	333	+ + + −	+ + − −	+ − − −	± − − −
		+ + + −	+ − − −	± − − −	− − − −
	357	+ + ± −	+ − − −	± − − −	− − − −
		+ + ± ±	+ − − −	− − − −	− − − −
	358	+ + + +	+ − − −	± − − −	− − − −
		+ + + +	± − − −	− − − −	− − − −
	359	+ + + ±	± − − −	− − − −	− − − −
		+ + + −	+ − − −	− − − −	− − − −

(continued)

TABLE IV *(continued)*

Treatment	No. of animal	Intima	Media: Internal	Media: Middle	Media: External
Adrenaline	391	+ + + −	+ + − −	+ − − −	± − − −
(1 hr)		+ + ± −	+ + − −	+ − − −	− − − −
	392	+ + + −	+ + − −	+ ± − −	+ ± − −
		+ + + −	+ ± − −	− − − −	− − − −
Adrenaline	372	+ + ± −	+ + ± −	+ + − −	+ ± − −
(3 hr)		+ + ± −	+ + ± −	+ ± − −	+ − − −
	395	+ + − −	+ + + −	+ + ± −	+ ± − −
		+ + + −	+ + − −	+ − − −	+ − − −
Adrenaline	371	+ ± − −	+ + − −	+ + − −	+ ± − −
(5 hr)		+ + ± −	+ + ± −	+ ± − −	+ − − −
Adrenaline	382	+ ± − −	+ ± − −	+ ± − −	± − − −
(7 hr)		+ ± − −	− − − −	− − − −	− − − −
Adrenaline	387	+ ± − −	± ± − −	− − − −	− − − −
(24 hr)		± ± − −	− − − −	− − − −	− − − −
Cholesterol	330	+ + ± −	+ ± − −	± − − −	± − − −
(2 hr)		+ + ± −	+ − − −	− − − −	− − − −
	331	+ + + −	+ ± − −	± − − −	− − − −
		+ + + −	± − − −	− − − −	− − − −
Cholesterol	354	+ + + −	+ + − −	± − − −	± − − −
(3 hr)		+ + + −	± − − −	− − − −	− − − −
	355	+ + + ±	± − − −	− − − −	− − − −
		+ ± ± −	+ − − −	± − − −	− − − −
	356	+ + + ±	+ + − −	+ ± − −	± − − −
		+ + + −	+ − − −	− − − −	− − − −
Cholesterol	351	+ + ± −	+ + − −	+ − − −	± − − −
(5 hr)		+ ± ± −	+ ± − −	± − − −	− − − −
	352	+ + − −	+ ± − −	+ − − −	− − − −
		+ + ± −	+ ± − −	+ − − −	− − − −
	353	+ + ± −	+ + ± −	+ ± − −	+ ± − −
		+ + ± −	+ − − −	+ − − −	− − − −
Cholesterol	393	+ + ± −	+ + ± −	+ + − −	+ ± − −
(6 hr)		+ ± − −	+ + − −	+ + − −	+ ± − −
	394	+ + − −	+ + − −	+ + − −	+ − − −
		+ + − −	+ − − −	+ − − −	+ − − −
Cholesterol	373	+ ± − −	± − − −	± − − −	± − − −
(7 hr)		+ − − −	+ − − −	± − − −	− − − −
Cholesterol	374	± ± − −	± ± − −	± − − −	− − − −
(24 hr)		± − − −	± − − −	− − − −	− − − −
	322	+ + + ±	± − − −	− − − −	− − − −
		+ + ± −	− − − −	− − − −	− − − −
Cholesterol	323	+ + + −	+ − − −	− − − −	− − − −
+		+ + + −	− − − −	− − − −	− − − −
adrenaline	341	+ + + ±	+ ± − −	± − − −	± − − −
(2 hr)		+ + ± −	+ ± − −	± − − −	− − − −
	343	+ + + ±	+ − − −	− − − −	− − − −
		+ + + ±	± − − −	− − − −	− − − −
	400	+ + + −	+ ± − −	− − − −	− − − −
		+ + ± ±	± − − −	− − − −	− − − −

(continued)

TABLE IV *(continued)*

Treatment	No. of animal	Intima	Media: Internal	Media: Middle	Media: External
	401	**+** + ± ±	**+** + − −	± − − −	− − − −
		+ **+** + ±	+ − − −	− − − −	− − − −
PDC	334	+ ± − −	+ − − −	− − − −	− − − −
(cholesterol		± ± − −	± − − −	− − − −	− − − −
+	335	+ ± ± −	± − − −	± − − −	− − − −
adrenaline)		+ ± − −	± − − −	− − − −	− − − −
(2 hr)	338	+ ± − −	± − − −	− − − −	− − − −
		+ ± − −	± − − −	− − − −	− − − −
	339	± ± − −	− − − −	− − − −	− − − −
		± ± − −	− − − −	− − − −	− − − −
	340	+ ± − −	± − − −	± − − −	− − − −
		± ± − −	± − − −	− − − −	− − − −

The whole transverse section of 1 ~ 2 μ of thickness of thoracic aorta, at the level of the orifice of the first intercostal artery, of all test animals was evaluated for the presence and intensity of the immunofluorescence of IgG, which are described in each column of the table, except cases receiving lanolin, olive oil, or ethanol which gave negative results: ± = faint fluorescence, + = weak fluorescence (mainly patchy), **+** = brilliant and definite fluorescence (sometimes patchy but sometimes extending continuously).

barrier structure in veins may, along with low venous pressure, explain the extreme rarity of atheromatous changes in veins. However, the same impairment of the repelling function of endothelial cells against platelets and leukocytes has been shown to be induced by atherogenic stresses (Shimamoto, 1960, 1963, 1969*a*; Shimamoto et al., 1959) and the acute infiltration of plasma and plasma proteins, as shown in this observation. This phenomenon is obviously related to the formation of venous thrombosis and phlebitis, and indicates the need for preventive substances against such impairment of endothelial cells — and hence for the prevention and treatment of venous thrombosis and inflammation.

In another experiment, the author (Shimamoto et al., 1972) observed the early atheromatous lesions of rabbits fed cholesterol over long periods. Wherever the internal elastic lamina was preserved, β-lipoprotein, fibrinogen, IgG and γ-globulin were present in the intimal lesion, showing the increased influx of plasma substances into fatty streaks. This is entirely consistent with the demonstration of increased plasma cholesterol infiltration into fatty streaks as shown by Lofland and Clarkson (1970) and also with the morphological changes of endothelial cells with marked contraction with pinches and blebbing, which were described above. In these lesions, the above-mentioned plasma proteins appeared to be limited by the intact internal elastic lamina. This is in contrast to atheromatous lesions in which the internal elastic lamina has been destroyed; in these cases, plasma proteins penetrate deeply into the medial layers. This finding suggests a possibly important barrier function of the internal elastic lamina, which may protect smooth muscle from the acute massive infiltration of active plasma substances, as suggested by Wilens (1951), besides promoting the stagnation of atheromatous substances such as β-lipoprotein in the intima.

III. THE HUMAN ARTERY UNDER TRAUMATIC STRESS

It is important to see whether the acute infiltration of β-lipoprotein and other plasma proteins into the human arterial wall is caused by atherogenic stress. In order to observe such responses of the human arterial wall, arterial specimens were obtained by surgical operation from patients undergoing traumatic stress.

Materials and methods

Specimens were obtained by surgical operation from the left femoral artery and vein of a 36-year-old male patient suffering from severe stress due to a bone fracture incurred as the result of an accident. The specimen obtained was immediately placed in a cryostat. The immunofluorescent methods described above with anti-human β-lipoprotein antibody, anti-human fibrinogen antibody and anti-human γ-globulin antibody were applied to the human vessels and routine histochemical staining with hematoxylin and eosin was also performed on these specimens.

Results

In these specimens, the infiltration of β-lipoprotein, fibrinogen and γ-globulin was clearly shown, occupying the whole subendothelial space and partly in patchy areas of the innermost medial layers. The hematoxylin and eosin stain of this segment was almost normal in appearance, without any atheromatous changes, but it showed definite subendothelial edema and patchy edema in the innermost medial layers, which corresponded well with the location of the plasma proteins mentioned above. In the vein a weak, diffuse infiltration of the above-mentioned plasma proteins was found in the subendothelial and inner layers of the media (Fig. 13).

Discussion

It has been shown by Haust (1968) that fibrinogen is not found by immunofluorescent techniques in the normal human artery. This evidence of the infiltration of plasma proteins including fibrinogen in the seemingly normal arterial and venous wall is important. It is a single case and should be confirmed by further observations in many cases. However, the acute infiltration of plasma proteins such as fibrinogen and β-lipoprotein due to traumatic stress and also some atherogenic stresses even in the human artery unaffected by atherosclerosis is strongly suggested by the author's studies on the rabbit and monkey.

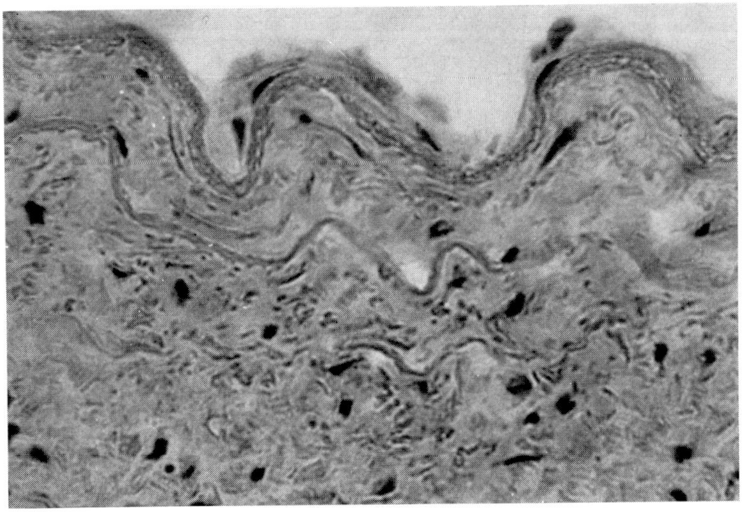

Fig. 13a. Section of femoral artery of accident patient. Hematoxylin and eosin stain shows diffuse subendothelial and patchy medial edema.

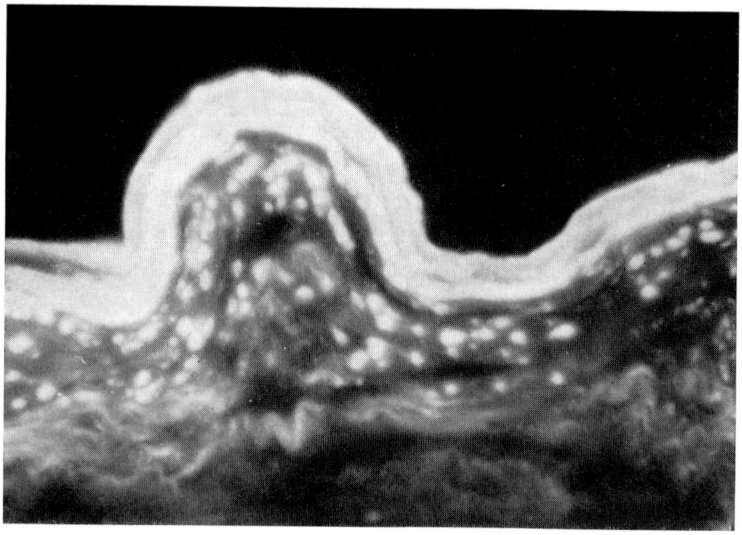

Fig. 13b. Section of femoral artery of accident patient. Immunofluorescence of β-lipoprotein is shown diffusely in the subendothelial layer and patchy in the innermost medial layer.

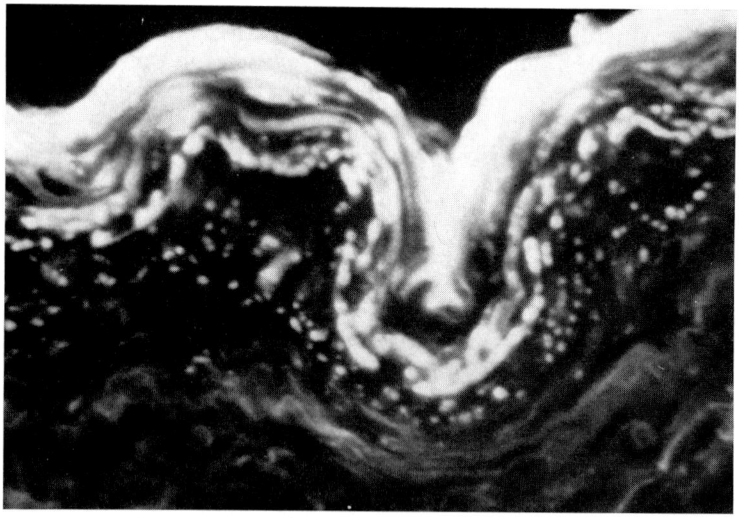

Fig. 13c. Section of femoral artery of accident patient. Immunofluorescence of fibrinogen is shown diffusely in the subendothelial layer and patchy in the innermost medial layer.

IV. SIGNIFICANCE OF THE FUNCTIONAL ALTERATION OR INJURY OF ENDOTHELIAL CELLS IN ATHEROGENESIS AND THROMBOGENESIS

The single administration of cholesterol, adrenaline or angiotensin in monkeys was also analysed at the author's Institute; preliminary data showed similar changes in the fine structure of endothelial cells compared with the arteries of rabbits and the immunofluorescent technique also showed similar results to those obtained in rabbits. It was again noted that the serum cholesterol level rose 1 ~ 3 mg/100 ml after a single administration of cholesterol but there is an acute and strong infiltration of large-sized plasma proteins into the arterial wall. The quantitative measurement will be performed in the future.

Agents such as adrenaline, angiotensin or cholesterol have been shown in this experiment to alter and reduce the physiological functions of vascular endothelial cells, such as the repelling function of the endothelial surface against formed elements of the blood as well as active, selective permeability which prevents the infiltration of an excessive amount of plasma substances or large plasma proteins such as γ-globulin, β-lipoprotein and fibrinogen. The experimental results suggest that these substances, by contracting the contractile protein of endothelial cells (Becker and Murphy, 1969), may be responsible for such an alteration of the physiological functions.

Such a contraction may widen the space at the intercellular junction, thereby admitting plasma proteins, and the concomitant formation of blebs may increase the adherence of platelets. Pyridinolcarbamate significantly inhibited the contraction of endothelial cells and at the same time inhibited the above-mentioned changes, i.e. the blebbing of endothelial cells, acute infiltration of plasma proteins into the arterial and venous wall, the enhancement of platelet aggregability, and blood coagulability, induced by adrenaline or cholesterol.

Agents inducing the above-mentioned changes in the functions of endothelial cells have also been known to induce atherosclerosis. On the other hand, a substance such as pyridinolcarbamate, which is capable of inhibiting these changes in the function of endothelial cells, has also been shown to inhibit experimental atherosclerosis (Shimamoto et al., 1966; Pick, 1969; Wu et al., 1969) and to enhance the regression of atheroma (Shimamoto et al., 1968). Pyridinolcarbamate has been extensively tested in human atherosclerotic and thrombotic disorders in Japan and abroad, and its clinical usefulness has already been established (Shimamoto, 1972*a*, *b*). This evidence may suggest the importance of the protection of the essential physiological function of vascular endothelial cells, such as the repelling function against blood-formed elements accompanied by enhancement of platelet aggregability and blood coagulability as well as the active, selective permeability of the endothelial lining in the prevention and treatment of atherosclerosis and thrombosis (Shimamoto 1960).

The above-mentioned evidence also suggests the importance of substances inhibiting the contraction of endothelial cells. Platelets and vascular endothelial cells have been shown to have immunologically similar contractile protein (Becker and Murphy, 1969; Nachman, 1968), and the application of contracting substances such as adrenaline has been well known to enhance the aggregability of platelets. Here again, pyridinolcarbamate inhibits the enhancement of platelet aggregability by adrenaline and cholesterol in vivo (Yamazaki et al., 1971, 1972) and by adrenaline in vitro (Didisheim et al., 1970; Yamazaki et al., 1972).

The correction of abnormal lipid metabolism is also important in atherogenesis, and this abnormality is no doubt an important risk factor. However, it should be remembered that most human atherosclerosis also appears without appreciable abnormality of the lipid metabolism; the experimental basis for this finding has already been shown by Constantinides (1965), as well as by the author's group (Shimamoto, 1960, 1963, 1969*a*; Shimamoto et al., 1959). The author feels that the rapid relaxation of strongly contracted endothelial cells covering atheroma is important in preventing the dangerous progress of atherosclerosis; therefore, he considers it necessary to conduct further research on the series of changes under discussion, the 'edematous arterial reaction' (Shimamoto, 1963), and to establish preventive procedures capable of protecting against this strong contraction of the endothelial cells (Shimamoto, 1972*a*, *b*).

SUMMARY

The combined scanning and transmission electron-microscopic observation of morphological changes in the endothelial cells of the aorta induced by single-dose treatment of rabbits with adrenaline (1 μg/kg i.v.) or cholesterol (1 g/kg p.o.) or angiotensin (1 μg/kg i.v.) was used to investigate the role of endothelial cells in the formation of the edematous arterial reaction and the reduction in the repelling function of endothelial cells to platelets and leukocytes induced by the above-mentioned challenges. The preventive effect of pyridinolcarbamate against such changes has also been investigated in this study.

Immunofluorescent observation has also been performed in rabbits to see whether plasma proteins such as β-lipoprotein, fibrinogen, γ-globulin and IgG enter into the subendothelial and medial layers through the endothelial lining after the above-mentioned challenges and also to see whether the pretreatment of animals with pyridinolcarbamate has an inhibitory effect. The same technique was also used to see whether plasma proteins such as β-lipoprotein, fibrinogen, γ-globulin and IgG diffuse into the arterial wall during traumatic stress in man.

1. In the scanning electron-microscopic analysis of the luminal surface of aorta, a statistically significant appearance of vertical lines at regular intervals of 0.6–1.8 μ and depths of 0.2–0.3 μ after administration of cholesterol and adrenaline was found ($p < 0.01$ in both cases), and also a statistically significant appearance of crater-like structures was observed after administration of cholesterol or adrenaline ($p < 0.01$ in both cases). Similar responses were also observed after angiotensin administration. The observations were performed on photographs taken at random of specimens sampled from the central portion of the thoracic aorta at the level of the orifice of the second intercostal artery, and also from the orifice itself. Pyridinolcarbamate pretreatment reduced significantly the appearance of the vertical lines and crater-like artifacts induced by the above-mentioned challenges ($p < 0.01$ in both cases). The crater-like structures appeared predominantly on or close to the boundaries of endothelial cells, and the majority of such structures was reasonably considered to represent blebs. On the basis of transmission electron-microscopic observation done at the same time, the vertical lines were found to represent the active contraction of the endothelial cells.

2. In the transmission electron-microscopic analysis, the appearance of subendothelial edema was confirmed to be induced by single-dose treatment of rabbits with adrenaline or with cholesterol. At the same time, the unevenness of endothelial cells, accompanied by strong indentations such as pinches ($p < 0.001$), which represent the contraction of endothelial cells, and also the formation of blebs, have been shown to be induced by the above-mentioned challenges. After the challenge with cholesterol the formation of blebs ($p < 0.01$), especially of large blebs with a diameter of over 1 μ, was induced ($p < 0.01$) and after the challenge with adrenaline the number of small blebs was increased ($p < 0.1$). Also, the sticking of platelets to blebs and the formation of fibrin by such platelets were often observed. In animals which received the same challenges after pretreatment with pyridinolcarbamate (10 μg/kg p.o.), the above-mentioned changes were significantly inhibited.

3. In the immunofluorescent analysis, the acute infiltration of plasma proteins was practically negative in the untreated animals, or those given commercial pellets, olive oil or alcohol, while the acute infiltration of β-lipoprotein, fibrinogen, IgG and γ-globulin into the blood vessel wall was found after the challenge either with adrenaline (1 μg/kg i.v.) or with cholesterol (1 g/kg p.o.). The plasma proteins entered the subendothelial space and then the medial layer, disappearing presumably through lymphatic ducts in the course of 7–24 hours after the challenges. The relative barrier function of the internal elastic lamina in causing stagnation of plasma proteins in the subendothelial space for several hours was visualized. This infiltration of plasma proteins was significantly inhibited by pretreatment of animals with pyridinolcarbamate (10 mg/kg p.o.). It is important to note that the so-called 'episodic insudation', inducing and aggravating atherosclerosis, was first visualized in this experiment.

In the caval veins of these animals, the acute infiltration of plasma proteins after adrenaline or cholesterol was found; however, it was diffuse and disappeared rapidly, and there was no temporal stagnation in the venous wall.

4. The femoral artery obtained by surgical operation from a 36-year-old man injured in an

accident showed infiltration of β-lipoprotein, fibrinogen, IgG and γ-globulin into the whole subendothelial space and in patchy areas of the media of his almost normal arterial wall. The areas showing the presence of plasma proteins also showed edematous features in the hematoxylin and eosin stained specimen. Diffuse infiltration of plasma proteins was also found in the subendothelial and inner medial layers of the femoral vein.

5. The characteristic response of the endothelial cells of the artery induced by cholesterol or adrenaline and also by angiotensin was shown in the present observations. It seemed to come from the contraction of their contractile proteins and his response has been proposed as the important trigger mechanism in atherogenesis and thrombogenesis.

REFERENCES

BECKER, C. G. and MURPHY, G. E. (1969): Demonstration of contractile protein in endothelium and cells of the heart valves, endothelium, intima, arteriosclerotic plaques, and Aschoff bodies of rheumatic heart disease. *Amer. J. Path., 55*, 1.

CHIANG, J., KAWADA, M., AMES III, A., WRIGHT, R. L. and MAJNO, G. (1968): Cerebral ischemia. III. Vascular changes. *Amer. J. Path., 52*, 455.

CONSTANTINIDES, P. (Ed.) (1965): *Experimental Atherosclerosis*. Elsevier Publ. Co., Amsterdam.

DIDISHEIM, P., STURM, R. E. and OWEN, Jr, C. A. (1970): Experiments on thrombosis and its prevention. In: *Current Concepts of Coagulation and Hemostasis*, pp. 177–185. Editors: R. Losito and B. Longpré. F. K. Schattauer, Stuttgart-New York.

FRENCH, J. E. (1966): Atherosclerosis in relation to the structure and function of the arterial intima, with special reference to the endothelium. *Int. Rev. exp. Path., 5*, 253.

GARBARSCH, C. and COLLATZ CHRISTENSEN, B. (1970): Scanning electron microscopy of aortic endothelial cell boundaries after staining with silver nitrate. *Angiology, 7*, 365.

HAUST, M. D. (1968): Electron microscopic and immuno-histochemical studies of fatty streaks in human aorta. In: *Progress in Biochemistry and Pharmacology, Vol. 4*, p. 249. Editors: C. J. Miras, A. Y. Howard and R. Paoletti. S. Karger, Basel-New York.

KAO, V. C. Y. and WISSLER, R. W. (1965): A study of the immunohistochemical localization of serum lipoproteins and other plasma proteins in human atherosclerotic lesions. *Exp. molec. Path., 4*, 465.

LOFLAND, H. B. and CLARKSON, T. B. (1970): The bi-directional transfer of cholesterol in normal aorta, fatty streaks, and atheromatous plaques. *Proc. Soc. exp. Biol. (N.Y.), 133*, 1.

MAJNO, G., SHEA, S. M. and LEVENTHAL, M. (1969): Endothelial contraction induced by histamine-type mediators. An electron microscopic study. *J. Cell Biol., 42*, 647.

NACHMAN, R. L. (1968): Platelet proteins. *Semin. Hemat., 5*, 18.

NELSON, E., SUNAGA, T. and SHIMAMOTO, T. (1972): Scanning and transmission electron microscopy of ischemic endothelium in the monkey carotid artery. In: *Proceedings, Princeton Conference*, in press.

PICK, R. (1969): The effect of pyridinolcarbamate on the induction and regression of aortic and coronary atherosclerosis in cholesterol-fed cockerels. In: *Atherogenesis. Proceedings, I International Symposium on Atherogenesis, Thrombogenesis and Pyridinolcarbamate Treatment, Tokyo 1969*, pp. 57–64. Editors: T. Shimamoto and F. Numano. ICS 201, Excerpta Medica, Amsterdam.

RYGAARD, J. and OLSEN, W. (1971): Determination of characteristics of interference filters. *Ann. N.Y. Acad. Sci., 177*, 430.

SHIMAMOTO, T. (1960): Damages to 'silicone-like property' of vascular endothelial cells and prevention by monoamine oxidase inhibitor, nialamide. *Asian med. J., 3*, 479.

SHIMAMOTO, T. (1963): The relationship of edematous reaction in arteries to atherosclerosis and thrombosis. *J. Atheroscler. Res., 3*, 87.

SHIMAMOTO, T. (1969*a*): Experimental study on atherosclerosis – an attempt at its prevention and treatment. *Acta path. jap., 19*, 15.

SHIMAMOTO, T. (1969*b*): An introduction to the investigation of atherogenesis, thrombogenesis and pyridinolcarbamate treatment – Visualization of the transendothelial passage through intercellular junctions and discovery of endothelial folds and intercellular bridges of vascular endothelium. In: *Atherogenesis. Proceedings, I International Symposium on Atherogenesis, Thrombogenesis and Pyridinolcarbamate Treatment, Tokyo 1969*, pp. 5–27. Editors: T. Shimamoto and F. Numano. ICS 201, Excerpta Medica, Amsterdam.

SHIMAMOTO, T. (1972*a*): A new concept in atherogenesis and treatment of atherosclerosis. *Z. Gefässkr.*, in press.
SHIMAMOTO, T. (1972*b*): A new attempt in the prevention and treatment of atherosclerosis and thrombosis. *Jap. J. Angiol.*, in press.
SHIMAMOTO, T., ATSUMI, T., NUMANO, F. and FUJITA, T. (1968): Treatment of atherosclerosis with pyridinolcarbamate. *Progr. Biochem. Pharmacol.*, *4*, 597.
SHIMAMOTO, T., KOBAYASHI, M. and NUMANO, F. (1972): Infiltration of γ-globulin, fibrinogen and β-lipoprotein into blood vessel wall by atherogenic stress visualized by immunofluorescence. *Proc. Jap. Acad.*, *48*, 336.
SHIMAMOTO, T., NUMANO, F. and FUJITA, T. (1966): Atherosclerosis-inhibiting effect of an anti-bradykinin agent, pyridinolcarbamate. *Amer. Heart J.*, *71*, 216.
SHIMAMOTO, T., YAMAZAKI, H., FUJITA, T., SUNAGA, T., ISHIOKA, T., IWAHARA, S. and YAJIMA, G. (1959): Method of finding the arteriosclerogenic substance and producing intimal arteriosclerosis on various species of animals. *Proc. Jap. Acad.*, *35*, 632.
SHIMAMOTO, T., YAMASHITA, Y., NUMANO, F. and SUNAGA, T. (1971): Scanning and transmission electron microscopic observation of endothelial cells in the normal condition and in initial stages of atherosclerosis. *Acta path. jap.*, *21*, 93.
WILENS, S. L. (1951): The nature of diffuse intimal thickening of arteries. *Amer. J. Path.*, *27*, 825.
WILLMS-KRETSCHMER, K. and MAJNO, G. (1969): Ischemia of the skin. *Amer. J. Path.*, *54*, 327.
WU, C., HUANG, T. and HSU, C. (1969): Prevention of experimental atherosclerosis with pyridinolcarbamate. *Amer. Heart J.*, *77*, 657.
YAMAZAKI, H., SANO, T., ODAKURA, T., TAKEUCHI, K., MATSUMURA, T., HOSAKI, S. and SHIMAMOTO, T. (1971): Appearance of thrombogenic tendency induced by adrenaline and its prevention by β-adrenergic blocking agent, nialamide and pyridinolcarbamate. *Thrombos. Diathes. haemorrh. (Stuttg.)*, *26*, 251.
YAMAZAKI, H., SANO, T. and SHIMAMOTO, T. (1972): Enhancement of ADP-induced platelet aggregation by adrenaline and cholesterol and its prevention. Paper presented at: III Congress, International Society on Thrombosis and Hemostasis, Washington, D.C. 1972.

DISCUSSION

Dr. CONSTANTINIDES: Dr. Shimamoto, I would like to say that I have been completely able to confirm your observations in the rabbit, and I think that I can propose one mechanism at least for it. Using quite larger doses of adrenaline than you did, we induced further junctions to stay open longer and also a greater number of endothelial junctions to open up, so that we could examine them under the microscope. I hope to show in my paper that there is a definite opening of endothelial junctions with high enough doses of adrenaline that one cannot see with small physiological doses. The only reason is that the small physiological doses only open up 1 in every 500 junctions and each is open for only a few microseconds. The statistical chances of seeing one under the microscope is very, very minimal. I also would like to say that I was very intrigued to see your blebs at the same sites at which they develop in response to all kinds of other insults, such as proteolytic enzymes. It seems that the junctional area is the weakest spot which is first injured.

Dr. SPECTOR Dr. Shimamoto, I would like to ask whether the effects that you see with cholesterol and adrenaline on the increased permeability are restricted to the vasculature or do you see this same increased permeability in other tissues?

Dr. SHIMAMOTO: No.

Dr. NELSON: Again, on the same topic of combined administration of adrenaline and cholesterol, it appeared from the micrographs, and I believe you stated, that there seemed to be an increasing stagnation of the fluorescent material as if it were dammed by the internal elastic lamina. Do you have any speculation as to why that occurs, with the combined treatment?

Dr. SHIMAMOTO: No, we have no idea at the moment.

Dr. NELSON: Was there, for example, an increase in the degree of contraction of the internal elastic lamina in such cases?

Dr. SHIMAMOTO: We saw no change in the internal elastic lamina itself but possibly there was change in the smooth muscle. If the smooth muscle swells, it could be that the protrusions through the fenestrations are disturbed. We have maybe a very delicate control of the transportation through these tiny structures.

INVESTIGATIONS INTO THE PATHOGENESIS OF ARTERIOSCLEROSIS: DRUG PROPHYLAXIS

H. FROST

Medizinische Poliklinik, University of Munich, Munich,
Federal Republic of Germany

If one reviews the published work on arteriosclerosis, it is not difficult to establish that the search for the location of the initial event in the pathogenesis of arteriosclerosis is still progressing.

More than 100 years ago, as a result of his investigations which he carried out with technically inferior instruments, the Viennese pathologist Karl Rokitansky reported that a vascular process of this kind arose from an 'excessive formation by the organism and coating of the

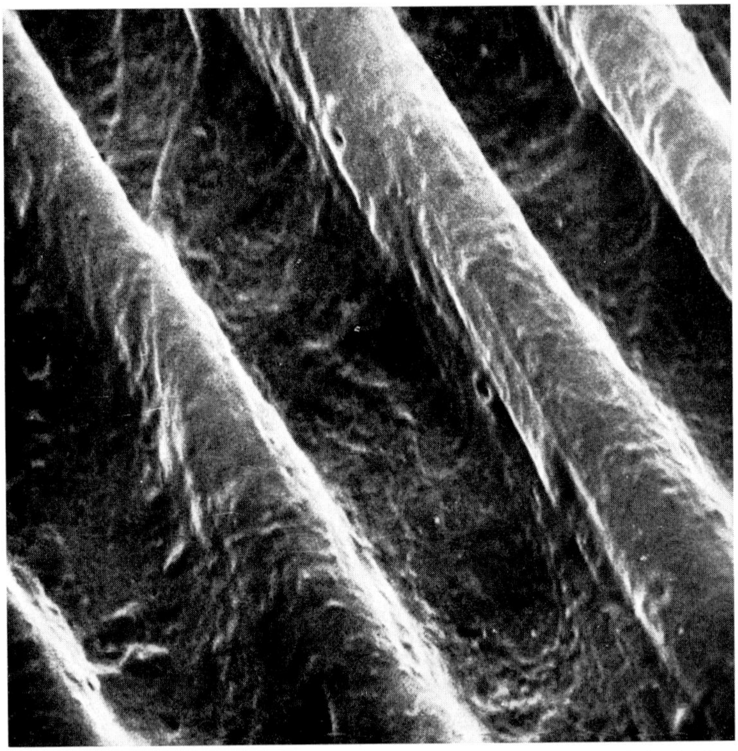

Fig. 1. Inner surface of abdominal aorta of a healthy rabbit. The outline of the folds corresponds to the course of the tunica elastica interna. × 5000.

→

Fig. 2. Desquamated endothelial cells, thrombocytes, fibrin and isolated trapped erythrocytes on the inner surface of the abdominal aorta of a rabbit exposed to the smoke of 17 cigarettes for 3½ hours. × 2000.

Fig. 3. Another section of the blood vessel shown in Fig. 2. × 5000.

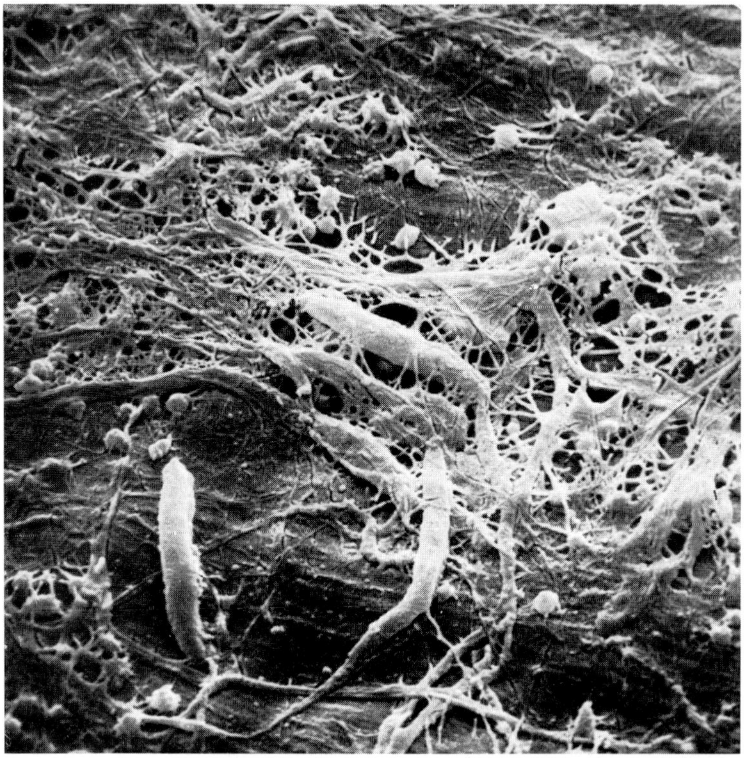

Fig. 2

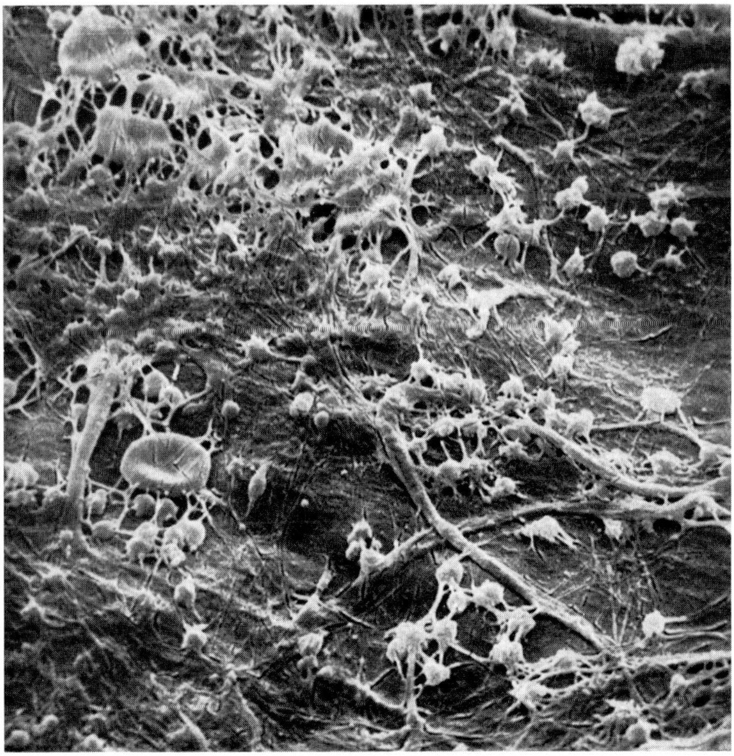

Fig. 3

internal membrane of the vessel from the mass of the blood'. He went on to point out that this vascular process 'did not originally represent a disease of the structure of the arterial membrane, but was soon followed by one'. At that time, as also today, other conflicting ideas were put forward. Virchow in particular, unlike Rokitansky, considered atheroma to be an inflammatory process and the thickening of the vessel wall to be the result of a reactive proliferation on the part of the connective tissue cells of the intima.

Recently, Rokitansky's ideas have been taken up again and given more sound support by Duguid. Duguid has shown that changes in the vessel wall which are morphologically identical to atherosclerosis can arise through arterial organization of a thrombus. Guided by the idea that this process can begin not in but on the inner surface of the vessel, we have followed up the question of the nature of the first morphological changes in animal experiments. For these investigations we used a scanning electron microscope which, as already seen from the work of Shimamoto, is ideally suited for the examination of surfaces (Fig. 1) and for detecting and following even the smallest changes, much less than 1 μ in size, of the inner surfaces of the vessels.

It is well known that a number of factors such as hypercholesterolaemia, inhalation of cigarette smoke, diabetes mellitus and hypertension can initiate the development of an arteriosclerotic vascular process, or at least favour it. Therefore, for the experimental animals, we have imitated conditions which are comparable to those injurious factors. It has been shown

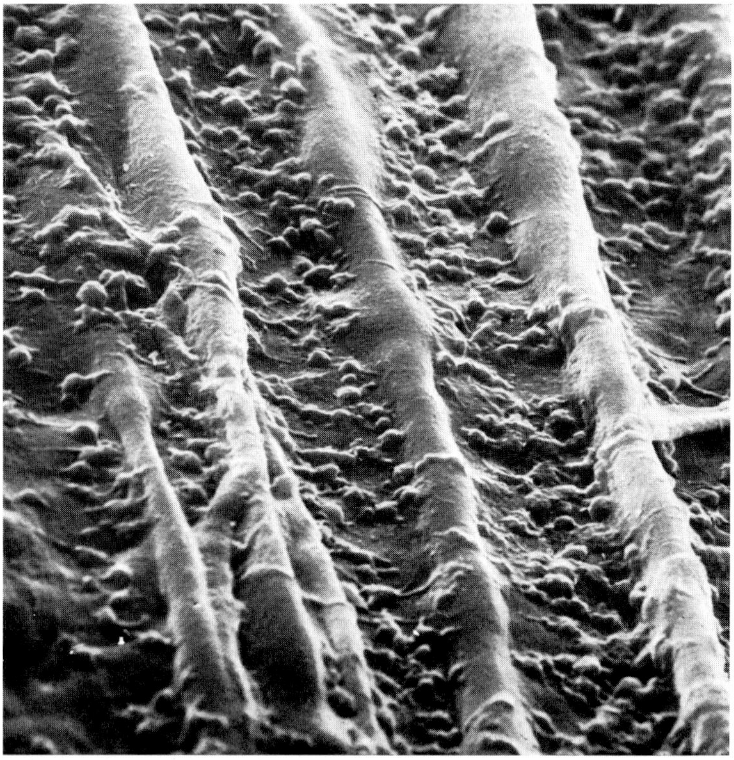

Fig. 4. Inner surface of the abdominal aorta of a rabbit fed on diet containing 2% cholesterol. Thrombocytes and desquamated endothelial cells. × 2000.

→

Fig. 5. Enlargement of Fig. 4. × 5000.

Fig. 6. Another section of the vessel shown in Figs. 4 and 5. × 5000.

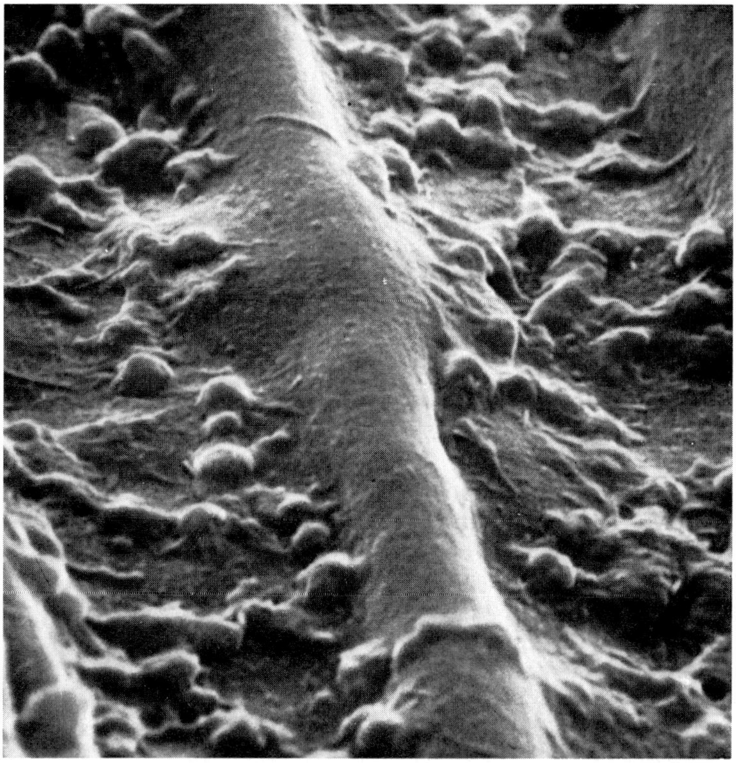

Fig. 5

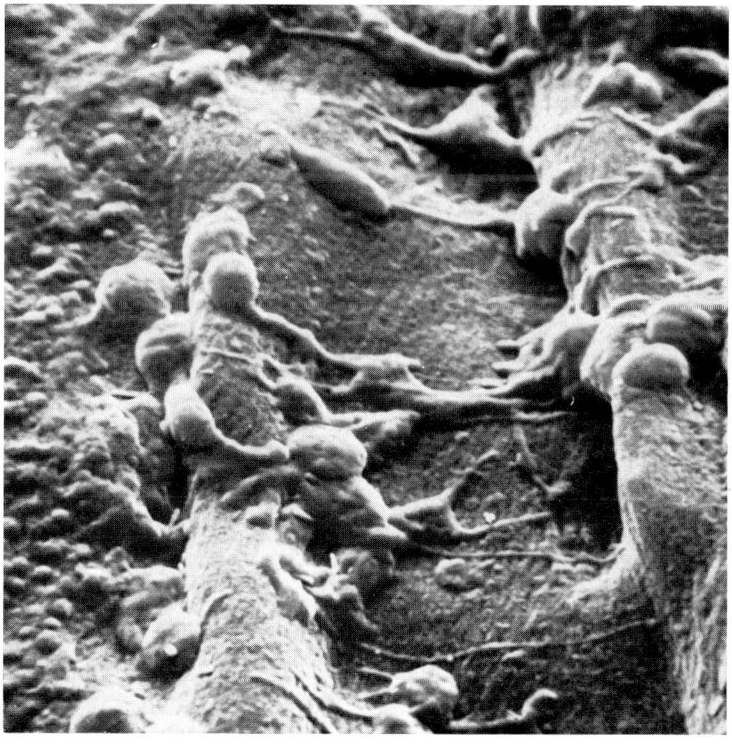

Fig. 6

that, independent of the kind of injurious agent, the first changes on the inner surface of the vessels become visible as platelet adhesions which are associated with disturbances of the endothelial structure.

I would like to give some examples of this. A rabbit which had been exposed for $3\frac{1}{2}$ hours to the smoke of 17 cigarettes, and which also received smoke through a simple apparatus in front of the mouth and nose while anaesthetized and during the surgical removal of the vessels, showed increasing changes on the internal surfaces of the arteries with increasing duration of the effects of the smoke. The abdominal aorta, therefore, as the last vessel to be removed from the animal, showed numerous desquamating or desquamated endothelial cells and numerous platelets sticking to the wall between them after a further $3\frac{1}{2}$ hours exposure to the effects of cigarette smoke (Fig. 2). Between the thrombocytes a rather dense network of fibrin threads extended with occasional trapped erythrocytes (Fig. 3).

If the rabbit is fed for 3 weeks on a diet containing 2% cholesterol, the serum cholesterol level increases considerably during this period. Up to now, we have measured levels of about 260 mg%. This corresponds to 4–5 times the normal level for a rabbit. We also find desquamated endothelial cells (Fig. 4) and an internal vascular wall with thrombocytes scattered over it (Figs. 5 and 6).

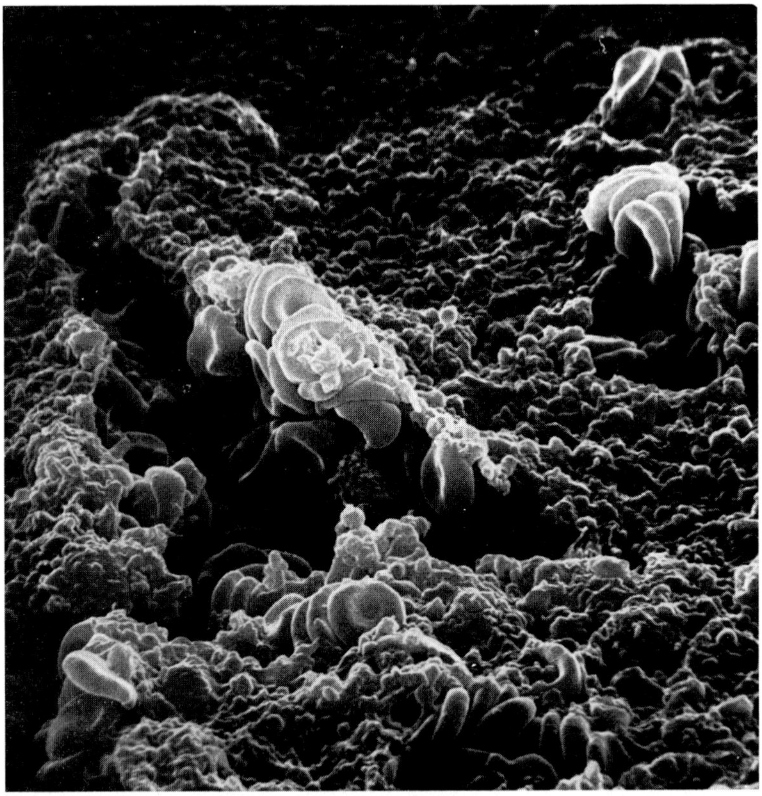

Fig. 7. Stratified thrombus in the lumen of human anterior tibial artery. × 2000.

→

Fig. 8. Enlargement of the stenosing thrombus seen in Fig. 7, with basal layer of thrombocytes on which the agglomerated erythrocytes are piled up. × 5000.

Fig. 9. Erythrocytes trapped in a network of fibrin from the stenosing thrombus seen in Figs. 7 and 8. × 5000.

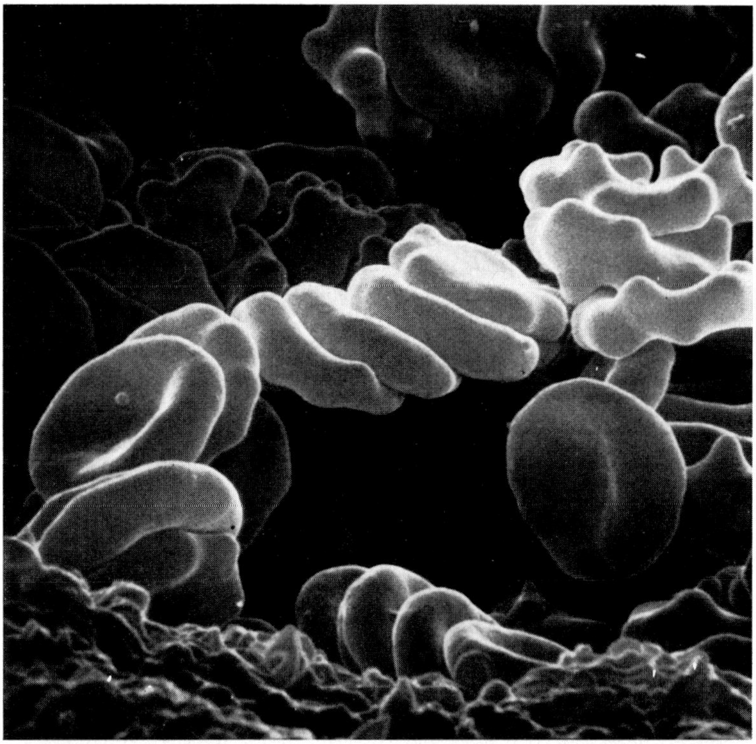

Fig. 8

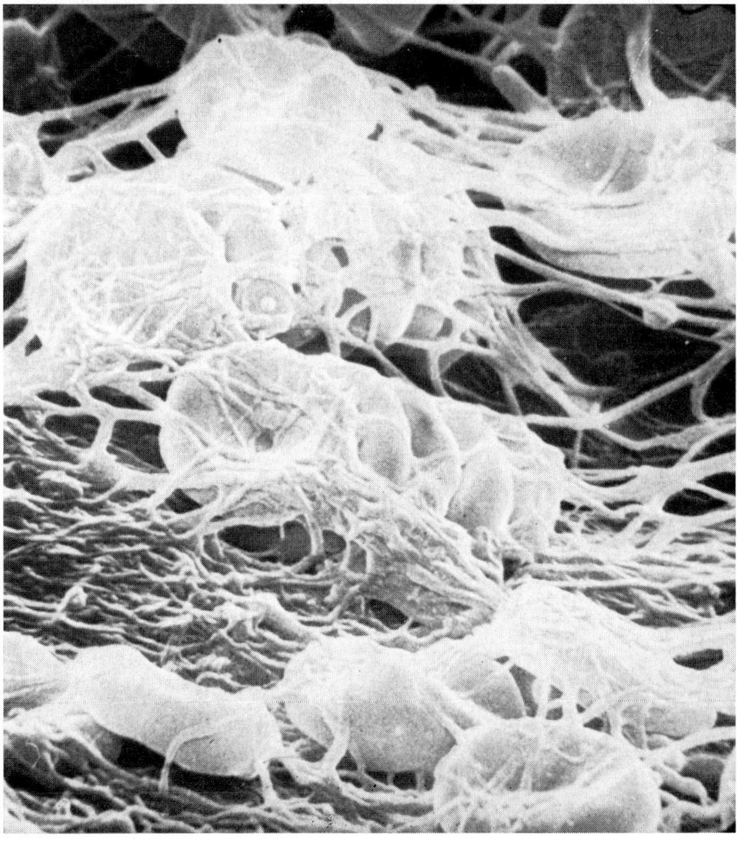

Fig. 9

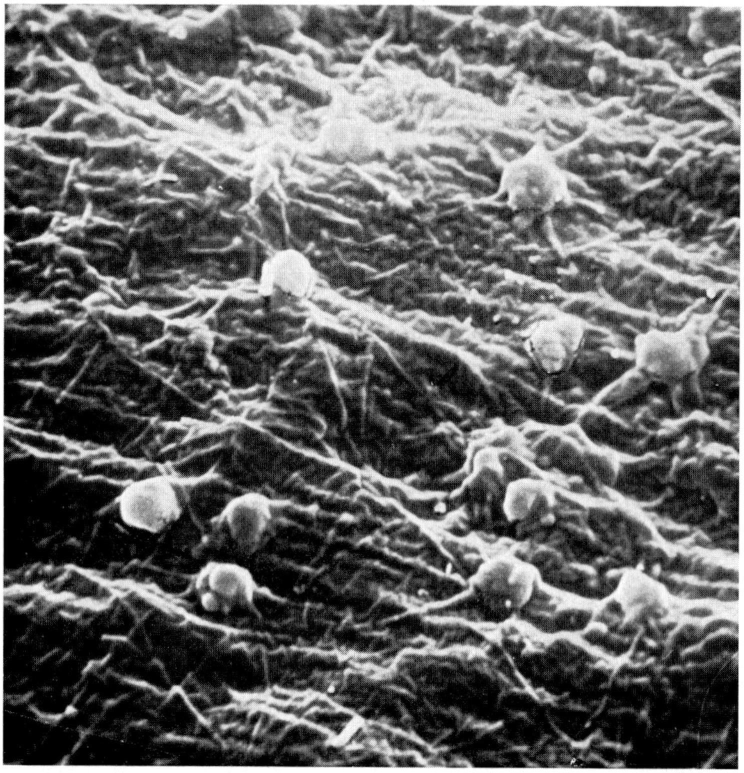

Fig. 10

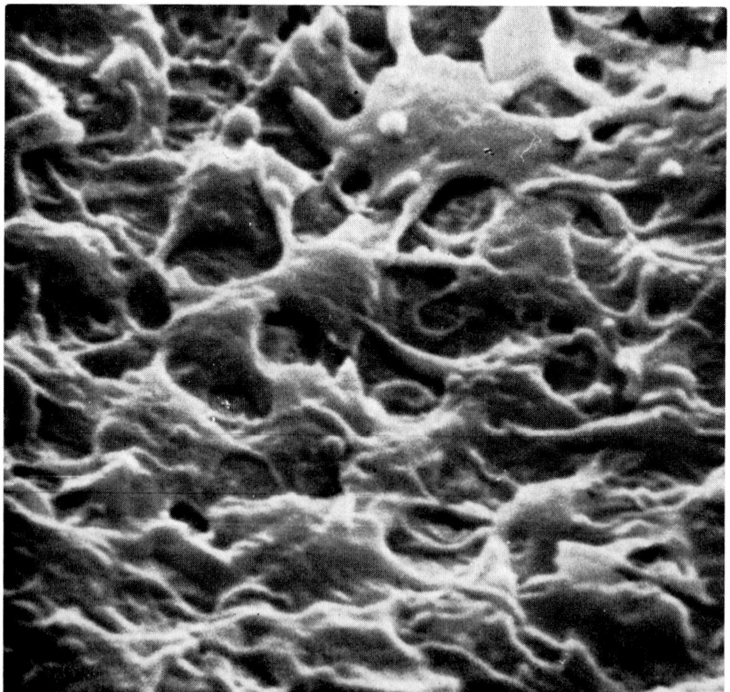

Fig. 11

The question of how far the results of animal experiments can be transferred to the actual course of the vascular process in man is not easy to answer. Similar observations in man and in suitable animal experiments, however, have led to the supposition that the important processes in the development of disease also proceed in the same way.

The right leg of a 69-year-old patient had to be amputated because of an obliterative angiopathy. He was a habitual smoker with hypercholesterolaemia. In the anterior tibial artery (Fig. 7), which was the only artery in the lower leg which still had a small residual lumen for a short distance, we found a stratified parietal thrombus consisting of dense layers of thrombocytes intermingled with erythrocytes and fibrin (Fig. 8). This finding corresponds, I think, to those of the animal experiment, which developed under the effect of the same injurious factors (Fig. 9).

To the question of what fate these deposits now undergo, and what significance they may possibly have for changes in the vessel wall with reference to arteriosclerosis, Duguid's investigations have already given an answer. As far as possible, I would like to describe briefly our observations on these points using the scanning electron microscope.

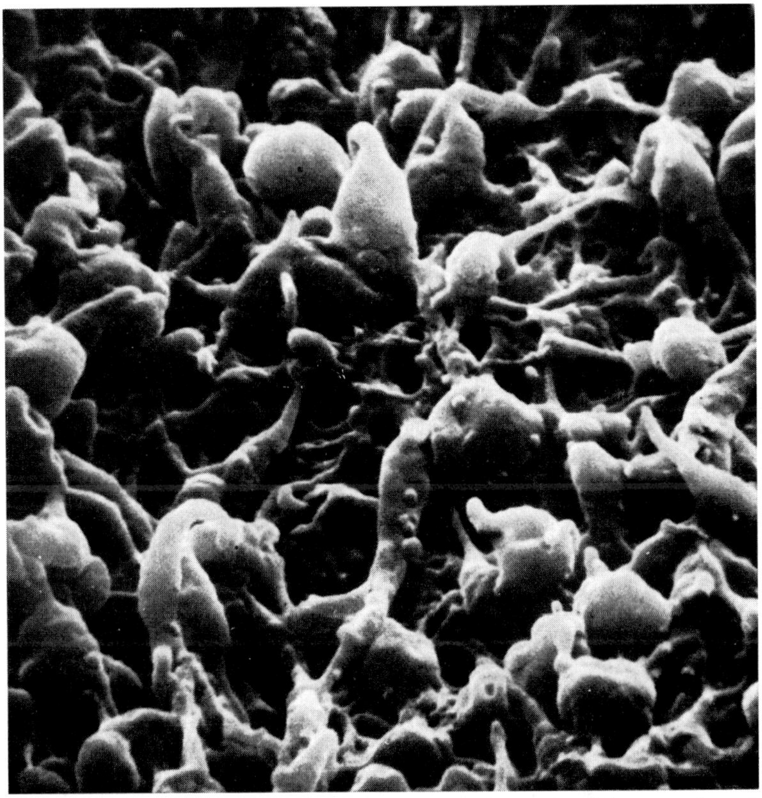

Fig. 12. 20 min after a local injury to the wall of the common carotid artery of a rabbit by an electric current (170 V/sec). A thick thrombocyte deposit covers the inner surface of the injured vessel. × 10,000.

←

Fig. 10. Inner surface of the common carotid artery of a rabbit 20 min after local cold stimulus. Numerous thrombocytes adhere to the inner surface of the vessel. × 5000.

Fig. 11. 1 hour after a cold stimulus to the common carotid artery. The inner surface of the vessel is covered with a carpet of mis-shapen, interwoven thrombocytes. × 10,000.

The concept of cold-induced angiitis is known, an arterial disease which finally can no longer be differentiated from endarteritis or arteriosclerosis. We have tried to produce such a vascular process by holding a small piece of ice on the exposed common carotid artery or abdominal aorta for 10 min without exerting any pressure on the artery. 20 min after the beginning of this cold stimulus, numerous desquamated endothelial cells and parietal thrombocytes (Fig. 10) were found on the internal surface of these vessels. An hour later, they had formed a thick, carpet-like layer (Fig. 11).

A similar result, but much more intense, can be seen on the internal surface of the arterial wall after passing a local current stimulus. With this method it is possible to form an accurately measured and reproducible lesion in the internal wall of the vessel, without damaging the vessel to a great extent. In a few seconds, countless thrombocytes are deposited on the endothelial lesion of the damaged vessel wall. The platelet carpet is already very thick 20 min after such a stimulus (Fig. 12). 2 hours later, obviously under the effect of the blood flow, the first deposits have been transformed into smooth coatings (Fig. 13) in which thrombocytes, erythrocytes and fibrin can be recognized. These deposits are then either endothelialized in a few days or a relatively extensive hyaline thrombus develops on the original deposit or on a

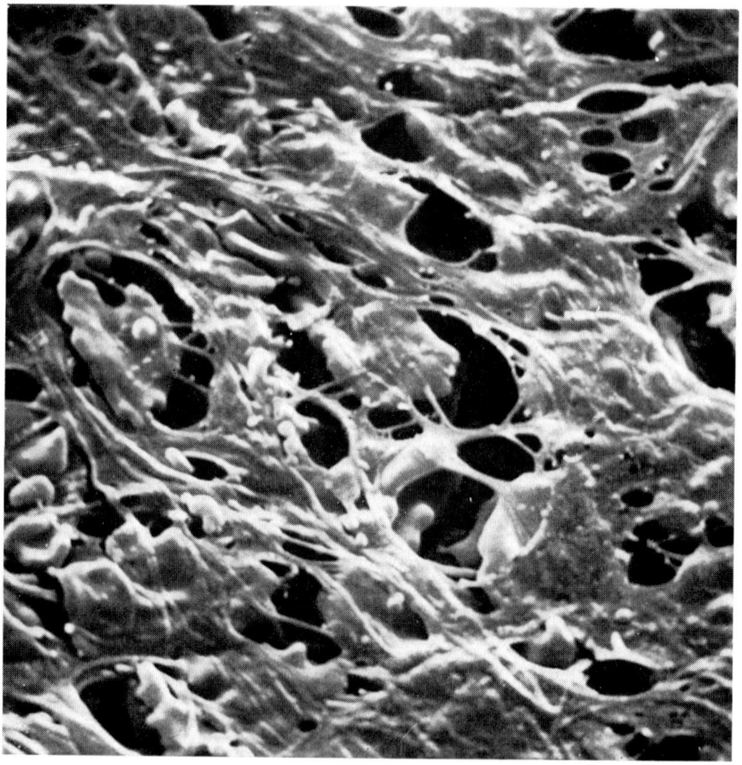

Fig. 13. Multilayered coating of thrombocytes and fibrin 2 hours after a local current stimulus to the common carotid artery of a rabbit. × 10,000.

→

Fig. 14. Longitudinal section of the common carotid artery of a rabbit 20 days after injury by a local current stimulus. × 100.

Fig. 15. Enlargement of Fig. 14 showing fibrous structures enclosing formed elements of the blood. × 10,000.

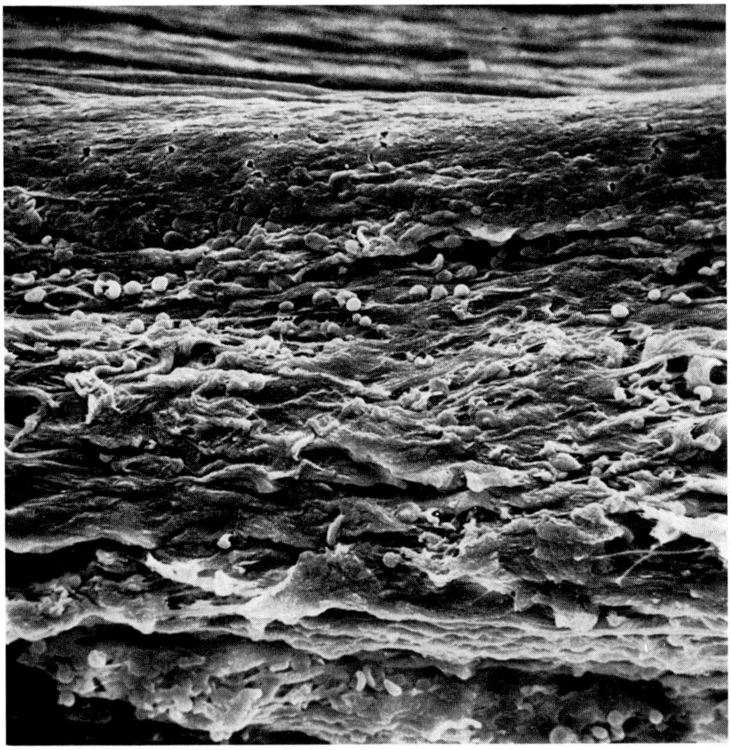

Fig. 14

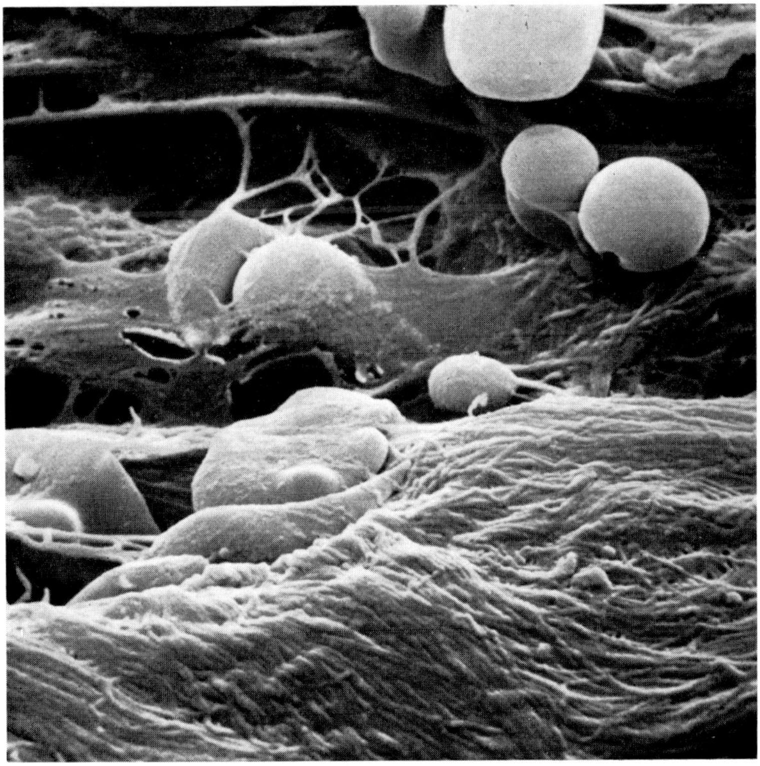

Fig. 15

new deposit, which also becomes very rapidly endothelialized if the vessel is not completely obliterated.

The next case shows such a result (Fig. 14). 20 days after the current stimulus which had produced an endothelial lesion 0.6 mm in size, the vessel wall was doubled in thickness to the extent of 2 cm. Microscopic examination shows that this increase in thickness occurs exclusively in the region of the intima. In the endothelial lesion a mural thrombus had formed at first, in the region of which fibrous structures were largely seen, in addition to isolated blood cells (Fig. 15). Laid over this is a broad hyaline thrombus of erythrocytes and fibrin which is covered with newly formed endothelium (Fig. 16).

Let us recall Duguid's investigations in which he was able to show that such incorporated deposits could no longer be distinguished from arteriosclerosis by light microscopy, after their organization.

Investigations with the scanning electron microscope have brought us a still further result. With an excessive increase in the serum cholesterol level during a 12-week diet rich in cholesterol, adhesions of cholesterol crystals also appear on the vessel wall in addition to platelet adhesions and disturbances of the endothelial structure. These can clearly be seen as a single deposit on the endothelial cells (Fig. 17) and as a surface covering (Fig. 18) or a massive deposit (Fig. 19) like thrombotic adhesions on the wall, covered with new endothelium and incorporated into the intima.

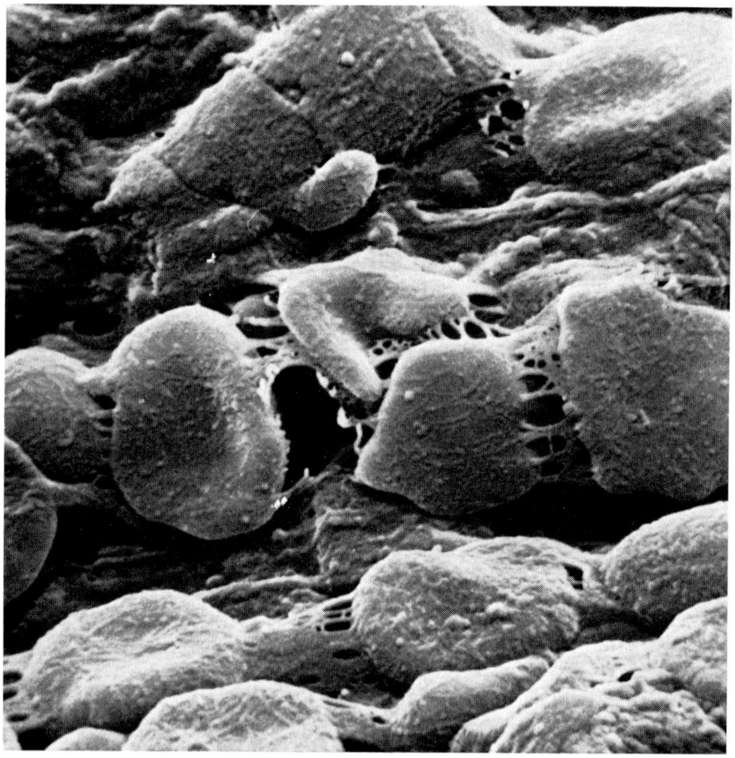

Fig. 16. Enlargement of Fig. 14 showing clumped erythrocytes and fibrin fibres. × 10,000.

→

Fig. 17. Inner surface of the abdominal aorta of a rabbit after 11 weeks on a cholesterol-enriched diet. Endothelial cell with prominent nucleus. × 10,000.

Fig. 18. Multilayered coating on the inner surface of the abdominal aorta of a rabbit after 11 weeks on a cholesterol-enriched diet. × 10,000.

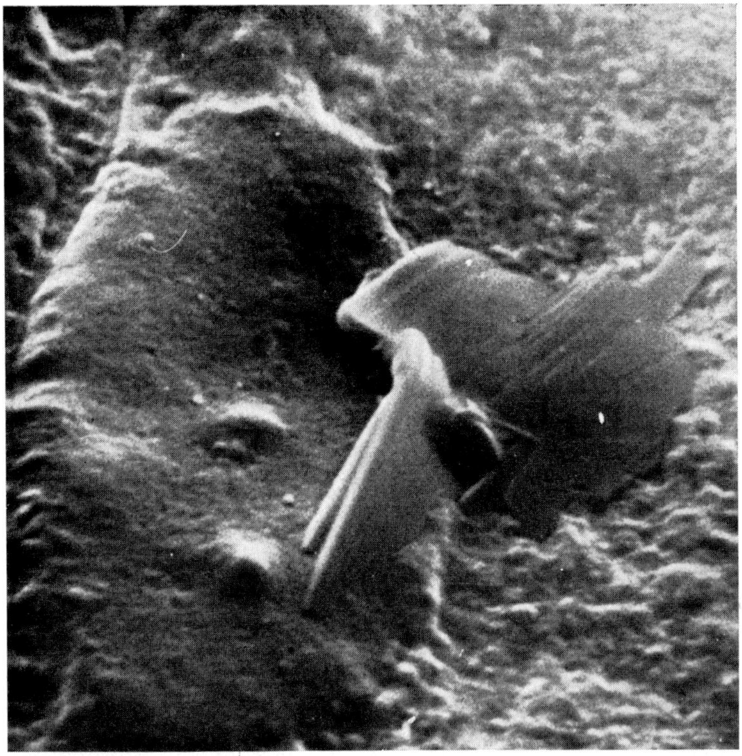

Fig. 17

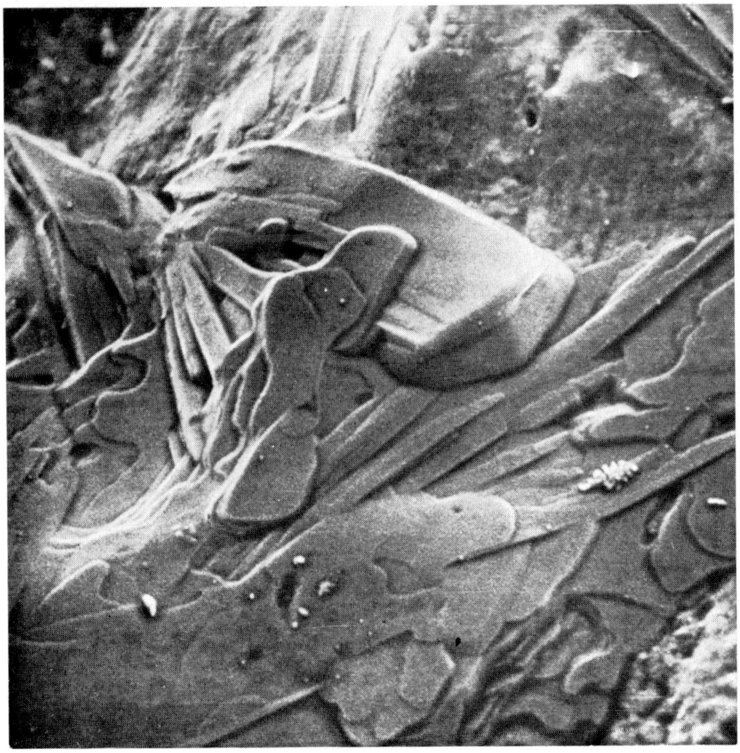

Fig. 18

Longitudinal sections of such a vessel show, e.g. in the descending branch of the left coronary artery, cholesterol crystals in several layers of a thickened intima (Fig. 20) which is covered by a wide layer of endothelium. Its basic structure is similar to those which we have also seen in already partly organized and incorporated parietal deposits and hyaline thrombi (Fig. 21). Only by such a method can an idea be actually obtained of the considerable reconstruction of the vascular intima which takes place in this relatively short period of time.

If one starts from the idea that endothelial lesions and platelet adhesions can play a primary role in the pathogenesis of arteriosclerosis, then an inhibiting effect on this process can also be expected from a drug which is supposed to be an antiarteriosclerotic agent. To test such effects it seemed to us that an experiment with local, easily reproducible and measurable vascular wall lesions provided by current stimulus or the effect of cold would be particularly suitable for a rapid test. We have also carried out this test with pyridinolcarbamate (Anginin) in 5 animals using the current stimulus method and in 3 animals using a local cold stimulus.

The rabbits under test weighed 2.5–3.2 kg and received a single intravenous injection of 10 mg pyridinolcarbamate per kg body weight. The vessels were removed in each case 20 min after the local current stimulus lesion or after the beginning of the cold stimulus and 30, 60

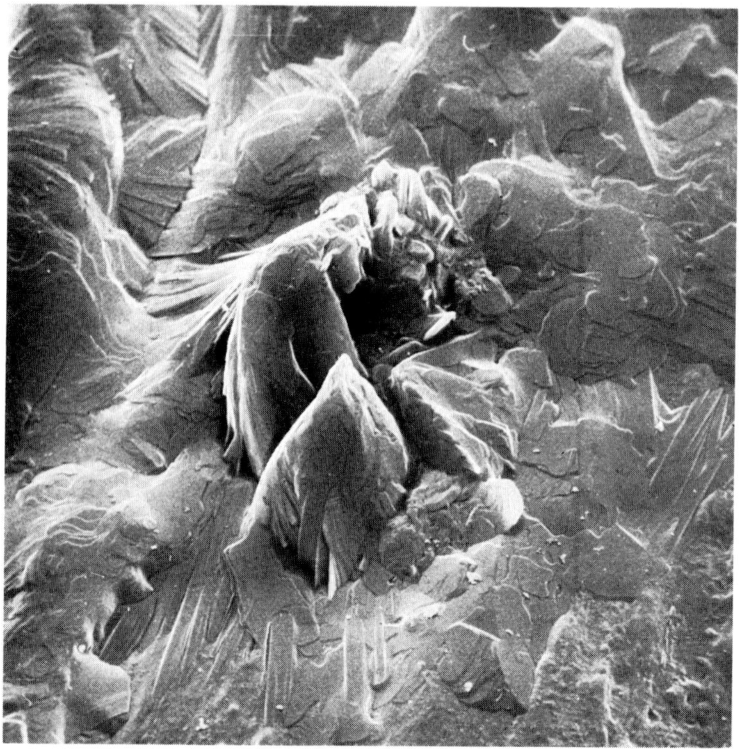

Fig. 19. Massive cholesterol deposit on the inner surface of the abdominal aorta of a rabbit after 11 weeks on a cholesterol-enriched diet. × 5000.

→

Fig. 20. Longitudinal section showing open lumen of the descending branch of the left coronary artery of a rabbit after 11 weeks on a cholesterol-enriched diet. Cholesterol crystals can be seen in the clefts of a thickened intima. × 500.

Fig. 21. Enlargement of Fig. 20. × 2000.

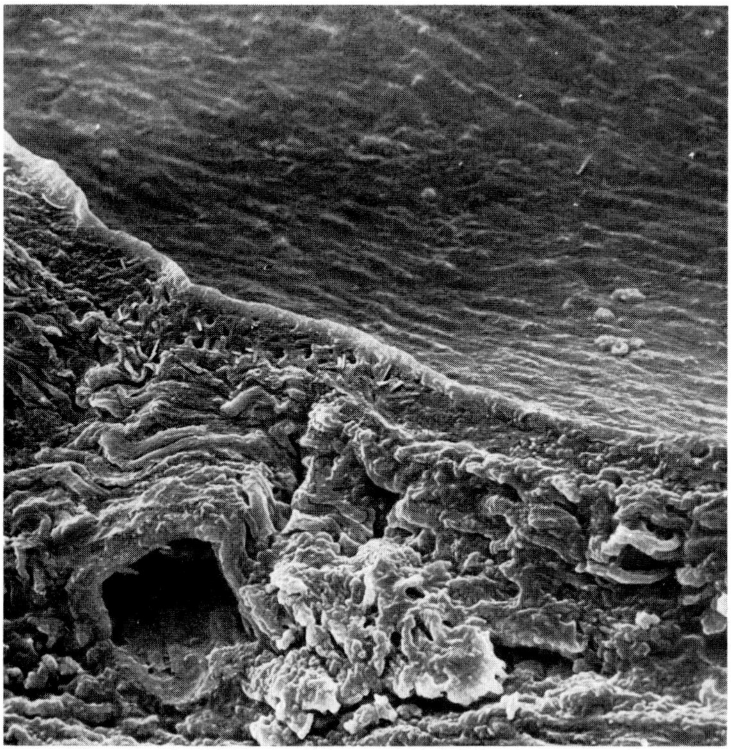

Fig. 20

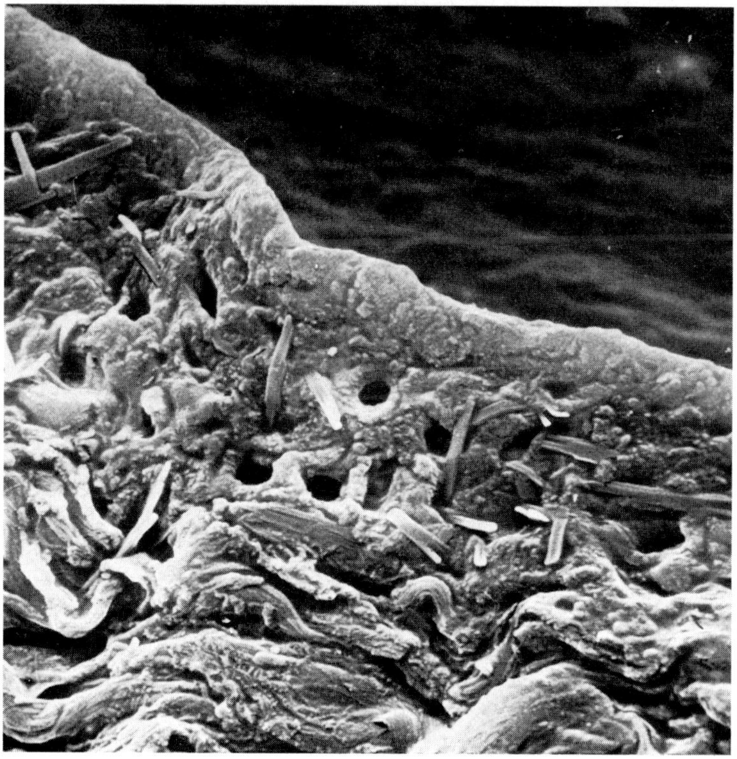

Fig. 21

and 90 min after the administration of Anginin. The animals treated with pyridinolcarbamate were compared with 6 control animals in the current stimulus test and 4 in the cold stimulus group.

In the control animals, as already described, it was found that a massive deposit of platelets occurred 20 min after passing a local current stimulus (170 V/sec) on the internal surface of the vessel under the positive electrode (Fig. 22). The animals previously treated with Anginin showed (Fig. 23) only isolated thrombocytes and fibrous structures (Fig. 24) lying on the inner surface in the region of the lesion of the vessel wall (Fig. 25) in addition to a thin marginal covering. Platelets were also found occasionally in small islands (Fig. 26) which clearly showed endothelial damage (Fig. 27) but there were no massive platelet adhesions as seen in the control animals.

After a local cold stimulus lasting 10 min, in the region of the lesion in the control animals there were numerous platelets surrounded by a border of desquamated endothelial cells.

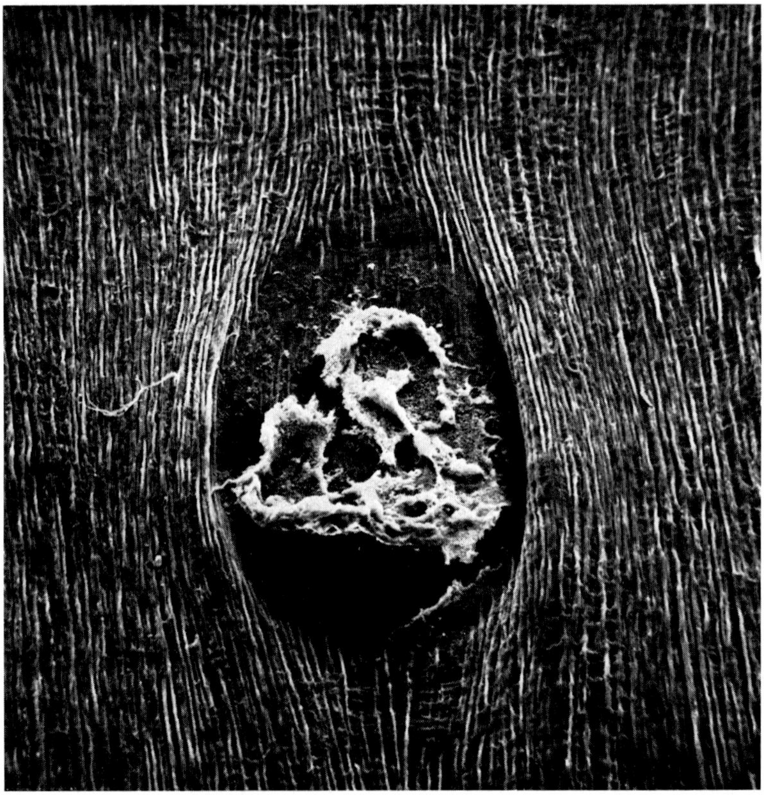

Fig. 22. Deposition thrombus on the inner surface of the common carotid artery after injury by local current stimulus (170 V/sec). × 50.

→

Fig. 23. Inner surface of the common carotid artery of a rabbit pretreated with pyridinolcarbamate 20 min after local current stimulus. Thrombocytes at different stages of metamorphosis adhere to the wall. × 10,000.

Fig. 24. Enlargement of Fig. 23. × 20,000.

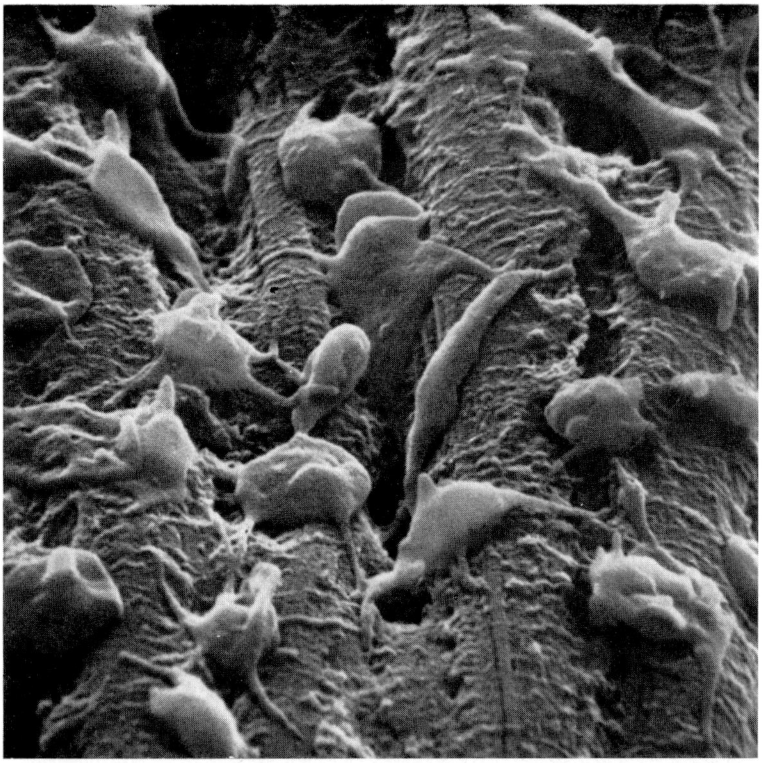

Fig. 23

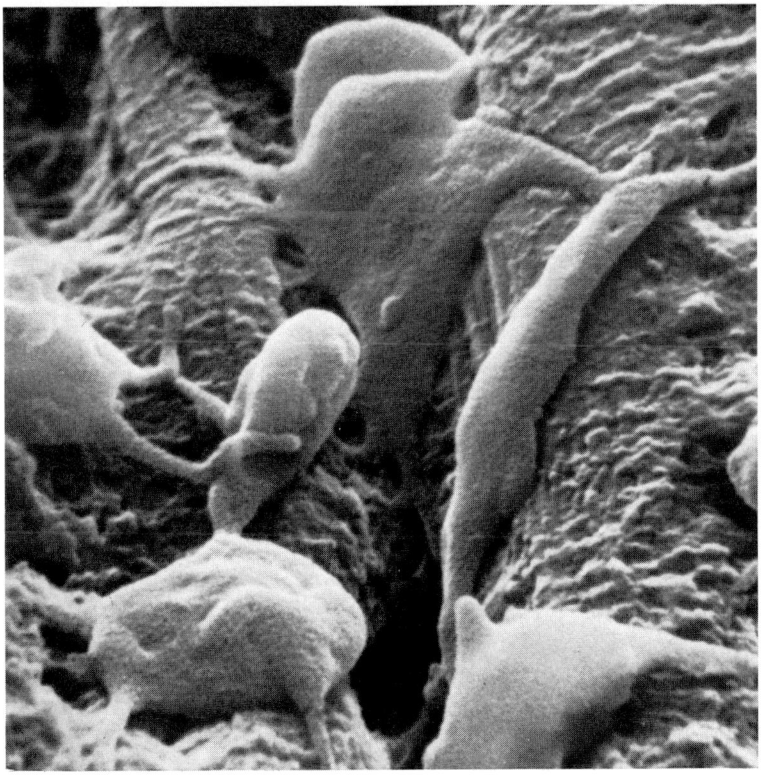

Fig. 24

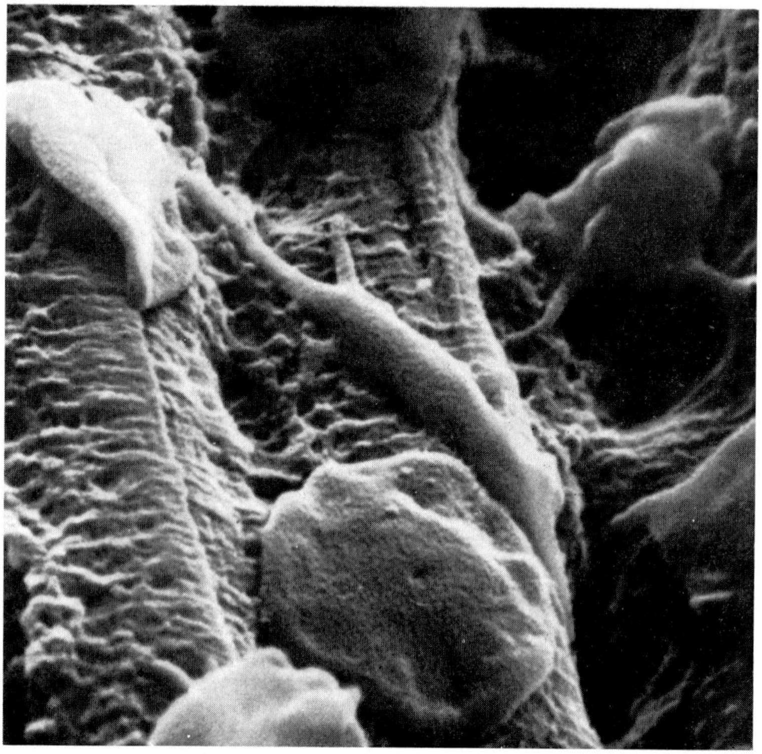

Fig. 25

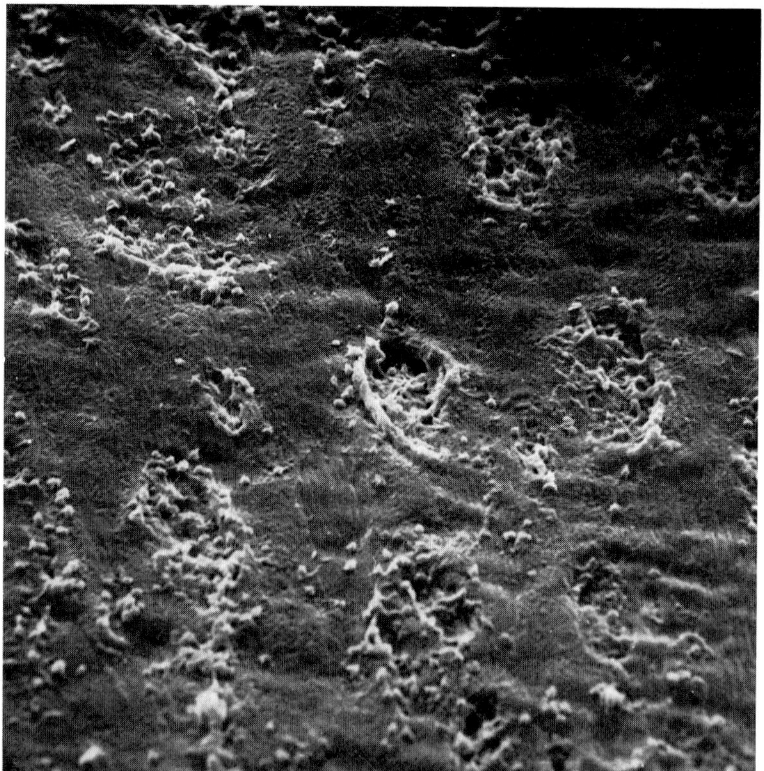

Fig. 26

The animals treated with Anginin showed a few desquamated endothelial cells but no parietal thrombocytes.

The number of these investigations may seem small, but the results clearly stand out so that on the basis of these results we may attribute a preventive effect to Anginin in both experiments which we used for the study of the pathogenesis of arteriosclerosis. The effect was visible in both the only partly recognizable damaged endothelial coat and the considerably smaller layers of platelets, which most of all do not show dense clumps on the damaged vessel wall.

SUMMARY

The appearance of endothelial damage and parietal thrombocytes in animal experiments a very short time after or during the effect of injurious factors considered significant for the development of arteriosclerosis suggests the initial or initiating part which they play in this vascular process. Both endothelial lesions and platelet adhesions, obviously associated with damaging stimuli, can appear independently of each other, or can mutually induce each other.

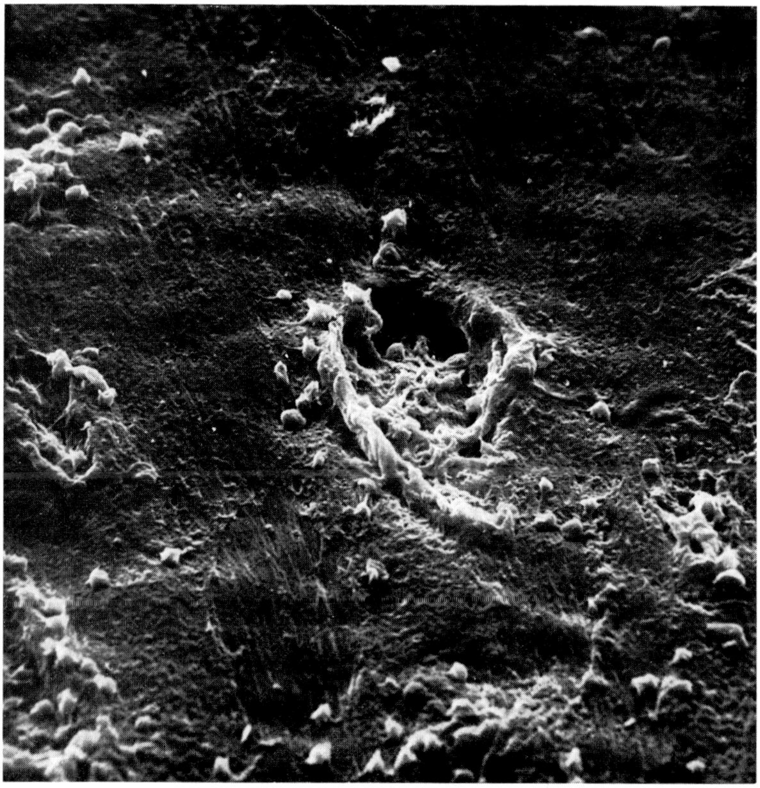

Fig. 27. Enlargement of Fig. 26. × 2000.

←

Fig. 25. Another section of the vessel shown in Fig. 23 showing thrombocytes on the inner surface. × 20,000.

Fig. 26. Islands of endothelial damage with thrombocyte deposit 20 min after local current stimulus (170 V/sec). Pretreatment with pyridinolcarbamate. × 1000.

The organization of incorporated deposits leads to a change in the vessel wall which cannot be differentiated from arteriosclerosis. It can be assumed from comparable findings in animal experiments and in arteriosclerotic patients that the process demonstrated here is also a possible pathway to arteriosclerosis in man. From this, an effect on these vascular processes is to be expected from drugs which reduce the harmful effect on the vascular endothelium and inhibit the adhesive tendency of platelets. Pyridinolcarbamate appears to fulfil this task to a certain degree.

REFERENCES

References for this paper will be supplied on application to the author.

DISCUSSION

Dr. AUSTIN: Dr. Frost, you mentioned that your animals were pretreated with pyridinolcarbamate. Do you have any experience in creating local lesions, and then later treating with pyridinolcarbamate?

Dr. FROST: No. We have not yet performed such experiments.

Dr. CONSTANTINIDES: One result of yours needs further investigation, namely the cholesterol crystal precipitation that you showed here. I wonder if this crystallization of cholesterol could be the result of cholesterol crystallizing during the procedure used in scanning microscopy. As you know, unless the artery is thoroughly perfused and washed of all plasma, a residual layer of plasma proteins may very often adhere to the endothelium, and if you have a very cholesterol-rich plasma, during the process of extreme dehydration and metal shadowing that are involved in scanning microscopy it may be that some of the cholesterol crystallizes inside during the procedure. The resolving power of 150 Å of the scanning microscope would never reveal small microfractures or changes in the plasma membrane of, e.g., 40, 50, or 60 Å width, which could very well be the expression of a microinjury in a certain spot of the cell.

Dr. FROST: This is correct. However, in another series of discoveries which I have not reported here, I have seen that damage to the whole cell is necessary.

THE IMPORTANT ROLE OF ENDOTHELIAL CHANGES IN ATHEROGENESIS*

PARIS CONSTANTINIDES
Department of Pathology, University of British Columbia,
Vancouver, Canada

INTRODUCTION AND METHODOLOGY

There is increasing evidence that endothelial injury, and therefore arterial injury, can play a very important role in promoting both atherogenesis and thrombogenesis (Constantinides, 1965).

Thus, to limit ourselves here only to the subject of atherogenesis, experimental atherosclerosis can be produced very quickly and with very little lipemia if the arteries are injured in any of a dozen ways, while it takes an extremely high lipemia and a very long time to accomplish the same result if the arteries are normal – apparently because injury produces gaps in the endothelial lining, as we have found in our calciferol experiments with the electron microscope (Constantinides, 1968).

We therefore proposed the following model of atherogenesis three years ago, on the occasion of the First Tokyo Symposium (Constantinides, 1969*a*):

We proposed that the endothelium of normal arteries represents a barrier that prevents the crossing of large protein and lipoprotein molecules into the arterial wall. Normally only small molecules, such as H_2O, electrolytes, glucose, small proteins (perhaps below 40 Å in diameter), and small hydrolysis products, e.g. amino and fatty acids, are transported across the endothelium to service the metabolic needs of the vessel wall.

The large molecules and particles would normally leave the vascular tree only through some of its finest twigs, namely through the perforated capillaries of the liver, the intestine, and the RES, and through the leaky post-capillary venules, in order to get to the tissue where they are needed. If we stop to think about this arrangement for a moment, it makes biological sense: Since the big molecules are destined for the tissues, nature does not want them to get lost in the walls of the arterial canals while they are in transit; it has therefore made the walls of arteries relatively impermeable to them.

When, however, an artery is injured, the permeability of its endothelium is pathologically increased; gaps are created in it through which not only the small but also the large molecules pour into the wall in such overwhelming quantities that they cannot be metabolized and, therefore, accumulate. In other words, injury 'opens the doors' for the lipids so they can enter the wall, and we have verified that this can happen with the electron microscope, using lipids as markers.

What type of injury can produce such ultrastructural changes?

Since we started studying this problem, we found that many agents produce gaps in the arterial endothelium – some by opening intercellular junctions and others by destroying cells and causing them to slough off (exfoliate) into the lumen, if their action is sufficiently violent (Constantinides, 1969*b*).

So far, of all these agents we studied, the following appear to have potential significance

* These investigations were supported mainly by the Medical Research Council of Canada and in part by the British Columbia Heart Foundation.

for human arterial disease: angiotensin, serotonin, tyramine and other amines, proteolytic enzymes, bile acids, calciferol, lysophosphatides and antigen-antibody complexes. And there are increasing indications, one of which I will present below, that even hyperlipemia itself can be an injuring agent, an idea which we elaborated in our monograph on experimental atherosclerosis and which is also supported by the earlier findings of Shimamoto in cholesterol-fed rabbits (Shimamoto et al., 1966).

Here, I would like to report on three new things: (1) on the effects of certain diabetes metabolites, of nicotine and of an alimentary lipid load on the endothelium of rat femoral arteries; (2) on the pharmacological modification of the effects of serotonin and angiotensin; and (3) on a species difference with regard to the sensitivity of the arterial endothelium to epinephrine and norepinephrine.

MATERIALS AND METHODS

Most materials tested were given by brief intra-arterial infusion into the superficial femoral artery of rats or rabbits, followed by glutaraldehyde perfusion and tissue processing for the transmission electron microscope as described in our previous studies of this type (Constantinides, 1969*b*). An exception was made in the case of nicotine, which was also given subcutaneously for 2 weeks, and in the case of linoleic acid which was given as a single shot by stomach tube. Most substances were dissolved in neutral Millonig's buffer (pH 7.2); their concentrations are quoted in the legends of the figures that document their effects. Male Wistar rats 350–450 g and male New Zealand White rabbits 3–4 kg were used. Each agent was given to 2 animals, with the exception of subcutaneous nicotine and oral linoleic acid, which were given to 4 rabbits and 6 rats, respectively.

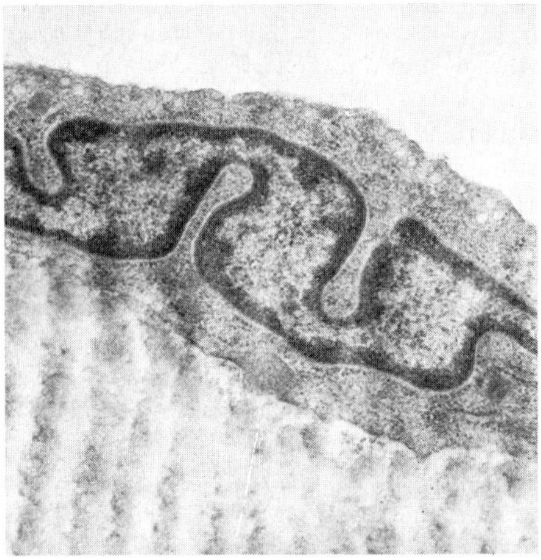

Fig. 1

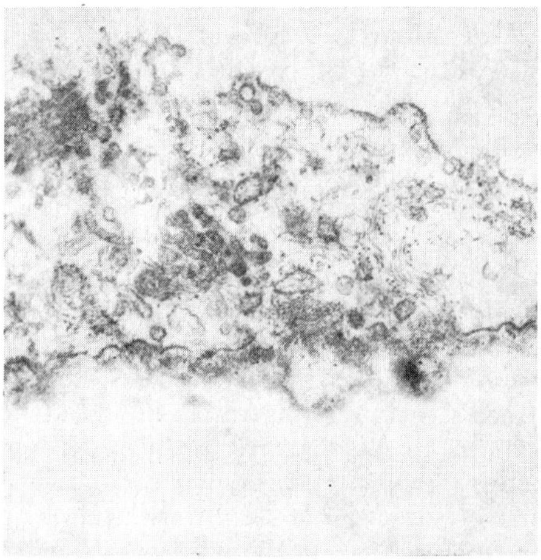

Fig. 2

* *Fig. 1. Normal endothelium* of a rat femoral artery that was perfused with Millonig's buffer (pH 7.2) 40 sec. Note, from top to bottom, the lumen, the normal endothelial cell with its dark cytoplasm and for its accordioned nucleus (with a dense peripheral and a dilute central chromatin component), the narrow subendothelial space with its short subendothelial fibrils, and the internal elastic lamella. × 18,150.

Fig. 2. Endothelium of a rat femoral artery that was perfused for 40 sec with a solution of 0.2 μM/ml *acetoacetic acid* in buffer. The endothelial cell has become very edematous (water-logged) and its superficial plasma membrane has begun to break up. × 28,875.

* All illustrations reduced 14% for reproduction.

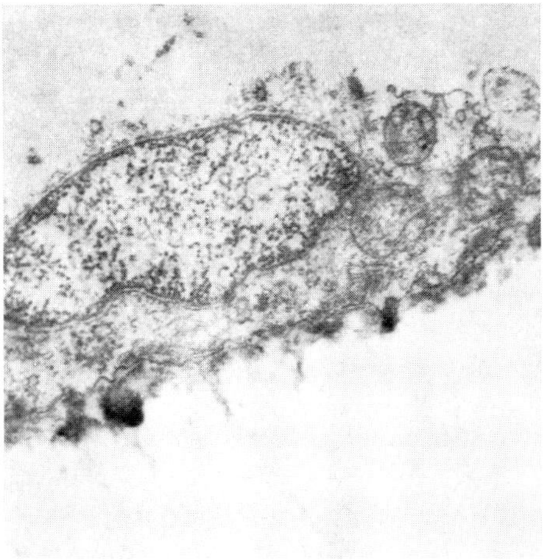

Fig. 3

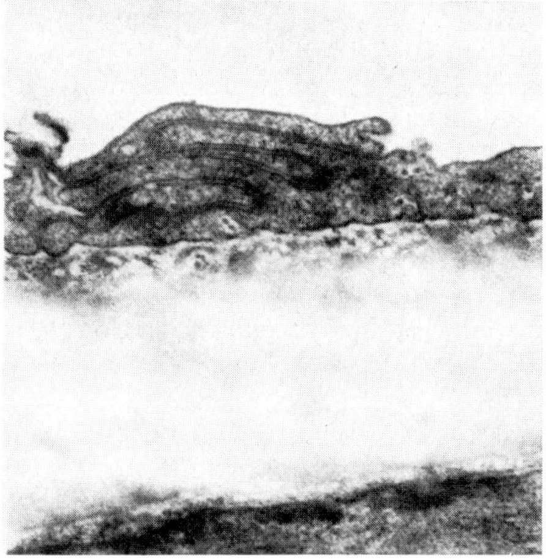

Fig. 4

Fig. 3. Endothelial cell of a rat femoral artery that was perfused for 40 sec with a solution of 0.2 μM/ml *acetoacetic acid* in buffer. The disintegration of the endothelial cell is more advanced here, leading to exposure of the nucleus to the lumen. Note the edema of the nucleus (that has led to an obliteration of its folds and to a homogenization of its chromatin) and the swelling of the mitochondria. It is evident that acetoacetic acid has increased the permeability of plasma membrane as well as of nuclear and mitochondrial envelopes. × 18,150.

Fig. 4. *Normal interendothelial junction* of a buffer-perfused rat femoral artery. Note the steady, approx. 200 Å wide, zig-zag gap of this junction. × 28,875.

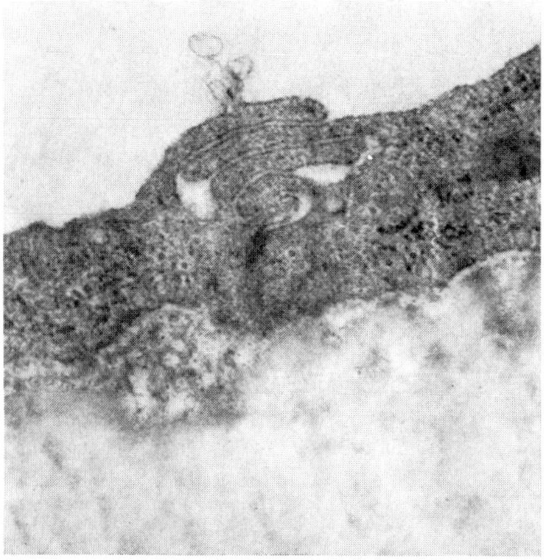

Fig. 5. Focal dilatation of the gap of the interendothelial junction of a rat femoral artery that was perfused with a solution of 1 μM/ml *β-hydroxybutyric acid* in buffer for 40 sec. × 28,875.

RESULTS AND CONCLUSIONS

First, the effects of *diabetes metabolites*:

We infused directly into the femoral artery of some rats, and i.v. into others, certain substances that accumulate in the blood of untreated diabetics, namely β-hydroxybutyric and acetoacetic acid.

We found that both acids tended to cause dilatation of the intercellular endothelial junctions (ICJ's) and, in addition, acetoacetic acid caused marked edema and rupture of endothelial cells (see Figs. 1–5 for effects of diabetes metabolites).

These findings lead to the intriguing hypothesis that diabetes may promote atherosclerosis not only because of its hypercholesterolemia, but also because some of the metabolites that accumulate in this condition damage the endothelium and increase its permeability to lipoproteins.

I have no idea at the moment through what mechanism acetoacetic acid damages the cell membranes of the endothelium, but I think it possible that the two anions we studied may have loosened the intercellular junctions by removing some of the calcium that seems to hold cells together at these sites; in other words, they may have acted like the chelating agent EDTA.

This is what we found *EDTA* does to the arterial endothelial junctions, as we presented it at the Anatomists' meeting in Dallas (Constantinides, 1972) (see Figs. 6 and 7 for effects of EDTA). It is probable that calcium atoms are lined up in the junction gap and that, being electropositive ions, they form bonds with the electronegative polysaccharide coats (glycocalyces) of the cells on both sides, thus creating 'chemical bridges' between them. It is also probable that, when one removes calcium ions, either through chelating agents or through acids, one 'unzips' the junctions by removing the chemical bridges between endothelial cells.

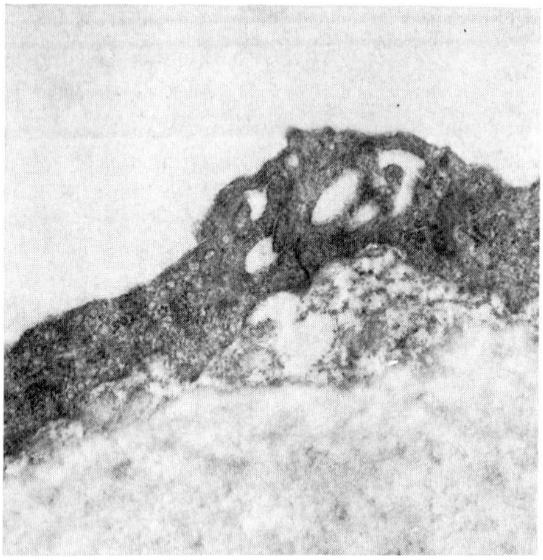

Fig. 6

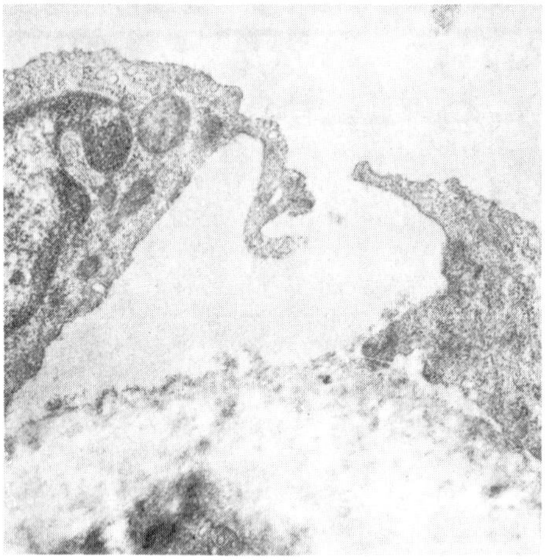

Fig. 7

Fig. 6. Focal dilatation of the gap of the interendothelial junction of a rat femoral artery that was perfused with a solution of 25 mM/l *EDTA* (ethylene diamine tetra-acetate) in buffer for 100 sec. The widened subendothelial space directly underneath the loosened junction is evidence of the increased permeability of the latter. × 18,150.

Fig. 7. Opened interendothelial junction of a rat femoral artery that was perfused with a solution of 25 mM/l *EDTA* in buffer for 100 sec. The wide gap created by the separation of the two endothelial cells has exposed to the lumen a large segment of the internal elastic lamella and its attached fibrils. × 18,150.

Next, I would like to summarize our experience with *nicotine*. We gave this alkaloid both acutely (by a single direct intra-arterial perfusion) and chronically (through daily subcutaneous injections for 2 weeks) to rats and to rabbits.

We found no effects in the rat, but definite effects in the rabbit! Nicotine, when given acutely (by arterial perfusion), caused injury in the form of endothelial cell edema and detachments ('lift-offs'); when given chronically (subcutaneously), it induced reactive proliferation in the form of the creation of a double or triple-layered intima, as an expression of repair; it also visibly stimulated protein synthesis in the rough endoplasmic reticulum of endothelial cells (see Figs. 8–12 for effects of nicotine).

These results may explain the previous findings of Hass et al. (1966) in rabbits that cholesterol feeding combined with nicotine causes much more atherosclerosis than cholesterol feeding alone; they may also offer an explanation for the recent epidemiological discovery that atherosclerotic complications of man such as heart attacks and strokes are much more frequent among smokers than among non-smokers (National Heart and Lung Institute, 1971).

Finally, we examined the ultrastructure of the femoral artery endothelium in the rat 6 hours after the administration of an acute oral load of 5 g *linoleic acid* and 1 g *phosphatidylethanolamine* (PE). These lipids were given by stomach tube and therefore reached the endothelium by a physiological route.

We found that PE had no effects apart from causing the appearance of occasional lipid droplets within endothelial cells, but *linoleic acid* caused significant structural changes in the endothelium of 5 out of the 6 animals to which it was given; these changes ranged from microvillus formation, and loosening of junctions in 2 animals to real injury with severe whole

text continued p. 60

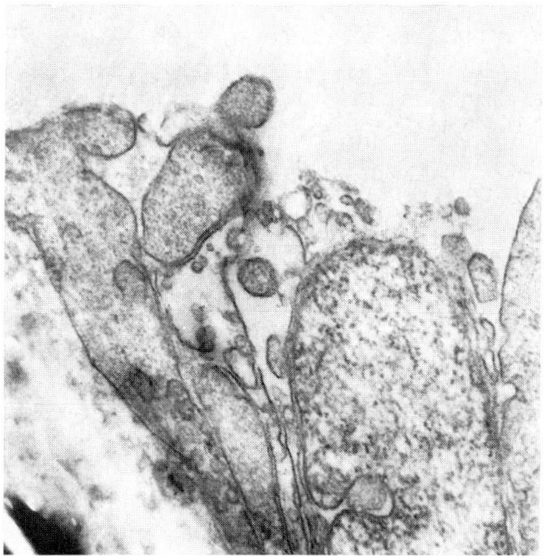

Fig. 8

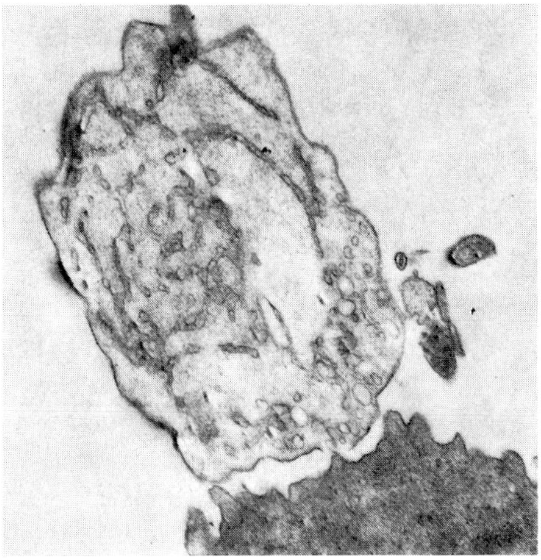

Fig. 9

Fig. 8. Rabbit femoral artery perfused for 40 sec by a solution of 100 μg/ml *nicotine* in buffer. Note the shingle-like overlapping of endothelial cell processes in this contracted artery. There is acute edema in some endothelial processes in mid-field and rupture of the plasma membrane with exposure of the nucleus to the lumen close to the right side of the field. This endothelial injury could well have caused the adhesion of platelets that Dr. Frost (*This Volume* pp. 32–50) found in the aorta of nicotine-treated rabbits. × 23,100.

Fig. 9. Rabbit femoral artery perfused for 40 sec by a solution of 100 μg/ml *nicotine* in buffer. Note a large endothelial bleb or blister (edematous cell process) that originates from a plane above or below that of this section and seems to adhere to the underlying denser endothelium. It may be that the excessively stretched plasma membrane of such edematous cell processes may lose its electronegatively charged coat (glycocalyx) – or may suffer a dilution of its negative charges due to stretching – and thus stop repelling the still negatively charged cell membrane of normal endothelium. A similar mechanism might explain the adhesion of intact blood cells (leukocytes, platelets and erythrocytes) to partly or totally edematous endothelial cells. × 14,850.

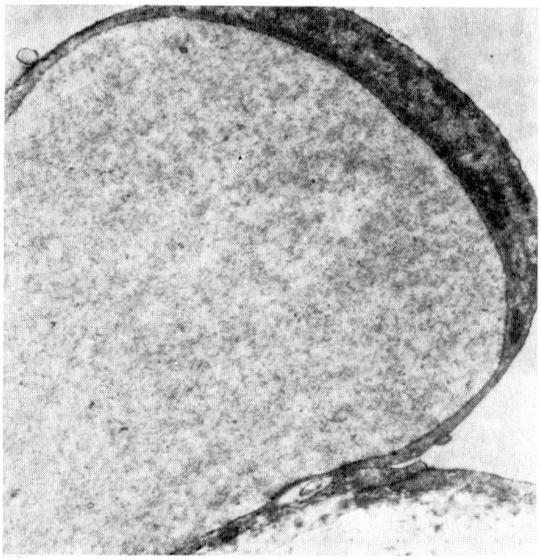

Fig. 10

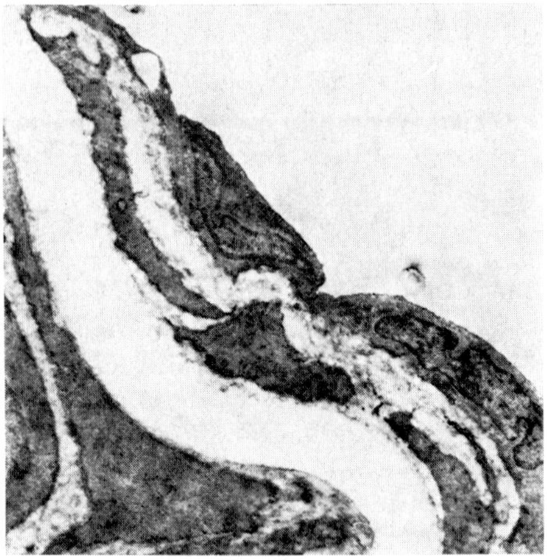

Fig. 11

Fig. 10. Rabbit femoral artery perfused for 40 sec by a solution of 100 μg/ml *nicotine* in buffer. Note the large amount of plasma that entered the subendothelial space and lifted an endothelial cell from its bed, ballooning it into the lumen. × 9,075.

Fig. 11. Rabbit femoral artery of an animal that was injected subcutaneously with 22 mg *nicotine* twice daily, for 2 weeks. Note the proliferation of the intima that has produced 2 cell layers (instead of the normal single layer) overlying the thick internal elastic lamella, as well as the formation of a new, much thinner elastic lamella between the 2 intimal cell layers. This is classical 'musculo-elastic intimal hyperplasia' as we get it whenever the arterial wall responds to a chronic injury. × 4,950.

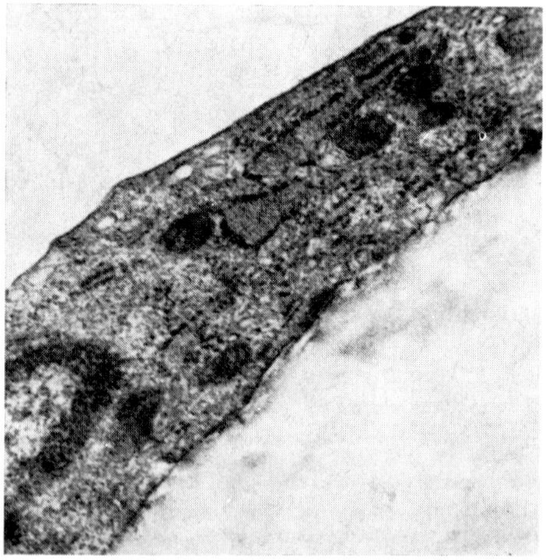

Fig. 12. Rabbit femoral artery endothelium of an animal that was injected subcutaneously with 22 mg *nicotine* twice daily, for 2 weeks. Note that the cisternae of the rough endoplasmic reticulum have been widened and filled with an amorphous dark material – which perhaps represents an adaptive enzyme produced by the endothelial cell in response to the nicotine insult. × 28,875.

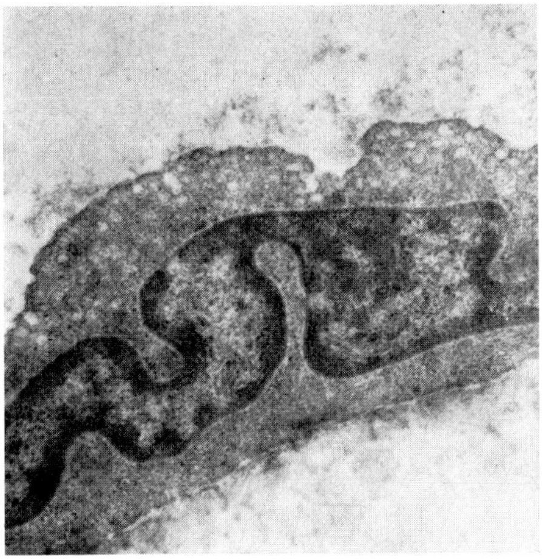

Fig. 13

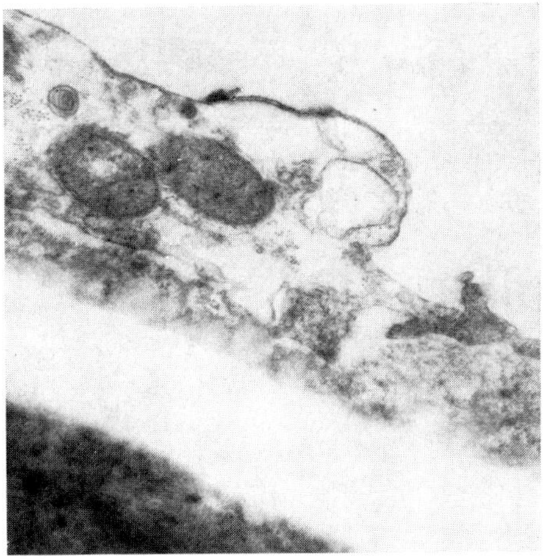

Fig. 14

Fig. 13. *Normal endothelium* of the femoral artery of a rat that received 5 ml tap water by stomach tube 6 hours before sacrifice. × 18,150.

Fig. 14. Endothelium of the femoral artery of a rat that received 5 g *linoleic acid* (liquid) by stomach tube 6 hours before sacrifice. Note the marked edema and beginning blister formation of an endothelial cell as well as the tremendous swelling of two of its mitochondria. Note also the apparent 'splitting' of certain segments of the superficial plasma membrane of the edematous cell which may represent a widening of the translucent middle lipid layer of the membrane due to the incorporation of fatty acid molecules from the lumen; such a structural disorganization of the plasma membrane could well interfere with its 'sodium pump' function and thus lead to the accumulation of electrolyte and water (edema) in the cell. It is interesting that the edematous change stops at the junction with the neighboring endothelial cell to the right, which has a dense cytoplasm; in other words, like all insults, the excessive rise of plasma fatty acid levels induced in these experiments has hit some endothelial cells while completely sparing their neighbors. × 23,100.

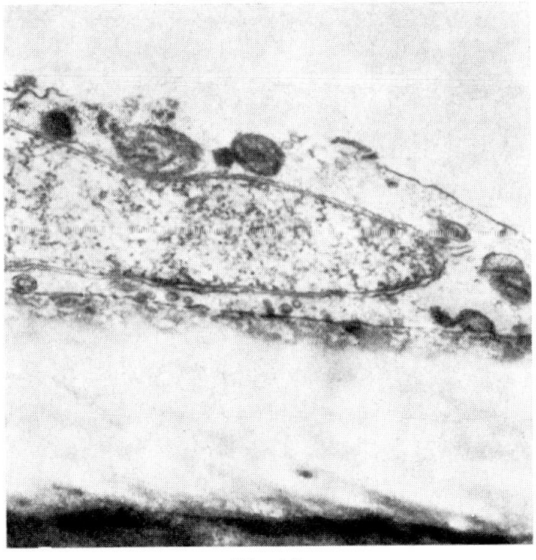

Fig. 15

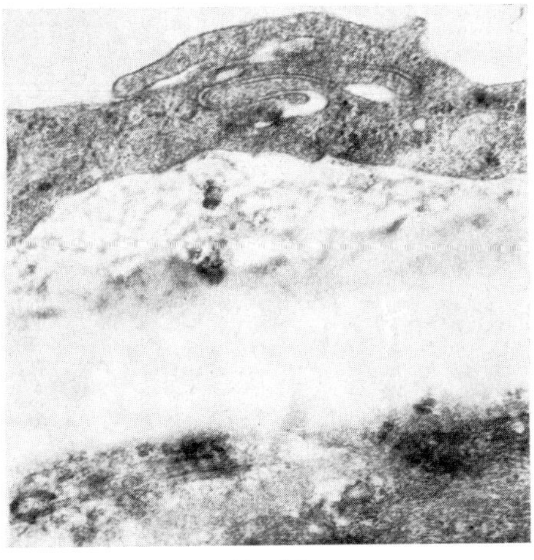

Fig. 16

Fig. 15. Endothelium of the femoral artery of a rat that received 5 g *linoleic acid* by stomach tube 6 hours before sacrifice. More severe injury: edema of an endothelial cell cytoplasm and nucleus accompanied by break and loss of a large segment of the superficial plasma membrane. × 18,150.

Fig. 16. Loosening of an interendothelial junction in the femoral artery of a rat that received 5 g *linoleic acid* by stomach tube 6 hours before sacrifice. × 28,875.

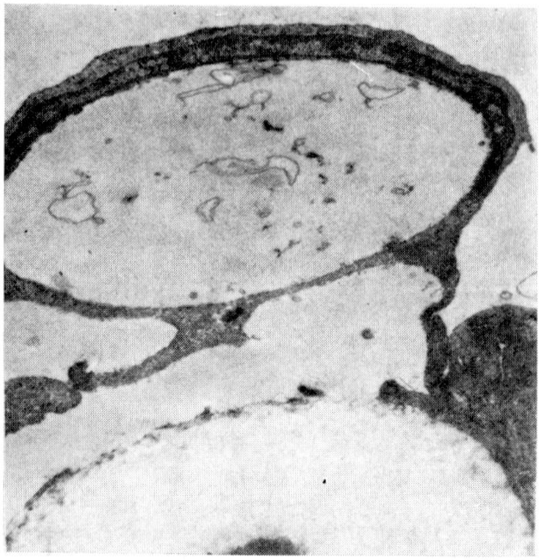

Fig. 17

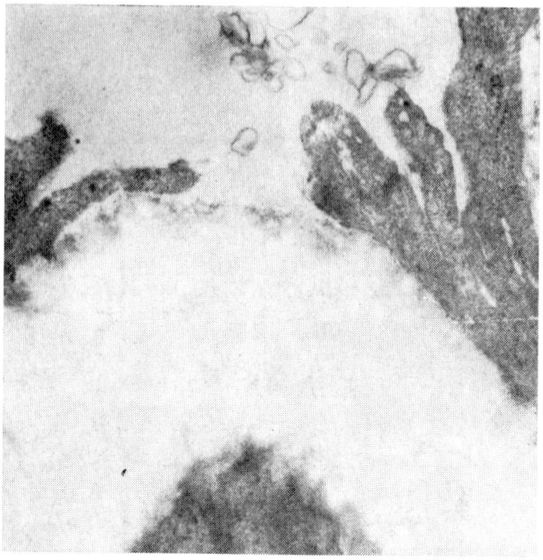

Fig. 18

Fig. 17. Endothelium of a rabbit femoral artery that was perfused with a solution of 10 μg/ml *serotonin* in buffer for 40 sec. Note the enormous cavity that developed within the endothelial cell and its detachment from the internal elastic lamella. × 11,550.

Fig. 18. Endothelium of a rabbit femoral artery that was perfused with a solution of 10 μg/ml *serotonin* in buffer for 40 sec. Note the wide gap in the endothelium which is probably due to an opened interendothelial junction. × 18,150.

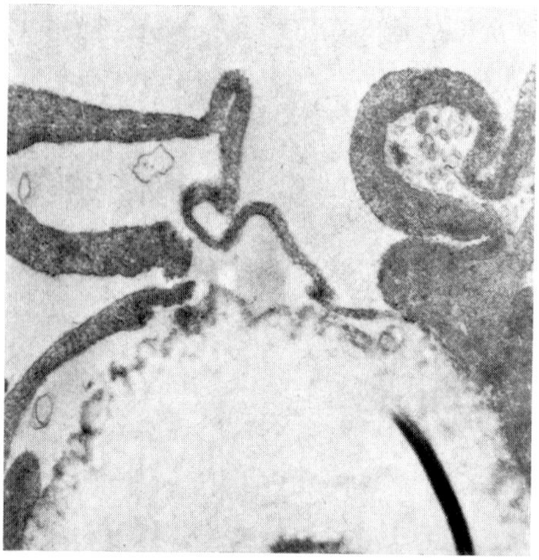

Fig. 19

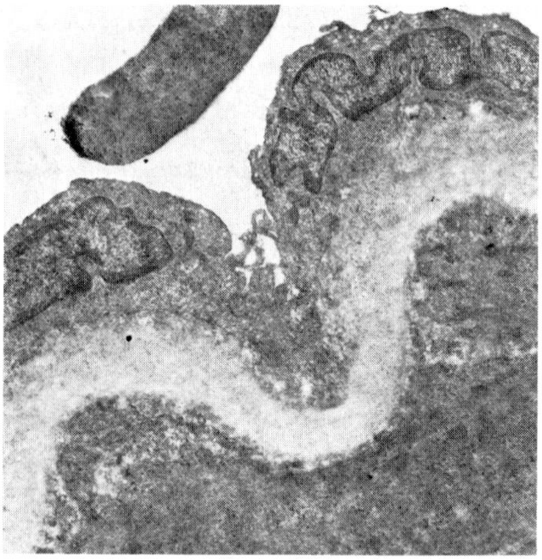

Fig. 20

Fig. 19. Endothelium of a rabbit femoral artery that was perfused with a solution of 10 μg/ml *serotonin* in buffer for 40 sec. Note the detachment and thinning of the endothelium as well the small fracture at left. × 14,850.

Fig. 20. Endothelium of a rabbit femoral artery that was perfused with a solution of 10 μg/ml *serotonin* combined with 200 μg/ml *lysergic acid* in buffer for 40 sec. Note the complete absence of serotonin-type injury, which is typical of all the sections examined in both the rabbits that received the above combined treatment. × 7,429.

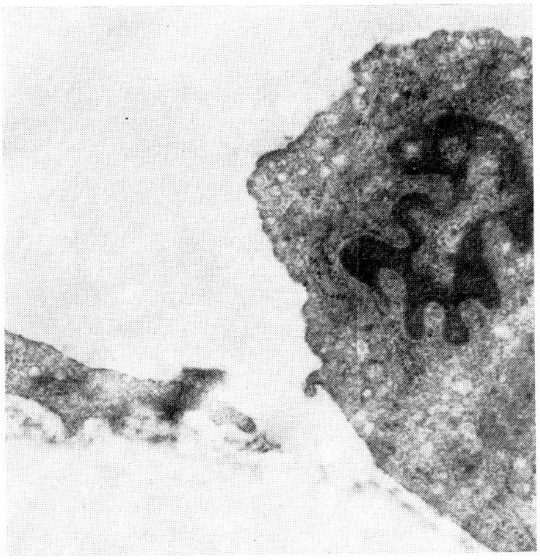

Fig. 21

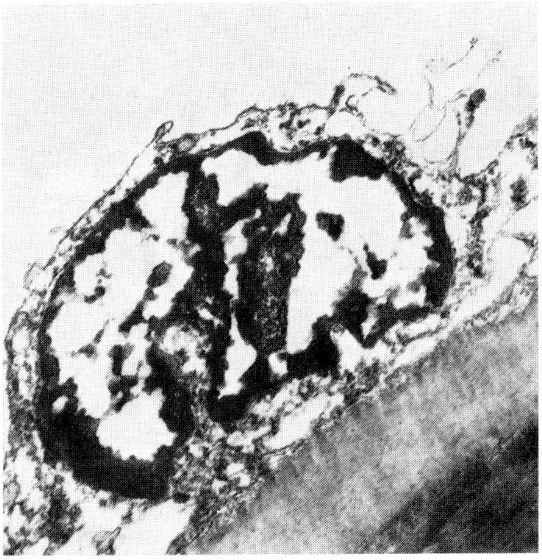

Fig. 22

Fig. 21. Endothelium of a rat femoral artery that was perfused with a solution of 10 μg/ml *angiotensin* for 40 sec. Note the creation of a gap due to opening of the junction between 2 endothelial cells; note also the evident contraction of the endothelial cell on the right and the absence of edema, plasma membrane breaks or other injury from both cells. × 23,100.

Fig. 22. Endothelium of a rat femoral artery that was perfused with a solution of 10 μg/ml *angiotensin* combined with 1 mg/ml dibenzyline for 40 sec. Note the dramatic endothelial injury that consists of cytoplasmic edema and the precipitation of most chromatin on the nuclear envelope. × 11,550.

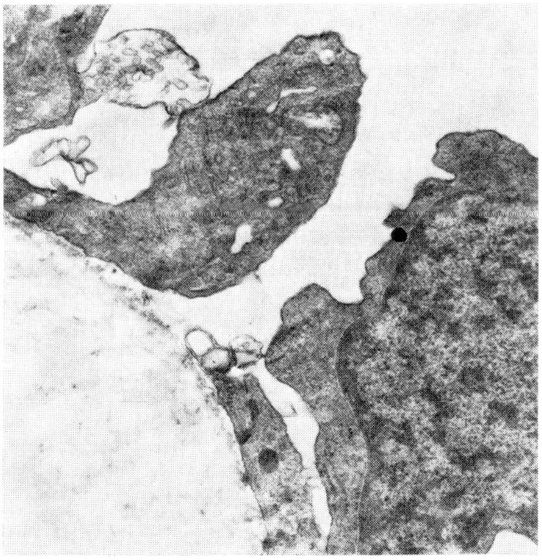

Fig. 23. Endothelium of a rabbit femoral artery that was perfused with a solution of 10 μg/ml *epinephrine* in buffer for 40 sec. Note the wide gap between 2 endothelial cells which is due to the opening of their junction and the absence of plasma membrane breaks along the apposed cell surfaces. Note also the development of a few small edematous cell processes or blisters. × 14,850.

cell edema and blister (bleb) formation in 3 animals, apparently as the result of cell membrane disorganization (see Figs. 13–16 for effects of oral fatty acid).

These results show that the endothelium of arteries can be injured within a few hours by a massive fatty acid intake, and thus provide direct support for the concept we expressed at the beginning, namely that hyperlipemia, when it is extreme or prolonged, can 'open its own doors' into the arterial wall. These findings may also help to explain the increased permeability of the cholesterol-fed arterial wall to ^{125}I-albumin as found by Adams et al. (1970) and by Gore et al. (1972), and the increased thymidine uptake that was found by the Albany group in the endothelium of pigs within 3 days of the commencement of a high fat diet (Florentin et al., 1969) – one would expect that destruction of cells would stimulate proliferation.

So much for new types of endothelial injury. Let us now turn our attention to some of the old types of endothelial injury and their chemical modifications.

First, *serotonin*. We discovered 4 years ago that this amine has very destructive effects on the lining of rat arteries since it causes the development of large intracellular and extracellular fluid pools, detachments ('lift-offs') and endothelial gaps; at first, we thought that all these gaps were due to opening of the junctions, but further morphological study suggested to us that many of them are due to fractures of a damaged cell membrane.

We have recently found an interesting thing about serotonin: Its destructive effects can be largely inhibited by the local anesthetic, procaine, and they can be completely blocked by lysergic acid! These findings support the idea that the primary target of serotonin is the endothelial cell membrane, and that its antagonists probably compete with it for receptor sites on this membrane (see Figs. 17–20 for the inhibition of serotonin by lysergic acid).

Next, we discovered that *angiotensin* can become an intensely destructive agent when combined with the sympatholytic drug, dibenzyline. Angiotensin, given alone, merely opens the junctions, without injuring the cells, as we found several years ago, but when it acts in the presence of dibenzyline, it causes massive endothelial necrosis and exfoliation. The implication of this result is interesting because it shows us that the endothelial effects of vasoactive agents depend greatly on their metabolic environment, and therefore even very low concentrations of such agents could suddenly become destructive under the right chemical condition (see Figs. 21 and 22 for the modification of the effect of angiotensin by dibenzyline).

In conclusion, I wish to report that we also observed a marked *species difference* between the sensitivity of the arterial endothelium of the rat and the rabbit towards certain vasoactive amines, which may explain some of the past conflicts in the literature in this area.

We found that the rat endothelium is very sensitive to serotonin but only slightly sensitive to norepinephrine and epinephrine, whereas the rabbit endothelium is very sensitive to all three.

Of particular interest was the effect of *epinephrine* in the rabbit where we found that just a few micrograms per milliliter of this catecholamine opened endothelial junctions and caused intraendothelial, subendothelial and subelastic edema in a few seconds.

We were thus able to confirm the provocation of an extracellular 'edema reaction' in the rabbit arterial wall by epinephrine, as postulated by Shimamoto several years ago (1961), and we think that this reaction is due largely to the opening of interendothelial junctions (see Fig. 23 for effects of epinephrine).

Norepinephrine briefly perfused through rabbit femoral arteries at 10 μg/ml in buffer caused intraendothelial, subendothelial and subelastic edema, like epinephrine.

SUMMARY

1. The brief intra-arterial perfusion of the *diabetes* metabolites acetoacetic acid and β-hydroxybutyric acid through rat femoral arteries caused loosening of some endothelial junctions and, in addition, acetoacetic acid caused marked edema and rupture of endothelial

cells. These findings suggest that diabetes may promote atherogenesis, at least in part, by increasing the permeability of arterial endothelium.

2. The brief intra-arterial perfusion of the chelating agent *EDTA* through rat femoral arteries loosened and opened several of their endothelial junctions. This indicates that calcium is a structural component of intercellular junctions in arterial endothelium.

3. The intra-arterial perfusion of a solution of *nicotine* through rabbit femoral arteries for a few seconds caused endothelial injury in the form of endothelial cell edema and detachment from the internal elastic lamina. The twice daily subcutaneous administration of nicotine to rabbits for 2 weeks induced musculoelastic intimal hyperplasia in their femoral arteries, i.e. it provoked a typical proliferative response to chronic injury. These results may help to explain the adjuvant role of nicotine in experimental and human atherogenesis.

4. The oral administration of a single large *fatty acid load* to rats caused, within a few hours, severe injury in the endothelial lining of their femoral arteries in the form of blisters (blebs), marked edema and rupture of many endothelial cells. This finding supports the concept that extreme hyperlipemia may damage the arterial lining.

5. The destructive effects of *serotonin* on rat arterial endothelium are largely inhibited by procaine and completely inhibited by lysergic acid.

6. In the presence of dibenzyline, *angiotensin* produces extremely destructive changes in rat arterial endothelium.

7. The brief intra-arterial perfusion of *epinephrine* through rabbit femoral arteries was found to open interendothelial junctions. The causation of edema in the inner arterial wall of the rabbit by this catecholamine (as previously reported by Shimamoto) was confirmed.

ACKNOWLEDGEMENTS

I wish to express my gratitude to Dr. Ken Wiggers and Miss Karen McDowell for their help in the execution of the studies. The excellent technical assistance of Miss Rosalee Watson is gratefully acknowledged.

REFERENCES

ADAMS, C. W. M., MORGAN, R. S. and BAYLISS, O. B. (1970): The differential entry of (I^{125})-albumin into mildly and severely atheromatous rabbit aorta. *J. Atheroscler. Res.*, *11*, 119.

CONSTANTINIDES, P. (1965): *Experimental Atherosclerosis*, pp. 49 and 66. Elsevier Publishing Co., Amsterdam–London–New York.

CONSTANTINIDES, P. (1968): Lipid deposition in injured arteries. *Arch. Path.*, *85*, 280.

CONSTANTINIDES, P. (1969*a*): The role of the endothelial barrier in atherosclerosis. In: *Atherogenesis. Proceedings, First International Symposium on Atherogenesis, Thrombogenesis and Pyridinolcarbamate Treatment, Tokyo, 1969*, pp. 99–102. Editors: T. Shimamoto and F. Numano. ICS 201, Excerpta Medica, Amsterdam.

CONSTANTINIDES, P. (1969*b*): Ultrastructural injury of arterial endothelium. *Arch. Path.*, *88*, 99.

CONSTANTINIDES, P. (1972): Opening of intercellular junctions in arterial endothelium by a chelating agent. *Anat. Rec.*, *172*, 295.

FLORENTIN, R. A., NAM, S. C., LEE, K. T., LEE, K. J. and THOMAS, W. A. (1969): Increased mitotic activity in aortas of swine after three days of cholesterol feeding. *Arch. Path.*, *88*, 463.

GORE, I., MIYASKI, T., KUROZUMI, T. and HIRST, A. (1972): Aortic permeability during atherogenesis in rabbits. *Amer. J. Path.*, *66*, 47a.

HASS, G. M., LANDERHOLM, W. and HEMMENS, A. (1966): Production of calcific atheroarteriosclerosis and thromboarteritis with nicotine, vitamin D and dietary cholesterol. *Amer. J. Path.*, *49*, 739.

NATIONAL HEART AND LUNG INSTITUTE (U.S.A.) (1971): Risk factors and prevention. In: *Task Force on Arteriosclerosis, Report*, p. 30. Publication No. (N.I.H.) 73–137, Department of Health, Education and Welfare, Washington, D. C.

SHIMAMOTO, T. (1961): Acute vascular endothelial reaction – in reference to atherogenesis. *Asian Med. J.*, *4*, 309.

SHIMAMOTO, T., MAEZAWA, H., YAMAZAKI, H., ISHIOKA, T., SUNAGA, T. and FUJITA, T. (1966): Edematous arterial reaction and its relationship to atherosclerosis and thrombosis. *Meth. Achiev. exp. Path.*, *1*, 337.

DISCUSSION

Dr. Spector: Dr. Constantinides' very provocative paper has led me to a number of both comments and questions.

The synergistic effects that you see between dibenzyline and angiotensin are readily explainable. First of all, dibenzyline is not an antagonist of angiotensin, but by the same token dibenzyline will stimulate formation of catecholamines, so here you have an explanation for your synergistic effect. With regard to nicotine and its stimulation of an enzyme, there is evidence that you can get a stimulation of the drug-metabolizing enzymes, so nicotine can stimulate certain of the enzymes. There are certain questions which I would like to pose. Firstly, in your opening points you commented that you thought the hydroxybutyrate perhaps might act as a chelator. I wonder whether you had administered any calcium to see whether you can antagonize the effects of the hydroxybutyrate. The other question I would like to ask is in regard to serotonin. What doses of serotonin do you use?

Dr. Constantinides: To answer your second question first, we used 10 μg/ml serotonin in this particular experiment. This is above the physiological level of serotonin, but such a concentration might occur directly underneath the platelets. The reason I used such high doses is that, if with a very low dose you cause an opening of, e.g., one in every 500 junctions, you have to start cutting many hundreds of sections and look at them all between now and next year, before you can find one open junction. If, however, you use a higher dose, you cause more gaps and then you can see them with the electron microscope in a few days or weeks. I have not tried to inhibit the hydroxybutyric effect as I am at the stage of having just discovered it, and therefore I have not yet attempted to investigate it in detail.

I have a counter-question to ask Dr. Spector, regarding the possibility that dibenzyline may have stimulated the production of a catecholamine. It is an interesting idea, and it might be true if we were dealing with nerve endings, but here we are dealing with an artery that was perfused for about 30 sec with dibenzyline, so I do not think that we have the time or even the tissue to produce catecholamines. In some species like the frog, the endothelium may produce catecholamine-like materials, but I do not think we have any evidence as yet that the rat endothelium behaves in the same manner.

Dr. Spector: But if you give a high enough dose, you may get a release, rather than having any synthesis as well. But the point that I would like to come back to is that people start to talk about adrenaline when perhaps they should talk about noradrenaline, and what effects noradrenaline has on this system is interesting.

Dr. Constantinides: In the rabbit it has the same effect as adrenaline. I have not seen an open junction yet, but perhaps this is because we have not studied enough sections – I suspect very much that one would find open junctions if one were to make a persistent search.

Dr. Shimamoto: As shown in the Figures which I presented in my paper (*This Volume*, pp. 3–31), the infiltration of IgG and γG was confirmed in the aorta of rabbits treated with 1 μg/kg of angiotensin, which may suggest that angiotensin opens up the junctions of endothelial cells, resulting in the infiltration of quite large molecular weight substances into the plasma. At the same time, I showed an electron-microscopic scan picture in my paper which exhibits a crater-like artefact, which may represent the bleb formation by angiotensin.

Dr. Constantinides: Dr. Shimamoto, I think that the crater formation most likely represents ruptured and collapsed blebs. The big balloons pop, and become holes or craters.

Dr. Numano: I should like to ask two primitive questions. Firstly, you mentioned the rather open junctions that may lead to atherosclerosis under pathological conditions. Do you think that open junctions can occur during physiological functions? The second one is that you mentioned the contraction of endothelial cells: Is that contraction the result of a total change of the endothelial cell, a physical change in endothelial cells or a change in some system of these cells?

Dr. Constantinides: In answer to the first question, I think that if you do nothing to the animal, if it lives well and happily and avoids things like gluttony and anger, nothing will happen to its endothelium. But if you insult that endothelium with hyperlipemia, amines, hypertension, nicotine, antigen-antibody complexes or diabetes, the arterial lining may be hit. This happens all the time; life is just an accumulation of stresses even when we do not suspect their existence. Antigen-antibody complexes, e.g., could accumulate very easily when we become sensitized to anything, such as additive agents in the diet. With regard to the second question, I think that endothelial cells contract directly and independently because of the contractile microfilaments that are in them. They are related to smooth muscle; they are cousins of the muscle cells of the media. The whole arterial wall (endothelium and muscle) develops from the same mesenchymal anlage. The endothelial cells have the same genomes as muscle, they can do the same things as muscle, but normally the muscle specializes in contracting, and the endothelium remembers how to contract only under extreme duress. Endothelial cells have microfilaments of myosin. Becker has shown that in Columbia University with fluorescent antimyosin antibodies.

Dr. HENRY: I would like to comment on your statement that there is a change in the electronegativity. Dr. Sawyer from New York has shown change of electronegativity in all forms of injury to one of electropositivity. We know also that in α-receptor site blockade there is a neutralization of charge, and the things that are essential for the interaction with an α-receptor site are a benzene ring, two carbon side-chains with a terminal methyl group. If we look at the molecule itself, we find that pyridinolcarbamate has a benzene ring, it has two side-chains, it does not have phenolic hydroxyl groups, but it does have a terminal amino group with the methyl substitution, and it has a carbon and oxygen rather than alcoholic hydroxyl group, thus making it a candidate for an α-receptor site blocker, which may explain some of these effects.

Dr. REDISCH: We see the overwhelming importance of catecholamine release on the small vessels. I wanted to ask if Dr. Constantinides feels that the effects of nicotine may also be similar since we know from the work of Burns that release of catecholamines is perhaps the most impressive action of nicotine.

Dr. CONSTANTINIDES: That is a very interesting thought, Dr. Redisch, and it may also apply to angiotensin, since pharmacologists tell us that one of the actions of angiotensin is to release catecholamines. But where do these things release the catecholamines from? They release them from nerve endings, and I think I would be intrigued with this possibility if I had given nicotine in vivo. But this effect was obtained almost in vitro. You take an artery and you flush it from the inside with nicotine or with angiotensin. So you do not have time to get these molecules to any adventitial nerve endings and release catecholamines, I think, unless some of the dense bodies that have been seen in the endothelium of several species may represent catecholamines, in which case the endothelium of some species may be just as catecholamine-discharging as nerve endings. But one would have to test this possibility through specially designed experiments in the rat and rabbit.

Dr. TERRY: We did actually study catecholamine contents in various vessel wall segments, and there is quite a lot in some of them which may be released with nicotine even when flushing the vessel.

Dr. CONSTANTINIDES: It may be so in the rabbit, yes. We obtained the effect of nicotine in the rabbit, now that I come to think of it.

Dr. BERKOWITZ: With respect to the suggestion that pyridinolcarbamate could be an α-blocker and antagonize catecholamines by that mechanism, we have looked directly at that and have found that it does not antagonize the effect of added noradrenaline on blood pressure in the rat.

Dr. BUSCH: Dr. Constantinides, the blebbing that you and Dr. Shimamoto have shown is a rather dramatic local change in an endothelial cell. Do you have any explanation as to why this remains so local, or is this just one stage in the process of becoming a diffuse cytoplasmic alteration?

Dr. CONSTANTINIDES: I believe the latter. I think that the degree of cell edema is a function of the concentration of the insulting molecules and of the time of action. If you hit the cell with just a few molecules for a short time, you will perhaps only destroy the sodium pump in a few microareas of the cell membrane, but if you hit with enough molecules over a longer time, you will hit the whole cell surface.

Dr. COTTON: We have considered nicotine and the effect on the endothelium. I was wondering if, in your experiment, you considered another factor in cigarette smoke, as Paul Astrop has, namely the effect of anoxia produced by carbon monoxide. He has demonstrated that with cigarette smoking the average cigarette smoker has 5–10% carboxyhemoglobin in the circulation, which is sufficient to produce a considerable shift of the hemoglobin dissociation curve to the left. He has noted also that in the cigarette smoke there are 400 parts per million of carbon monoxide. Now, if the rabbits are exposed to only 100–150 parts per million of carbon monoxide, then subintimal edema is produced and bleb formation is seen with the electron microscope. If the rabbit is then treated with cholesterol, the deposition is increased 5 times, and in those same cholesterol-fed rabbits hyperoxia eliminates this increased deposition. So, it is conceivable that in man this may be a factor as well as nicotine.

Dr. CONSTANTINIDES: You are building up quite an interesting and impressive case, Dr. Cotton. It may well be that cigarette smoke, at least when it is administered in vivo by inhalation and chronically, may partly act through carbon monoxide production and anoxia. One would have to demonstrate, of course, independently that carbon monoxide introduced into the blood at levels that are absorbed under smoke inhalation would have similar effects, and also that anoxia per se simulates such effects. So far, anoxia has been found to be a very drastic factor. We know that it increases the permeability of the endothelium, but I do not think we have sufficient information yet on the structural changes it causes beyond variable cell edema. While cyanide opens junctions, I do not think we have convincing evidence yet of endothelial junction opening due to low blood oxygen concentrations, but we will hear more about it in one of the next papers I hope.

Dr. AUSTIN: I would like to follow up your remark about rabbits and rats having a different response to nicotine. The question is a clinical one. Do rats and rabbits behave differently clinically after you give them an injection of nicotine?

Dr. CONSTANTINIDES: I am afraid that I do not know. I am ashamed to say so, but I did not observe them clinically myself. I had a graduate student working on this, and he had a look at them. I do know, however, that one of the rabbits died after 2 nicotine injections on the second day, while the others carried on for 2 weeks until we killed them.

Dr. AUSTIN: Is it possible, therefore, that the rabbits are having a more profound pressure response or some other response involving catecholamines to the nicotine?

Dr. CONSTANTINIDES: It is quite possible and cannot be excluded from these in vivo results. Blood pressure, carbon monoxide – anything could be a mediator.

Dr. CAMERINI-DAVALOS: I wonder if you would like to make some comments about Dr. Robert Lee's findings? You mention that hyperlipemia is a very significant factor in these changes. Dr. Lee seems to believe that, regardless of the values of the lipids or even of very low density lipoprotein, the most significant factor seems to be the protein moiety in these compounds. I wonder if you have any experience of that?

Dr. CONSTANTINIDES: In what type of experiments? In cholesterol feeding experiments or in human atherosclerosis?

Dr. CAMERINI-DAVALOS: In relation to vascularity in human subjects.

Dr. CONSTANTINIDES: No, I have really no personal experience with lipoprotein in this area. All I can say is that certain insults can open the doors for any big lipoprotein or protein molecules that normally find the doors shut in the healthy wall. Injury opens the doors for them to enter the wall.

Dr. KRITCHEVSKY: I have one comment and one question. The comment is in relation to your work with linoleic acid and phosphatidylethanolamine. We have done experiments on the uptake of cholesterol by cells in tissue culture and found that almost all of the phospholipids inhibit cholesterol uptake, which would be in line with the tightening, you might say, of the cell wall, whereas the fatty acids, when added at a very low concentration, increased cholesterol uptake and at a higher concentration caused cell death, so again that confirms what you have shown. But my question is in relation to the mode of perfusion or administration of the acetoacetic and hydroxybutyric acids. Did you put them in buffer or in plasma?

Dr. CONSTANTINIDES: Well, first, I find your comment very interesting – perhaps the fatty acids in your experiments also affected the cell membrane, but as far as the mode of administration is concerned, I gave the ketoacids dissolved in buffer at pH 7.2 to exclude other plasma components and to exclude an effect of acidity per se, which is known to exist.

Dr. SPECTOR: An interesting offshoot to your data and the data presented by Dr. Shimamoto is that both adrenaline and serotonin are capable of modifying the endothelial lining of the arteries. There are drugs that are being employed as antihypertensive agents which are potent releasers of both these agents. You have an agent like reserpine, which is capable of releasing both of these biogenic amines, which would have just the reverse effect that one desires by the administration of the drug itself. As a consequence, I then ask whether reserpine itself modifies the endothelial lining as seen with serotonin and adrenaline. Have you ever looked at that?

Dr. CONSTANTINIDES: No, it would be interesting to get the right species, and see what reserpine does to the amine-like granules contained within secreting endothelium. As far as the other comment is concerned, I may add something to it. As you know, several years ago people who were taking antihypertensive treatment in the form of monoamine oxidase inhibitors and at the same time happened to eat cheese (which contains much tyramine), got vascular accidents, some were blinded, others got strokes. We repeated this human accident in the form of an animal experiment: we gave tyramine and a monoamine oxidase inhibitor, both separately and combined, and found a tremendous potentiation of the endotheliotoxic effect of tyramine by the oxidase inhibitor. So, indeed, there are all kinds of parameters that can increase these amine effects.

UNIDENTIFIED SPEAKER: A very short answer to Dr. Spector. The release by reserpine is so slow that the catecholamine released is physiologically ineffective.

ENDOTHELIAL ISCHEMIA AS STUDIED BY CORRELATED SCANNING AND TRANSMISSION ELECTRON MICROSCOPY AND BY FLUORESCENT ANTIBODY STAINING

E. NELSON

Department of Neurology, School of Medicine, University of Maryland, Baltimore, Md., U.S.A.

The effect of ischemia on endothelium has received surprisingly little ultrastructural attention, although there has been light-microscopic evidence for the presence of alterations in vessels of various organs and species.

It occurred to me that this might be a fruitful area for further study. Ischemia of vessels must, after all, precede ischemia of the organs they supply; it might be expected to be associated with an increase in permeability; this might well be followed by extravasation of fluid which in some organs, e.g. the brain, produces a clinically highly significant state – cerebral edema. In addition, ischemic alteration of endothelium might be of interest as one of the several varieties of stress which could be of significance in the production of so-called 'degenerative' vascular disease or atherosclerosis.

Some work has been done in this area. The perfusion of visible particulate matter provided evidence for the existence of endothelial changes in vessels of several organs. This was emphasized by Ames and his collaborators in an ultrastructural study of cerebral vessels as a phenomenon of potential significance in the pathogenesis of cerebral ischemia (Chiang et al., 1968) and by Wilms-Kritschmer and Majno (1969) in ischemia of the skin.

Inherent difficulties in the investigation of fine structural changes of endothelial cells with transmission microscopy have been that only small samples can be examined; there could be an effect associated with parenchymal change, and the so-called 'no reflow' phenomenon seen in vessels of small caliber might be expected to preclude adequate fixation, thus making it difficult to distinguish between ischemic changes and alterations due to delayed or incomplete fixation. The no-reflow phenomenon, as you know, consists of the failure of circulation to be uniformly re-established in a tissue previously rendered ischemic.

About the time that I was thinking these thoughts, it had come to pass that I had completed 6 years of hard labor at the University of Maryland and therefore was eligible for a sabbatical leave. I was familiar with Professor Shimamoto's work and had visited Doctor Sunaga and was aware of their considerable experience in fine structure of endothelium with both scanning (SEM) and transmission (TEM) electron microscopy. They kindly allowed me to work in their laboratory, and this presentation is the result of our collaborative work.

There are two different methods that I would like to present by which we studied the effects of ischemia on endothelium. The first is an ultrastructural study and the second utilizes a fluorescent technique. In order to avoid the problems of transmission microscopy that I mentioned and with the unproven but reasonable assumption that endothelium of large and small vessels is probably similar in its reaction to ischemia, it was decided to render a large vessel ischemic, perfuse under direct observation, and study with SEM and TEM.

Figure 1 shows our rather simple experiment. The monkey carotid artery was clamped on one side, utilizing the opposite side as a control. Specimens were fixed by direct perfusion of the anesthetized animal. Material for SEM was air-dried or freeze-dried and coated with

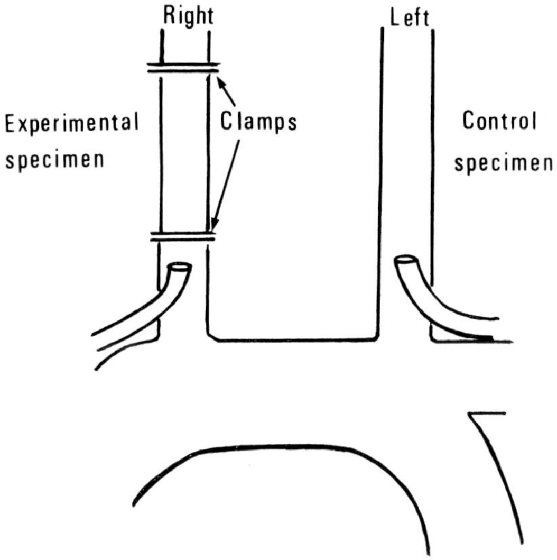

Fig. 1. Diagrammatic representation of the technique: (1) Both carotid arteries dissected free. (2) Right carotid clamped for varying periods of time. (3) Both carotids catheterized. (4) Perfusion with McEwen's solution followed by glutaraldehyde.

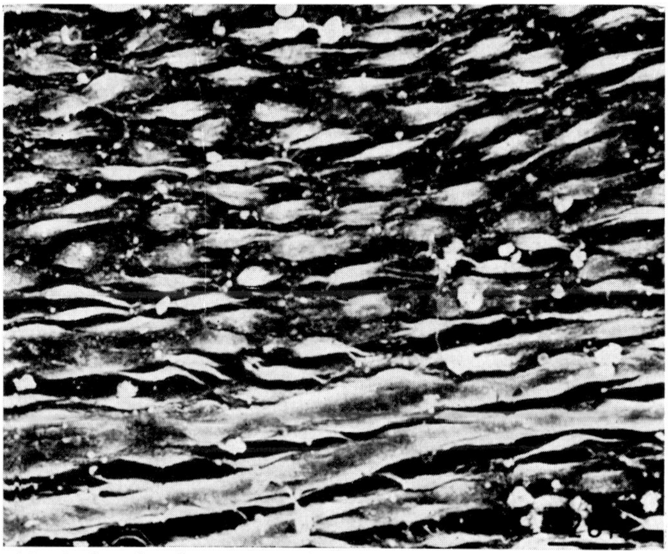

Fig. 2. Normal luminal surface from a control specimen. The folds in the lower portion are due to contraction of the internal elastic lamina.

gold palladium in a vacuum evaporator. Material for TEM was prepared in the usual manner.

Figure 2 shows the variable appearance of normal endothelial surface from a control specimen. The bridge-like structures seen in the lower portion of the micrograph have been shown by Sunaga and Shimamoto (1972), using combined SEM and TEM on the same area of a single specimen, to represent that portion of the endothelial cell which contains the nucleus.

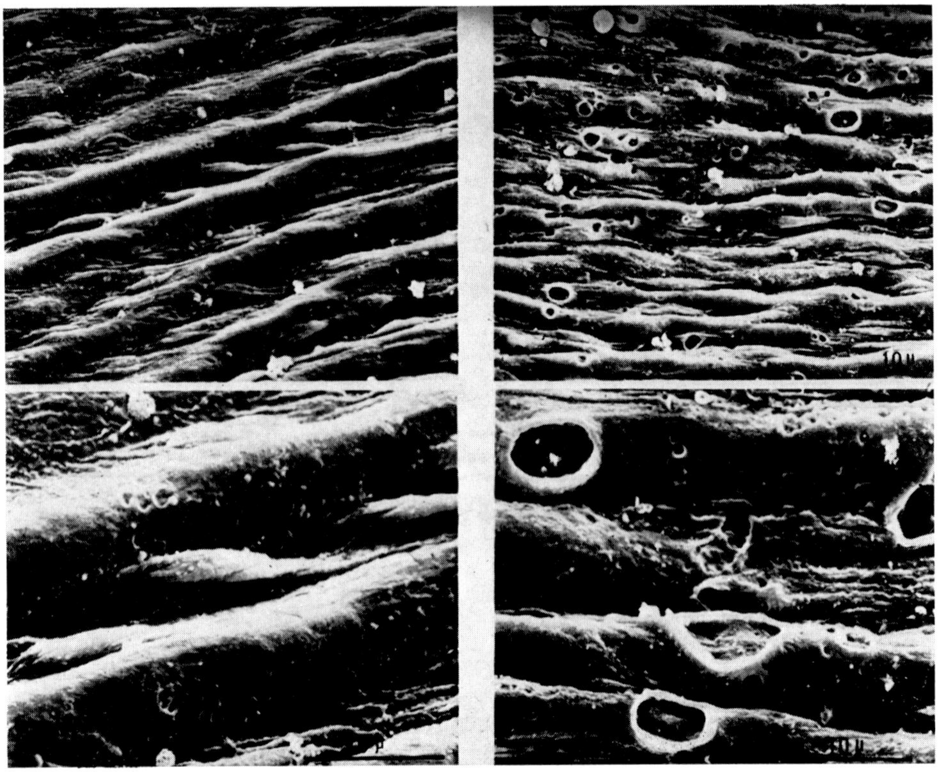

Fig. 3. On the left is the control at low and higher magnification. The right-sided panel is from the experimental side, ischemic for 2 hours.

Figure 3 shows the most striking abnormality as seen frequently in all ischemic specimens and significantly less frequently or not at all in the controls, with the 2-hour ischemic specimen on the right and the control on the left. Here, then, after 2 hours of ischemia there are numerous holes in the endothelial surface of varying sizes and shapes but most of which are round or oval. This is clearly different from the control shown at the same magnification on the left. The control, however, is not quite normal. You can see that there are a few very small craters or holes also in the control specimen. In addition to the difference in number and appearance of the holes, the ischemic vessel usually shows an irregularity of the endothelial surface so that there may be an absence of well-defined nuclear parts.

The specimen shown in Figure 4 was tilted to a 45° angle to show the neck and crater-like appearance of some of these holes as seen with the scanning microscope.

Figure 5 shows a transmission micrograph of a 4-hour specimen and illustrates what may be the TEM equivalent of the numerous holes seen with SEM. These blebs appear predominantly at or near marginal folds. Their origin from endothelium seems definite since at least some retain their attachment by a stalk or neck. In addition, they contain vesicles which, while swollen, are clearly the same as the pinocytic vesicles in the underlying endothelial cell. It is postulated that in the preparatory process for SEM, blebs may indeed rupture, producing a crater-like appearance.

Now, while there are some ultrastructural differences between these blebs and those published by Ames and others (Chiang et al., 1968; Wilms-Kretschmer and Majno, 1969), they probably represent the same phenomenon. However, a difference from other reports

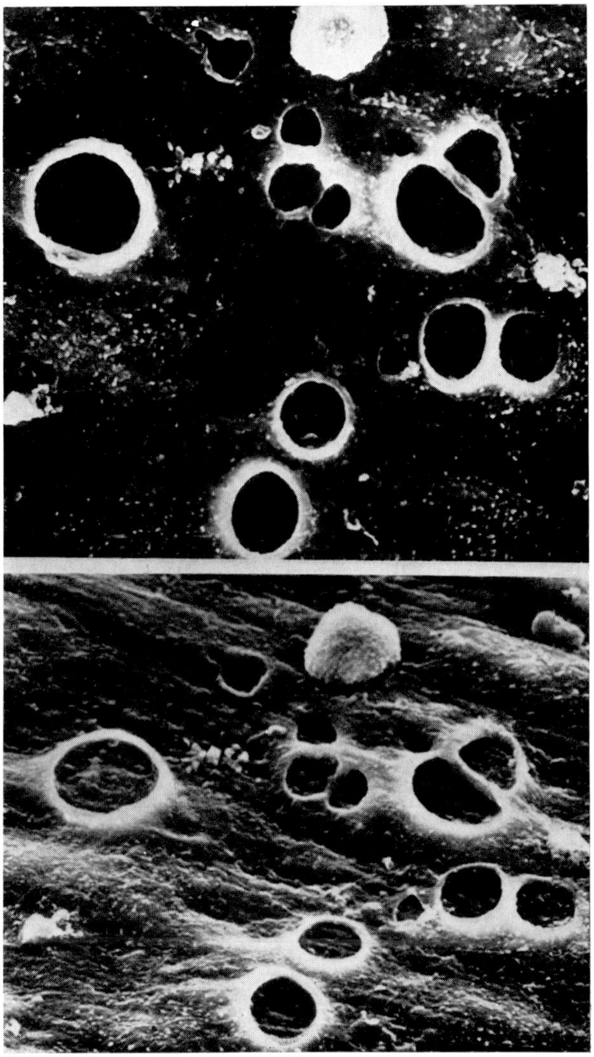

Fig. 4. Ischemic endothelial surface (same field) with specimen tilted 45° to show 'neck' of craters.

which so far seem consistently true in our experiments is the unexpected relative normality of the endothelial fine structure except for the bleb. Cytoplasmic swelling, enlargement of endoplasmic reticulum, enlargement of the perinuclear space and mitochondrial swelling reported by others have not been seen in this perfused material. There may be some loosening of the endothelial tight junctions and there were occasional cytoplasmic 'vacuoles'.

With this model, then, we have demonstrated the appearance by SEM and TEM of well-perfused, well-fixed ischemic and non-ischemic endothelium. However, it is not entirely satisfactory since some of the alterations seen in the ischemic specimen were present in the control, although to a lesser degree. It is probable that the technique, including the trauma of dissection and exposure, can also produce what are non-specific changes in a cell which has only a very limited number of ways to react to the injury. It should also be

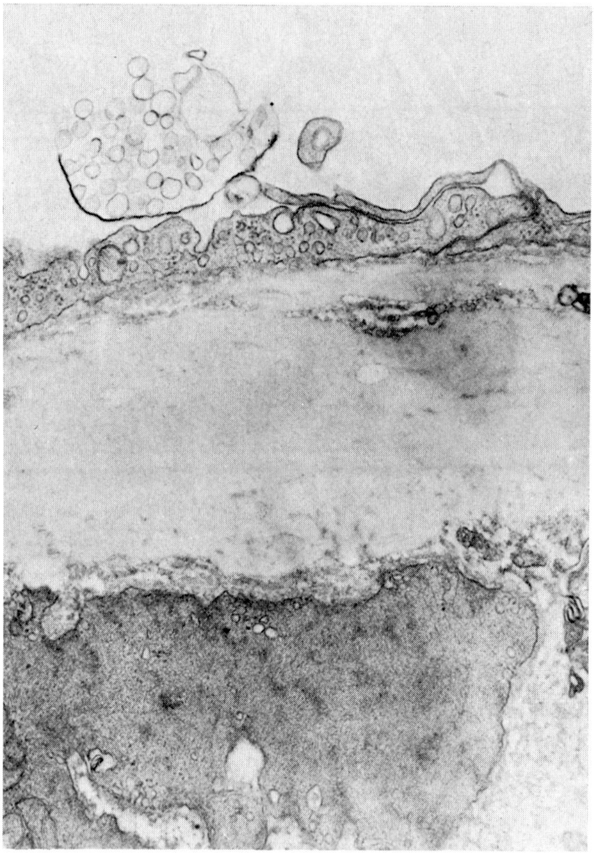

Fig. 5. Transmission micrograph of a bleb-like structure. Note loss of the luminal membrane of the bleb and its content of swollen vesicles. As is usual, the bleb is near the junction between 2 endothelial cells.

noted that SEM information on most biological specimens including endothelium is limited, especially in a pathological state.

Many questions remain unanswered; e.g. what is the earliest time that bleb or crater formation occurs after ischemia; exactly where do the blebs occur; what therapeutic measures will reduce or eliminate it and the basic question of why this particular response to injury and why do not all endothelial cells show the same change? It is hoped that a refined model and further studies with combined SEM and TEM may answer some of these questions.

Figure 6 shows an effort to combine SEM and TEM studies on the same specimen, this being a low-magnification scanning micrograph. In the square you can see the specimen shown at higher magnification in the middle panel. This area was then dissected out and embedded, and a section taken through this crater at the level shown here, with the lowest panel showing the crater in TEM. One can identify the vessel lumen, endothelium, internal elastic lamina, and what gives the impression of a ruptured bleb.

The second series of experiments which I would like to relate very briefly have to do with a simple but perhaps more dynamic way of studying effects of ischemia on endothelium.

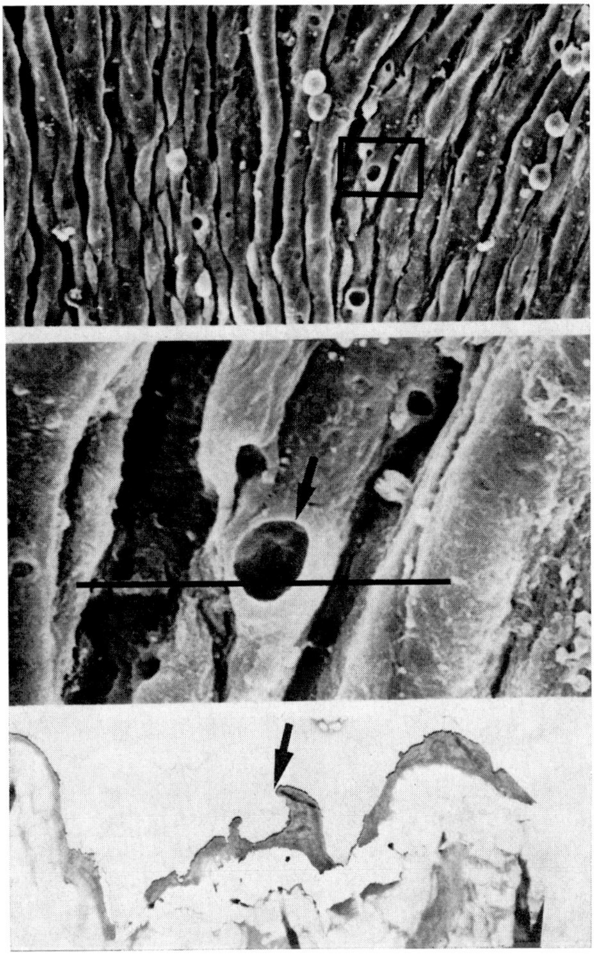

Fig. 6. The upper 2 panels are scanning micrographs with the lowest panel being a transmission micrograph with the plane of section through the hole (arrow) shown by the line in the middle panel.

Using a somewhat similar technique, we clamped the carotid artery of rabbit, using the opposite side as control. After washing, freezing, and cutting unfixed sections and staining with fluorescinated rabbit anti-rabbit gammaglobulin, one can investigate changes in endothelial permeability and, specifically, the infiltration of gammaglobulin into the vessel wall.

Figure 7 is from the control side of an animal whose opposite carotid was clamped for 10 min. Figure 8 shows the experimental side. After 10 min, one can see definite fluorescinated material within the intima but still not passing through the internal elastic lamina. After 30 min of clamping, the fluorescinated gammaglobulin penetrates quite deeply, albeit in a spotty fashion, into the media.

This, then, is a simple means of studying the effect of ischemia on endothelial permeability using a physiological marker. From these preliminary studies, there appears to be a definite time sequence of penetration of the plasma protein depending on the duration of the ischemia.

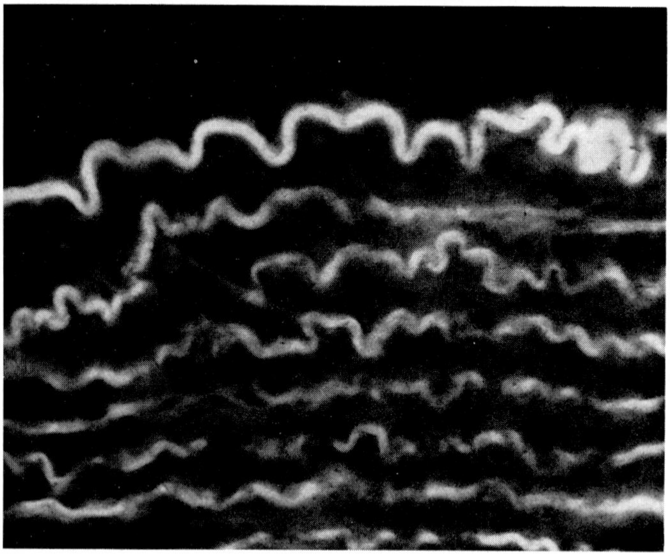

Fig. 7. Control side treated with fluorescinated rabbit anti-rabbit gammaglobulin with vessel lumen at the top.

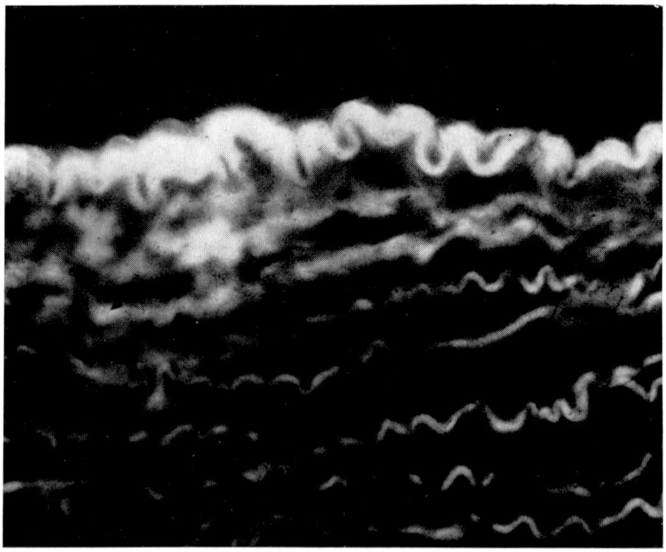

Fig. 8. Experimental side with clamping for 10 min. Note fluorescinated gammaglobulin penetrating the internal elastic lamina into the underlying media.

REFERENCES

CHIANG, J., KOWADA, N., AMES, A., WRIGHT, R. L. and MAJNO, G. (1968): Cerebral ischemia. III. Vascular changes. *Amer. J. Path.*, *52*, 455.
SUNAGA, T. and SHIMAMOTO, T. (1972): Unpublished observations.
WILMS-KRETSCHMER, K. and MAJNO, G. (1969): Ischemia of the skin. Electron microscopic study of vascular injury. *Amer. J. Path.*, *54*, 327.

DISCUSSION

UNIDENTIFIED SPEAKER: During ischemia, the vascular wall tissue produces many substances. These substances are different in different periods of ischemia; they are different in normal subjects and in patients. I think that these substances are very important in producing the injury in the vessel wall. My question is: Have you seen different conditions?

Dr. NELSON: All I can report is what happened in situations where there has been exclusion of segments of the vessel from the remainder of the circulation. There are several ways we have done this, not just the way I have shown you with clamping, but using other techniques. It has essentially all been related to the exclusion of vessels from the remainder of the circulation. We have not, for example, used only one clamp; we have not allowed reflow, and we have not yet utilized pharmacological techniques to see whether the lesions can be prevented or decreased in frequency or size.

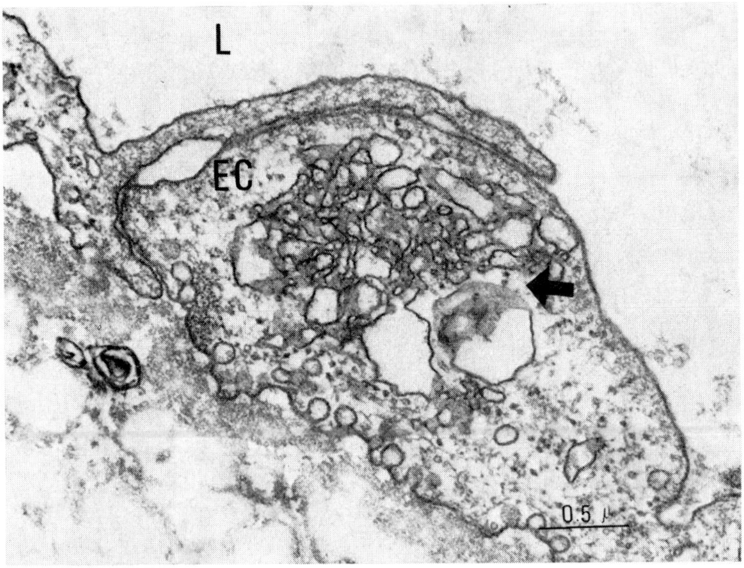

Fig. 1. Swelling of probable Golgi tubes. L = lumen, EC = endothelial cytoplasm.

Dr. PICK: How long can ischemia be maintained and still be reversible? Have you performed any experiments on this, e.g. after 30 min?

Dr. NELSON: We have not done that, but it is planned and is certainly clearly the next thing to do. There are some experiments during which the investigators excluded the circulation from the brain for prolonged periods, and it was found that, if circulation was re-established, important things happened, e.g. brain death did not occur after a period of only a few minutes. In fact, animals, after having a flat EEG, could have return of electrical and physiological function for prolonged periods.

Dr. PICK: What is prolonged?

Dr. NELSON: I am not sure, but I believe that circulation was stopped completely for much longer than previously had been thought compatible with recovery.

Dr. SUNAGA: As Dr. Nelson mentioned, there are many problems about bleb formation in ischemia and other conditions. Figure 1, from the cholesterol feeding experiment, shows swelling of what are probably Golgi tubes. Perhaps some of the blebs are the result of pouching of or out-pouching from such structures. Figure 2 shows blebs that might have such an origin. However, in ischemic studies the fine structure of the endothelium is often normal, except for the blebs themselves. Furthermore, as shown in Figure 2, they contain vesicles which, although often swollen, are clearly the same as the pinocytic vesicles of the endothelial cytoplasm. Finally, studies so far indicate that most of the blebs seem to be located at or near the intercellular junctions and as shown in Figure 2, often arise from the marginal folds. One might speculate that such changes at this site might be related to changes in endothelial permeability.

Dr. COLMAN: It would be really interesting to do the experiment with one clamp, thus simulating stasis. For example, it has been shown by Wessler and others that this situation allows for thrombosis formation after activation of the clotting system in the area which lies behind the clamp. This would be an interesting model for venous disease and possibly for certain types of disease in the arterial system, e.g. in the atrium, where stagnant circulation is present rather than the really extreme ischemia of the sort that you produce with the double clamp.

Dr. NELSON: You are quite right, and such investigations are what we are all concerned with, namely what happens in human disease. The next study will be on the effects of clamping and then reopening the middle cerebral artery using the techniques developed by Garcia

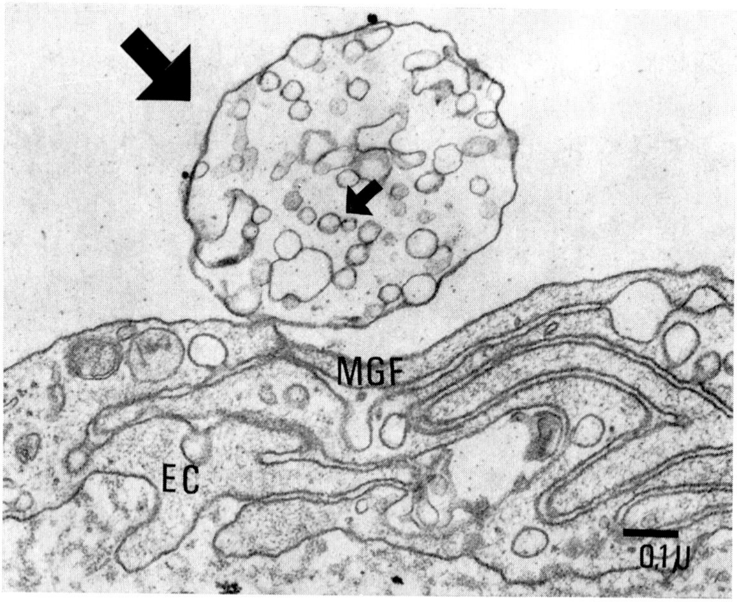

Fig. 2. Bleb formation. Large arrow, bleb; small arrow, vesicle. EC = endothelial cytoplasm, MGF = marginal fold.

and colleagues, but the reason why we chose this model first was basically to exclude the possibility of collateral circulation.

UNIDENTIFIED SPEAKER: After your beautiful study, may I ask a layman's question? I am sure that immunofluorescence has come a long way within the past 10–15 years. Is it now entirely specific?

Dr. NELSON: I believe that at least this technique is entirely specific.

Dr. CONSTANTINIDES: I would like to congratulate you on the enormous amount of labor that is required when doing such experiments. Most people who have not worked with the artery under the electron microscope do not realize how much is involved. Firstly, I should like to ask you, Dr. Nelson, if I got it right. How did you give the immunofluorescent stain? Did you inject it systemically, intravenously, prior to the clamping?

Dr. NELSON: No, this was done in vitro, flooding the specimen after it was removed.

Dr. CONSTANTINIDES: The second point has a bearing on the comments of Dr. Colman and your future work. A few years ago, we did clamp with only one clamp the femoral artery of the rat at various time intervals, and we did not use, of course, a fancy microscope. We found definite evidence of increased permeability of the junction by the fact that plasma accumulated underneath the junction and lifted it, not after 2, 4 or 8 min, but after 16 min, after just one clamp.

Dr. NELSON: Did you find bleb formation?

Dr. CONSTANDINIDES: Yes, there were blebs. I did not pay much attention to it at the time because I was looking for something at the junctions, but in retrospect it fits in with what is now being found.

Dr. NELSON: With regard to your first comment, I must pay tribute, not only to Dr. Sunaga's and Dr. Shimamoto's industry, but also to the incredible efforts of his band of inspired technicians.

THE ROLE OF PYRIDINOLCARBAMATE IN THE PREVENTION AND REVERSAL OF THE DEVELOPMENT OF EXPERIMENTAL CHOLESTEROL ATHEROSCLEROSIS

N. N. KIPSHIDZE, L. K. TKESHELASHVILI, G. A. VADACHKORIA, D. CHKHATARASHVILI and N. JAVAKHISHVILI

Institute of Therapy, Ministry of Health of Georgian S.S.R., Tbilisi, U.S.S.R.

The aim of the present investigation was to investigate the role of Anginin in the prevention and reversal of cholesterol-induced atherosclerosis.

MATERIAL AND METHODS

The experiments were carried out on 54 rabbits in which experimental atherosclerosis was produced according to the method of Anitschkov (1933). The animals were given cholesterol (0.3 g/kg animal weight) for 100 days. 15 rabbits were given Anginin together with the cholesterol (10 mg/kg), 10 rabbits received only cholesterol, 17 rabbits after the experimental atherosclerosis induction received Anginin for a month (20 mg/kg), and 12 rabbits were used as controls (on normal diet).

Before and after treatment some indices of lipid metabolism were determined in blood (cholesterol, lecithin, β-lipoproteins, phospholipids, triglycerides, non-esterified fatty acids). Some coagulation tests were also performed. Whole-blood coagulation time by the method of Lee et al. (1913), adhesive index of thrombocytes by the method of Mootton and Froman (1949), and blood coagulation activity were determined. The haemostatic changes in the first phase were determined by measuring plasma recalcification time. The second phase was determined by measuring the activity of prothrombin complex components by Quick's technique (1935). Changes in the third phase were determined by measuring the fibrinogen level in blood by Rutberg's method (1957). Together with the quantitative determination of fibrinogen levels in blood, qualitative changes were observed using the fibrinogen B test of Lyons. Some of the observed animals underwent thromboelastography. Blood anticoagulative activity was determined using the indices of thrombin time, blood-free heparin, and fibrinolytic activity. The degree of aortic damage by the atherosclerotic process was estimated by a direct planimetric technique. Microscopic investigations of the aorta were carried out.

RESULTS

The degree of aortic damage by atherosclerosis is shown in Table I. The data show that under the influence of Anginin the degree of aortic damage by atherosclerosis is diminished in the prophylactic group and that there is reversal of the development of atherosclerosis. The results of investigations of lipid metabolism changes in the blood serum of rabbits which had been given Anginin after cholesterol are shown in Tables II and III. The data show that, in control animals on a normal diet for 1 month after they have been given cholesterol for 100 days, cholesterol, phospholipids, and β-lipoproteins were considerably decreased ($p<0.05$, <0.01 and <0.05, respectively). In the group of animals with experimental atherosclerosis which have been given Anginin for 1 month, cholesterol and phospholipid levels were also decreased ($p<0.05$ and <0.01, respectively); however, the β-lipoproteins did not decrease significantly ($p>0.1$). Comparison of the indices of lipid metabolism in the animals with

TABLE I

*Degree of aortic damage by atherosclerosis (%)**

Statistical indices	Animals with experimental atherosclerosis: Control	Animals with experimental atherosclerosis: Anginin	Injection for 100 days: Cholesterol + Anginin	Injection for 100 days: Cholesterol
	Damaged regions of aorta			
M	37.0	9.0[a]	4.0	20.0[b]
SD	±14.0	±6.71	±3.32	±7.75
SE	± 6.20	±3.35[a]	±1.17	±3.16[b]

*) All values are mean (M) ± standard deviation (SD) ± standard error (SE).
[a]) Comparison between control and Anginin-treated animals is statistically significant: $p < 0.01$.
[b]) Comparison between cholesterol + Anginin and cholesterol-treated animals is statistically significant: $p < 0.01$.

TABLE II

*The effect of Anginin on the quantitative content of β-lipoproteins, lecithin and serum cholesterol in animals with experimental atherosclerosis**

Animals	Statistical indices	Cholesterol (mg %) Before	Cholesterol (mg %) After	Phospholipids (mg %) Before	Phospholipids (mg %) After	β-Lipoproteins (mg %) Before	β-Lipoproteins (mg %) After
Experimental	M	573.0	101.0[a]	228.0	101.0[a]	1047.0	247.0[a]
atherosclerosis	SD	±444.7	± 39.8	± 91.2	± 31.8	± 836.4	± 91.0
(control)	SE	±168.4	± 16.2	± 34.4	± 13.0	± 316.8	± 37.1
Atherosclerosis +	M	455[b]	157[ab]	220.0[b]	80.0[ab]	798.0[b]	433.0[ab]
Anginin (test)	SD	271.8	137.7	80.4	69.2	450.6	383.7
	SE	102.6	56.2	30.4	28.9	170.3	156.6

*) All values are mean (M) ± standard deviation (SD) ± standard error (SE).
[a]) Comparison between values before and after cholesterol treatment is statistically significant: $p < 0.05$ (for cholesterol and β-lipoproteins); $p < 0.01$ (for phospholipids) in control group and Anginin-treated group; not statistically significant: $p > 0.1$ (for β-lipoproteins).
[b]) Comparison between values in control group and Anginin-treated animals is not statistically significant: $p > 0.5$; $p > 0.2$.

experimental atherosclerosis and those which had been given Anginin for 1 month showed no statistically significant differences in the levels of cholesterol, phospholipids and β-lipoproteins. In this connection, cholesterol and β-lipoproteins remain at a higher level after Anginin treatment in spite of their lower initial level in comparison with the control group. The change in phospholipid level in both groups of animals is nearly identical.

In control animals on a normal diet for 1 month after they have been given cholesterol, total lipid content and non-esterified fatty acids were considerably decreased ($p < 0.02$ and 0.01, respectively). Triglyceride level does not change. As the data of Table III show, Anginin administration for 1 month does not lead to considerable changes in total lipids, triglycerides and non-esterified fatty acids in spite of the fact that the total lipid content diminishes to 31.7%.

In comparing the data of the control experiments with those following Anginin administra-

TABLE III

*The effect of Anginin on the quantitative content of total lipids, triglycerides, and non-esterified fatty acids in experimental atherosclerosis**

Animals	Statistical indices	Total lipids (mg%)		Triglycerides (mg%)		Non-esterified fatty acids (mg%)	
		Before	After	Before	After	Before	After
Experimental atherosclerosis (control)	M	452.0	252.0[a]	82.0	80.0	3.0	1.3[a]
	SD	±163.80	±558.0	±18.02	±28.91	± 1.00	±0.93
	SE	± 61.90	± 27.90	± 6.81	±11.80	± 0.38	±0.38
Atherosclerosis + Anginin (test)	M	425[b]	290[ab]	80.0[b]	84.0[a]	2.8[b]	2.1[ab]
	SD	±205.30	±104.40	±19.80	±23.21	± 2.26	±0.79
	SE	± 77.70	± 52.20	± 7.50	±10.40	± 0.92	±0.32

*) All values are mean (M) ±standard deviation (SD) ±standard error (SE).
[a]) Comparison between values before and after cholesterol treatment is statistically significant: $p < 0.02$ (for total lipids); $p < 0.01$ (for non-esterified fatty acids); not statistically significant: $p > 0.5$ (for triglycerides); not statistically significant in Anginin-treated group: $p > 0.1$ (for total lipids); $p > 0.5$ (for triglycerides and non-esterified fatty acids).
[b]) Comparison between values in control group and Anginin-treated animals is not statistically significant: $p > 0.5$; $p < 0.1$ for all parameters.

tion no large differences were found. However, in the test group, total lipid and non-esterified fatty acid levels as well as the level of cholesterol and β-lipoproteins remained at a higher level than in the control animals. Also, considerable improvement in the rabbits' clinical state following Anginin treatment should be taken into consideration. Thus the positive influence of Anginin on reversing the development of experimental atherosclerosis manifests itself in the considerable decrease in the degree of aortic damage by atherosclerosis and in the improvement of the animals' clinical state without considerable shifts in blood lipids.

The data on the investigations into the prophylactic effect of Anginin on experimental atherosclerosis are shown in Table IV. The data show that cholesterol and Anginin given by

TABLE IV

*Changes in the content of serum lipids in rabbits which had been given cholesterol and Anginin simultaneously**

Animals	Statistical indices	Total lipids (mg%)	β-Lipoproteins (mg%)	Triglycerides (mg%)	Cholesterol (mg%)	Phospholipids (mg%)	Non-esterified fatty acids (mg%)
Cholesterol	M	340.0	502.0	71.0	237.0	152.0	3.5
	SD	±138.30	±257.70	± 7.00	± 83.80	± 34.40	±1.25
	SE	± 56.40	±105.20	± 2.85	± 34.20	± 14.04	±0.51
Cholesterol + Anginin	M	371.0[b]	708.0[b]	93.0[a]	329.0[b]	210.0[b]	1.5[a]
	SD	±129.70	±319.00	±22.80	±172.80	±109.60	±0.62
	SE	± 34.70	± 85.00	± 6.09	± 46.20	± 29.60	±0.16

*) All values are mean (M) ±standard deviation (SD) ±standard error (SE).
[a]) Comparison between cholesterol and Anginin-treated animals is statistically significant: $p < 0.02$ (for triglycerides); $p < 0.001$ (for non-esterified fatty acids).
[b]) Not statistically significant: $p > 0.1$ for other parameters.

TABLE V

*Changes in coagulation indices in animals with experimental atherosclerosis**

Animals	Statistical indices	Blood coagulation time (sec)		Tolerance of plasma to heparin (sec)		Plasma recalcification time (sec)		Thrombin time (sec)		Free heparin (sec)		Fibrinogen quantity (mg%)		Fibrinolytic activity (days)	
		Before	After	Before	After	Before	After	Before	After	Before	After	Before	After	Before	After
	M	151.0	185.8	184.00	222.50	150.00	118.33	27.20	28.83	2.80	4.33	440.0	382.50	5.00	4.67
Cholesterol only	SD	± 14.33	± 58.59	± 47.30	± 25.75	± 17.35	± 17.86	± 2.16	± 2.41	±0.83	±0.82	± 41.9	± 30.73	±0.70	±0.81
	SE	± 6.40	± 23.91	± 21.12	± 10.51	± 7.74	± 7.29	± 0.96	± 0.98	±0.37	±0.33	± 18.70	± 12.54	±0.31	±0.33
	M	175.00[b]	383.33[a]	158.00[b]	325.00[a]	129.40[a]	190.83[a]	27.60[b]	36.67[a]	3.80[b]	8.33[a]	460.00[b]	316.67[b]	4.60[b]	2.83[a]
Cholesterol +	SD	± 24.01	±128.55	± 27.79	± 37.97	± 12.52	± 32.75	± 4.33	± 2.34	±0.83	±2.27	±114.22	± 93.46	±1.34	±0.77
Anginin	SE	10.72	± 52.47	± 12.41	± 15.50	± 5.59	± 13.37	± 1.93	± 0.95	±0.37	±0.93	± 50.93	± 38.15	±0.60	±0.31

*) All values are mean (M) ± standard deviation (SD) ± standard error (SE).

a) Comparison between values in control group and Anginin-treated animals is statistically significant: $p < 0.008$ (for blood coagulation time); $p < 0.000$ (for tolerance of plasma to heparin and for thrombin time); $p < 0.001$ (for recalcification time); $p < 0.003$ (for free heparin time and for fibrinolytic activity); $p < 0.035$ for plasma recalcification time).

b) Not statistically significant for all other parameters ($p > 0.05$).

simultaneous injection for 3 months cause considerable changes mainly in triglycerides and non-esterified fatty acids. In this connection the level of triglycerides and non-esterified fatty acids decreased. Total lipid, β-lipoprotein, cholesterol and phospholipid levels increase slightly. Thus in the prophylactic administration of Anginin all the parameters studied except for non-esterified fatty acids were increased.

In the aortae of rabbits which have been given cholesterol, atheromatous lesions of various sizes and shapes were macroscopically visible on the surface of the intima, mainly situated in the ascending aorta, the arch and in the thoracic part of the descending aorta. In the microscopic investigations a large quantity of sudanophilic material and cholesterol in the swollen intima was observed in large, medium and small droplets. A small quantity of fatty droplets was found in the media. A large quantity of atheromatous cells was found in the intima. A large increase in intracellular material was observed in the intima as well as in the media. The elastic fibres were swollen and were mostly destroyed.

In the group of rabbits in which the animals were killed on the 30th day after cholesterol feeding was stopped, atherosclerotic changes were also observed macroscopically. In the microscopic investigations of atherosclerotic changes sudanophilic substances and cholesterol were observed in much less quantity than in the previous series. Intracellular material was increased as well as in the previous group. In the group of tests where the animals were given Anginin together with cholesterol, atherosclerotic damage of the intima, intercellular material, increase, swelling and destructive change in elastic fibres etc. were also found. However, the amount of sudanophilic material and cholesterol in the intima was found in much less quantity than in the control group. A large number of small drops of sudanophilic material and cholesterol was found in the media, thus indicating the transport of these substances through it. The swelling of the intima in this group was much less than in the control group.

In the cholesterol-fed group in which Anginin was given for the purposes of treatment, we observed quite a different picture. White spots of various sizes and shapes on the surface of the intima of the ascending aorta, the arch, as well as of the thoracic part of the descending

TABLE VI

*Changes in coagulation indices in the prophylactic group of animals**

Animals		Statistical indices	Blood coagulation time (sec)	Tolerance of plasma to heparin (sec)	Plasma recalcification time (sec)	Thrombin time (sec)	Free heparin (sec)	Fibrinolytic activity (days)
Injection for 1 month	Cholesterol	M	151.00	117.50	73.75	26.50	3.50	5.75
		SD	± 50.39	± 12.54	± 9.43	± 3.09	±0.58	±0.95
		SE	± 22.50	± 6.27	± 4.71	± 1.54	±0.29	±0.47
	Cholesterol + Anginin	M	188.46[b]	170.38[a]	97.69[a]	28.08[a]	4.00[b]	5.15[b]
		SD	± 50.47	± 15.59	±17.56	± 4.00	±1.62	±1.15
		SE	± 14.02	± 12.66	± 4.88	± 1.11	±0.45	±0.32

*) All values are mean (M) ± standard deviation (SD) ± standard error (SE).

[a]) Comparison between values in control group and Anginin-treated animals is statistically significant: $p < 0.003$ (for tolerance of plasma heparin); $p < 0.004$ (for plasma recalcification time and thrombin time).

[b]) Not statistically significant: $p = 0.185$ (for blood coagulation time); $p = 0.384$ (for free heparin); $p = 0.291$ (for fibrinolytic activity).

TABLE VII

*Changes in coagulation indices in the prophylactic group of animals**

Animals		Statistical indices	Blood coagulation time (sec)	Tolerance of plasma to heparin (sec)	Plasma recalcification time (sec)	Thrombin time (sec)	Free heparin (sec)	Fibrinogen quantity (mg%)	Fibrinolytic activity (days)
Injection for 2 months	Cholesterol	M	129.17	154.17	59.67	23.33	2.33	395.83	5.50
		SD	± 63.76	± 27.75	± 10.06	± 2.08	± 0.12	± 103.41	± 1.65
		SE	± 26.02	± 11.33	± 4.11	± 0.85	± 0.05	± 42.21	± 0.67
	Cholesterol + Anginin	M	326.36[a]	147.73[b]	91.18[a]	36.27[a]	6.18[b]	340.01[b]	4.09[a]
		SD	± 113.54	± 26.89	± 22.54	± 8.03	± 1.79	± 306.60	± 0.94
		SE	± 34.20	± 8.10	± 6.79	± 2.84	± 0.54	± 92.35	± 0.28

*) All values are mean (M) ± standard deviation (SD) ± standard error (SE).

[a]) Comparison between values in control group and Anginin-treated animals is statistically significant: $p = 0.000$ (for blood coagulation time and fibrinolytic activity); $p = 0.002$ (for plasma recalcification time); $p = 0.001$ (for thrombin time).

[b]) Not statistically significant: $p = 0.625$ (for tolerance of plasma to heparin); $p = 0.438$ (for free heparin time); $p = 0.625$ (for fibrinolytic activity).

TABLE VIII

*Changes in coagulation indices in the prophylactic group of animals**

Animals		Statistical indices	Blood coagulation time (sec)	Tolerance of plasma to heparin (sec)	Plasma recalcification time (sec)	Thrombin time (sec)	Free heparin (sec)	Fibrinogen quantity (mg %)	Fibrinolytic activity (days)
Injection for 3 months	Cholesterol	M	163.67	138.89	60.00	28.00	3.50	509.17	5.17
		SD	± 28.97	± 25.81	± 12.91	± 2.73	±2.27	± 69.22	±0.74
		SE	± 11.82	± 8.60	± 5.27	± 1.11	±0.93	± 28.25	±0.30
	Cholesterol + Anginin	M	353[a]	148.33[b]	107.78[a]	31.00[b]	5.33[b]	244.44[a]	4.22
		SD	±117.80	± 40.74	± 31.01	± 3.04	±1.23	± 29.50	±0.68
		SE	± 39.27	± 16.63	± 10.34	± 1.01	±0.41	± 9.83	±0.23

*) All values are mean (M) ± standard deviation (SD) ± standard error (SE).

[a]) Comparison between values in control group and Anginin-treated animals is statistically significant: $p = 0.000$ (for blood coagulation time and fibrinogen quantity); $p = 0.001$ (for plasma recalcification time).

[b]) Not statistically significant: $p = 0.438$ (for tolerance of plasma to heparin); $p = 0.067$ (for thrombin time); $p = 0.095$ (for free heparin).

aorta were seen macroscopically. In the microscopic investigations no sudanophilic material or cholesterol were observed in the intima. Intercellular material was increased moderately but much less than in the control group.

As mentioned above, together with the biomorphological investigations, the study of blood coagulative activity was carried out in animals with experimental atherosclerosis which had been given Anginin. Blood coagulation time, plasma recalcification and thrombin time were increased as was free heparin and blood fibrinolytic activity. Plasma tolerance to heparin and the adhesive index were increased. Decrease in blood coagulation activity was also observed in the thromboelastogram. The prothrombin index in both control and experimental groups was not changed. The fibrinogen B test in untreated rabbits was often positive, which is why the results of this test have not been taken into consideration. When comparing the indices of the control and experimental groups of rabbits, statistically significant changes in all indices except fibrinogen level were found, while the initial data of both groups of rabbits were only slightly different (Table V). Treated and untreated rabbits which were given Anginin together with cholesterol for 1 month showed lengthening of plasma recalcification and thrombin times. Tolerance of plasma to heparin was decreased. Changes in blood coagulation time, fibrinogen level, fibrinolytic activity and free heparin were not significant (Table VI). Anginin injection together with cholesterol for 2 months caused greater changes in the blood coagulation system: blood coagulation time, plasma recalcification and thrombin time were prolonged, blood fibrinolytic activity was increased, fibrinogen level slightly decreased and free heparin ranged between wide limits with a tendency to increase. Plasma tolerance to heparin and the prothrombin index remained unchanged (Table VII). After Anginin had been given for 3 months the changes in the blood coagulation system were expressed greatly in rabbits with atherosclerosis. The lengthening of blood coagulation time and plasma recalcification was found. The amount of fibrinogen decreased and fibrinolytic activity increased. Changes in plasma tolerance to heparin, thrombin time, free heparin and the prothrombin index were observed but were not statistically significant (Table VIII).

The experiments to study Anginin prophylaxis and its therapeutic effect in cholesterol-induced atherosclerosis have shown that Anginin has a strong antiatherogenic effect. It protects the arterial wall from the deposition of cholesterol. The mechanism of the anti-atherogenic action of Anginin is to antagonize the action of kinins. From our investigations, Anginin revealed considerable therapeutic and prophylactic effects in experimental atherosclerosis and its clinical application in prevention and treatment of the various complications of atherosclerosis may be recommended.

REFERENCES

ADAMS, C. W. M., BAYLISS, O. B. and IBRAHIM, M. Z. M. (1971): Effects of nialamide on cholesterol induced atheroma in the rabbit. *J. Atheroscler. Res.*, *2*, 493.

ANITSCHKOV, N. N. (1933): Experimental atherosclerosis in animals. In: *Arteriosclerosis, A Survey of the Problem*, p. 271. Editor: E. V. Cowdry. New York.

CUMMINE, H. G. and LYONS, R. N. (1948): *Brit. J. Surg.*, *35*, 337.

HENRY, R. L. (1969): Effects of pyridinolcarbamate on specific components of hemostasis in Cruz's model. In: *Atherogenesis. Proceedings, I International Symposium on Atherogenesis, Thrombogenesis and Pyridinolcarbamate Treatment, Tokyo 1969*, pp. 75–80. Editors: T. Shimamoto and F. Numano. ICS 201, Excerpta Medica, Amsterdam.

LEE, R. J., WHITE, P. D. et al. (1913): *Amer. J. med. Sci.*, *145*, 495.

MARTINS DE OLIVEIRA, J. M. (1969): The effects of pyridinolcarbamate on experimental atherosclerosis. In: *Atherogenesis. Proceedings, I International Symposium on Atherogenesis, Thrombogenesis and Pyridinolcarbamate Treatment, Tokyo 1969*, pp. 53–55. Editors: T. Shimamoto and F. Numano. ICS 201, Excerpta Medica, Amsterdam.

MOOTTON, S. E. and FROMAN, R. (1949): *Amer. J. clin. Path.*, *19*, 701.

PICK, R. (1969): The effect of pyridinolcarbamate on the induction and regression of aortic and

coronary atherosclerosis in cholesterol-fed cockerels. In: *Atherogenesis. Proceedings, I International Symposium on Atherogenesis, Thrombogenesis and Pyridinolcarbamate Treatment, Tokyo 1969*, pp. 57–62. Editors: T. Shimamoto and F. Numano. ICS 201, Excerpta Medica, Amsterdam.
QUICK, A. J. (1935): *J. biol. Chem.*, *73/74*, 109.
ROCHA E SILVA, M. and GARCIA LEME, J. (1963): Antagonists of bradykinins. *Med. exp. (Basel)*, *8*, 287.
RUTBERG, R. A. (1957): *Probl. Gemat.*, *2/13*, 25.
SCHULDER, W. and ALBRECHT, W. (1962): Einfluss bekannter Hypertensiva auf die experimentelle Kaninchenatheromatose. *Schweiz. med. Wschr.*, *33*, 1007.
SHIMAMOTO, T., NUMANO, F. and FUJITA, T. (1966): Atherosclerosis-inhibiting effect of an anti-bradykinin agent, pyridinolcarbamate. *Amer. Heart J.*, *71*, 2216.
SHIMAMOTO, T., NUMANO, F., FUJITA, T., ISHIEKA, T. and ATSUMI, T. (1965): Treatment of experimental and human atherosclerosis with pyridinolcarbamate. *Asian med. J.*, *8*, 12.
YAMAZAKI, H. (1969): Changes in blood coagulability, platelet count and platelet aggregation induced by endotoxin or exercise and the prevention of these by pyridinolcarbamate. In: *Atherogenesis. Proceedings, I International Symposium on Atherogenesis, Thrombogenesis and Pyridinolcarbamate Treatment, Tokyo 1969*, pp. 93–95. Editors: T. Shimamoto and F. Numano. ICS 201, Excerpta Medica, Amsterdam.

DISCUSSION

Dr. KRITCHEVSKY: Was the Anginin administered by injection? Was the cholesterol fed with added fat, or was it just added to the diet as cholesterol?

Dr. KIPSHIDZE: Anginin was administered orally, not by injection. Pure cholesterol was administered, 0.3 g in 10% solution of sunflower-seed oil.

Dr. AUSTIN: You said there was no effect on free fatty acids. This is in contrast to what we have seen in our laboratory where we have found some. Could you comment on how you measured the free heparin level?

Dr. KIPSHIDZE: In our investigations blood-free heparin was determined by Sirmai's technique.

Dr. COTTON: I should like to make a comment about blood coagulation changes. We investigated a number of patients with intermittent claudication who were receiving pyridinolcarbamate from 4 to 6 months. We found no effect on the prothrombin time or partial thromboplastin time. We did, however, see a trend towards a reduction in the increased plasma antiheparin activity, i.e. a reduction in heparin tolerance, but this was not statistically significant. After 4 months of treatment there was a significant reduction in the levels of plasma fibrinogen.

Dr. DE SOLDATI: A few years ago we tried to see what happened to blood coagulation in a patient treated with pyridinolcarbamate, and we also could not find any change which was statistically significant. We also could not find any change in cholesterol level. We feel that the action is not through this mechanism.

Dr. KIPSHIDZE: As a matter of fact, it is very difficult to explain because we have the same lipid metabolism but more or less with atherosclerotic damage.

CHAIRMAN (Dr. Constantinides): I do not think it is yet proven that the cholesterol is really sedimenting on the arterial wall because nobody has yet really convincingly proven that this is a sediment on the outer surface.

Dr. KIPSHIDZE: After 4 months of pyridinolcarbamate treatment we have also observed a significant reduction in the level of plasma fibrinogen.

Dr. COLMAN: I would be very interested in some further definition of the bradykinin antagonism that you noted, in particular in the methods that you used to demonstrate it, and what its mechanism might be. Is this a potentiation of the kinases that destroy bradykinin? What do you think it is that you are observing?

Dr. KIPSHIDZE: I have not performed any experiments about this point. It is just a speculation. As far as I know, nobody has yet shown any increment in bradykinin activity in lipemic rabbits, either systemically or locally.

Dr. HENRY: If I recall correctly, in studies in vitro with blood coagulation we did not find a change with Anginin. I do not want to put Dr. Yamazaki on the spot, but I believe he did report no change in prothrombin time or recalcification time in his studies with humans.

Dr. KIPSHIDZE: We have observed the same with no change in the clinical condition.

Dr. YAMAZAKI: I measured one-stage prothrombin time in humans after a short treatment with pyridinolcarbamate and in this case I could not find any change in prothrombin time. The human subjects were injected with 0.1 μg/kg of adrenaline or given a fatty meal. However, the shortening of one-stage prothrombin time induced by adrenaline or fatty meal was inhibited by pyridinolcarbamate treatment.

THE ANTIATHEROGENIC EFFECT OF PYRIDINOLCARBAMATE

M. R. PARWARESCH
University Institute of Pathology, Kiel, Federal Republic of Germany

In order to investigate the preventive and therapeutic effect of pyridinolcarbamate (PDC) on experimentally induced atherosclerosis, the following experiments were performed.

A total of 168 non-inbred, male rabbits about 6 months old with an average weight of 3200 g were divided into 5 groups (I–V). Group I received a cholesterol-rich (3.5 g %), atherogenic diet for 6 weeks. Group II was fed a normal diet. Atherosclerosis was induced by exposing the animals to repeated hypoxia ($P_N = 95\ \%$, $P_{O_2} = 5\ \%$, 2×1 min; 2 times daily for 3 weeks). Group III received a normal diet and was treated with daily injections of noradrenaline (i.v.) and L-thyroxine (s.c.) for 3 weeks. The animals of Group IV were put on an atherogenic diet (1 g % cholesterol). The development of atherosclerosis was accelerated by a combination of the above-mentioned agents plus histamine. Experimental Group V served as control and showed no signs of arterial damage.

All groups were divided into 2 subgroups of which one received placebo (starch) and the other PDC (30 mg/kg daily p.o.).

The extent of the experimental atherosclerosis was expressed in terms of the percentage of the aortic surface affected. Comparing both subgroups, we could not find any significant differences between the PDC and placebo treated animals for experimental Groups I, II and III, whereas the extent of atherosclerosis in the PDC treated animals of Group IV was significantly lower than that in the corresponding placebo treated subgroup (Table I).

TABLE I

Experimental group	Percentage of aortic surface involved	
	Placebo	PDC
Control (n = 20)	0	
I. Cholesterol diet (3.5 g %) (n = 39)	60 ± 10	57 ± 11
II. Normal diet, hypoxia (n = 38)	32 ± 6	34 ± 8
III. Normal diet, noradrenaline, L-thyroxine (n = 35)	44 ± 7	40 ± 7
IV. Cholesterol diet (1 g %), hypoxemia, noradrenaline, L-thyroxine and histamine (n = 37)	48 ± 5*	24 ± 9*

* $p < 0.01$.

In other experiments we tried to study the so-called curative or therapeutic effect of PDC on experimentally induced atherosclerosis in rabbits (80 atherosclerotic rabbits of which 40 animals were put on PDC for 8 weeks and sacrificed at a rate of 5 animals weekly). These experiments revealed no convincing differences between the experimental groups.

Our results can be summarized as follows: (1) In the case of methods commonly used to induce atherosclerosis in rabbits, no convincing preventive effect could be seen following PDC medication. (2) The preventive effect of PDC on histamine-induced atherosclerosis

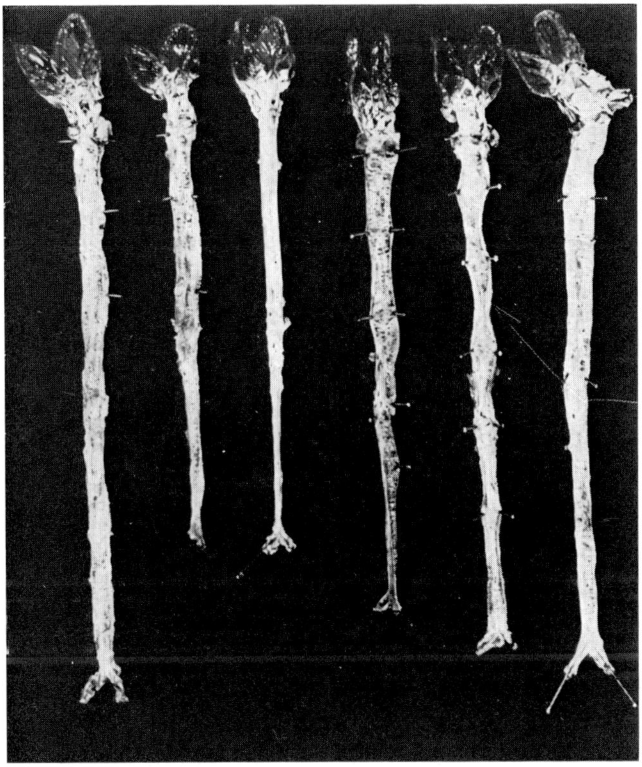

Fig. 1. Photographs of 6 rabbit heart-aorta preparations with severe cholesterol-induced atherosclerosis. All animals were treated with PDC for 6 weeks at the onset of the atherosclerogenic treatment (Group I).

speaks in favour of the view that PDC has an effect on transmural transport mechanisms, and supports the results gained by other authors in acute experiments. (3) According to the studies reported, PDC shows no convincing therapeutic effect on experimentally induced atherosclerosis regardless of the technique applied.

Figure 1 shows a gross view of heart-aorta preparations of the cholesterol-fed and PDC-treated animals. The so-called experimental atherosclerosis is highly developed in spite of PDC treatment. Figure 2 shows coronary arteries with massive deposition of lipid-laden macrophages in the vessel wall from a rabbit fed a cholesterol diet and PDC for 6 weeks.

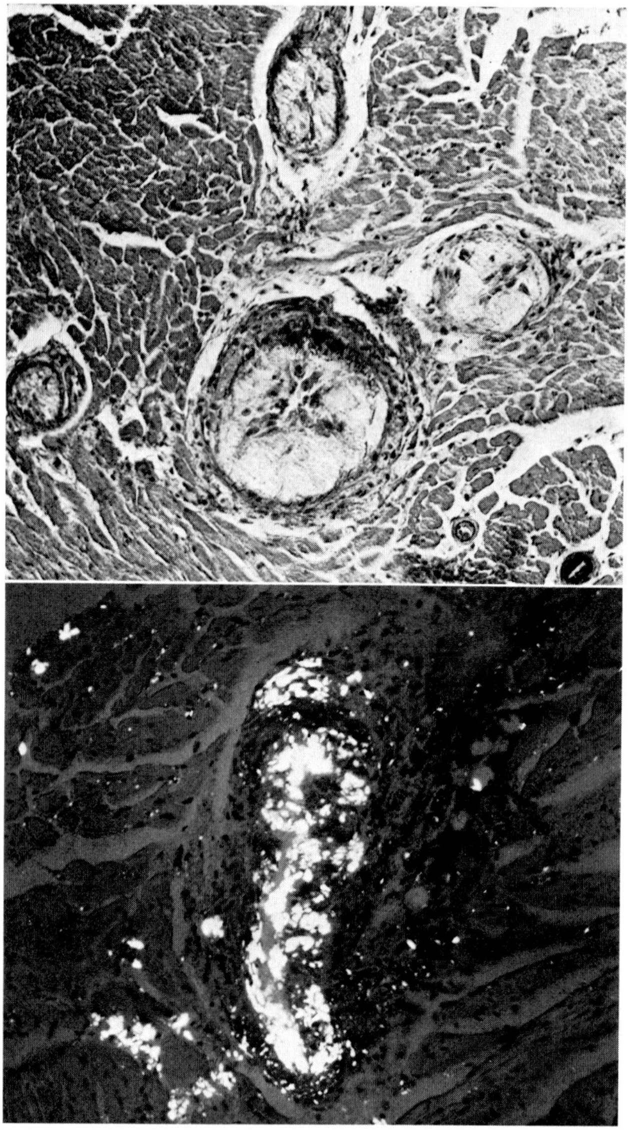

Fig. 2. Severe coronary atherosclerosis with deposition of lipid-laden macrophages from a rabbit of Group I after 6 weeks of PDC treatment. H and E, polarization; ×250.

DISCUSSION

Dr. Kipshidze: We get much more severe atherosclerosis in our experiments when we give 0.3 g cholesterol for 3 months.

Dr. Parwaresch: I wonder – a greater degree of atherosclerosis than that achieved in these experiments is hardly thinkable, even compared to severe human atherosclerosis. This is a very extreme degree of atherosclerosis. As you see, we had to keep the aortae unfolded by attaching them to the underlying surface by means of needles, otherwise the rolling up of the aortae would not allow visual access to the inner surface. In these preparations none of the aortae is stained, as the lesions are so easily seen. I confess that for some observers the magnification might be too low. In Figure 2 you see severe coronary atherosclerosis which is unambiguous. This also confirms the severity of the aortic lesions, as a selective coronary

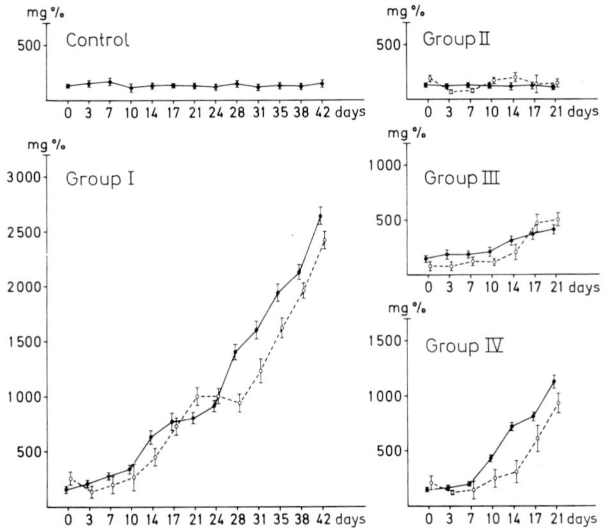

Fig. 3. Serum cholesterol in the 5 experimental groups during the experimental period (——— = placebo, ------ = PDC-treated subgroups).

atherosclerosis is not usual. In Figure 3 the serum cholesterol of pyridinolcarbamate and placebo treated animals in the course of the induced atherosclerosis is matched. There is no significant difference. As a consequence of the massive hyperlipidemia in spite of pyridinolcarbamate treatment you see in Figure 4 a massive accumulation of lipid-laden macrophages in the lymph nodes resembling a lipid storage disease.

In Figure 5 a higher magnification of aortic lesions in a cholesterol fed and pyridinolcarbamate treated animal is shown. This is a most severe atherosclerosis which does not need any staining to render the lesions visible.

Chairman (Dr. Constantinides): Dr. Parwaresch, I think you would strengthen your case if you could show that you studied this difference with a quantitative method. For example, either quantitative planimetry as Dr. Kipshidze did, or the total cholesterol content of the aorta, and express the results statistically. What were the quantitative and statistical methods you used to arrive at your conclusion?

Dr. Parwaresch: I am sorry not to have stressed these details more clearly. Of course, all points stated are strictly based on statistical analysis. As I mentioned, the degree of atherosclerosis was expressed in terms of the percent of aortic surface affected, which is only possible by planimetric measurement. The means of the individual values were then compared by Student's t-test, assuming a normal distribution.

CHAIRMAN: In 5 or 6 weeks most people would be glad to obtain just the very beginning of atherosclerosis – some slight streaks in the ascending aortae, perhaps less than 7, 6 or 5 % of the surface. It might help if you had extracted the cholesterol of the aorta because some people may quarrel with you.

Dr. PARWARESCH: Of course, at the same time all aortae were studied histologically.

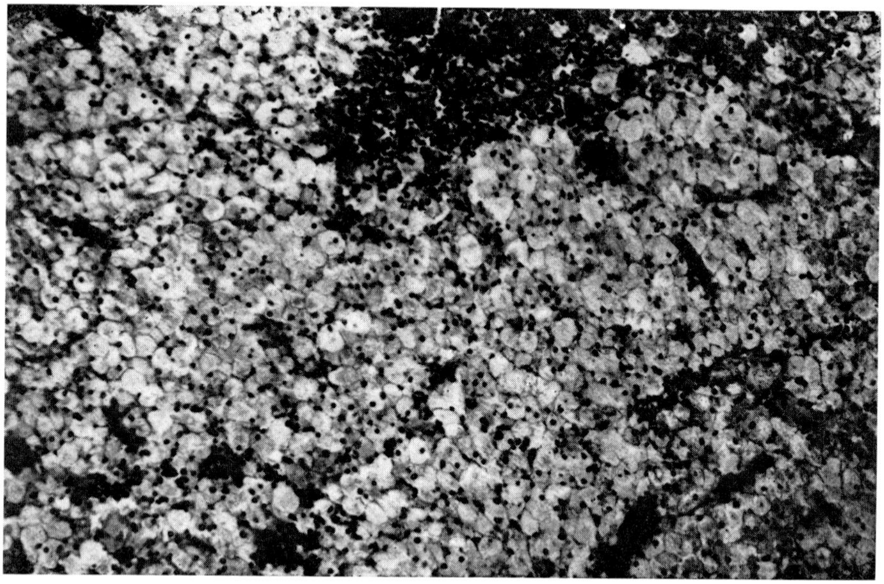

Fig. 4. Accumulation of lipid-laden macrophages in a para-aortic lymph node resembling lipid storage disease (Group I).

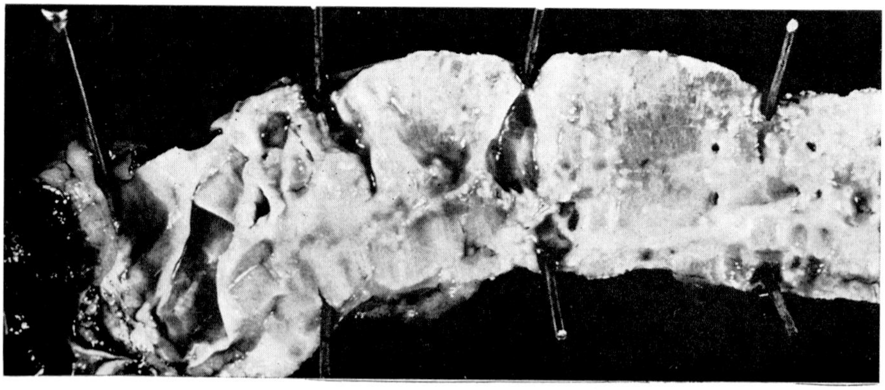

Fig. 5. Photograph of an atherosclerotic aorta after 6 weeks of cholesterol feeding and PDC treatment.

CHAIRMAN: Yes, but this is a qualitative test. If you say that you get 60 % of the area of the aorta occupied by plaques after 5 weeks of cholesterol feeding, then this is very unusual. Most people get less than 10 % in 5 or 6 weeks or even nothing at all.

Dr. PARWARESCH: That is right, but you have also our quantitative planimetric results. The percentage of the aortic surface involved depends on the total dose of cholesterol. This can be regulated by the duration of the experimental period as well as by the daily amount of cholesterol fed. We have been using 3–4 g cholesterol per 100 g diet for 6 weeks. As we heard, Dr. Kipshidze gave 0.3 g per 100 g, which is about the dosage reported in the literature. For the quantitation of arterial lesions it is more exact to evaluate the lesions planimetrically or even to assess them from a gross view than to estimate the mural cholesterol content of the aortae, since the latter does not by any means correlate with the extent and intensity of all arteriosclerotic lesions. Further, in experiments using cholesterol concentrations of less than 2 g per 100 g diet the standard deviations are so high that it is unjustifiable to assume a normal distribution for the samples. This last point especially is very often overlooked in the literature. I think that falsely conceived statistics cause more harm than simple quantitative and perhaps not very exact evaluations.

FURTHER STUDIES ON THE EFFECT OF PYRIDINOLCARBAMATE ON CHOLESTEROL-INDUCED ATHEROSCLEROSIS IN COCKERELS

RUTH PICK

Experimental Atherosclerosis Section, Cardiovascular Institute,
Michael Reese Hospital and Medical Center, Chicago, Ill., U.S.A.

Since the First International Symposium on Atherogenesis, Thrombogenesis and Pyridinolcarbamate Treatment, a large body of work has been carried out with this interesting compound resulting in numerous publications. For reasons still unknown, the results with pyridinolcarbamate or Anginin are still contradictory, not only between laboratories but also within a given laboratory, as our results will demonstrate.

Since the last meeting, we have carried out 2 further experiments in cockerels, giving Anginin in one experiment during the induction of atherosclerosis and in another during the regression period. In the second induction experiment we not only compared but also combined Anginin with natural conjugated equine estrogens (Premarin).

MATERIALS AND METHODS

Young, growing male chicks (cockerels) were used throughout. In the first experiment (designated S102) 2 groups of 20 birds each were used. Both groups were fed on a diet of chick starter mash supplemented with 1% cholesterol and 5% cottonseed oil. Group 1 served as control; Group 2 received Anginin 500 mg/bird/day, 7 days a week orally in a gelatin capsule. The experiment lasted 5 weeks and the birds were 10 weeks of age at the beginning of the experiment. Two additional groups (40 birds) were fed the same cholesterol-supplemented diet for 10 weeks. After 10 weeks the cholesterol-oil supplement was stopped and they were continued on unsupplemented mash for the next 5 weeks.

Twenty of these animals were given Anginin at the same doses and the same schedules as during the induction period. At the end of each experiment the birds were bled for plasma cholesterol and lipid phosphorus determinations. They were then killed, comb index was measured (expressed as the length times height of the comb in centimeters) and the testes were weighed, giving an indication of sexual development. Aorta atherosclerosis was graded grossly by 2 independent observers on a scale of 0 (no lesion) to +4 (most severe involvement) and the mean value for each group was calculated. Coronary atherosclerotic involvement was determined microscopically on 2 standard blocks from each heart and again the mean for a group was calculated.

In a further experiment (designated S109) induction was studied exactly as in Groups 1 and 2 of Series S102. In addition to these 2 groups however, 2 additional groups were added. Group 3 received 7.5 mg Premarin per day in the drinking water and Group 4 Premarin and Anginin as above in combination. At the end of 5 weeks the same procedures were followed as described in experiment S102.

RESULTS

Table I shows the biological effects and thoracic aorta atherogenesis. It can be seen that Anginin-treated birds ate less, gained less weight and showed feminization as determined by the size of the testes and the comb. The p-values are given at the bottom. Thoracic aorta

TABLE I

Biological effects and thoracic aorta atherogenesis of Anginin in cholesterol-fed cockerels (S102)

Group*	Δ Body weight (g)	Food intake (g/bird/day)	Testes weight (g)	Comb index	Thoracic aorta lesions: Incidence	Thoracic aorta lesions: Grade	Plasma cholesterol (mg%)
1. Control	566		4.72	62.1	20/20	1.28	1506
	±24**	67	±0.70	±3.7	100%	±0.07	±92
2. Anginin	134		1.55	34.7	18/18	1.15	864
	±31	46	±0.62	±6.2	100%	±0.11	±70
p-values							
	<0.001	–	<0.005	<0.001	–	NS	<0.001

* Both groups on 1% cholesterol, 5% cottonseed oil, low protein diet.
** Standard error of the mean.
NS = not significant

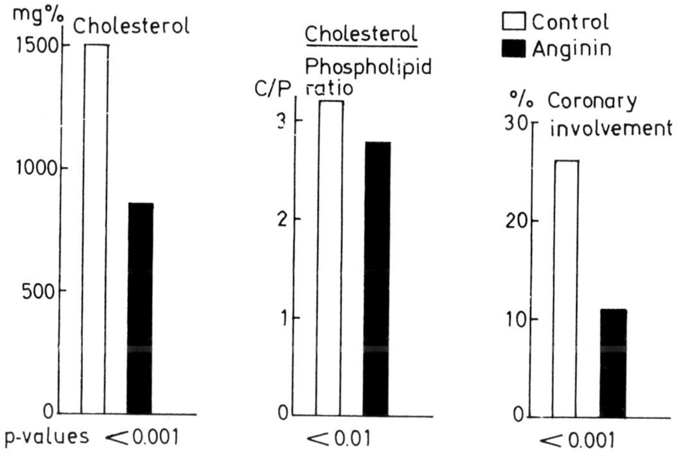

Fig. 1. Effects of Anginin in cholesterol-fed cockerels (S102).

atherosclerosis was slightly lower in the Anginin-treated birds, but the difference was not statistically significant. Plasma cholesterol was statistically significantly lower in the Anginin-treated birds than in the controls.

In Figure 1 the cholesterol values are once more presented. The cholesterol/phospholipid ratio is also significantly lower than in the controls, and a highly significant decrease in coronary atherosclerotic involvement can be seen.

Table II shows that, during the regression period, Anginin had no beneficial effect in accelerating regression of coronary lesions over the regression occurring due to the withdrawal of the cholesterol supplement.

In this experiment we also tested, on paraffin sections of coronary, thoracic and abdominal aorta stained with hematoxylin and eosin and resorcin fuchsin for elastic fibers, the occurrence of fibrosis and calcification, in the control as compared with Anginin-treated regression

TABLE II

Effect of Anginin on regression of lesions (S102)

Group	Plasma cholesterol (mg %)	Thoracic aorta lesions		Coronary lesions	
		Incidence	Grade	Incidence	Grade
1. Control*	1506	20/20	1.28	20/20	26.2
1 CO 5 weeks	±92**	100%	±0.07	100%	±2.0
2. →RM control	188	18/18	1.49	18/19	15.7
(10 weeks)	±14	100%	±0.21	95%	±2.1
3. →RM + Anginin	251	19/19	1.21	20/20	19.5
(10 weeks)	±41	100%	±0.12	100%	±2.1
		p-values			
1 vs 2	<0.001	–	NS	–	<0.005
1 vs 3	<0.001	–	NS	–	<0.05

* 1 CO = 1% cholesterol, 5% cottonseed oil, low protein diet.
** Standard error of the mean.
NS = not significant. RM = regular mash.

TABLE III

Effects on secondary changes during regression — regular mash (RM) and regular mash + Anginin

S102	Fibrosis (≧ 2 +)			Calcium		
	Coronary	Thoracic	Abdominal	Coronary	Thoracic	Abdominal
	5/19	11/19	9/19	6/19	2/19	1/19
→RM control*	26 %	58 %	47%	32 %	11 %	5 %
	4/20	8/20	7/20	6/20	0/20	1/20
→RM + Anginin**	20 %	40 %	35 %	30 %	0 %	5 %

* 1 CO = 1 % cholesterol, 5 % cottonseed oil 10 weeks, regular mash 5 weeks.
** To regular mash + Anginin 500 mg.

animals. The results are shown in Table III. It can be seen that there was no difference between the control and the Anginin-treated groups. Anginin neither accelerated nor prevented the occurrence of fibrosis or calcification in these lesions.

Table IV gives the effect on biological parameters and thoracic aorta atherogenesis of cholesterol-fed cockerels in Premarin, Anginin and Premarin + Anginin treated birds. In this series of birds weight gain was not different in any of the groups, neither was food intake. Both Premarin and Premarin + Anginin significantly decreased testis weights and comb indices, while Anginin alone in this group of birds had no effect on these 2 parameters. Thoracic aorta atherosclerosis was, as usual, higher in Premarin-treated animals and as high in Premarin + Anginin treated animals, while Anginin and control animals were similar.

Figure 2 shows the effects of these combinations on cholesterol/phospholipid ratio and on coronary atherosclerosis. The values for cholesterol have already been described. The cholesterol/phospholipid ratio showed a typical estrogen effect in the Premarin group and in the Anginin + Premarin group. Premarin as usual significantly protected the cockerels against coronary involvement. However, in experiment S109, Anginin did not protect the coronaries

TABLE IV

Biological effects and thoracic aorta atherogenesis of Premarin and Anginin in cholesterol-fed cockerels (S109)

Group	Δ Body weight (g)	Food intake (g/chick/day)	Testes weight (g)	Comb index	Thoracic aorta lesions Incidence	Thoracic aorta lesions Grade	Plasma cholesterol (mg%)
1. Control	530		5.67	78.6	18/19	1.14	1215
1 CO	±23	99	±0.76	±2.4	95 %	±0.12	±109
2. Premarin	606		1.09	23.8	19/19	2.07	901
1 CO	±26	107	±0.54	±2.7	100 %	±0.20	±52
3. Anginin	490		4.20	70.1	19/20	1.04	1470
1 CO	±23	98	±0.61	±4.2	95 %	±0.14	±114
4. Anginin +	548		0.86	0.86	20/20	2.12	1418
Premarin	±24	105	±0.28	±0.28	100 %	±0.18	±115
1 CO							
			p-values				
1 vs 2	NS	–	< 0.001	< 0.001	–	< 0.001	< 0.02
1 vs 3	NS	–	NS	NS	–	NS	NS
1 vs 4	NS	–	< 0.001	< 0.001	–	< 0.001	NS

NS = not significant.

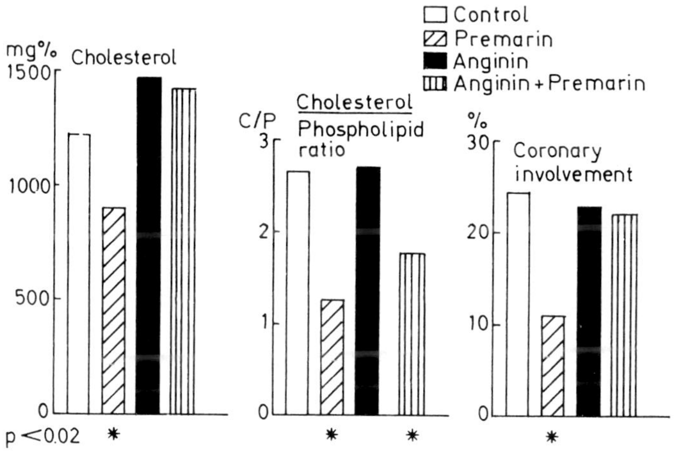

Fig. 2. Effects of Anginin and Premarin in cholesterol-fed cockerels (S109). The asterisks denote statistical significance.

against cholesterol-induced atherogenesis and, surprisingly, it prevented the Premarin effect on coronary atherosclerosis. A summary of the 2 different experiments, a routine usually followed in our laboratory in handling data, is given in Figure 3. The Anginin groups of the positive and the negative experiment combined still show a significant difference between the controls and the Anginin-treated animals in the involvement with coronary atherosclerosis.

Figure 4 shows the lipid pattern on paper electrophoresis. It can be seen that in the Premarin and in the Anginin groups there is a similar pattern, different from the controls, in that there

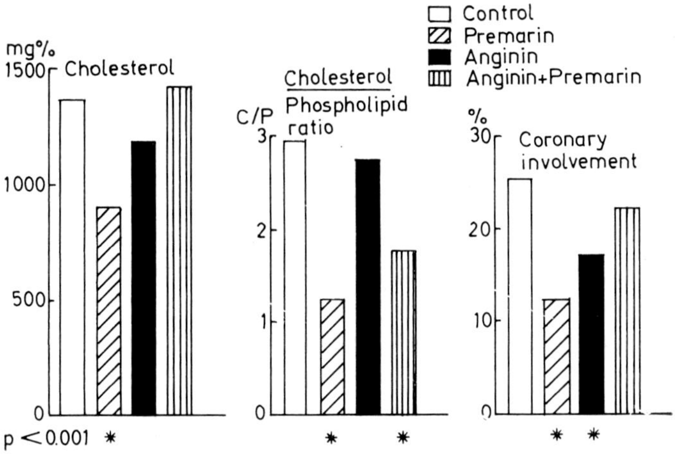

Fig. 3. Effects of Anginin and Premarin in cholesterol-fed cockerels (S102 + S109). The asterisks denote statistical significance.

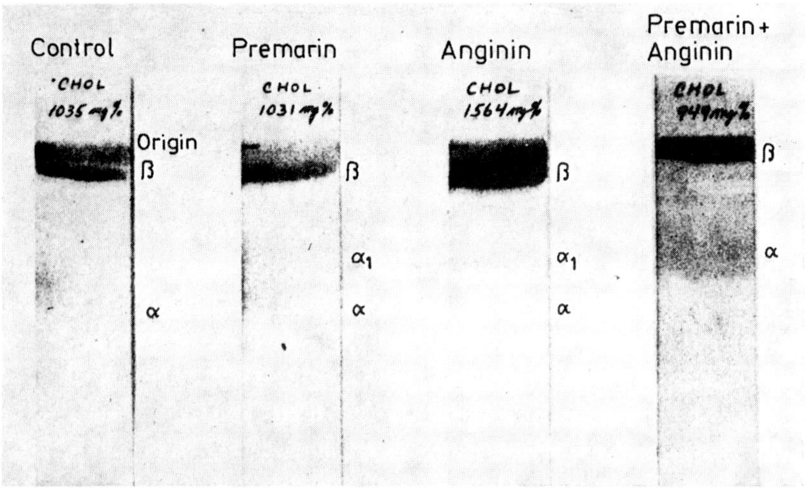

Fig. 4. Paper electrophoresis showing lipid pattern.

are 2 α-peaks. When Premarin and Anginin were combined (the last strip) the pattern resembles the controls; the 2 α-peaks are not visible. The meaning of this finding is not understood at present.

DISCUSSION AND CONCLUSION

Anginin protects cockerels against cholesterol-induced thoracic and coronary atherosclerosis. The effects are not consistent between experiments, which is not unusual in experiments of this type and this species. This type of finding has happened previously with dietary as well as hormonal regimens. Despite our long experience with this species, we do not know why there is a difference, nor can we predict which group of chicks will react in which way. However, Anginin has given consistently negative results as an accelerating factor during regression of lesions. The counteraction of the protective effect of estrogens on coronary atherosclerosis without counteracting the lipid effects or the feminizing effects of Premarin has come as a surprise and warrants intensive further studies including combination with other hormones such as testosterone and adrenal hormones. Furthermore, the question that remains unanswered at the moment is whether in a group of birds, reacting to Anginin with a significant protection of coronary atherosclerosis, the results would be the same as shown here.

In summary, Anginin is of value in the protection of coronary atherosclerosis in cholesterol-fed cockerels. Anginin does not accelerate regression of lesions. Anginin counteracted estrogen-induced protection of coronary arteries against diet-induced atherosclerosis without preventing the effect of estrogens on serum lipids and on feminization of secondary sex characteristics. This latter experiment has been carried out so far in only one experiment and these findings have to be confirmed by further studies. We have no explanation for these surprising results and I hope to get some indication of what you think about them.

ACKNOWLEDGEMENTS

I wish to thank Professor Shimamoto and Dr. Numano for making available, through Banyu Pharmaceutical Co., Tokyo, an ample supply of Anginin for our experiments.

THE SEARCH FOR ANTIATHEROSCLEROTIC AGENTS

Histological and Biochemical Analysis of the Preventive Effect of Estrogen, Progesterone and Pyridinolcarbamate on Experimentally Induced Atherosclerosis

FUJIO NUMANO, MIKIO TAKENOBU, ATSUSHI SAGARA, MASAHIKO KOBAYASHI, KINYA MORIYA, TOMOE KUROIWA, SHOKO YAMAZAWA, TAKIO SHIMAMOTO, HIROYOSHI HIDAKA[1] and KIKUO MOHRI[2]

Institute for Cardiovascular Diseases, Tokyo Ika-Shika National University, Tokyo, [1]Department of Biochemistry, Nagoya University, Nagoya and [2]Department of Surgery, Kansai Medical College, Kansai, Japan

INTRODUCTION

Pyridinolcarbamate, which was synthetized in 1962 by Shimamoto and Ishikawa, was found to be a substance capable of inhibiting the acute vascular injury of the arterial wall induced by chemical stresses such as cholesterol, epinephrine, and saturated fatty acid and by traumatic stress (Shimamoto, 1963, 1969*a*). It has been reported to inhibit experimental atherosclerosis by us (Shimamoto et al., 1966), Pick (1969), De Oliveira (1969) and other reseachers (Noda, 1966; Perrin and Loire, 1969; Wu et al., 1969). Nowadays it has been used successfully in the treatment of many patients suffering from atherosclerotic disorders (De Soldati et al., 1969; Heisig et al., 1970; Kanaya and Horie, 1969; Shimamoto et al., 1970). Parallel to these experimental and clinical studies, many studies have been undertaken to seach for its mode of action from the pharmacological, biochemical, physiological and histochemical points of view.

On the other hand, it has been well known for a long time that women live longer than men and since 1951, when Pick et al. first described the preventive effect of estrogen on cholesterol-induced atherosclerosis, the mechanism of its effect has been studied from all angles. Estrogen also exerts a preventive effect on acute vascular response as does pyridinolcarbamate, but recently we observed in a histoenzymatic study that both substances showed a different effect on enzyme activities in the aortic wall (Numano et al., 1971*a*, *b*, 1972*a*).

The present study deals with the comparative histological, histoenzymatic and biochemical analyses of the enzyme activities in the aortic wall of rabbits treated with pyridinolcarbamate, estrogen and progesterone, the last of which was used to compare its antiatherosclerotic effect with estrogen and also to study the combined effect of both hormones. At the same time, the catecholamines in the arterial wall were measured in this series of experiments both biochemically and histochemically, the results of which are presented in the papers by Hidaka and Mohri (*This Volume*, pp. 145–146, 147–151).

MATERIALS AND METHODS

Fifty-five male albino rabbits were selected for this study. The rabbits were all 5 or 6 months old and came from the same strain. They were born and bred together on our farm: 50 rabbits were divided equally into 5 groups. Each of them was treated every morning with 10 mg/kg of pyridinolcarbamate (Banyu Co.) (PDC), 1 mg/kg of diethylstilbestrol (Mann Research Laboratories) (EST), 1 mg/kg of chlormadinone acetate (Shionogi Co.) (PGT), 1 mg/kg of EST and 1 mg/kg of PGT (EST + PGT) alternate weekly, or potato starch as a placebo together with 150 g/day of commercial diet (Oriental Ltd., RC-5) mixed with 1% of cholesterol (l'Industrie Biologique Française) (Numano et al., 1971*a*; Shimamoto et al.,

1966). Five rabbits were simultaneously given 150 g/day of commercial diet as a normal group. During the experiment, the food consumption of each rabbit was measured every day, body weight every week and serum cholesterol level every 2 weeks by the method of Zak as modified by Henry. After the completion of a 15 week regimen, they were all sacrificed and geographical, pathological, histological, histoenzymatic and microbiochemical analyses were performed on the aortae of each group.

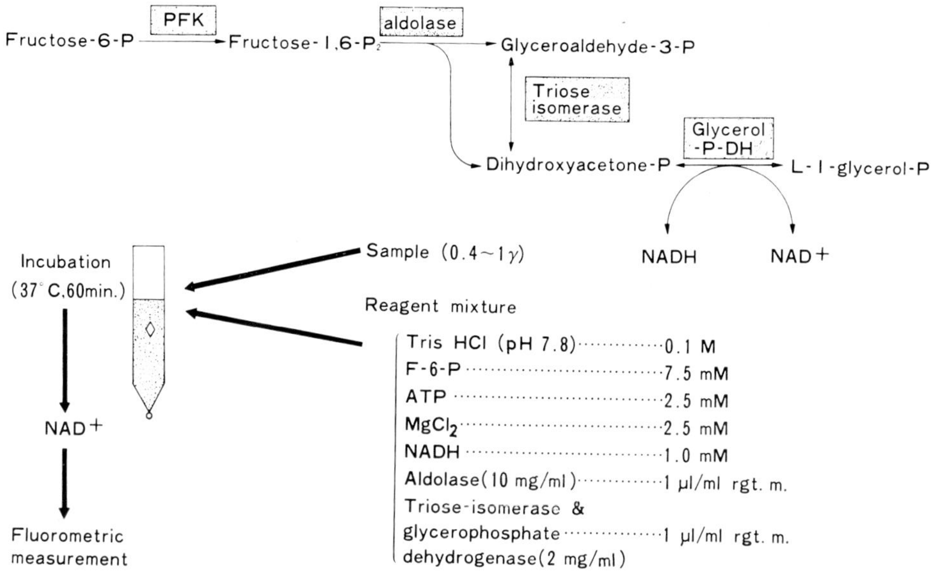

Fig. 1. Microbiochemical assay of phosphofructokinase (PFK) activity.

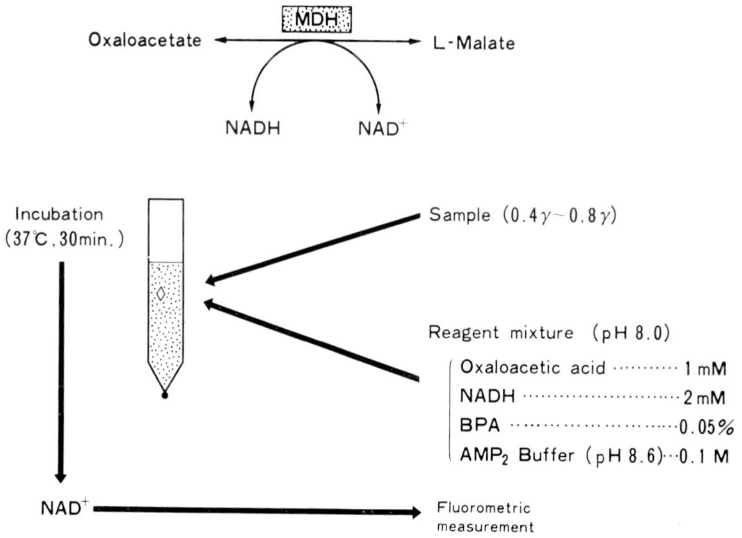

Fig. 2. Microbiochemical assay of malic dehydrogenose (MDH) activity.

Percent surface area involved by atheromatous lesions was calculated in thoracic aorta stained with Sudan IV (Shimamoto et al., 1966). Glycolytic and hydrolytic enzyme activities in the aortic wall of each treated rabbit were compared histoenzymatically with a 10 μ thick specimen of the aortic arch segment using previously described methods under double-blind conditions (Numano et al., 1971*a*). Phosphofructokinase (PFK) and malic dehydrogenase (MDH) activities were measured by our modification of Lowry's microbiochemical method in the intima, media and atheromatous lesions of the aortae (Numano et al., 1973*a*, *b*). Figures 1 and 2 give a summary of the microbiochemical procedures. The methods of these geographical, histoenzymatic and microbiochemical studies have been precisely described previously (Numano et al., 1971*a*, *b*, 1973*a*, *b*; Shimamoto et al., 1966).

RESULTS

Analysis of the course of the experiment

In the course of the 15 weeks, 1 rabbit on placebo control, 2 on PDC, 5 on EST, and 3 on EST + PGT died of infectious disease, diarrhea or accidents. In this experiment, the EST treated group exhibited the highest mortality, but it should be noted that the combined EST + PGT treated group exhibited a low mortality. All rabbits treated with progesterone completed the experimental course.

TABLE I

Findings in the experiments

Group	Body weight (kg)		Total food consumption (g)
	Before	15th week	
Placebo control	3.3470 ± 0.1044	3.0000 ± 0.1077	8448.5 ± 754.2
Pyridinolcarbamate (10 mg/kg)	3.3620 ± 0.0959	2.9871 ± 0.0911	9073.1 ± 392.9
Diethylstilbestrol (1 mg/day)	3.3830 ± 0.1019	3.1340 ± 0.0685	8800.8 ± 344.8
Alternate weekly diethylstilbestrol and chlormadinone	3.3610 ± 0.0806	3.2740 ± 0.0741	9463.2 ± 330.8
Chlormadinone acetate (1 mg/day)	3.2980 ± 0.0774	3.2520 ± 0.0994	8984.2 ± 239.8

Group	Serum cholesterol level (mg/100 ml)		Fatty streak involvement (%)
	Before	15th week	
Placebo control	32.49 ± 1.49	1569.8 ± 145.7	46.1 ± 9.0
Pyridinolcarbamate (10 mg/kg)	32.36 ± 2.37	1416.4 ± 200.7	25.3 ± 4.7*
Diethylstilbestrol (1 mg/day)	29.86 ± 2.36	1789.6 ± 179.3	10.9 ± 3.2*
Alternate weekly diethylstilbestrol and chlormadinone	34.78 ± 4.26	1669.2 ± 216.6	19.9 ± 6.6*
Chlormadinone acetate (1 mg/day)	31.97 ± 2.91	1803.4 ± 194.4	54.6 ± 9.2

* $p < 0.05$

Table I is a summary of body weight, total food consumption and serum cholesterol level before and after treatment in rabbits who completed the entire 15 weeks. Every group exhibited a slight decrease in body weight without any significant difference among them and they also showed almost the same food consumption. Figure 3 shows the level of serum cholesterol. A steady increase in serum cholesterol level was found in all the cholesterol fed groups in the course of the experiment and at 12 weeks the highest cholesterol levels of more than 2000 mg/100 ml were reached. Although a small decrease was observed by the last week, the level in 4 groups remained at more than 1500 mg/100 ml and there was no statistically significant difference between these groups.

Pathological and geographical analysis

Table II summarizes the organ weight of the 5 treated groups fed the cholesterol diet. In this analysis it was found that hepatosplenomegaly occurred in the sex hormone treated groups. The weight of the liver of the PGT treated group and the spleen of all 3 groups exhibited a statistically significant increase over those on placebo control rabbits. However, histological study revealed remarkable differences between EST treated and PGT treated rab-

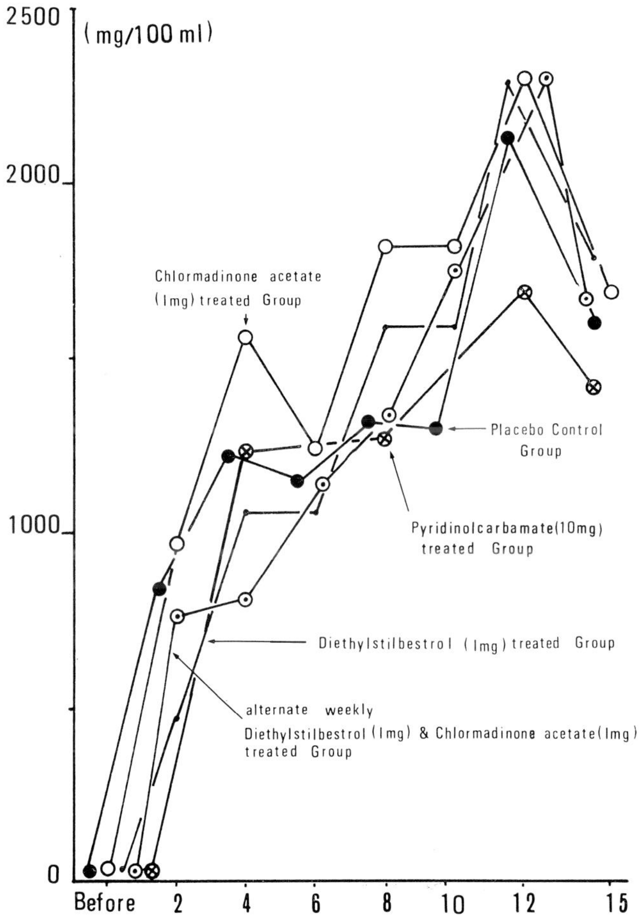

Fig. 3. Serum cholesterol level.

TABLE II

Organ weight

Organ weight (g) \ Group		Placebo control	Estrogen treated	Progesterone treated	Estrogen and progesterone treated	Pyridinol-carbamate treated
Liver		137.3 ± 11.8	166.4 ± 9.0	178.7 ± 11.8*	175.0 ± 12.0	145.4 ± 12.8
Lung		15.4 ± 1.2	14.7 ± 1.1	21.9 ± 3.4	15.2 ± 1.3	14.6 ± 1.5
Heart		9.5 ± 0.2	9.8 ± 0.3	9.3 ± 0.1	9.6 ± 0.2	9.2 ± 0.3
Brain		7.9 ± 0.5	7.8 ± 0.6	7.3 ± 0.5	7.7 ± 0.5	7.5 ± 0.9
Spleen		2.2 ± 0.3	5.9 ± 1.9*	4.3 ± 0.8*	6.0 ± 0.8*	2.4 ± 0.4
Kidney	R	10.1 ± 0.4	10.4 ± 1.0	10.8 ± 1.1	9.1 ± 0.3	9.8 ± 0.6
	L	10.2 ± 0.4	8.7 ± 1.1	11.0 ± 1.1	9.2 ± 0.3	10.1 ± 0.6
Testis	R	5.1 ± 0.3	2.1 ± 0.2*	4.6 ± 0.5	3.5 ± 0.3*	5.2 ± 0.5
	L	4.9 ± 0.4	2.1 ± 0.2*	4.4 ± 0.6	3.4 ± 0.3*	4.7 ± 0.4

* Placebo control vs treated group, $p < 0.05$.

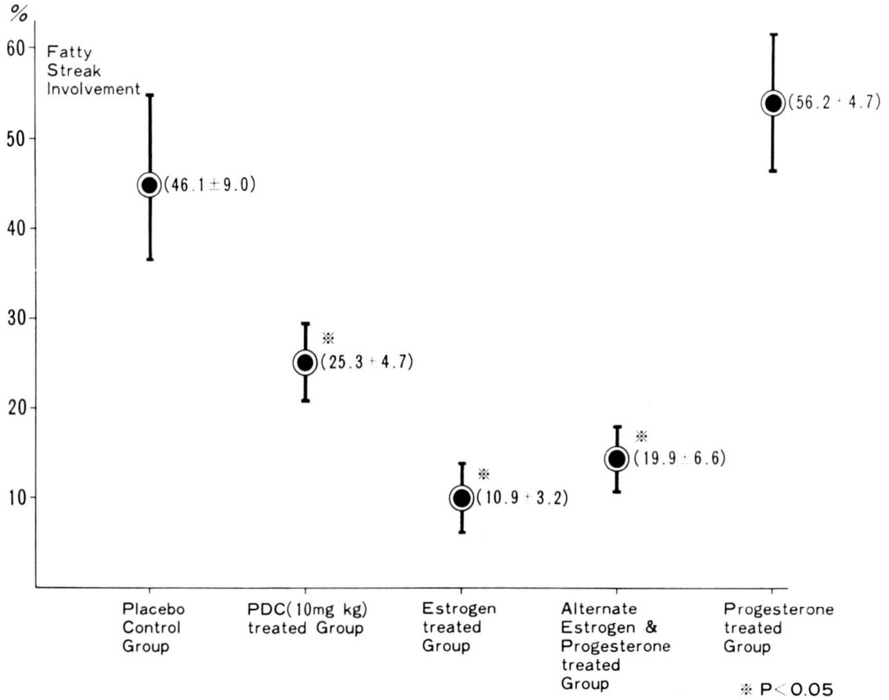

Fig. 4. Fatty streak involvement.

→

Fig. 5. Histological features of atheromatous lesions of rabbit aorta.

a. Placebo control group (H and E stain; × 120). Note: typical accumulation of foam cells with fatty degeneration and calcification.

b. Estrogen treated group (H and E stain; × 210). Note: small atheromatous lesion characterized by fibrosis.

c. Progesterone treated group (H and E stain; × 210). Note: typical foam cells and marked fatty infiltration into media.

d. Cyclic treated group with estrogen and progesterone (H and E stain; × 210). Note fibrosis in center of atheroma.

bits, i.e. fatty liver was characteristic of PGT treated rabbits, whereas the liver of EST treated rabbits exhibited cirrhotic features with large amounts of fibrous tissue invading from Glisson's capsule into the lobuli. Splenomegaly in PGT treated rabbits was also characterized

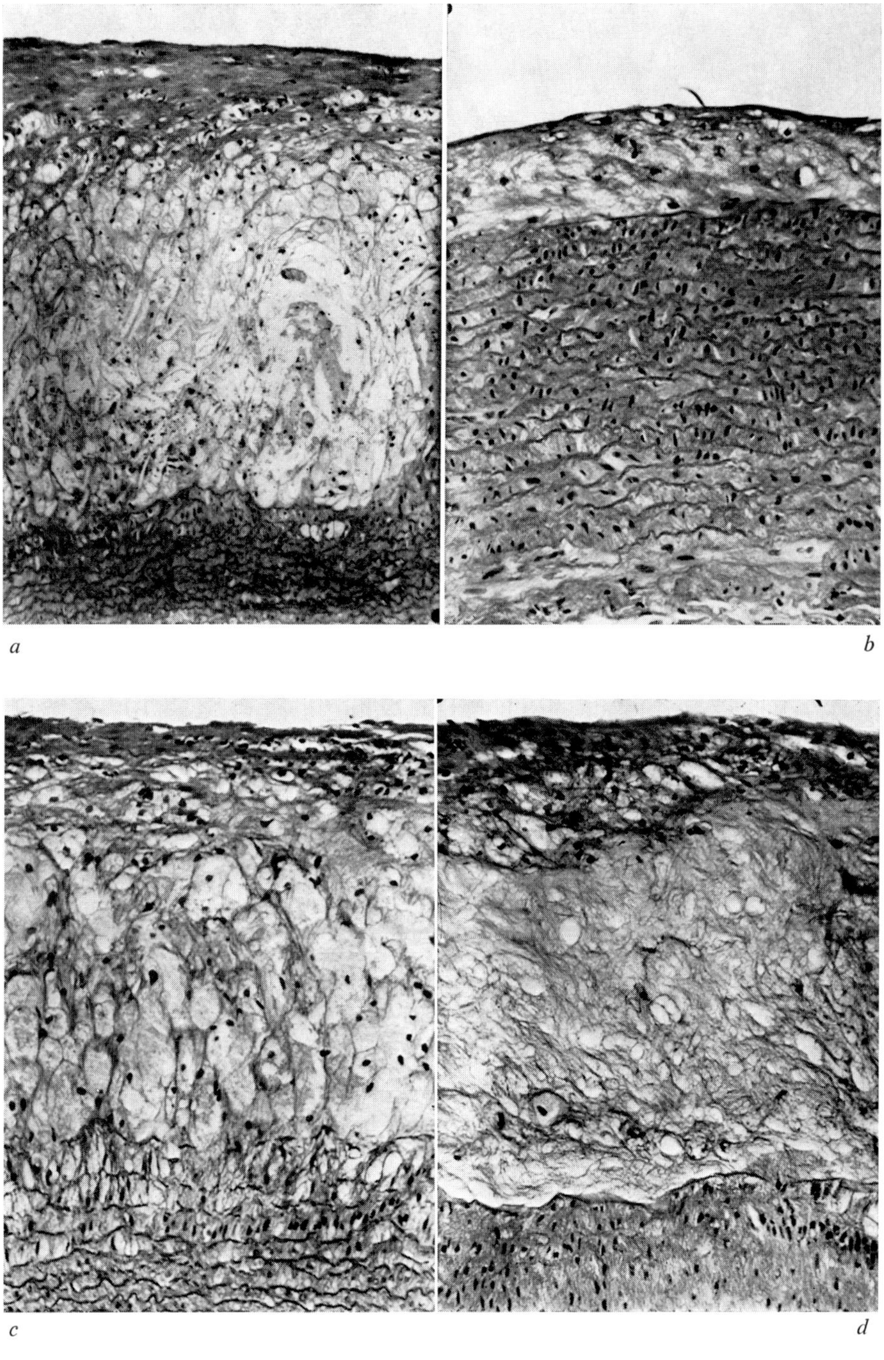

a *b* *c* *d*

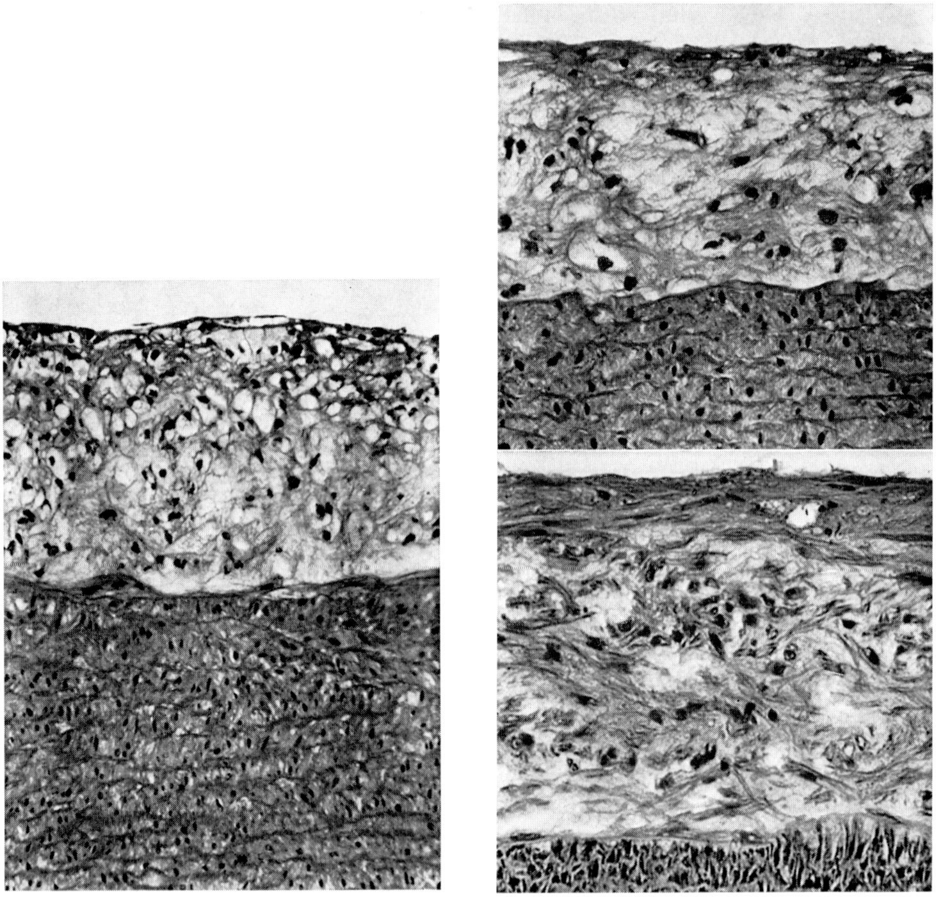

e *f*

Fig. 5. *e.* Cyclic treated group with estrogen and progesterone. Note: fibrosis and small-sized foam cells are missing.
f. Pyridinolcarbamate treated group. Note: atheroma with scanty foam cells and fibrosis (upper) occasionally occupied by many smooth muscle fibers (lower).

by fatty infiltration similar to Niemann-Pick disease, in contrast with EST treated rabbits which were characterized by fibrosis or sinus hyperplasia of Banti's disease (Numano et al., 1969, 1971*c*). Ascites was found in 3 rabbits of the EST treated group. Atrophy of the testes was severe in the EST and EST + PGT treated rabbits.

Gastric xanthomatous polyposis was sometimes encountered in the cardia of stomachs of PGT treated rabbits (Katsu et al., 1972) and typical severe atheromatous changes were also frequently observed in the gastric, coronary and other vessels of PGT treated rabbits.

With continuous cholesterol feeding for 15 weeks, the aortae of rabbits treated with placebo had $46.1 \pm 9.0\,\%$ of their surface covered with fatty streaks. However, in spite of hypercholesterolemia the 3 groups of PDC, EST and combined EST + PGT treated rabbits showed only a small percentage of fatty streak involvement, which was statistically significant compared to the placebo control group. PGT treated rabbits, on the contrary, revealed a higher percentage of fatty streaks than the control group (Fig. 4).

Histological analysis of aorta

Histological observation of aortae and atheromatous lesions revealed the same characteristic features in PDC and EST treated rabbits as previously described (Numano et al., 1971*b*). As shown in Figure 5, placebo control rabbits exhibited typical atheromatous changes characterized by large amounts of foam cells, scanty fibrous and muscle fibers, and fatty infiltration into the medial layer which were accompanied by necrotic foci in the middle portion of atheroma. In contrast to this typical cholesterol-induced atheroma, atheromatous lesions in EST treated rabbits were thin and characterized by fibrous or amorphous changes with almost no foam cells.

On the other hand, PDC treated rabbits exhibited an atheroma rich in smooth muscle and collagen fibers and poor in small-sized foam cells. At the same time, it should be noted that the aorta of EST treated rabbits exhibited very few atheromatous changes and it became so thin that histological diffuse atrophy of smooth muscle cells was observed, sometimes accompanied by necrotic foci or calcification.

PGT treated rabbits exhibited typical atheromatous lesions similar to those of placebo control rabbits. Many large foam cells accumulated in the arterial layers, accompanied by fatty degeneration in the central portions which were covered by a thin, fragile, fibrous cap. Fatty infiltration was observed in the inner and sometimes the middle third of the media in almost all cases. These typical atheromatous changes were frequently encountered in coronary, mesenteric and other arteries, but atrophy of smooth muscles or calcifications or necrotic foci in the media were scarcely encountered in comparison with EST treated rabbits.

In general, atheroma in the aorta of alternate weekly EST and PGT treated rabbits was histologically similar to the atheroma of EST treated rabbits. Fibrous elements were rich, and scanty small foam cells were occasionally found. A few necrotic foci or areas of calcification were seen in both atheromatous lesions and medial layers and, what is more important, the atrophy of smooth muscle was not as marked as in EST treated rabbits.

Histoenzymatic analysis

Table III gives a comparison of the glycolytic enzyme activities in the medial layers of

TABLE III

Comparative histoenzymatic study of the aortic wall of cholesterol fed rabbits treated with estrogen (1 mg/kg), progesterone (1 mg/kg) and pyridinolcarbamate (10 mg/kg)

Group / zyme	Normal	Placebo control	Estrogen treated	Progesterone (1 mg) treated	Alternate weekly estrogen and progesterone	Pyridinol-carbamate (10 mg/kg)
ɔsphorylase	++	+	⇓	~↓	⇓	⇑
xokinase	++	+	~↓	~↑	~↑	⇑
ɪcose-6-phosphate dehydrogenase	+	±	⇓	~	~	⇑
ɔsphofructokinase	++	+~++	~↓	~	~↓	~
:tic dehydrogenase	++	+~++	~↓	~↑	~↓	⇑
:cinic dehydrogenase	++	+~++	~↓	~	~	~
.late dehydrogenase	++	+	~↓	~	~	~↑

+ = marked reaction   ⇑⇓ = marked change
= moderate reaction   ↑↓ = moderate change
= slight reaction   ~ = no change
= no reaction

: enzyme activities in each treated group were compared with those in the placebo control group.

TABLE IV

Comparative histoenzymatic study of the aortic wall of cholesterol fed rabbits treated with estrogen (1 mg/kg), progesterone (1 mg/kg) and pyridinolcarbamate (10 mg/kg)

Group / Enzyme	Normal	Placebo control	Estrogen treated	Progesterone (1 mg) treated	Alternate weekly estrogen and progesterone	Pyridinol-carbamate (10 mg/kg)
Acid phosphatase	±	++	⇓	~	⇓	⇓
Alkaline phosphatase	—	± ~ +	~ ↑	⇑	~	~
β-Glucuronidase	±	+	⇓	~ ↓	⇓	~
ATPase	++	+	⇓	~	~	⇑
5′-Mononucleotidase	++	+	~ ↓	~	~ ↓	~
Esterase	+	++	~ ↓	⇓	~ ↓	~ ↓
Lipase	+	++	~ ↓	⇓	~ ↓	~ ↓

++ = marked reaction ⇑⇓ = marked change
+ = moderate reaction ↑↓ = moderate change
± = slight reaction ~ = no change
— = no reaction

The enzyme activities in each treated group were compared with those in the placebo control group.

aortae in each treated rabbit with those in the placebo control group. The placebo group exhibited decreased activities in almost all glycolytic enzymes compared with normal rabbits fed on the commercial diet.

As has already been described (Numano et al., 1971*b*), EST treated rabbits generally showed a much greater decrease in activity of glycolytic enzymes than placebo control rabbits. Phosphorylase and glucose-6-phosphate dehydrogenase activities decreased strikingly in the former group. In comparison, PGT treated rabbits did not show any striking characteristic change in these enzymes, although a few rabbits had increased activity of hexokinase and lactic dehydrogenose.

On the other hand, the activities of enzymes in PDC treated rabbit aortae were found to be almost the same as in rabbits fed on a normal diet. Combined EST + PGT treated rabbits were observed to have generally the same change in activities as those in EST treated rabbits.

A comparison of hydrolytic enzyme activities of all 4 treated groups exhibited almost the same lowered activity compared to placebo control rabbits (Table IV). The increase in ATPase activity in PDC treated rabbits, the lowering of both lipase and esterase activities, and the increase in alkaline phosphatase activity in PGT treated rabbits were characteristic of their respective groups.

Microbiochemical analysis

Table V shows PFK activity in the intima, media and atheromatous lesions of aortae in each treated group. Placebo control rabbits fed on the cholesterol diet exhibited a statistically significant decrease in activity in both intima and media compared with the normal groups which were fed on commercial diet for the same duration.

On the other hand, the intima of aortae of rabbits which were treated with PDC or EST exhibited almost the same PFK activities as that in the normal diet group. Thus, a statistically significant difference was recognized between these treated groups and placebo control rabbits. On the contrary, in PGT treated rabbits the activity decreased as much as that in placebo control rabbits. Combined EST + PGT treated rabbits also showed decreased activity in the intima.

TABLE V

Microbiochemical analysis of phosphofructokinase activity in the rabbit aorta

Group \ Specimen	Aortic wall: Intima	Aortic wall: Media	Atheromatous lesion
Normal	0.887 ± 0.117	1.572 ± 0.193	—
Placebo control	0.676 ± 0.068*	1.223 ± 0.130*	0.456 ± 0.059
Pyridinolcarbamate treated	0.800 ± 0.078†	1.343 ± 0.152	0.318 ± 0.048
Diethylstilbestrol treated	0.828 ± 0.137†	1.027 ± 0.198*	0.242 ± 0.063†
Chlormadinone acetate treated	0.526 ± 0.137*	1.500 ± 0.145†	0.457 ± 0.070
Alternate diethylstilbestrol and chlormadinone treated	0.64 ± 0.09	1.15 ± 0.15†	0.33 ± 0.05

* Normal vs treated group, $p < 0.05$.
† Placebo vs treated group, $p < 0.05$.
Enzyme activity is expressed as moles of NAD^+ converted from NADH per kg dry weight tissue per hour.

In the media, however, PGT treated rabbits showed high activity as did the PDC treated rabbits. EST treated and combined EST + PGT treated rabbits showed a statistically significant decrease in PFK activity compared with the normal diet group. The PFK activity in atheromatous lesions was low in EST treated rabbits.

Table VI shows the MDH activity in each group. Activity in placebo control rabbits decreased in the intima and is inclined to increase in the media. In the intima only PDC treated rabbits exhibited an increase in activity greater than that of placebo control rabbits ($p < 0.05$). On the other hand, the activity in the media of both EST treated and PDC treated rabbits increased more than that of the normal diet group.

TABLE VI

Malate dehydrogenase activity in the rabbit aorta

Group \ Specimen	Aortic wall: Intima	Aortic wall: Media	Atheromatous lesion
Normal	13.65 ± 0.62	14.71 ± 0.58	—
Placebo control	11.34 ± 0.73*	15.65 ± 0.49	12.27 ± 0.92
Pyridinolcarbamate treated	14.17 ± 0.94†	16.76 ± 0.48*	15.29 ± 0.73†
Diethylstilbestrol treated	12.52 ± 0.60	17.00 ± 0.58*	10.63 ± 1.88
Chlormadinone treated	13.69 ± 1.50	15.65 ± 0.74	16.58 ± 2.80
Alternate diethylstilbestrol and chlormadinone acetate treated	14.72 ± 1.26	16.2 ± 2.00	16.5 ± 2.6

* Normal vs treated group, $p < 0.05$.
† Placebo control vs treated group, $p < 0.05$.
Enzyme activity is expressed as moles of NAD^+ converted from NADH per kg of dry weight tissue per hour.

DISCUSSION

At the First International Symposium on Atherogenesis held in 1969 (Shimamoto and Numano, 1969) vascular permeability became the main topic in relation to atherogenesis. The anti-atherosclerotic effect of estrogen and pyridinolcarbamate was much discussed from the point of view of the permeability-inhibiting effect. In fact, both estrogen and pyridinolcarbamate are well known for their ability to inhibit acute vascular response and pharmacological studies and microcirculatory observation have revealed their inhibiting effect against the permeability-increasing phenomenon induced by various stresses and inflammatory substances (Ishikawa et al., 1969; Shimamoto, 1968; Spector and Willoughby, 1968). At the same time, Shimamoto (1969*b*) demonstrated the infiltration of serous substances across the endothelial lining and into the arterial wall under the scanning and electron microscope using peroxidase and afterwards by the immunofluorescence method, using anti-γ-globulin and anti-β-lipoprotein (Shimamoto et al., 1972). He also showed that pyridinolcarbamate protects the arterial wall from this plasma infiltration through the endothelium.

Our comparative histoenzymatic study revealed the different activities of enzymes, especially the glycolytic enzymes, in the aortic wall of rabbits treated with estrogen or pyridinolcarbamate while being fed on a cholesterol diet, which suggested to us a different approach in studying the common pharmacological characteristics of the permeability-inhibiting effect on the arterial wall. However, before pursuing this possibility, we must clarify the effect of these substances on the metabolism of endothelial cells, because the histoenzymatic comparison was performed on the activities of enzymes in the vessel wall and not in the endothelial cells. Recently the metabolism and function of endothelial cells have been highlighted in relation to vascular permeability and atherosclerosis and many papers on these problems have been published (Adams, 1967; Hess and Stäubli, 1963; Shimamoto, 1968, 1969*b*; Sandler and Bourne, 1963). Most of these studies were performed from the histoenzymatic point of view and very few with biochemical analysis (Adams et al., 1969; Chobanian, 1963; Smith, 1965) due to the anatomical difficulty of studying endothelial cells biochemically.

Our microbiochemical analysis performed in this study showed that both estrogen and PDC increased the activity of PFK in the aortic intima in contrast to the decreasing effect of estrogen on PFK in the media. This agreed with our histoenzymatic findings. MDH activity also showed the same effect of both substances in the intima. These findings suggest that further analysis of the metabolic effect of these substances on endothelial cells should be carried out separately from smooth muscles in the media. Chobanian (1963) has already reported that estrogen has an effect in increasing protein and RNA metabolism in the intima and several tissue culture studies or in vivo studies showed rather active metabolism in endothelial cells (Koide and Pollak, 1963; Wright, 1972). In fact, our microbiochemical analysis on glycolytic and TCA cycle enzyme activities in the intima and media of the pig aorta showed rather high enzyme activities in the intima and suggested a different metabolic pattern in the glycolytic pathway between the intima and media (Numano, unpublished data).

These findings permit us to speculate again on the possibility of a common effect of estrogen and PDC on the vascular permeability-inhibiting effect and further research will follow centering on the function and metabolism of endothelial cells. In contrast to the common effect on endothelial cells, the different characteristic effect of estrogen and PDC on the metabolism of smooth muscle cells should be noticed. This may produce the different histological features of atheromatous lesions and sometimes may induce atrophy, necrosis and calcification in the media of estrogen treated rabbits.

In these experiments another female sex hormone, progesterone, was studied to compare its effect on the vessel wall with that of estrogen. In our previous studies progesterone exhibited neither an acute vascular response-inhibiting effect nor any anti-inflammatory activity and the present experiment showed no preventive effect on cholesterol induced atherosclerosis (Shimamoto, 1963, 1969*a*). Histologically, the atheromatous lesion exhibited an accumulation of larger amounts of foam cells and the fatty infiltration in the medial layer was sometimes more severe than in the placebo control rabbits. This histological characteristic was also recognized in other organs. Liver and spleen of rabbits treated with progesterone, which has phagocytic activity, showed a statistically significant increase in weight and the histological features revealed fatty change similar to Niemann-Pick disease. Galletti and Klopper (1964) reported that progesterone treatment led to the accumulation of fat in tissue which could produce a typical fat-accumulated atherosclerosis in the vessel wall. In fact, xanthomatous polyposis was also observed in the stomachs of rabbits treated with progesterone. In connection with this phenomenon, it is interesting that the activity of esterase and lipase in the vessel wall is decreased in progesterone treated rabbits.

Recently, Wolinsky (1972) reported a comparative study on the effect of both hormones on the aorta of hypertensive rats. He found that estrogen has a distinctly inhibitory effect and progesterone a slightly stimulatory effect on the aortic wall response to hypertension. Danforth (1964), observing histological changes of the arterial wall in pregnancy, reported that gestational changes appear to occur in smooth muscle which is increased in amount, and in reticulin which is lacy and greatly fragmented. Kang-Jey (1970) studied the changes in connective tissue metabolism in the aortic wall of rabbits treated with alternate weekly cyclic treatment of estrogen and progesterone but he did not get any characteristic results.

Our cyclic treated rabbits exhibited generally the same characteristic features as estrogen treated rabbits, which may suggest difficulties in dose combination. However, the biochemical analysis and histological findings allow us to suppose that progesterone protects the vessel wall from damage induced by estrogen, which increases the usefulness of combined sex hormones as antiatherosclerotic agents. The comparison of PDC and combined sex hormones will become one new aspect of further study.

SUMMARY

Comparative histological, histoenzymatic and microbiochemical studies on the antiatherosclerotic effect of pyridinolcarbamate (PDC) (10 mg/kg), estrogen (EST) (diethylstilbestrol 1 mg/day), progesterone (PGT) (chlormadinone acetate 1 mg/day) and combined estrogen and progesterone (EST + PGT) were performed on the aortae of rabbits which had been fed on a cholesterol diet for 15 weeks.

Three groups of PDC, EST and combined EST + PGT treated rabbits showed a statistically significant lower percentage of surface area of aorta involved by fatty streaks. The PGT group showed as great an area of fatty streaks as the placebo control rabbits and histologically the atheromatous lesion of rabbits treated with PGT showed typical fat-accumulated atherosclerosis.

Histoenzymatically, PDC treated rabbits showed increased activity of glycolytic enzymes in the aortic wall in contrast to decreased activity in EST treated rabbits. On the other hand, microbiochemical analysis of phosphofructokinase (PFK) and malic dehydrogenase (MDH) activities revealed statistically increased activities in the intima of both PDC and EST treated rabbits, compared with those in placebo control rabbits. In aortic media, PFK activity increased in the PDC and decreased in the EST treated group and MDH increased in both groups. The permeability-inhibitory effect on the intima was discussed as a common effect of both antiatherosclerotic agents.

PGT did not have any preventive effect on cholesterol induced atherosclerosis and histologically was characterized by lipoidosis in the tissues. However, combined cyclic treatment of EST and PGT also prevented the appearance of fatty streaks in the aortic wall and protected smooth muscles in the medial layers from atrophy or necrosis which would be induced by treatment with EST alone. These findings suggest a beneficial effect of the combined cyclic treatment which should be compared with the antiatherosclerotic effect of PDC.

REFERENCES

ADAMS, C. W. M. (1967): *Vascular Histochemistry*. Lloyd-Luke Ltd., London.

ADAMS, C. W. M., BAYLASS, O. B., ABDULLAR, Y. H., MAHLER, F. R. and ROOT, M. A. (1969): Lipase, esterase and triglyceride in the ageing human aorta. *J. Atheroscler. Res.*, *9*, 87.

CHOBANIAN, A. V. (1963): Effects of sex hormones on phospholipid RNA, and protein metabolism in the arterial intima. *J. Atheroscler. Res. 8*, 763.

DANFORTH, D. F. (1964): The effect of pregnancy and of Enovid on the rabbit vasculature. *Amer. J. Obstet. Gynec.*, *88*, 952.

DE OLIVEIRA, J. M. (1969): The effect of pyridinolcarbamate on experimental arteriosclerosis. In: *Atherogenesis. Proceedings, I International Symposium on Atherogenesis, Thrombogenesis and Pyridinolcarbamate Treatment, Tokyo 1969*, pp. 53–54. Editors: T. Shimamoto and F. Numano. ICS 201, Excerpta Medica, Amsterdam.

DE SOLDATI, L., CASTRO, C. H., GRILLI, H. and REUSSI, J. (1969): Ensayo clínicos con piridinolcarbamato sobre la circulación arterial y la coagulación de la sangre en pacientes con aterosclerosis obliterante. *Pren. med. argent.*, *56*, 12.

GALLETTI, F. and KLOPPER, A. (1964): The effect of progesterone on the quantity and distribution of body fat in the female rat. *Acta. endocrinol. (Kbh.)*, *46*, 379.

HEISIG, N., WESTERMANN, K. W., STOLTERFOHT, C. A. and ZAKI, J. (1970): Die Wirkung von Pyridinolcarbamate bei peripheren arteriellen Durchblutungsstörungen. *Med. Klin.*, *65*, 2289.

HESS, R. and STÄUBLI, W. (1963): The development of aortic lipoidosis in the rat. *Amer. J. Path.*, *18*, 301.

ISHIKAWA, T., HONDA, Y., SAGARA, A. and SHIMAMOTO, T. (1969): The effect of estrogens on bluing lesions by bradykinin and histamine. *Acta endocrinol. (Kbh.) 60*, 177.

KANAYA, H. and HORIE, Y. (1969): Statistical observation of the effects of pyridinolcarbamate on cerebrovascular diseases in Japan. In: *Atherogenesis. Proceedings, I International Symposium on Atherogenesis, Thrombogenesis and Pyridinolcarbamate Treatment, Tokyo 1969*, pp. 229–238. Editors: T. Shimamoto and F. Numano. ICS 201, Excerpta Medica, Amsterdam.

KANG-JEY, HO (1970): Female sex hormones. Effect on aortic acid mucopolysaccharides and atherosclerosis in rabbits. *Arch. Path.*, *90*, 129.

KATSU, K., SHIMAMOTO, T., NUMANO, F., MAEZAWA, S. and SHIMAMOTO, T. (1972): Gastric xanthomatous polyposis in cholesterol fed rabbits induced by progesterone. *Jap. J. Gastroenterol.*, *69*, 559.

KOIDE, R. and POLLAK, O. J. (1963): Cytochemical studies of rabbit aortic cells in tissue culture. *J. Histochem. Cytochem.*, *11*, 265.

NODA, K. (1966): Studies on the treatment and prophylaxis of arteriosclerosis – effect of pyridinolcarbamate on the development of experimental atherosclerosis. *Bull. Inst. constit. Med. Kumamoto Univ.*, *17*, 136.

NUMANO, F.: Unpublished data.

NUMANO, F., KATSU, K., KITTA, T. and SHIMAMOTO, T. (1969): Banti-like syndrome induced by estrogen and cholesterol. *Acta hepato-splenol. (Stuttg.)*, *16*, 77.

NUMANO, F., KATSU, K., TAKENOBU, M., SAGARA, A. and SHIMAMOTO, T. (1971*a*): Comparative studies on the preventive effect of pyridinolcarbamate and estrogen against aortic and coronary atherosclerosis of cholesterol-fed rabbits. I. Topographic and pathological studies. *Acta. path. jap.*, *21*, 177.

NUMANO, F., KATSU, K., TAKENOBU, M., SAGARA, A. and SHIMAMOTO, T. (1971*b*): Comparative studies on the preventive effect of pyridinolcarbamate and estrogen against aortic and coronary atherosclerosis of cholesterol-fed rabbits. II. Histoenzymatic studies. *Acta path. jap.*, *21*, 93.

NUMANO, F., KATSU, K., TAKENOBU, M. and SHIMAMOTO, T. (1971*c*): Increased urinary excretion of total estrogens in Banti's and aortic arch syndrome. *Jap. J. clin. Med.*, *10*, 42.

NUMANO, F., KUROIWA, T., KOBAYASHI, M., YAMAZAWA, S. and SHIMAMOTO, T. (1973*a*): Phosphorylase activity in vessel wall. *Atherosclerosis*, in press.

NUMANO, F., SAGARA, A., TAKENOBU, M., YAMAZAWA, S. and SHIMAMOTO, T. (1973*b*): Microbiochemical analysis of vessel wall. I. Phosphofructokinase. *Atherosclerosis*, in press.

PERRIN, A. and LOIRE, R. (1969): Bilan d'une première expérience clinique et expérimentale avec le pyridinolcarbamate. In: *Atherogenesis. Proceedings, I International Symposium on Atherogenesis,*

Thrombogenesis and Pyridinolcarbamate Treatment, Tokyo 1969, pp. 71–74. Editors: T. Shimamoto and F. Numano. ICS 201, Excerpta Medica, Amsterdam.
PICK, R. (1969): The effect of pyridinolcarbamate on the induction and regression of aortic and coronary atherosclerosis in cholesterol-fed cockerels. In: *Atherogenesis. Proceedings, I International Symposium on Atherogenesis, Thrombogenesis and Pyridinolcarbamate Treatment, Tokyo 1969*, pp. 57–62. Editors: T. Shimamoto and F. Numano. ICS 201, Excerpta Medica, Amsterdam.
PICK, R., STAMLER, J., RODBARD, S. and KATZ, L. N. (1951): The inhibition of coronary atheromas in cholesterol-fed chickens receiving estrogen. *Circulation, 4*, 468.
SANDLER, M. and BOURNE, G. H. (1963): Histochemistry of atherosclerosis. In: *Atherosclerosis and its Origin*, pp. 515. Editors: M. Sandler and G. H. Bourne. Academic Press, New York, N.Y.
SHIMAMOTO, T. (1963): The relationship of edematous arterial reaction in arteries to atherosclerosis and thrombosis. *J. Atheroscler. Res., 3*, 87.
SHIMAMOTO, T. (1968): Microcirculating aspects of atherogenesis, thrombogenesis and antiatherosclerotics. *Amer. Heart J., 76*, 105.
SHIMAMOTO, T. (1969*a*): Experimental study on atherosclerosis – An attempt at its prevention and treatment. *Acta path. jap., 19*, 15.
SHIMAMOTO, T. (1969*b*): An introduction to the investigation of atherogenesis, thrombogenesis and pyridinolcarbamate – Visualization of the transendothelial passage through intercellular junctions and discovery of endothelial folds and intercellular bridges of vascular endothelium. In: *Atherogenesis. Proceedings, I International Symposium on Atherogenesis, Thrombogenesis and Pyridinolcarbamate Treatment, Tokyo 1969*, pp. 5–27. Editors: T. Shimamoto and F. Numano. ICS 201, Excerpta Medica, Amsterdam.
SHIMAMOTO, T., ATSUMI, T., YAMASHITA, S., MOTOMIYA, T., ISOKANE, N., ISHIOKA, T. and SAKUMA, A. (1970): Clinical pharmacologic evaluation of the antiatherosclerotic agent pyridinolcarbamate. A double-blind cross over trial in the treatment of atherosclerosis obliterans. *Amer. Heart J., 79*, 5.
SHIMAMOTO, T., KOBAYASHI, M. and NUMANO, F. (1972): Infiltration of γ-globulin, fibrinogen and β-lipoprotein into blood vessel wall by atherogenic stress visualized by immunofluorescence. *Proc. Jap. Acad., 48*, 336.
SHIMAMOTO, T. and NUMANO, F. (Eds.) (1969): *Atherogenesis. Proceedings, I International Symposium on Atherogenesis, Thrombogenesis and Pyridinolcarbamate Treatment, Tokyo 1969*. ICS 201, Excerpta Medica, Amsterdam.
SHIMAMOTO, T., NUMANO, F. and FUJITA, T. (1966): Atherosclerosis-inhibiting effect of an antibradykinin agent, pyridinolcarbamate. *Amer. Heart J., 71*, 261.
SMITH, E. B. (1965): The influence of age and atherosclerosis on the chemistry of aortic intima. *J. Atheroscler. Res., 5*, 224.
SPECTOR, W. G. and WILLOUGHBY, D. A. (1968): *The Pharmacology of Inflammation*, pp. 111. Engglish University Press, Ltd., London.
WOLINSKY, H. (1972): Effects of estrogen and progesterone treatment on the response of the aorta of male rats to hypertension. *Circulat. Res., 30*, 341.
WRIGHT, H. P. (1972): Mitosis patterns in aortic endothelium. *Atherosclerosis, 15*, 93.
WU, C. C., HUANG, T. S. and HSU, C. J. (1969): Prevention of experimental atherosclerosis with pyridinolcarbamate. *Amer. Heart J., 77*, 657

DISCUSSION

Dr. BERKOWITZ: Dr. Numano, one of the puzzling things, at least to me, from this morning's session is the apparent disappearance of the therapeutic effect as the dose of Anginin is increased. Do any of your enzyme studies suggest that, as the dose of Anginin is increased, there is any alteration in the direction of changes in enzyme activity? That is, is there a biphasic effect on any of the enzyme activities in the blood vessel walls?

Dr. NUMANO: I am sorry, I do not have any data on the relationship between dose and activity of enzymes in arterial walls.

CHAIRMAN (Dr. Pick): Did I understand, Dr. Numano, that you combined pyridinolcarbamate and estrogens, or did you always separate them?

Dr. NUMANO: We have not performed experiments with pyridinolcarbamate and estrogen combined.

CHAIRMAN: I hope you will.

Dr. KRITCHEVSKY: Dr. Numano, what substrates did you use for the lipase and esterase assays? The reason I ask this is because in atherogenesis one of the things that increases in the aortic wall is the cholesterol esters, so you would expect that, if the drug affected the course of the establishment of atherosclerosis, the esterase activity should go up rather than down. But this may be true if the substrates were cholesterol ester rather than just a non-specific ester.

Dr. NUMANO: Thank you for your comment. I used β-naphthol acetate. However, in this study we emphasized studies of glycolytic enzymes. In future I will study such lipolytic enzymes.

METABOLIC EFFECTS OF PYRIDINOLCARBAMATE ON THE VASCULAR WALL OF RATS

OLGA MRHOVÁ, TAKIO SHIMAMOTO and FUJIO NUMANO
Research Centre of Cardiovascular Diseases, Institute of Clinical and Experimental Medicine, Prague, Czechoslovakia, and Institute for Cardiovascular Diseases and Department of Medicine, Tokyo Ika-Shika National University, Tokyo, Japan

Our present knowledge of the enzymes of the vascular wall allows us to conclude that metabolism in the vascular wall is a sensitive indicator of changes which accompany the onset and development of atherosclerosis, and unimpaired metabolism of the vascular wall is one of the important mechanisms which protect the artery against lipid accumulation and atherosclerotic changes.

Table I shows our results obtained from years of study of the enzymes of the vascular wall with the use of numerous models of experimental atherosclerosis and of arterial injury, as well as from investigations on enzyme activities in human arteries and in the arteries of animals which are prone to the development of atherosclerosis. As can be seen, the states which predispose to the onset of this disease are accompanied by a decrease in the activity of some enzymes of the Krebs cycle and of anaerobic glycolysis, together with increased activity of phosphomonoesterases.

Logically, the question follows from these findings whether it might be possible to affect favourably the metabolism of the vascular wall by pharmacological means and thus increase its resistance to the accumulation of lipids and to the development of atherosclerotic changes. Our attention was drawn to pyridinolcarbamate (PDC) which was synthetized by Shimamoto and Ishikawa in 1962, the preventive and therapeutic antiatherosclerotic effects of which have become well known.

MATERIALS AND METHODS

The effect of PDC on the enzymes of the vascular wall of rats kept either on a standard pellet diet, or on a high-fat diet containing 40 % soy oil and 5 % cholesterol was investigated. Rats with experimentally induced hypervitaminosis D were also studied. We measured the activities of lactate dehydrogenase (LDH), malate dehydrogenase (MDH), acid phosphatase (ACP), 5′-mononucleotidase (5′-Nu), adenylpyrophosphatase (APP), carboxylic esterase and β-glucuronidase in the aortic wall. As far as methodology is concerned, I cannot go into great details here. Sufficient to say that the enzyme activities were measured in saline extracts obtained by extraction of the homogenates of intima-media preparations of the aortae. All activities, determined either by classical or by our own methods, were always expressed on the basis of the protein content of each extract. In the figures to be presented, activities were expressed as a percentage for the purpose of easy comparability. Daily administrations of PDC were made into the oesophagus using a needle with a rounded tip which was attached to a syringe.

RESULTS

Table II shows that 8 weeks of PDC administration in daily doses of 30 mg/kg led to an increase in the activity of LDH, MDH and carboxylic esterase in the aorta. We observed this favourable effect of PDC on the same enzymes in rats which were kept on the diet rich in fat

TABLE I

Pattern of results obtained in our laboratory

	Tricarboxylic acid cycle enzymes	Phosphomono-esterases
Activity in human thoracic aortae* compared with pulmonary arteries	↘	↗
Activity in human abdominal aortic segment* compared with ascending aortic segment	↘	↗
Activity in human femoral arteries* compared with brachial arteries	↘	↗
Activity in pig abdominal aortic segment* compared with ascending aortic segment	↘	→
Activity in aortae of rats on Hartroft diet (accumulation of lipids produced in endothelial macrophages, without connective tissue reaction)	↘	↗
Activity in aortae of calciferol-fed rats (connective tissue changes produced)	** ↘	↗
Renal artery clamping in rats compared with normal controls	↘	↗
DOCA + NaCl hypertension in rats compared with non-treated animals	↘	↗

* Arterial segment in which the extent and severity of atherosclerosis is greater.
** Decrease in later stages of calciferol-induced mineralization of aortae.
DOCA = desoxycorticosterone acetate.

and cholesterol. However, PDC showed no effect on the activity of phosphomonoesterases.

Further experiments performed in vitro showed that addition of either 150 or 300 μg PDC per ml of incubation medium increased the activity of aortic LDH and MDH and decreased the activity of 5′-Nu. The activity of the other enzymes studied in vitro, i.e. ACP, APP, carboxylic esterase and β-glucuronidase, was not influenced to any significant extent. It follows from these results that PDC exerted a favourable effect on the metabolism of the vascular wall. We also studied the effect of PDC in rats with experimentally induced hypervitaminosis D, which, according to Gillman (Gillman, 1957, 1958; Gillman et al., 1960), is accompanied by histochemical changes typical of scar tissue and forms an ideal basis for lipid accumulation and for the development of atherosclerotic changes. Our earlier work led to the conclusion that calciferol intoxication is accompanied by an early increase in the activity of phosphomonoesterases and in the latter stages by a decrease in the activity of enzymes participating in the Krebs cycle and anaerobic glycolysis (Zemplényi and Mrhová, 1965). According to Martins de Oliveira (1969) PDC was effective in slowing down the formation of

TABLE II

The effect of pyridinolcarbamate on aortic enzyme activities in rats on either a standard diet or a high-fat diet

	Pyridinolcarbamate	Pyridinolcarbamate + high-fat diet
Adenylpyrophosphatase	→	→
Acid phosphatase	→	→
Carboxylic esterase	↗ $P<0.025$	→
5′-Mononucleotidase	→	→
Adenylpyrophosphatase	→	→
Lactate dehydrogenase	↗ $P<0.005$	↗
Malate dehydrogenase	↗	↗ $P<0.01$
β-Glucuronidase	→	↗

arterial lesions in rats fed a diet to which cholesterol and vitamin D_3 were added. The question arose, therefore, whether the administration of PDC would favourably reverse enzyme changes brought about by calciferol intoxication.

Hypervitaminosis D was induced by the daily administration of 30,000 U vitamin D (Calciferol Spofa forte) for 5 or 9 days. Vitamin D was administered into the oesophagus as before. Half of the vitamin D treated experimental animals were given PDC in the same way at a dose of 25 mg/kg/day for 3 or 9 weeks. The control group of animals was given tap water.

The increase in the activity of aortic ACP and 5′-Nu brought about by calciferol intoxication was not influenced by PDC administration after either 3 or 9 weeks of the experiment

(Fig. 1). Similarly, the activity of adenylpyrophosphatase and of carboxylic esterase was lower in both experimental groups compared with the control group after 3 and 9 weeks (Fig. 2). However, the activity of LDH and MDH was significantly higher after 9 weeks of PDC administration compared with that in the calciferol-intoxicated rats which were not treated with PDC (Fig. 3).

This means that the administration of PDC prevented the decrease in LDH and MDH activities which, as already mentioned, occurs during calciferol intoxication. When studying the LDH isoenzymes in this experimental model of the vascular wall injury, we used both DEAE-Sephadex and paper electrophoresis combined with the nitroblue monotetrazolium chloride (NBMT) reaction and subsequent photometric evaluation of acetone eluates (Mrhová, 1971). We found a higher content of the LDH M-isoenzyme in the aortae of cal-

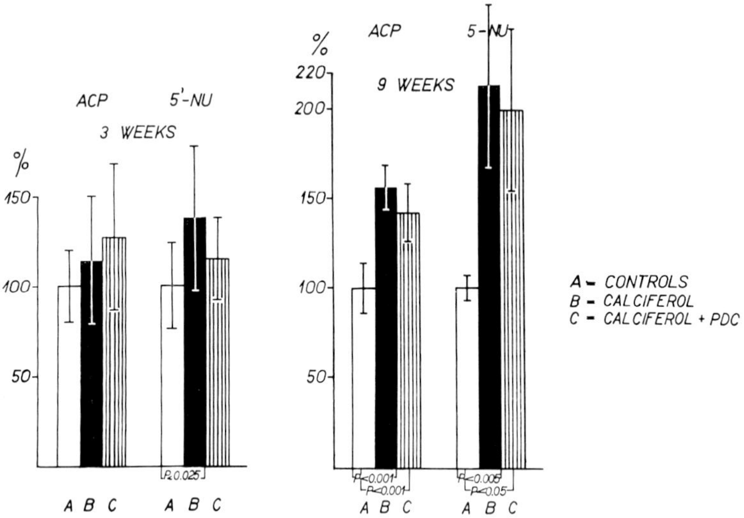

Fig. 1. Activity of acid phosphatase (ACP) and 5′-nucleotidase (5′-Nu) in the aortae of calciferol-intoxicated rats, 3 and 9 weeks after treatment with pyridinolcarbamate (PDC).

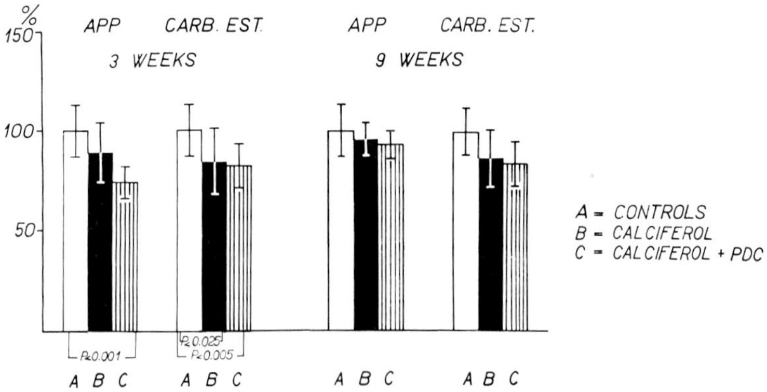

Fig. 2. Activity of adenylpyrophosphatase (APP) and carboxylic esterase (carb. est.) in the same aortae as in Fig. 1.

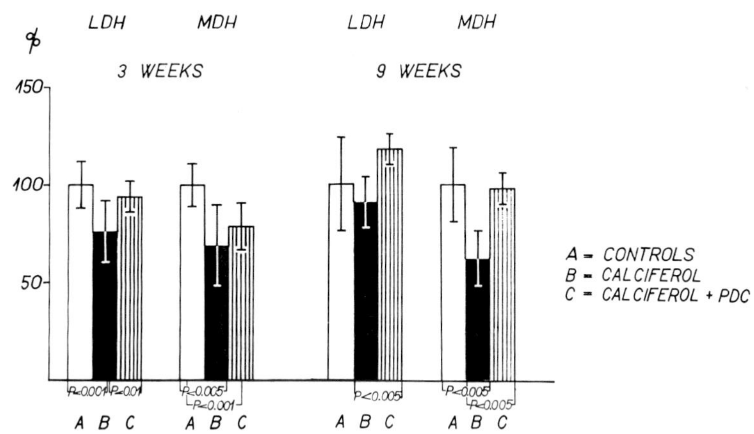

Fig. 3. Activity of lactate dehydrogenase (LDH) and malate dehydrogenase (MDH) in the same aortae as in Fig. 1.

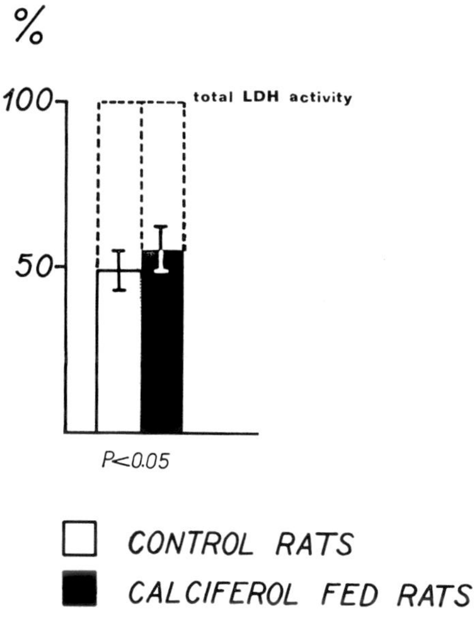

Fig. 4.

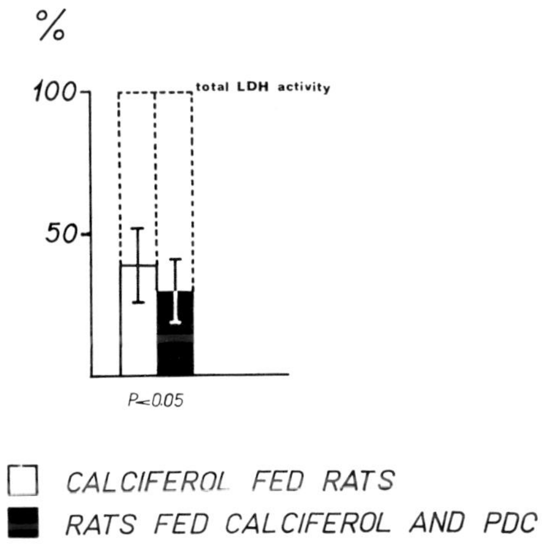

Fig. 5.

Fig. 4. M (anaerobic) fractions of lactate dehydrogenase (LDH) in the aortae of calciferol-intoxicated rats compared with controls.

Fig. 5. M (anaerobic) fractions of lactate dehydrogenase (LDH) in the aortae of calciferol-fed rats and in the aortae of rats fed calciferol and pyridinolcarbamate (PDC).

ciferol-intoxicated rats compared with the controls (Fig. 4). In the other experiment, calciferol-intoxicated rats were compared with rats which had also PDC in addition to vitamin D for 7 weeks. As can be seen from Figure 5, PDC caused a decrease in the M-isoenzyme fraction.

Figure 6 shows the electrophoretic separation of LDH isoenzyme fractions in the aortae of the same rats. PDC brought about a marked increase in the H-fractions of LDH (α_2, α_3)

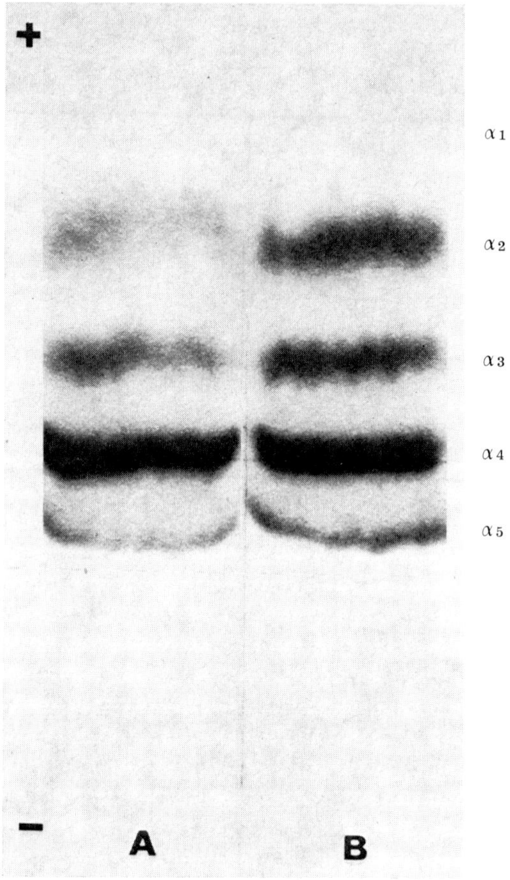

Fig. 6. Electrophoretic separation of lactate dehydrogenase isoenzymes in the aortae of the same animals as in Fig. 5.

A = Calciferol-fed rats.
B = Rats fed calciferol and pyridinolcarbamate.

(Fig. 7). This agrees with the results obtained by the Sephadex technique. The action of PDC on the LDH isoenzyme fraction was also studied in vitro by the addition of 0.5, 1.0, and 1.5 mg PDC per ml to the incubation medium after electrophoretic separation. As is apparent from Figure 8, the concentrations of PDC used activated the anodal H-fractions (α_2, α_3), while in the M-fractions no difference could be detected (Fig. 9).

DISCUSSION

It is known that LDH is a tetrameric molecule made up of 4 subunits of the 2 principal or 'parent' forms of LDH, i.e. of the H (heart) and M (muscle) forms, according to the tissues in which they predominate. According to Dawson et al. (1964) low oxygen tension apparently favours the synthesis of the M-type which is the form assumed to be best suited to anaerobic metabolism. On the other hand, higher oxygen tension appears to favour synthesis of the H-type, the form supposed to predominate in aerobic tissues. If so, the LDH isoenzyme pattern could be used to indicate hypoxia in insufficiently vascularized tissues. This is probably

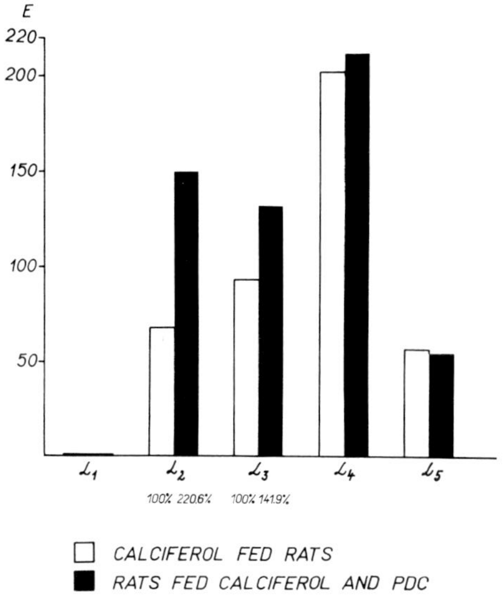

Fig. 7. Quantitative evaluation of fractions shown in Fig. 6. Lactate dehydrogenase isoenzymes in the aortae of rats fed with calciferol, and calciferol with pyridinolcarbamate (PDC).

the case in the aorta damaged by calciferol intoxication, where a higher content of the M-fraction of LDH was found. The activation of the aerobic fractions of LDH by PDC seems to be of major importance, as the effect of PDC in the artery damaged by calciferol prevents overdomination of the M-fraction of LDH which could otherwise lead to a greater dependence of the tissue on less effective anaerobic glycolysis.

Our results, therefore, allow the conclusion that PDC affects the entire metabolism of the vascular wall mainly by influencing the enzymes of the Krebs cycle and of anaerobic glycolysis. This is in good agreement with the histochemical findings of Numano (1971) who detected a higher activity of glycolytic enzymes (including glucose-6-phosphate dehydrogenase) in the vascular wall of rabbits which were kept on a diet containing cholesterol and PDC.

Study of enzymes of the Krebs cycle indicates that probably the most important defence mechanism in the vascular wall is intact oxidative metabolism together with intact production of high-energy phosphate bonds and with unimpaired capacity to synthetize proteins including enzymes. Impairment of this defence might finally cause a complete failure of all other mechanisms protecting the vessel wall against the accumulation of lipids. Considering the influence of PDC on the metabolism of the vascular wall, one could assume that the retardation of the development of arterial lesions in rats with hypervitaminosis D, as observed histologically (Martins de Oliveira, 1969), is at least in part due to the favourable influence of PDC on the metabolism of the vascular wall. However, the activity of phosphomonoesterases, which is already increased on the 4th day of calciferol intoxication, is not affected by PDC. The activity of these enzymes is connected with tissue calcification in a way which has not been completely clarified and its increase may be the result of modified metabolism of the connective tissue in the artery. The early stages of calciferol intoxication are characterized by the production and depolymeration of mucoproteins and by damaged collagen structures. According to Gillman et al. (1960), conditions for later accumulation of lipids are created in this way. Therefore, it may be assumed that PDC plays a role mainly in the later stages of calciferol intoxication, when lipids might already be accumulating, and the activity of the enzymes of the Krebs cycle and of glycolysis decreased.

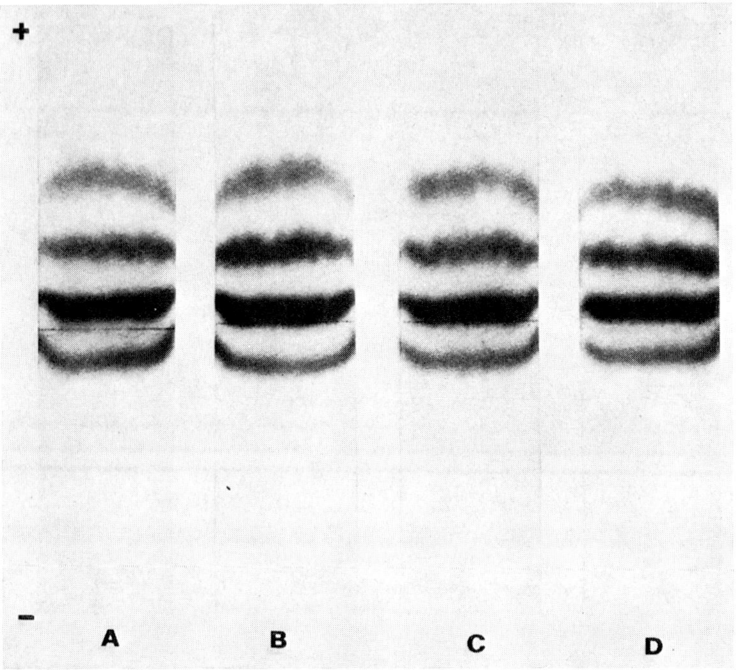

Fig. 8. In vitro effect of pyridinolcarbamate (PDC) on lactate dehydrogenase isoenzymes in the aortae of rats.

A = controls;
B = 1.5 mg PDC per ml;
C = 1.0 mg PDC per ml;
D = 0.5 mg PDC per ml.

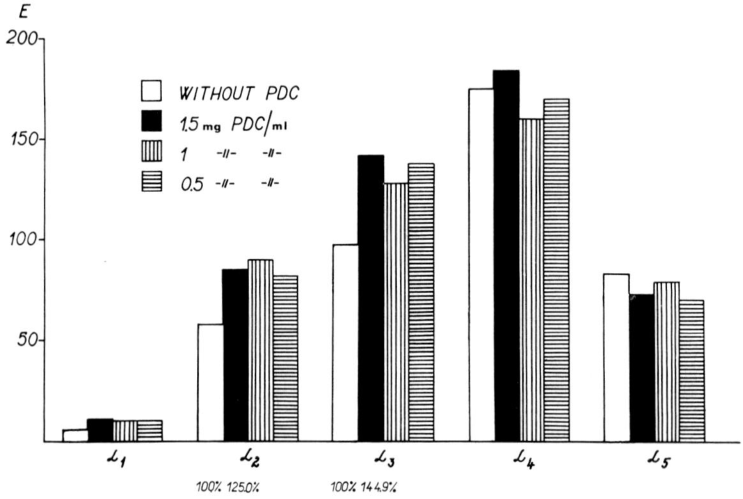

Fig. 9. In vitro effect of pyridinolcarbamate (PDC) on lactate dehydrogenase isoenzymes in the aortae of rats. Quantitative evaluation of fractions shown in Fig. 8.

It is well known that the arterial wall, i.e. the organ of atherosclerosis development, has a special blood supply and exerts specialized functions connected with the transport of blood. The problem of the origin and treatment of atherosclerosis cannot be studied without reference to these facts. Whatever the pathogenesis of atherosclerosis, the participation of the arterial wall in the development of pathological changes is certainly one of the most important factors. Therefore, it is necessary to look for the means by which the metabolic disorders in the vessel wall, accompanying the onset of atherosclerosis, could be prevented or at least limited. Our results indicate that the activity of certain enzymes and thus probably of whole metabolic cycles can be influenced pharmacologically in the vascular wall. It seems necessary, in the treatment of atherosclerosis, to look for drugs which would be able to affect favourably the metabolism of the vessel wall and thus increase its resistance to the development of the disease.

REFERENCES

DAWSON, D. M., GOODFRIEND, T. L. and KAPLAN, N. O. (1964): Lactic dehydrogenases: functions of the two types. *Science, 143*, 929.

GILLMAN, I. (1957): Coronary artery diseases – a possible pathogenesis. *Lancet, 2*, 1117.

GILLMAN, I. (1958): Arterial injury repair and degeneration. *Lancet, 2*, 901.

GILLMAN, I., GRANT, R. A. and HATHORN, M. (1960): Histochemical and chemical studies of calciferol induced vascular injuries. *Brit. J. exp. Path., 41*, 1.

MARTINS DE OLIVEIRA, J. (1969): The effects of pyridinolcarbamate on experimental arteriosclerosis. In: *Atherogenesis. Proceedings, I International Symposium on Atherogenesis, Thrombogenesis and Pyridinolcarbamate Treatment, Tokyo 1969*, pp. 53–56. Editors: T. Shimamoto and F. Numano. ICS 201, Excerpta Medica, Amsterdam.

MRHOVÁ, O. (1971): Sexual differences in the cathodic (anaerobic) 'M' fraction of lactic dehydrogenase in the rat aorta. *Čas. Lék. čes., 110*, 62.

NUMANO, F. (1971): Comparative studies on the preventive effect of pyridinolcarbamate and estrogen against aortic atherosclerosis of cholesterol-fed rabbits. *Acta path. jap., 21*, 182, 210.

ZEMPLÉNYI, T. and MRHOVÁ, O. (1965): Vascular enzyme activity changes accompanying the induction of experimental atherosclerosis. II. Rats fed excess vitamin D. *J. Atheroscler. Res., 5*, 548.

DISCUSSION

Dr. PARWARESCH: Did you relate the enzyme activities to the total protein content?

Dr. GRAFNETTER: Everything was calculated strictly on the protein basis content of the extract, which was measured by the Lowry method.

Dr. PARWARESCH: Did you have any trouble with hemoglobin contamination?

Dr. GRAFNETTER: Hemoglobin contamination in the aorta?

Dr. PARWARESCH: Yes.

Dr. GRAFNETTER: Aortic tissue was carefully cleaned and washed by saline before it was used, so I doubt whether there would be any significant amount of it.

BLOOD AND TISSUE LIPIDS DURING THE TREATMENT OF RATS WITH HIGH-FAT DIET, CALCIFEROL AND PYRIDINOLCARBAMATE

D. GRAFNETTER[1], TAKIO SHIMAMOTO[2] and FUJIO NUMANO[2]

[1] Institute of Clinical and Experimental Medicine, Prague, Czechoslovakia and [2] Institute for Cardiovascular Diseases and Department of Medicine, Tokyo Ika-Shika National University, Tokyo, Japan

INTRODUCTION

On the basis of studies in which blood lipids have been measured, it might be assumed that no large hypolipaemic effects can be attributed to pyridinolcarbamate. However, some changes in lipids have been observed as a result of treatment with pyridinolcarbamate both in blood and the tissues. Firstly, a decreased cholesterol content was found in the aortae of atheromatous rabbits treated with pyridinolcarbamate in the experiments of Shimamoto (Shimamoto, 1969; Shimamoto et al., 1966). Goto and Nakamura (1969) showed that pyridinolcarbamate can lower plasma free fatty acids in humans, and Kritchevsky and Tepper (1971) demonstrated a decrease in plasma and liver triglycerides in pyridinolcarbamate-fed rats as well as an increased rate of cholesterol oxidation by liver mitochondria. In view of these facts, it seemed interesting to carry out studies on the metabolic effects of pyridinolcarbamate under conditions which would cause injuries to the vessel wall or lead to the increased danger of lipid deposition, due to enhanced blood lipid levels.

METHODS

A synthetic diet with a high content of fat and cholesterol and calciferol intoxication were used in the study. White female rats (weight 200–240 g) were divided into 4 groups (Table I)

TABLE I

Experimental design

Group I	Controls	Standard laboratory diet
Group II	PDC	Standard laboratory diet + pyridinolcarbamate
Group III	HFD	High-fat diet
Group IV	HFD + PDC	High-fat diet + pyridinol-carbamate

in the first set of experiments. Rats of Group I (controls) and of Group II (PDC) were fed a standard laboratory diet for 8 weeks, but in addition the rats of Group II were given daily 30 mg/kg of pyridinolcarbamate orally. Rats of Group III (HFD) and of Group IV (HFD + PDC) were fed a high-fat diet containing 40 % soy oil as a vehicle for the 5 % content of cholesterol. The rats of Group IV had 30 mg/kg of pyridinolcarbamate daily in addition. Pyridinolcarbamate in the form of a suspension in tap water was given by direct injection into the oesophagus by using a round-tipped needle attached to a syringe.

The second experiment concerned the effects of pyridinolcarbamate during calciferol intoxication. All rats were kept on a standard laboratory diet. Rats of the control group had no treatment. All other rats received 30,000 IU of calciferol (Spofa, Czechoslovakia) daily for 9 days. Half of the calciferol-intoxicated rats were then treated with 25 mg/kg of pyridinolcarbamate (PDC) daily for 28 days. The rest were sham-treated with tap water.

All results are expressed as means ± SD.

RESULTS AND DISCUSSION

Serum cholesterol was markedly increased (Fig. 1) due to the high-fat diet at the end of the experiment compared to the controls. PDC, whether given with the high-fat diet or with the normal diet, did not significantly affect serum cholesterol. Only a slight decrease was observed when the normal diet was combined with PDC. There was also no striking effect of PDC on serum phospholipids, on esterified fatty acids or on glucose.

We also analysed lipids in the heart, liver and aorta and obtained results similar to those in serum. Table II shows tissue cholesterol contents. Cholesterol increased significantly in the heart and liver tissue with high-fat diet feeding with a tendency to increase in the aorta. However, PDC did not significantly affect tissue cholesterol at 8 weeks. On the other hand (Fig. 2), PDC showed a significant effect on total protein, calcium and free fatty acids (FFA) in the serum. These 3 metabolites decreased when PDC was fed in addition to the standard laboratory diet and the animals sacrificed 2 hours after the last dose.

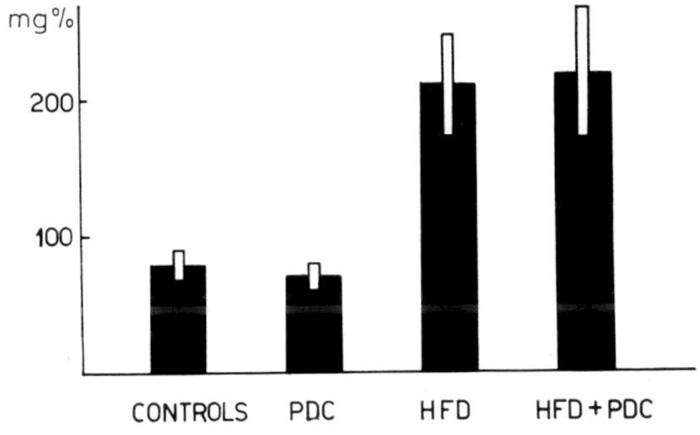

Fig. 1. Serum cholesterol

TABLE II

Tissue cholesterol

Tissue	Controls	PDC	HFD	HFD + PDC
Heart (mg/g wet weight)	1.55 ± 0.08 (9)	1.51 ± 0.08 (9)	1.88 ± 0.10 (10)	1.33 ± 0.08 (10)
Liver (mg/g wet weight)	2.32 ± 0.08 (9)	2.30 ± 0.13 (9)	31.3 ± 6.7 (10)	26.5 ± 4.3 (10)
Aorta (mg/100 mg fat-free dry weight)	0.65 ± 0.08 (8)	0.62 ± 0.05 (9)	0.68 ± 0.06 (10)	0.68 ± 0.06 (10)

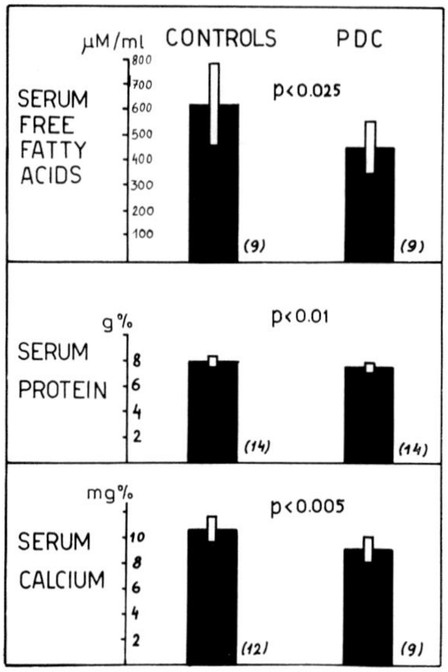

Fig. 2. Effect of PDC on serum total proteins, FFA and calcium.

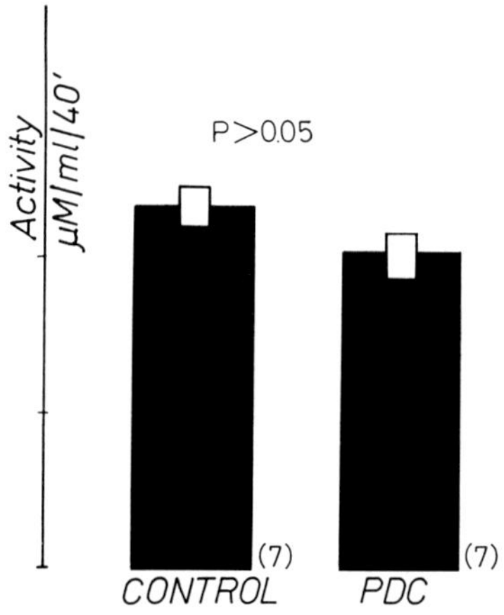

Fig. 3. Cardiac lipoprotein lipase in female rats, 200 g weight, given PDC 30 mg/kg/day for 8 weeks.

We also measured the lipoprotein lipase activity. This enzyme activity was not significantly altered by PDC when measured in either in vivo or in vitro experiments (Fig. 3, Table III).

The weight of animals decreased about 25 % during 9 days of calciferol treatment. However, this weight difference compared to controls disappeared before the experiment was concluded. Serum cholesterol levels, measured in 2 independent experiments, are shown in Table IV. The animals treated with calciferol + PDC had virtually the same serum cholesterol as controls, while calciferol alone tended to cause an elevated cholesterol level. Although the difference of the means was not statistically significant, this indication may be of use in planning periods of observation in future experiments.

TABLE III

Effect of PDC on post-heparin plasma lipolytic activity in vitro

PDC in substrate (mg/ml)	Inhibition (%) at	
	Ediol concentration 3,000 mg%	Ediol concentration 600 mg%
1.00	7	10
0.10	7	10
0.01	4	6

Ediol (Schen Labs Pharmaceuticals, Inc.), commercial triglyceride emulsion as substrate after activation with serum.

TABLE IV

Serum cholesterol

Experiment	Controls	Calciferol	Calciferol + PDC
I	84.3 ± 9.0 (10)	91.5 ± 13.3 (10)	85.2 ± 10.4 (10)
II	70.5 ± 7.3 (10)	78.0 ± 8.2 (7)	73.6 ± 11.7 (10)

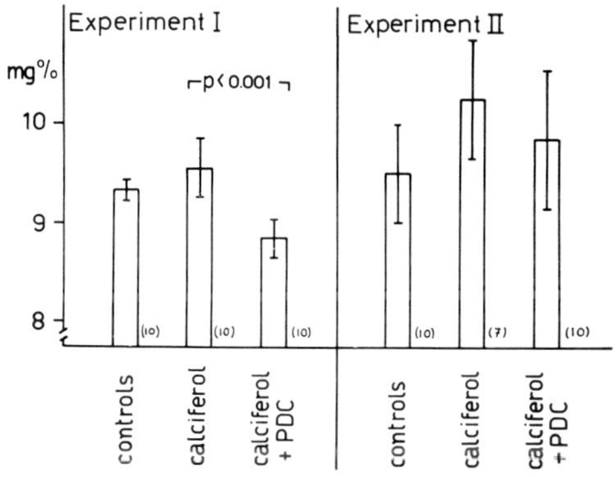

Fig. 4. Serum calcium.

Serum calcium (Fig. 4) was higher in the calciferol group compared to controls and lower in the calciferol + PDC group.

Calciferol feeding caused a small but significant rise in the heart cholesterol content (1.54 ± 0.1 mg/g compared to 1.42 ± 0.09 mg/g in controls). This increase was not found when PDC was fed at the same time. No effect of PDC on cardiac total lipids was observed. On the other hand, liver total lipids were significantly increased by calciferol feeding (49.3 ± 7.5 mg/g compared to 43.3 ± 4.6 mg/g in controls), but was not increased when PDC was fed (44.3 ± 2.3 mg/g). Liver cholesterol content remained unchanged.

Aortic cholesterol, when expressed on a wet weight basis, was slightly but significantly increased by calciferol feeding (0.196 ± 0.017 mg/100 mg) compared to controls (0.171 ± 0.012 mg/100 mg). Although a lower mean value was observed after PDC feeding (0.186 ± 0.017

mg/100 mg) the difference did not reach statistical significance. A similar tendency was seen if the results were calculated on the fat-free dry weight basis.

As a whole, the results of our studies confirm that PDC is not a primary hypolipaemic drug. The accelerated removal of aortic cholesterol as earlier observed (Shimamoto, 1969; Shimamoto et al., 1966) can therefore be considered as secondary and linked to the long-term action of PDC, which has been reported to accelerate the reparative processes in the vessel wall. In the present experiments PDC was tested for a possible protective action. Similar experiments in the future with a modified design and extended to longer periods of observation may show whether lipid deposition could be reduced in the vessel wall by PDC.

PDC shows an interesting effect, namely the ability to lower serum FFA, in humans (Goto and Nakamura, 1969) and as shown by us in the rat. Therefore, we attempted to analyse whether the observed in vivo fall in blood FFA could be caused by inhibition of lipolysis in fat tissue. Rat epididymal fat pads were incubated in vitro in calcium and magnesium free Krebs-Ringer phosphate buffer. No albumin was added so that FFA produced by lipolysis had to accumulate inside the fat tissue. Fat tissues were analysed for FFA at the end of incubation. Where necessary, the incubation media were enriched with various concentrations of PDC, adrenaline or of both. We believed that the blood FFA lowering effect of PDC could be due to inhibition of lipolysis in fat tissue. To our surprise, the presence of 1.0 mg/ml of PDC caused a significant accumulation of FFA inside the tissue (Fig. 5). When both adrenaline and PDC were present, the increase was approximately the sum total of accumulations produced by PDC or adrenaline, respectively. This effect was present in epididymal fat of both fed and fasted or starved rats. However, the effect of PDC was weaker when fat tissue FFA had already been increased by fasting or starving. It was also clear that the effect of PDC was much weaker than the strong lipolytic effect of adrenaline since approximately a 4,000 times higher concentration of PDC was necessary to bring about a similar result. It seemed improbable, therefore, that PDC would act on fat tissue lipolysis at its low in vivo concentrations. Its blood FFA lowering effect is probably due to some other mechanism. The first of these to be considered was the property of PDC to affect cell permeability. The following experiments were designed to investigate this possibility. Fat pads were incubated in the presence of PDC and also of adrenaline for the purpose of comparison. This time, however, the buffer contained bovine serum albumin. FFA were measured at the end of incubation in the medium and in the tissue. The residual post-incubation concentration of FFA inside the fat tissue was higher and paralleled by release of FFA into the incubation medium in the case of adrenaline-treated fat pads. In the case of PDC, the increase observed inside the tissue was not paralleled by a FFA release into the incubation medium. This result suggests that PDC may act on the transport of FFA from fat tissue.

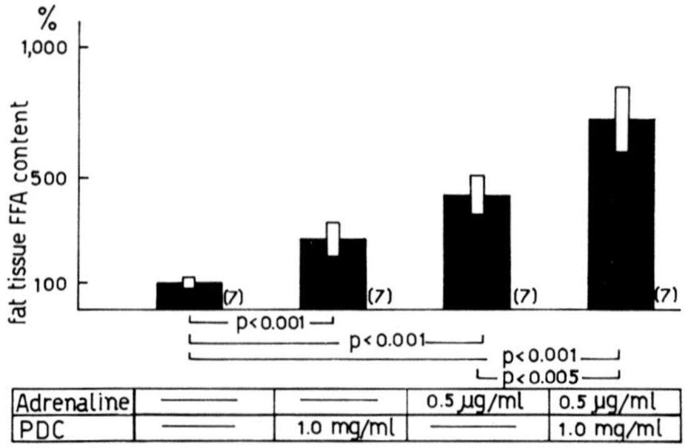

Fig. 5. Free fatty acid content in fat tissue. Fed rats, weight 390 g. 100% = 2.13 ± 0.45 µM/g.

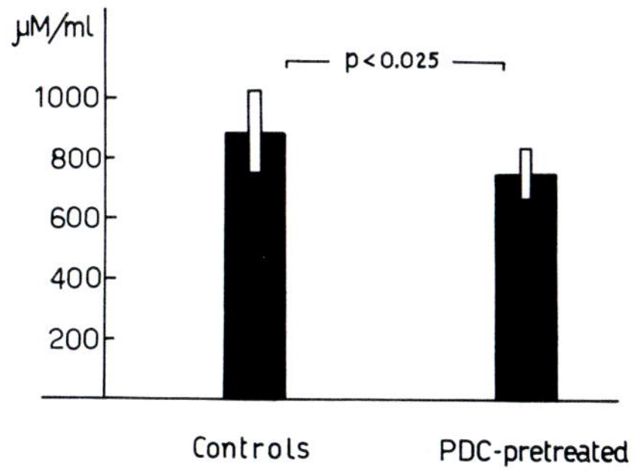

Fig. 6. Serum free fatty acids after injection of adrenaline (20 µg/rat).

We then measured serum FFA in rats pretreated for 3 or 5 days with PDC and injected with adrenaline 1 hour prior to killing. The level of FFA was compared with FFA in rats injected with adrenaline but without pretreatment with PDC. If a high dose (100 µg) of adrenaline was used, FFA was the same in both groups. This dose, which drastically influenced lipolysis, also caused glucose release. However, if a lower dose of only 20 µg adrenaline per rat was used, the level of serum FFA was significantly lower in the rats pretreated with PDC. This result seems to support the hypothesis that permeability changes may play a role in the mechanism of the PDC-induced decrease in FFA. However, we are aware that further data are needed to validate this hypothesis. For example, it will be interesting to see whether PDC would also be able to prevent or diminish in a similar way the uptake of FFA from a fatty acid–albumin complex in the incubation medium.

The decrease in serum FFA observed after administration of PDC should result in a decreased rate of triglyceride synthesis by the liver. In fact, Kritchevsky and Tepper (1971) observed a decreased liver and plasma triglyceride concentration when feeding rats with PDC. A lower level of serum FFA gives a smaller concentration gradient between their blood and tissue level and thus lowered entry into tissues and peripheral utilization. The switch to preferential utilization of endogenous tissue energy sources, together with the favourable enzyme activity changes reported by Numano et al. (1971) and Mrhová et al. (1972*a*, *b*) to occur in the oxidative and glycolytic cycles of the vessel wall due to the PDC treatment, might at least in part explain the mechanism of the antisclerotic action of the drug.

REFERENCES

GOTO, Y. and NAKAMURA, H. (1969): Effect of pyridinolcarbamate on the plasma lipids and glucose in vivo. In: *Atherogenesis. Proceedings, I International Symposium on Atherogenesis, Thrombogenesis and Pyridinolcarbamate Treatment, Tokyo 1969*, pp. 119–120. Editors: T. Shimamoto and F. Numano. ICS 201, Excerpta Medica, Amsterdam.

KRITCHEVSKY, D and TEPPER, S. A. (1971): Influence of pyridinolcarbamate on oxidation of cholesterol by rat liver mitochondria. *Arnzneimittel-Forsch.*, *21*, 146.

MRHOVÁ, O., SHIMAMOTO, T. and NUMANO, F. (1972*a*): The metabolic effect of pyridinolcarbamate in rats. *Acta path. jap.*, *22/2*, 353.

MRHOVÁ, O., SHIMAMOTO, T. and NUMANO, F. (1972*b*): Metabolic effect of pyridinolcarbamate on the vascular wall of rats with hypervitaminosis D. *Atherosclerosis*, *16/1*, 1.

NUMANO, F., KETSU, K., TAKENOBU, M., SAGARA, A. and SHIMAMOTO, T. (1971): Comparative studies on the preventive effect of pyridinolcarbamate and estrogen against aortic and coronary atherosclerosis of cholesterol-fed rabbits. *Acta path. jap.*, *21/2*, 193.

SHIMAMOTO, T. (1969): Experimental study on atherosclerosis. An attempt at its prevention and treatment. *Acta path. jap.*, *19*, 15.

SHIMAMOTO, T., NUMANO, F. and FUJITA, T. (1966): Atherosclerosis-inhibiting effects of an antibradykinin agent, pyridinolcarbamate. *Amer. Heart J.*, *71*, 216.

DISCUSSION

Dr. PARWARESCH: How much adrenaline in your in vivo studies would you need to increase free fatty acids? The dose you used was 20 μg per rat. What is the least amount of adrenaline that will give you a decent measurable rise in free fatty acids?

Dr. GRAFNETTER: As you have seen, 20 μg adrenaline caused a free fatty acid level which is unusual because, in the rat, if you use a specific method, normal free fatty acids would be something between 200 and 400 μM/ml. This was doubled. I think 20 μg per rat would certainly enhance the free fatty acids in 1 hour. In fact, we performed studies some years ago in which we used various concentrations up to 100 μg and there was a rise in free fatty acids in 1 hour.

Dr. PARWARESCH: I was implying by the question, not that it would not, but that it was really a tremendous amount of catecholamine. Would you see similar blocking effects if you used a smaller amount, if it was possible to show your biochemical effects? Not that it did not occur at such high amounts.

Dr. GRAFNETTER: I think it is a good question and we may have to use a lower dose. We started with 100 μg. Then I went lower to 20 μg per rat, which I thought would be a dose suitable for the rats to raise free fatty acids in 1 hour. There was a lowering effect of pyridinolcarbamate on the raised free fatty acids.

Dr. SPECTOR: It might be that you could use a much lower dose of catecholamine if you incorporated methylxanthine into your assay, so that you would block phosphodiesterase, stimulate adenylcyclase and get the cyclic AMP effects that the catecholamine may well produce.

Dr. GRAFNETTER: What I spoke about here was a hypothesis concerning permeability from the fat tissue and it will need confirmation. But I was also thinking in terms of performing further experiments with adenylcyclase, which I think would be very important in this case.

Dr. PICK: You have shown in your paper that pyridinolcarbamate decreases serum free fatty acids and increases them in the tissue. Did I understand you correctly? Do you think there is a change in the pool?

Dr. GRAFNETTER: Well, as far as my results are concerned, I cannot answer 'yes' or 'no' because I have no direct evidence. Our results showed decrease in vivo and increase in vitro. I am not sure whether I can combine it only on that basis.

Dr. PARWARESCH: Are the peripheral effects of adrenaline due to α- or β-activity?

Dr. GRAFNETTER: I think this has been much studied. I am a chemist, so from the pharmacological point of view I could not answer you very well. Perhaps Dr. Spector could help me.

Dr. SPECTOR: Normally, one thinks of the metabolic effects as β-effects which will be blocked by propranolol.

INFLUENCE OF PYRIDINOLCARBAMATE ON CHOLESTEROL METABOLISM IN RATS AND RABBITS*

DAVID KRITCHEVSKY, JANE T. KOLIMAGA,
HONG K. KIM and SHIRLEY A. TEPPER
The Wistar Institute of Anatomy and Biology, Philadelphia, Pa., U.S.A.

Shimamoto and his co-workers (1965, 1966, 1968) have reported that 2,6-bis(hydroxymethyl)-pyridine di-*N*-methylcarbamate (pyridinolcarbamate; PYC) relieves the complications of arteriosclerosis in man and inhibits development of experimental atherosclerosis in rabbits. There are few data pertaining to the influence of this compound on cholesterol metabolism in rats. We have studied the influence of PYC on cholesterol synthesis by rat liver slices (Kritchevsky and Tepper, 1967) and degradation by rat liver mitochondria (Kritchevsky and Tepper, 1971; Kritchevsky et al., 1959). More recently we have studied the influence of PYC on cholesterol absorption. We have also studied the influence of PYC (30 mg/day) on the development of cholesterol-induced atherosclerosis in rabbits.

The rat and rabbit studies are summarized in this report.

MATERIALS AND METHODS

Male Wistar rats were fed a diet consisting of mixed cereal (70%), wheat germ (7%), skim milk powder (22%) and vitamin mix (1%). Test compounds were added at the expense of the cereal. In the experiments on cholesterol synthesis PYC was fed at the level of 0.3%; in the other experiments it was fed as 1% of the diet.

The biosynthesis experiments were carried out using male Wistar rats which had been maintained on 0.3% PYC for 3 weeks. After 3 weeks the rats were decapitated, and the livers excised and washed in chilled phosphate buffer. Liver slices (0.5 g) were incubated for 3 hours under 100% oxygen in 5 ml of phosphate buffer (pH 7) containing 0.006 M $MgCl_2$, 0.03 M nicotinamide and either 1 μCi of sodium acetate-1-^{14}C or 0.5 μCi of mevalonic acid-2-^{14}C. The reaction was stopped by the addition of hot 15% alcoholic KOH; the cholesterol was extracted from the saponification mixture and isolated as the digitonide. The radioactivity of the cholesterol digitonide was then assayed by liquid scintillation spectrometry. Another portion of the liver was saponified in 15% alcoholic KOH and the cholesterol then extracted. The total serum and liver cholesterol levels were determined by the method of Mann (1961).

The oxidation of 26-^{14}C-cholesterol by rat liver mitochondria was studied in rats which had been fed 1% PYC for 10 days. Results were compared with those obtained from control rats and from rats fed 1% nicotinic acid. The procedure for preparation of the liver mitochondrial and supernatant fractions has been described in detail (Whitehouse et al., 1959; Kritchevsky et al., 1959). Incubations were carried out in stoppered Erlenmeyer flasks containing center wells. Each incubation mixture consisted of: 1 ml of the mitochondrial preparation (corresponding to 2–2.5 g liver); 1 ml of a solution containing ATP (25 mg), NAD (5 mg), AMP (8 mg), reduced glutathione (15 mg), sodium citrate monohydrate (30 mg), Mg $(NO_3)_2 \cdot 6H_2O$ (10 mg), potassium penicillin G (2000 U) and streptomycin sulfate (1 mg);

* This work was supported, in part, by United States Public Health Service Research Grants HL-03299 and HL-05209 and Research Career Award HL-0734 from the National Heart and Lung Institute.

4 ml of 26-^{14}C-cholesterol emulsion ($2.6–6.7 \times 10^{-2}$ nmoles; $4.48 \times 10^4–11.4 \times 10^4$ dpm) in 0.25 M tris (hydroxymethyl)aminomethane · HCl, pH 8.5; and 5 ml of boiled 104,000 *g* supernatant fluid (cytosol). The incubation mixture was shaken at 37°C for 18 hours, at which time 2.5 ml of a 1 M methanolic solution of Hyamine® (*p*-(diisobutylcresoxyethoxy-ethyl)dimethylbenzylammonium hydroxide) was injected into the center well through the sleeve stopper. The solution was acidified with 25% trichloroacetic acid solution (2.5 ml) or in H_2SO_4 (2.5 ml), and shaking was continued for 3 hours at 37°C to displace $^{14}CO_2$. The Hyamine solution was removed from the center well which was rinsed with 0.5 ml of Hyamine and enough toluene to give a 5 ml solution. One ml of this solution was taken for radioactive assay by liquid scintillation spectrometry.

Plasma free fatty acids (FFA) were determined by the method of Dole (1956) with minor modifications (Bizzi et al., 1969). Liver aliquots were homogenized in chloroform-methanol (2:1) and the extract used for lipid analysis. Plasma and liver cholesterol were determined by the method of Mann (1961) and triglycerides by the method of Van Handel and Zilversmit (1957).

In the cholesterol absorption experiments, male Wistar rats were fed 1% PYC for 14 days. At this time each rat was given 0.5 μCi of 4-^{14}C-cholesterol in 0.2 ml propylene glycol by gavage. After 24 hours the rats were killed and sera and livers taken for analysis of lipid content and cholesterol radioactivity.

In the atherosclerosis experiments, two groups of 25 male rabbits of the Dutch belted strain (1500 g) were maintained for 8 weeks on a diet of laboratory chow augmented with 2% cholesterol and 6% corn oil.

One group of rabbits was fed 30 mg/day (20 mg/kg) of PYC in 0.5 ml of 95% ethanol. The control rabbits were given 0.5 ml ethanol alone.

At the end of the feeding period the rabbits were bled by cardiac puncture, killed by injection of sodium pentothal, and the liver and aorta were removed. Serum was assayed for total cholesterol and triglyceride. A sample of liver was homogenized in chloroform-methanol (2:1) and the lipid extract was used for determination of total cholesterol and triglyceride. Aortas were graded for atheromata using a 0–4 scale (Duff and McMillan, 1949).

The aortas from each group were pooled and extracted with chloroform-methanol 2:1. Aortic free and total cholesterol were determined by the method of Sperry and Webb (1950).

Aortic lipids were also subjected to thin-layer chromatography on silica gel G (developing solvent, petroleum ether: ether: acetic acid, 74:25:1) in order to separate cholesteryl esters and triglycerides. These lipid classes were eluted from the adsorbent, transesterified with BF_3-methanol, and the component fatty acids were determined by gas-liquid chromatography on 16% diethylene glycol succinate supported on Chromasorb. All chemicals used were of reagent grade. Labeled substrates were purchased from the New England Nuclear Corp., Boston, Mass. The PYC was generously supplied by Professor T. Shimamoto.

RESULTS AND DISCUSSION

A. Cholesterol biosynthesis in rat liver

The results of two experiments are summarized in Table I. In these studies PYC showed no effect upon serum or liver cholesterol. Although liver weights were somewhat lower in PYC-fed rats, the differences were not significant.

Incorporation of 1-^{14}C-acetate into cholesterol by rat liver slices was significantly reduced in the PYC-fed rats ($p > 0.02$ in Experiment 1 and $p > 0.001$ in Experiment 2). There was no effect observed in the experiment involving cholesterol biosynthesis from 2-^{14}C-mevalonate.

B. Oxidation of cholesterol by rat liver mitochondria

The effects of PYC and nicotinic acid on serum and liver lipids are summarized in Table II.

TABLE I

Influence of pyridinolcarbamate (PYC) (0.3 %) on serum and liver cholesterol and hepatic cholesterogenesis in rats (compound fed for 3 weeks)

	Experiment 1		Experiment 2	
	PYC	Control	PYC	Control
Number	6	6	5	5
Weight gain (g)	42	52	106	112
Liver weight (g)	8.7	10.0	11.8	12.4
Liver as % body weight	3.97	4.48	3.75	3.93
Cholesterol				
Serum (mg/dl)	38.9 ± 1.8[a]	33.2 ± 4.3	43.2 ± 9.8	47.3 ± 3.6
Liver (mg/100 g)	370 ± 31	384 ± 21	364 ± 30	299 ± 8
Serum-liver pool (g)	38.8	40.6	47.1	41.6
Conversion (%)				
1-^{14}C-acetate	0.37 ± 0.02[b]	0.93 ± 0.24	0.82 ± 0.20	3.40 ± 0.69[c]
2-^{14}C-mevalonate	1.06 ± 0.13	1.14 ± 0.12	–	–

[a] Standard error
[b] $p < 0.05$
[c] $p < 0.01$

TABLE II

Influence of 1 % pyridinolcarbamate (PYC) and nicotinic acid (NA) on plasma and liver lipids in rats (10 day feeding)

	Group		
	PYC	NA	Control
Number	6	6	6
Weight gain (g)	38 ± 5[a]	49 ± 8	46 ± 2
Liver weight (g)	8.1 ± 0.3	8.2 ± 0.3	8.2 ± 0.3
Liver as % body weight	4.30 ± 0.07	4.02 ± 0.13	4.08 ± 0.09
Plasma FFA (mEq/l)	479 ± 22[b]	378 ± 29	473 ± 42
Cholesterol (mg/dl)	46.0 ± 3.4	46.5 ± 3.4	41.8 ± 6.9
Triglyceride (mg/dl)	39.3 ± 2.9	43.1 ± 4.2	49.7 ± 4.9
Liver			
Cholesterol (mg/100 g)	187 ± 14	180 ± 6	185 ± 7
Triglyceride (mg/100 g)	490 ± 83	432 ± 41	620 ± 106
Serum-liver pool			
Cholesterol (mg)	18.2	17.6	17.7
Triglyceride (mg)	43.0	38.0	55.5

[a] Standard error
[b] PYC vs NA, $p < 0.02$

The test compounds did not affect weight gain, liver weight or plasma and liver cholesterol levels. Nicotinic acid lowered plasma FFA but PYC did not. Both PYC and nicotinic acid lowered plasma and liver triglyceride levels.

The extent of oxidation of 26-^{14}C-cholesterol to $^{14}CO_2$ by suitably fortified liver mitochondrial preparations from rats fed PYC is higher than that observed in similar preparations from livers of either control rats or rats fed nicotinic acid. In rats fed PYC, oxidation of

TABLE III

Oxidation of 26-^{14}C-cholesterol to $^{14}CO_2$ by liver mitochondria of rats fed 1 % pyridinolcarbamate (PYC) or 1 % nicotinic acid (NA) for 10 days (average of 6 experiments)

	% Oxidation		
	PYC	NA	Control
Oxidation (per mg N)	11.6 ± 1.8*	8.8 ± 2.6	8.5 ± 1.7
Oxidation (per g liver)	1.43	1.07	1.04
Oxidation (per mg liver cholesterol)	0.77	0.60	0.56

* Standard error

cholesterol was 38 % higher than that by the control mitochondria whether calculated on the basis of mg mitochondrial N, g liver or mg liver cholesterol (Table III). The differences are not statistically significant, however.

C. Cholesterol absorption

Rats were fed 1 % PYC for 2 weeks, fed one dose of 0.5 μCi of 4-^{14}C-cholesterol and killed 24 hours later. The serum and liver lipid levels are summarized in Table IV. Livers of the rats fed PYC were significantly larger in relation to body size than were those of controls. Liver cholesterol levels in the test rats were lower on the basis of mg/100 g liver. The actual

TABLE IV

Influence of 1 % pyridinolcarbamate (PYC) on serum and liver lipids in rats (2 week feeding) *

	PYC	Control
Number	7	7
Weight gain (g)	52	54
Liver weight (g)	9.8 ± 0.5[a]	8.6 ± 0.4
Liver as % body weight	4.39 ± 0.17[b]	3.82 ± 0.09
Cholesterol		
Serum (mg/dl)	44.6 ± 2.9	42.3 ± 3.1
Liver (mg/100 g)	110 ± 4[b]	136 ± 8
Serum-liver pool (mg)	13.8	14.6
Triglyceride		
Serum (mg/dl)	52.6 ± 3.5	65.0 ± 7.7
Liver (mg/100 g)	403 ± 26	489 ± 89
Serum-liver pool (mg)	43.0	46.4
Recoverable ^{14}C-cholesterol		
Serum (dpm × 10^3)	1.35 ± 0.11[c]	2.19 ± 0.12
Liver (dpm × 10^4)	1.43 ± 0.10[c]	2.20 ± 0.11
Serum plus liver (dpm × 10^4)	1.57 ± 0.11[c]	2.42 ± 0.12

* Rats were fed 0.5 μCi 4-^{14}C-cholesterol 24 hours before termination of experiment.

[a] Standard error

[b] $p < 0.01$

[c] $p < 0.001$

liver cholesterol content was PYC 10.8 mg and control 11.7 mg. Serum and liver triglycerides in the PYC-fed rats were lower than those of the control rats by 19 and 18%, respectively. Due to the wide variation, the results were not statistically significant. The radioactive cholesterol recovered from the serum after 24 hours was $1.35 \pm 0.11 \times 10^3$ dpm in the test rats and $2.19 \pm 0.12 \times 10^3$ dpm in the controls ($p < 0.001$). The radioactive cholesterol in 1 ml of serum was isolated and assayed. The total serum content was calculated as 3% of the body weight (D'Amour and Blood, 1954) and used to calculate the total recoverable ^{14}C-cholesterol. Total liver cholesterol was extracted, an aliquot precipitated as the digitonide and assayed for radioactivity. The ^{14}C-cholesterol recoverable from liver was $1.43 \pm 0.10 \times 10^4$ dpm in the rats fed PYC and $2.20 \pm 0.11 \times 10^4$ dpm in the controls ($p < 0.001$). Total recoverable radioactivity was $1.57 \pm 0.11 \times 10^4$ dpm in the PYC group and $2.42 \pm 0.12 \times 10^4$ dpm in the controls ($p < 0.001$).

PYC feeding in rats results, generally, in reductions in serum and liver triglycerides, a drop in liver cholesterol but no discernible effect on serum cholesterol levels. PYC inhibits cholesterol biosynthesis and cholesterol absorption, so that one might expect this compound to lower cholesterol levels in cholesterol-fed rats. PYC enhances oxidation of cholesterol by rat liver mitochondria to a slight extent.

D. Experimental atherosclerosis

It can be seen from Table V that, when administered at a level of 30 mg/day to rabbits fed 2% cholesterol, PYC does not significantly affect serum or liver lipid levels and has no effect on the severity of induced atherosclerosis. The PYC was administered in 0.5 ml alcohol. Kritchevsky and Moyer (1960) have shown that alcohol (9.5% of drinking water) does not influence the course of experimental atherosclerosis in rabbits, so that the levels of alcohol administered weekly (3.5 ml/wk) could not have affected our results. The triglyceride and cholesterol levels in aortas of rabbits fed cholesterol with and without PYC were comparable (Table VI). Patterns of total aortic fatty acids and cholesteryl ester fatty acids in the two groups were also comparable (Table VII).

The effect of PYC on cholesterol-induced atherosclerosis has been studied in the chicken, monkey and rabbit. Pick (1969) and Martins de Oliveira (1969) fed relatively large doses of PYC to chickens (50 and 500 mg/day, respectively) and the latter author reported a statistically significant reduction in atherosclerosis. Pick found that, in cockerels fed 1% cholesterol and 500 mg PYC daily, thoracic lesions were present in all birds but the severity (1.16) was lower than that observed in controls (1.36). Serum cholesterol levels were also lower (868 vs

TABLE V

Effect of pyridinolcarbamate (PYC) (30 mg/day) on cholesterol-induced atherosclerosis in rabbits

Group	PYC	Control
Number	21/25	18/25
Weight gain (g)	124	157
Liver weight (g)	107.2 ± 3.0	114.9 ± 3.9
Serum cholesterol (mg/dl)		
4 weeks	708 ± 54	849 ± 115
8 weeks	1739 ± 138	1448 ± 178
Serum triglyceride (mg/dl)	144 ± 19	125 ± 14
Liver cholesterol (g/100 g)	4.45 ± 0.37	4.73 ± 0.28
Liver triglyceride (g/100 g)	1.86 ± 0.18	2.15 ± 0.18
Average atheromata		
Arch	1.21 ± 0.14	1.39 ± 0.16
Thoracic	0.88 ± 0.10	0.83 ± 0.09

TABLE VI

Aorta lipids of rabbits fed atherogenic regimen $\pm$30 mg/day of pyridinolcarbamate (PYC)

	PYC	Control
Triglyceride (mg/g)	122	106
Cholesterol		
Total (mg/g)	2.62	2.52
Free (mg/g)	1.68	1.70
Ester (mg/g)	0.94	0.82
Ester/free	0.56	0.48

TABLE VII

Aorta fatty acids of rabbits fed atherogenic regimen $\pm$30 mg/day of pyridinolcarbamate (PYC)

Acid	PYC		Control	
	TFA*	CEFA**	TFA	CEFA
14:0	1.2	tr	1.2	tr
16:0	31.6	31.1	33.0	29.1
16:1	1.7	tr	1.4	1.7
18:0	4.4	11.8	4.2	7.2
18:1	27.4	44.3	27.4	48.2
18:2	33.7	12.8	32.8	13.7
18:1/18:2	0.81	3.46	0.84	3.52

* Total fatty acid
** Cholesteryl ester fatty acid

1044 mg/dl). Coronary involvement was 18.3% in controls and 15.2% in treated birds. All the differences were significant at the 5% level.

Malinow et al. (1968, 1972) found that PYC failed to protect female squirrel or cynomolgus monkeys against atherosclerosis induced by a butter-cholesterol diet. The squirrel monkeys were given 10–16 mg/kg PYC and the cynomolgus monkeys received 400–2000 mg/kg of food. Shimamoto and co-workers (Shimamoto, 1969; Shimamoto et al., 1966) reported that, when PYC was fed to cholesterol-fed rabbits at a level of 10 mg/kg, there was a distinct reduction in extent of aortic fatty streaking. Serum cholesterol levels were higher in the treated group. Wu et al. (1969) also found that a daily dose of 10 mg/kg of PYC protected rabbits against the fatty streaking produced by a diet containing 1.5% cholesterol. Sanwald and Wagener (1971), however, have reported that administration of PYC to cholesterol-fed rabbits does not affect the chemistry or metabolism of the arterial wall.

Möttönen et al. (1972) have also found no effect of PYC on the aortic metabolism of cholesterol-fed rabbits. These authors administered 100 mg/kg of PYC daily for 8 weeks to rabbits being fed 1% cholesterol. They found no effect of the compound on aortic ATPase or lactate-NAD-tetrazolium reductase. There were no differences in atherosclerosis between rabbits fed PYC plus cholesterol or those fed cholesterol alone.

The differences between our results and those of Shimamoto, Wu and their co-workers cannot be due to differences in the level of dietary cholesterol.

Three differences are evident: the mode of administration of the drug, the apparent lack of added fat in their diets and the strain of rabbit. Of the three, the difference in level of dietary fat seems to be the most relevant and may be worth examining further.

REFERENCES

Bizzi, A., Veneroni, E. and Tepper, S. A. (1969): Effect of sugars and sugar derivatives on plasma free fatty acid in rats. *Biochem. Pharmacol.*, *18*, 688.

D'Amour, F. E. and Blood, F. (1954): *Manual for Laboratory Work in Mammalian Physiology.* University of Chicago Press, Chicago, Ill.

Dole, V. P. (1956): A relation between non-esterified fatty acids in plasma and the metabolism of glucose. *J. clin. Invest.*, *35*, 150.

Duff, G. L. and McMillan, G. C. (1949): The effect of alloxan diabetes on experimental cholesterol atherosclerosis in the rabbit. *J. exp. Med.*, *89*, 611.

Kritchevsky, D., Kitagawa, M., Tepper, S. A. and Davidson, L. M. (1971): Influence of nicotinic acid and its derivatives on oxidation of cholesterol by rat liver mitochondria. In: *Metabolic Effects of Nicotinic Acid and its Derivatives*, p. 585. Editors: K. F. Gey and L. A. Carlson. Hans Huber Verlag, Bern.

Kritchevsky, D., Kolman, R. R., Whitehouse, M. W., Cottrell, M. C. and Staple, E. (1959): Oxidation of cholesterol by rat liver mitochondria: effect of dietary fat. *J. Lipid Res.*, *1*, 83.

Kritchevsky, D. and Moyer, A. W. (1960): Effect of alcohol on experimental atherosclerosis in rabbits. *Naturwissenschaften*, *47*, 138.

Kritchevsky, D. and Tepper, S. A. (1967): Influence of pyridinolcarbamate on hepatic cholesterogenesis in rats. *Experientia (Basel)*, *23*, 1006.

Kritchevsky, D. and Tepper, S. A. (1971): Influence of pyridinolcarbamate on oxidation of cholesterol by rat liver mitochondria. *Arzneimittel-Forsch.*, *21*, 146.

Mann, G. V. (1961): A method for measurement of cholesterol in blood serum. *Clin. Chem.*, *7*, 275.

Malinow, M. R., McLaughlin, P. and Perley, A. (1972): The effects of pyridinolcarbamate on induced atherosclerosis in cynomolgus monkeys (*Macaca ira*). *Atherosclerosis*, *15*, 13.

Malinow, M. R., Perley, A. and McLaughlin, P. (1968): The effects of pyridinolcarbamate on induced atherosclerosis in monkeys. *J. Atheroscler. Res.*, *8*, 455.

Martins de Oliveira, J. (1969): The effects of pyridinolcarbamate on experimental atherosclerosis. In: *Atherogenesis*, pp. 53–56. Editors: T. Shimamoto and F. Numano. ICS 201, Excerpta Medica, Amsterdam.

Möttönen, M., Pantio, M. and Nieminen, L. (1972): Enzyme histochemical observations on the effect of pyridinolcarbamate on cholesterol-induced atherosclerosis. *Atherosclerosis*, *15*, 77.

Pick, R. (1969): The effect of pyridinolcarbamate on the induction and regression of aortic and coronary atherosclerosis in cholesterol-fed cockerels. In: *Atherogenesis*, pp. 57–64. Editors: T. Shimamoto and F. Numano. ICS 201, Excerpta Medica, Amsterdam.

Sanwald, R. and Wagener, H. (1971): The effect of pyridinolcarbamate (Anginin) on arterial wall metabolism. In: *Abstracts, IV International Symposium on Drugs Affecting Lipid Metabolism, 1971*, p. 98.

Shimamoto, T. (1969): Experimental study on atherosclerosis – an attempt at its prevention and treatment. *Acta path. jap.*, *19*, 15.

Shimamoto, T., Atsuni, T., Numano, F. and Fujita, T. (1968): Treatment of atherosclerosis with pyridinolcarbamate. *Progr. Biochem. Pharmacol.*, *4*, 597.

Shimamoto, T., Numano, F. and Fujita, T. (1966): Atherosclerosis inhibiting effect of an antibradykinin agent, pyridinolcarbamate. *Amer. Heart J.*, *71*, 216.

Shimamoto, T., Numano, F., Fujita, T., Ishioka, T. and Atsumi, T. (1965): Treatment of experimental and human atherosclerosis with pyridinolcarbamate. *Asian med. J.*, *8*, 825.

Sperry, W. M. and Webb, M. (1950): A revision of the Schoenheimer-Sperry method for cholesterol determination. *J. biol. Chem.*, *187*, 97.

Van Handel, E. and Zilversmit, D. B. (1957): Micromethod for the direct determination of serum triglyceride. *J. Lab. clin. Med.*, *50*, 152.

Whitehouse, M. W., Staple, E. and Gurin, S. (1959): Catabolism *in vitro* of cholesterol. I. Oxidation of the terminal methyl groups of cholesterol to carbon dioxide by rat liver preparations. *J. biol. Chem.*, *234*, 276.

Wu, C. C., Huang, T. S. and Hsu, C. J. (1969): Prevention of experimental atherosclerosis with pyridinolcarbamate. *Amer. Heart J.*, *77*, 657.

DISCUSSION

Dr. NUMANO: Your effect of decrease in synthesis of cholesterol from acetate was done in the rat. Have you performed similar studies in the rabbit?

Dr. KRITCHEVSKY: No. It is paradoxical that investigators in this field measure cholesterol metabolism in rats, but study atherosclerosis in rabbits. Possibly this is because the rat is small enough and available enough for metabolic studies but is not susceptible to easy induction of atherosclerosis.

Dr. NUMANO: Regarding the choice of the rat for the determination of serum cholesterol, it was my impression that the rat has an unlimited supply of cholesterol and therefore would be somewhat unsuitable to measure serum cholesterol.

Dr. KRITCHEVSKY: The rat has very good control of his cholesterol level, so unless you take outrageous measures you cannot raise serum cholesterol level in rats easily. All the measurements that you saw on the slides were carried out ancillary to the point of the experiments, which in one case was the synthesis of cholesterol and another its degradation.

Dr. AUSTIN: In your rabbit experiments you mentioned that the rabbits were fed daily with 30 mg of pyridinolcarbamate. Was that in one oral dose by tube?

Dr. KRITCHEVSKY: Yes, there was one single dose dissolved in 0.5 ml of 95% alcohol, and administered in much the same way as Dr. Grafnetter has described. We use a syringe with a blunt-end needle, put it deep against the esophagus and just squirt it in.

Dr. AUSTIN: How long does the blood level of pyridinolcarbamate last when given in this manner?

Dr. KRITCHEVSKY: I could not tell you. I wonder if Professor Shimamoto has some data on this?

Dr. SHIMAMOTO: I am sorry, but I do not have the precise data here but later I should like to show the blood level in rabbits and man.

Dr. AUSTIN: Did I understand earlier that pyridinolcarbamate was absorbed rather rapidly?

Dr. SHIMAMOTO: We got the highest level 2 or 3 hours after administration orally.

Dr. AUSTIN: How long is the pyridinolcarbamate, once it has been absorbed, at an effective pharmacological level in the systems that are being measured?

Dr. SHIMAMOTO: From our study, the highest level is reached 2 or 3 hours after administration and for 4 or 6 hours continues at a high level, although about 50%. After that, the level goes down rather rapidly, so I think that hypercholesterolemia continues for 14 hours. In our experiments we gave pyridinolcarbamate twice a day: in the morning and in the afternoon, or in the evening, and I advise this dose regime.

Dr. AUSTIN: This is my point. I think those giving it only once a day may perhaps not be giving enough – not at a sustained level appropriate for the metabolic problem.

Dr. KRITCHEVSKY: Our method of drug administration was chosen to ensure that each animal received the prescribed dose of pyridinolcarbamate. The alternative was to have the compound milled directly into the diet, but rabbits waste a large amount of their feed, so we would have no idea of the exact dosage administered, although it would have been a sustained dose.

Dr. SHIMAMOTO: I should like to know how you give pyridinolcarbamate to rabbits. In alcohol? By putting it in a capsule?

Dr. KRITCHEVSKY: Dissolved in alcohol and injecting it from a syringe, into the back of the mouth.

Dr. SHIMAMOTO: To get a 'model' for various antiatherosclerotic substances, we have to go to a lot of trouble. Since there are individual variations in feeding which have proved troublesome over the last few years we looked at the 'strain' of rabbits. Our rabbits have been kept for almost 50 years without contamination from other strains. The amount of cholesterol given to produce arteriosclerosis may be a big problem so that with a large amount we cannot see any preventive effect with various antiatherosclerotic substances. The dose of cholesterol may also be a big problem. We have reduced the daily dose to approximately 1 g. At first, the quantity administered to each rabbit had to be given by mouth, but recently we have been using a 1% pellet of cholesterol. Every day we measure the amount of cholesterol and if there is any tremendous difference we reject these rabbits.

Anyhow, we have to get more reliable models for the investigation of preventive substances.

Dr. KRITCHEVSKY: This is perfectly true. We need a means of normalizing the experiments – same strain of rabbits, same diet, same means of drug administration. But even under ideal conditions there are variations. I should like to remind you of the experiments of Lofland and Clarkson who fed cholesterol to monkeys of the same strain under similar conditions, yet found that the hypercholesteremic response was not the same.

Dr. KIPSHIDZE: I should like to ask about the dosage of alcohol. In my experiments I am studying the influence of alcohol in atherosclerosis and I find antiatherogenic agents in alcohol.

Dr. KRITCHEVSKY: We gave just 0.5 ml of 95% alcohol, but the rabbits drink several hundred milliliters of water a day. Thus, the amount of alcohol they got in this particular case was really very small and the controls got the same amount; so I do not think that the alcohol was a factor here.

Dr. KIPSHIDZE: I gave 21 g alcohol per 3 kg rabbits every day for 6 months together with 1 g/day cholesterol. We have not seen any changes yet.

Dr. KRITCHEVSKY: We reported a similar experiment in 1960 (*Naturwissenschaften*, *47*, 1960, 138). We fed rabbits 3% cholesterol and put 10% of 95% alcohol into their drinking water. Thus their drinking water was 9.5% ethanol. They may have died happier, but their average atheromata were no different from those of the control rabbits.

THE EFFECTS OF PYRIDINOLCARBAMATE ON BLOOD VESSELS, HEART AND BRAIN BIOGENIC AMINES

S. SPECTOR and B. A. BERKOWITZ
Rochester Institute of Molecular Biology, Nutley, New Jersey, U.S.A.

This Session has made it quite apparent that the biogenic amines, serotonin and catechols, have a vital and dynamic role in the etiology of atherosclerosis. Tanabe et al. have also shown that pyridinolcarbamate likewise can exert an effect on some peripheral vascular diseases. A number of agents capable of eliciting such an effect on the peripheral vascular system exert this effect by affecting the neurotransmitter of the sympathetic nervous system. The vascular system not only possesses catecholamines but also possesses the enzymatic machinery to synthetize it. As a consequence, we asked the following questions: What effect does pyridinolcarbamate have on catecholamine in various tissues? What effect does pyridinolcarbamate have on blood vessels and cardiac catecholamines? What effect does it have on the adrenal catecholamines in the brain? Also, if it impinges on these systems, one is obliged to look at catecholamines in the brain. My colleague, Dr. Berkowitz, will discuss the effect of atherogenesis on vascular and adrenal catecholamines, and he will present his data following this presentation.

The biosynthetic pathway in the synthesis of norepinephrine involves the following steps: tyrosine→dopa→dopamine→norepinephrine. The immediate precursor of norepinephrine is tyrosine. Tyrosine is hydroxylated to form a catechol, namely dihydroxyphenylalanine (dopa). Dopa is then decarboxylated to form dihydroxyphenylethylamine (dopamine). Dopamine is a very interesting compound because it can serve as a precursor for norepinephrine by being hydroxylated in the β-position of the side-chain to form norepinephrine. It has also been shown that dopamine itself has a role as a neurotransmitter. Thus, dopamine has to be considered when one discusses catecholamines. In the adrenal, there is one more step, namely methylation by the enzyme phenylethyl-*N*-methyltransferase which transfers a methyl group to norepinephrine to form epinephrine. We shall concern ourselves primarily with the sequence from tyrosine to norepinephrine as this is the sequence occurring in the nervous system. The sequence that transpires is that tyrosine is taken up into the nerve by an amino acid transport mechanism. Once it gets into the nerve, it goes through this enzymatic machinery to be converted to norepinephrine. Norepinephrine can effect its own synthesis, so that end-product inhibition occurs. The step that it will block will be the rate-limiting step, tyrosine hydroxylase.

When one measures norepinephrine one is looking at a composite of a number of phenomena or processes that are going on. We see both synthesis and degradation.

Table I indicates what happens if one gives pyridinolcarbamate to a rat at a dose of 50 mg/kg for 3 days. Animals were sacrificed 4 hours after the last dose. If one looks at the norepinephrine content (μg/g of tissue), the site that is particularly modified is the mesenteric artery. There is an appreciable elevation in the endogenous content of noradrenaline. There is likewise an elevation in the endogenous norepinephrine content in the heart. One can obtain an increase in the endogenous content if synthesis is stimulated. One can also find an increase in the endogenous content if the catabolic enzymes are inhibited. The other possibility, and I will just allude to this toward the end, is that the compound can prevent efflux of the amine.

One can speculate that pyridinolcarbamate elevates endogenous norepinephrine levels as a

TABLE I

Effect of Anginin on norepinephrine concentration in the rat cardiovascular system*

Tissue	Norepinephrine (μg/g)
Control aorta	0.20 ±0.05
Anginin aorta	0.27 ±0.18
Control mesenteric artery	2.99 ±0.42
Anginin mesenteric artery	4.32 ±0.81**
Control mesenteric vein	1.86 ±0.24
Anginin mesenteric vein	1.88 ±0.20
Control heart	1.00 ±0.17
Anginin heart	1.30 ±0.26**

* Anginin 50 mg/kg for 3 days i.p. Rats were sacrificed 4 hours after last dose.
** Statistically significant, $p < 0.05$.

TABLE II

Effect of in vitro pyridinolcarbamate on adrenal tyrosine hydroxylase activity

Pyridinolcarbamate molarity	Tyrosine hydroxylase activity
0	6.15 ±6.39
1×10^{2}	5.57 ±0.15
1×10^{-3}	6.50 ±0.37
1×10^{-4}	6.14 ±0.0
1×10^{-5}	7.15 ±0.44*

Rat adrenal tyrosine hydroxylase activity is expressed as mμmoles/15 min/mg protein ± standard deviation.
* Statistically significant, $p < 0.05$.

TABLE III

Effect of pyridinolcarbamate on adrenal tyrosine hydroxylase

Drug*	Activity**
Control	6.17 ±0.58
Pyridinolcarbamate	8.5 ±1.42***

* Pyridinolcarbamate 75 mg/kg was administered twice daily for 3 days and once on day 4 and rats killed 4 hours later.
** Tyrosine hydroxylase activity is expressed as mμmoles dopa/mg protein/hour. Results are the average ± standard deviation obtained from 3 control and 4 pyridinolcarbamate treated rats.
*** Statistically significant, $p < 0.05$.

consequence of an effect on the synthetic machinery. The one enzyme that one would initially think of is tyrosine hydroxylase since this is the rate-limiting step. In an in vitro study in which we incubated varying concentrations of pyridinolcarbamate and measured tyrosine hydroxylase activity, even at very high concentrations, there is no effect on this enzyme (Table II). At low concentrations, there may be an indication of an effect; however, we are highly skeptical of the results and our feeling is that we must do many more studies because it is difficult to understand why very low concentrations of the material would modify tyrosine hydroxylase while the high concentrations do not.

We decided to look at the effect of pyridinolcarbamate in vivo (Table III). Pyridinolcarbamate was administered to animals for a period of time and then we measured tyrosine hydroxylase activity and now we are beginning to see changes. This becomes an interesting possibility, as it might imply that continuous administration of the compound can increase or cause compensatory changes in the enzyme. There need not be an increase in the protein synthesis, but there may be some compensatory mechanism for an increase in tyrosine hydroxylase activity, to form more norepinephrine. As to whether this is a consequence of the vasodilating effect of pyridinolcarbamate, it is a possibility.

One could look at the effect of this material by measuring the endogenous content following pyridinolcarbamate. A more effective way of getting an insight as to what the compound does to catecholamines is to analyse the system. Using an inhibitor of tyrosine hydroxylase, we block the synthetic pathway. Since synthesis is not a component, one is looking at the other end of the equation, namely utilization.

When pyridinolcarbamate and α-methyltyrosine are combined, pyridinolcarbamate blocks the reduction caused by α-methyltyrosine. It may protect by affecting monoamine oxidase (a degradative enzyme) or by preventing the efflux of the catecholamine (Table IV).

Table V shows that in the brainstem there is an appreciable amount of catecholamine. Pyridinolcarbamate elicited a statistically significant elevation of catecholamine in the brain. Again, a blockade of synthesis caused a marked reduction in the endogenous content of the amine. However, when tyrosine hydroxylase inhibitor is combined with pyridinolcarbamate, there is an inhibition in the reduction. It almost resembles the type of picture that one sees with monoamine oxidase inhibitors. Dr. H. Hidaka (personal communication) has looked at the effect of pyridinolcarbamate on monoamine oxidase. He found that, in vitro, high concentrations of pyridinolcarbamate may have a slight inhibitory action on monoamine oxidase.

TABLE IV

Effect of pyridinolcarbamate on heart norepinephrine following inhibition of norepinephrine synthesis

Drug*	Dose (mg/kg)	Norepinephrine (mg/g)
Saline	–	1.25 ± 0.07
Pyridinolcarbamate	75, 75	1.12 ± 0.04
α-MPT	250	0.89 ± 0.06**
α-MPT + pyridinolcarbamate	250 + 75, 75	1.14 ± 0.07***

* α-MPT was given i.p. and rats killed 4 hours later; pyridinolcarbamate was given i.p., 2 hours apart, and rats killed 3 hours after the first dose. When both drugs were administered, α-MPT was given 1 hour prior to pyridinolcarbamate. Results are the average of 5 determinations ± standard error of the mean.

** Significantly different from saline injected rats, $p < 0.05$.

*** Significantly different from α-MPT injected rats, $p < 0.05$.

TABLE V

Effect of pyridinolcarbamate on brainstem norepinephrine following inhibition of norepinephrine synthesis

Drug*	Dose (mg/kg)	Norepinephrine (μg/g)
Saline	–	0.52 ± 0.03
Pyridinolcarbamate	75, 75	0.77 ± 0.03**
α-MPT	250	0.25 ± 0.04**
α-MPT + pyridinol-carbamate	250 + 75, 75	0.42 ± 0.01***

* α-MPT was given i.p. and rats killed 4 hours later; pyridinolcarbamate was given twice i.p., 2 hours apart, and rats killed 3 hours after the first dose. When both drugs were administered, α-MPT was given 1 hour prior to pyridinolcarbamate. Results are the average of 5 determinations ± standard error of the mean.

** Significantly different from saline injected rats, $p < 0.05$.

*** Significantly different from α-MPT injected rats, $p < 0.05$.

If one looks at the cortex (Table VI), this becomes an interesting area because here one finds not only norepinephrine but also dopamine. Again, the same pattern appears, namely pyridinolcarbamate will reverse the reduction of endogenous catecholamines caused by the administration of α-methyltyrosine.

The other biogenic amine that was of interest was serotonin. Previous speakers in this session have alluded to the fact that serotonin has a potent effect on the endothelial system and may cause alteration of permeability. If one looks at the effect of pyridinolcarbamate on the serotonin content, the same pattern emerges as with the catecholamine, namely an elevation in serotonin (Table VII). A possibility for the elevated serotonin content is that the precursor pool, namely tryptophan, may be altered by pyridinolcarbamate. However, the tryptophan content following pyridinolcarbamate is not altered. Thus, the elevation of serotonin is not a consequence of an alteration of the pool size of its precursor. Again, it might indicate an effect on monoamine oxidase. There are various possibilities that one might

TABLE VI

Effect of pyridinolcarbamate on cortex catecholamines following inhibition of catecholamine synthesis

Drug*	Dose (mg/kg)	Norepinephrine (μg/g)	Dopamine (μg/g)
Saline		0.38 ± 0.04	1.17 ± 0.20
Pyridinolcarbamate	75, 75	0.44 ± 0.05	1.02 ± 0.22
α-MPT	250	0.11 ± 0.01**	0.33 ± 0.08**
α-MPT + pyridinol-carbamate	250 + 75, 75	0.29 ± 0.02***	0.57 ± 0.17

* α-MPT was given i.p. and rats killed 4 hours later; pyridinolcarbamate was given i.p. twice and rats killed 3 hours after the first dose. When both drugs were administered, α-MPT was given 1 hour prior to pyridinolcarbamate. Results are the average of 5 determinations ± standard error of the mean.

** Significantly different from saline injected rats, $p < 0.05$.

*** Significantly different from α-MPT injected rats, $p < 0.05$.

TABLE VII

Effect of pyridinolcarbamate on brainstem serotonin and tryptophan

Drug*	Serotonin (μg/g)	Tryptophan (μg/g)
Saline	0.56 ±0.03	4.10 ±0.34
Pyridinolcarbamate	1.01 ±0.06**	4.77 ±0.20

* Pyridinolcarbamate was given in 2 doses of 75 mg/kg, 2 hours apart, and rats killed 3 hours after the first dose.
** Results are the average of 5 determinations ± standard error of the mean.

consider. The elevation of the biogenic amines reported may be the consequence of a blockade of an enzyme that degrades amines intraneuronally, namely monoamine oxidase. The other possibility is that pyridinolcarbamate prevents the efflux of the amines from the nerve ending. There are some interesting compounds that are now being used. One of the compounds that exerts an effect in this manner is lithium which has application in psychiatric conditions. The question might be raised as to whether pyridinolcarbamate acts like lithium. I raise this question because administration of pyridinolcarbamate can cause behavioral changes. However, you may never see behavioral changes unless pyridinolcarbamate is administered to a patient suffering from a particular affective mental disorder analogous to that for which lithium is used. My colleague, Dr. Berkowitz, will discuss another aspect of this problem.

REFERENCE

TANABE, T., TAKAGI, M., KATO, K. and WATANABE, S.: In: *Proceedings, II Symposium on Effect of Anginin on Peripheral Vascular Diseases.* Banyu Pharmaceutical Co., Ltd., Tokyo.

For discussion, see p. 146.

THE EFFECTS OF PYRIDINOLCARBAMATE ON BLOOD VESSELS, HEART AND BRAIN BIOGENIC AMINES (DISCUSSION)

B. A. BERKOWITZ, H. HIDAKA and S. SPECTOR
Roche Institute of Molecular Biology, Nutley, N.J., U.S.A.

It is important to emphasize that a drug which has an ability to improve peripheral vascular blood flow may do so by a number of possible mechanisms.

Our studies demonstrate that pyridinolcarbamate can influence blood vessels directly by affecting the norepinephrine content of heart and blood vessels. Since the pyridinolcarbamate is a weak monoamine oxidase inhibitor, blockade of this enzyme may be important in the cardiovascular effects produced. It is interesting to recall that one of the classes of drugs which have been used to treat hypertension is monoamine oxidase inhibitors. The possibility that pyridinolcarbamate, like some monoamine oxidase inhibitors, can decrease release of neuronal norepinephrine should also be explored further.

Increasing attention is being given to central nervous system regulation of blood pressure and the potential of drugs to modify cardiovascular activity by an action on the brain. Pyridinolcarbamate was shown by us to raise the levels of brain norepinephrine and serotonin. Drugs which modify the disposition of central nervous system neurotransmitters may thus exert effects not only on behavior but also on peripheral systems modulated by central control centers. A future area of investigation might also consider drug effects on any central control of lipid metabolism and free fatty acid mobilization.

We know that behavioral stress and hypertension facilitate atherogenesis. Shimamoto and colleagues have demonstrated that application of catecholamines as well as other biogenic amines produces marked atherogenic-like effects on vascular smooth muscle. Nothing, however, is known of the effects of atherogenesis on the nervous system in blood vessels or other areas. We have begun studies to answer this question and have obtained some interesting preliminary results.

We fed rabbits a diet containing 1 % cholesterol for 6 weeks and then analyzed the tissues for catecholamines. Heart and brain norepinephrine levels were unchanged, although

TABLE I

Effect of cholesterol feeding on rabbit blood vessel and adrenal tyrosine hydroxylase activity

Tissue	Treatment	Tyrosine hydroxylase activity
Adrenal	Control	1.63 ± 0.02
	Cholesterol	0.95 ± 0.04*
Mesenteric artery	Control	0.55 ± 0.06
	Cholesterol	1.69 ± 0.35*
Mesenteric vein	Control	0.30 ± 0.10
	Cholesterol	1.05 ± 0.33*

* Significantly different from control, $p < 0.05$.

vascular norepinephrine content may have been diminished. Vascular tyrosine hydroxylase activity was increased several fold. In contrast, no increase occurred in adrenal tyrosine hydroxylase activity. The specific effects of a high cholesterol diet on the vascular sympathetic nervous system are of interest and we are continuing our studies in this area (Table I).

To summarize our findings, pyridinolcarbamate may influence biogenic amines in many organs including the heart, blood vessels, adrenals, and brain. Cholesterol feeding and subsequent vascular plaques may alter the disposition and regulation of the vascular neurotransmitter, norepinephrine.

For discussion, see p. 146.

EFFECT OF PYRIDINOLCARBAMATE AND CHOLESTEROL ON THE CONCENTRATION OF TISSUE NOREPINEPHRINE AND SEROTONIN IN THE RABBIT

H. HIDAKA

Section of Neurochemistry, Institute of Development Research,
Aichi Prefecture Colony, Aichi-ken, Japan

I would like to show the results of our study which was done in collaboration with Dr. Shimamoto, Dr. Numano and Dr. Spector. Table I shows the effect of pyridinolcarbamate and cholesterol on the concentration of norepinephrine and serotonin in the mesenteric arteries and the brains of rabbits which were fed on 1% cholesterol for 3 months. Pyridinolcarbamate was administered orally, 10 mg/kg, once a day. Details are given in the paper by Numano et al. (*This Volume*, pp. 98–112). The most interesting phenomenon is the reduction in norepinephrine after the administration of cholesterol. This reduction in norepinephrine in the mesenteric arteries was prevented by the administration of pyridinolcarbamate. But the levels of norepinephrine and serotonin in the brain remained unchanged, and the reduction in norepinephrine occurred only in the blood vessels. This is not so surprising, because arterial walls were badly damaged and nerve terminals had probably degenerated. It should be noticed that administration of pyridinolcarbamate prevents the reduction in norepinephrine in blood vessels.

TABLE I

The effect of pyridinolcarbamate (PDC) on the content of noradrenaline and serotonin in various tissues of cholesterol-fed rabbits

Tissue	Drug	NA (μg/g)	Serotonin (μg/g)
Heart	Control	1.57 ± 0.09	–
	Cholesterol	1.22 ± 0.15*	–
	Cholesterol + PDC	1.60 ± 0.22	–
Mesenteric artery	Control	1.90 ± 0.29	–
	Cholesterol	0.90 ± 0.18*	–
	Cholesterol + PDC	2.27 ± 0.32	–
Brain	Control	0.197 ± 0.03	0.148 ± 0.02
	Cholesterol	0.165 ± 0.03	0.160 ± 0.01
	Cholesterol + PDC	0.180 ± 0.04	0.165 ± 0.02

* Rabbits were treated with placebo or 10 mg/kg/day of pyridinolcarbamate under cholesterol feeding for 15 weeks (see Numano et al., *This Volume*, pp. 98–112).

As far as serotonin levels in the rat brain are concerned, Dr. Spector showed increase in serotonin after administration of pyridinolcarbamate. I have no answer to the question why rabbit brain is different from rat brain with regard to the effect of pyridinolcarbamate.

DISCUSSION

Dr. CRAIG: I was fascinated by Dr. Spector's suggestion that pyridinolcarbamate may cause behaviour changes. During a clinical trial in which we gave it to 33 patients, several of them complained of lethargy and depression and early waking. This was a spontaneous comment. One elderly man with a history of depression became suicidal on a high dose.

Dr. TERRY: Did you, by any chance, also try to determine norepinephrine in plasma?

Dr. SPECTOR: The difficulty with this is that we really lack a very good method for measuring plasma levels of norepinephrine.

Dr. AUSTIN: Dr. Spector, I wonder if in addition you considered the possibility that pyridinolcarbamate was producing an increase in the reuptake of norepinephrine? One might test this by giving, say, labelled norepinephrine and seeing if more were taken up.

Dr. SPECTOR: Pyridinolcarbamate does not block norepinephrine uptake. We have not looked at the reuptake mechanism, and our general feeling is that it is not involved here.

HISTOCHEMICAL ANALYSIS OF TISSUE CATECHOLAMINE IN THE ARTERIES OF CHOLESTEROL-FED RABBITS TREATED WITH PYRIDINOLCARBAMATE, ESTROGEN AND PROGESTERONE

KIKUO MOHRI[1] and FUJIO NUMANO[2]
[1] Department of Surgery, Kansai Ika-daigaku Medical School and Second Department of Surgery, Medical School, Kyoto University, Kyoto and [2] Department of Medicine, School of Medicine, Tokyo Ika-Shika National University, Tokyo, Japan

The antiatherosclerotic effects of pyridinolcarbamate and estrogen, both of which have a preventive effect on the acute edematous vascular injury of cholesterol-fed rabbits, have been studied by Numano et al. (1971). Comparative fluorescent histochemical changes in adrenergic innervation or noradrenaline content of the acute injured artery of cholesterol-fed rabbits and the artery of pyridinolcarbamate- and estrogen-treated rabbits, were studied in this report.

MATERIALS AND METHODS

40 healthy albino rabbits, 6 months old, were used in this series. The diet (RC-5) was prepared by the Oriental Yeast Co., Ltd. and contained 1% of cholesterol by weight. The rabbits were divided into 4 equal groups. The first group received a placebo capsule, the second received daily doses of estrogen 1 mg/kg and the third received daily doses of progesterone 1 mg/kg. The fourth group received pyridinolcarbamate in daily doses of 10 mg/kg.

After medication, all rabbits were given water and 100 g of the cholesterol-containing diet. The diet was continued for 15 weeks, then all rabbits were sacrificed. The daily food consumption of rabbits, body weight and the serum cholesterol level were checked. The aortas and the superior mesenteric arteries of the rabbits were studied by the fluorescent histochemical techniques of Falck and Fujiwara. Immediately after excision, the specimens were freeze-dried, treated with paraformaldehyde, embedded in paraffin, sectioned (5–7.5 μ) and mounted in Entellan for fluorescence microscopy. Sections adjacent to those for fluorescence microscopy were stained with hematoxylin-eosin.

RESULTS

Superior mesenteric artery

Normal distribution of adrenergic nerves to the superior mesenteric artery is in the outer layer of the media and also in the adventitia. Specific noradrenaline fluorescence is observed in the outer layer of the media of the artery in normal rabbits (Fig. 1). On the other hand, there were significant differences in the fluorescent histochemical features of the noradrenaline fluorescence of the superior mesenteric artery between the control cholesterol-fed rabbits and the normal rabbits. Little noradrenaline fluorescence was found in the media of the artery in the controls (Fig. 2).

Noradrenaline fluorescence in the smooth muscle layer of the media of the artery was not so greatly affected by cholesterol feeding in the rabbits treated with pyridinolcarbamate, and it was significantly seen in the smooth muscle layer of the media of the artery. No marked difference in noradrenaline fluorescence was observed between the artery of the

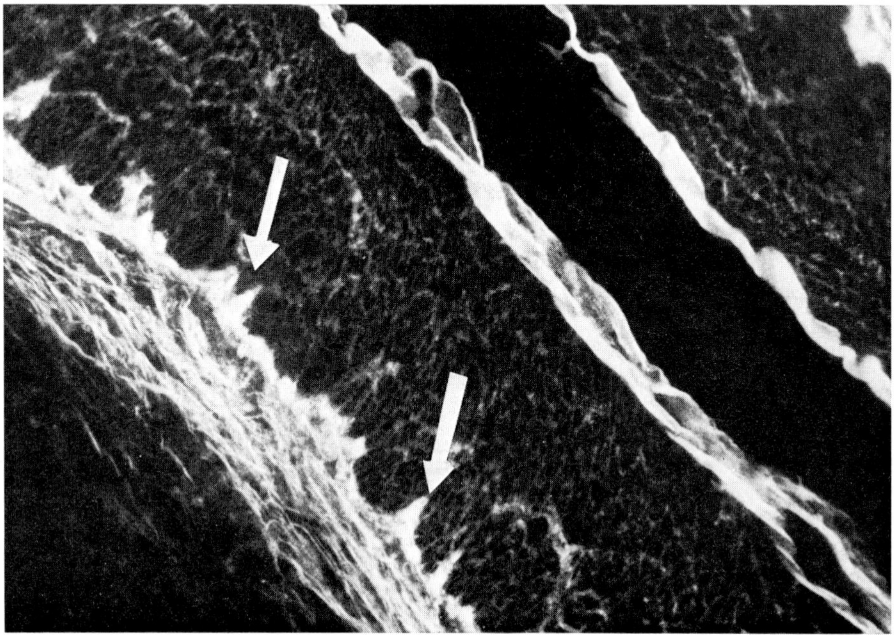

Fig. 1. Noradrenaline fluorescence (↓) in the superior mesenteric artery of a normal rabbit. × 128.

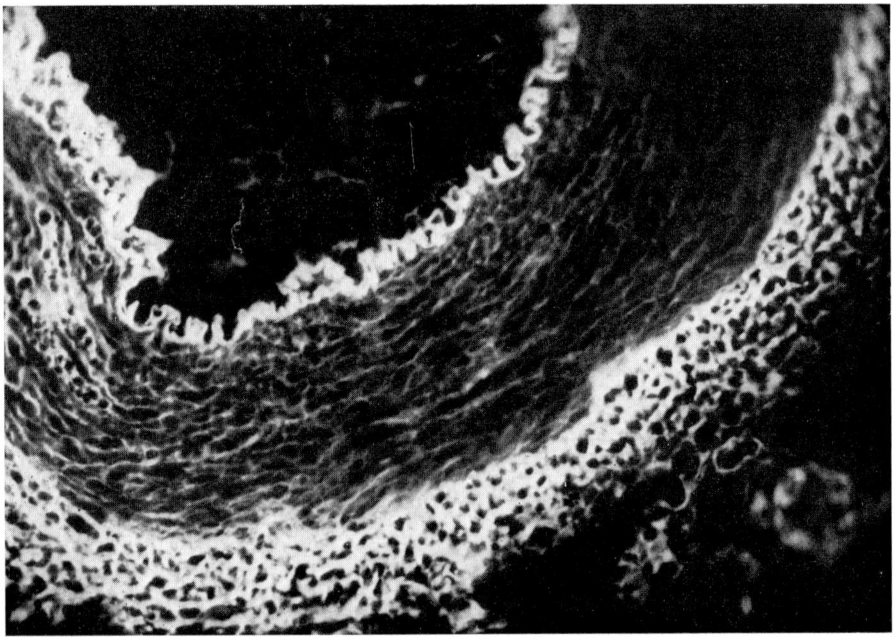

Fig. 2. No noradrenaline fluorescence in the superior mesenteric artery of a control cholesterol-fed rabbit. × 128.

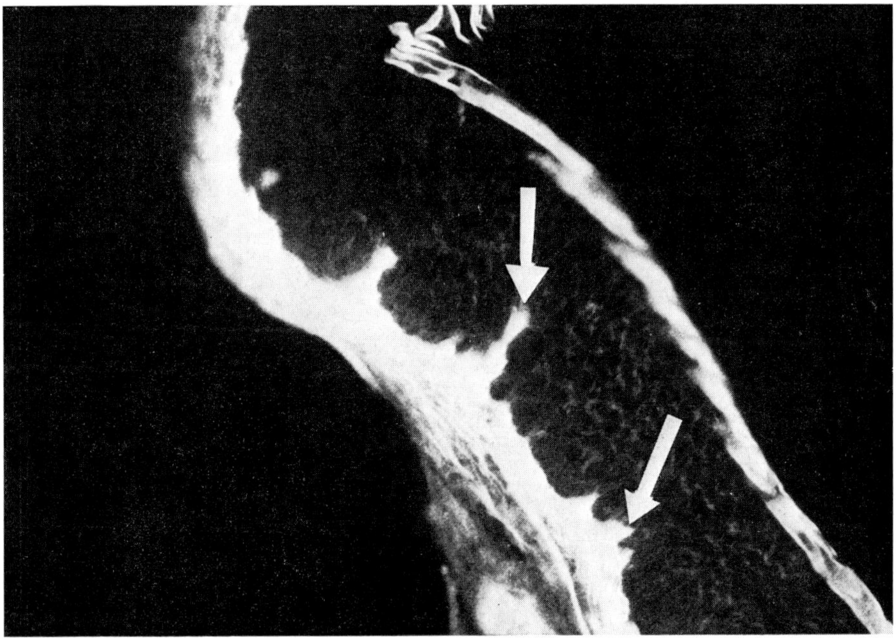

Fig. 3. Noradrenaline fluorescence (↓) in the superior mesenteric artery of a pyridinolcarbamate-treated rabbit, fed on a cholesterol-containing diet. × 128.

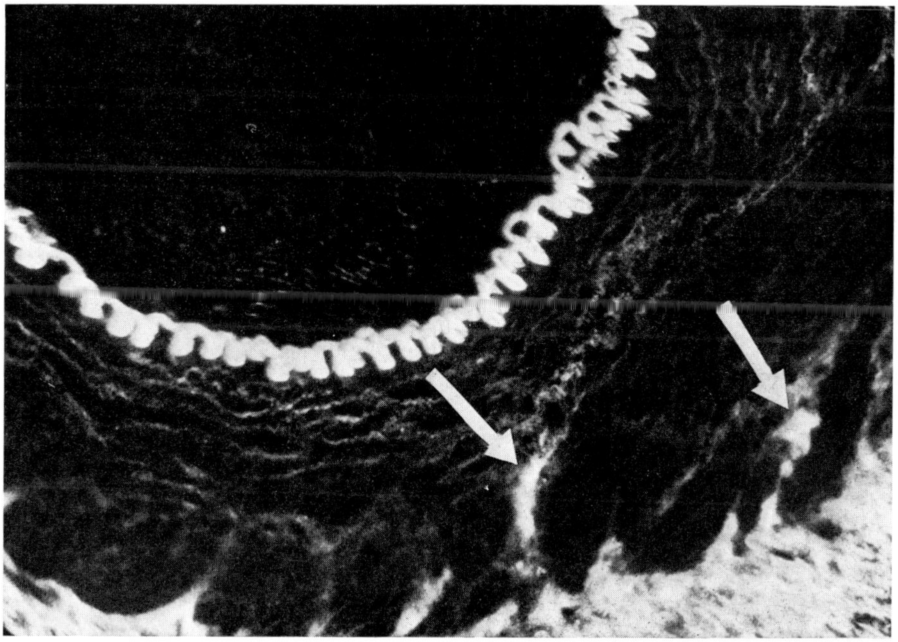

Fig. 4. Noradrenaline fluorescence (↓) in the superior mesenteric artery of an estrogen-treated rabbit, fed on a cholesterol-containing diet. × 128.

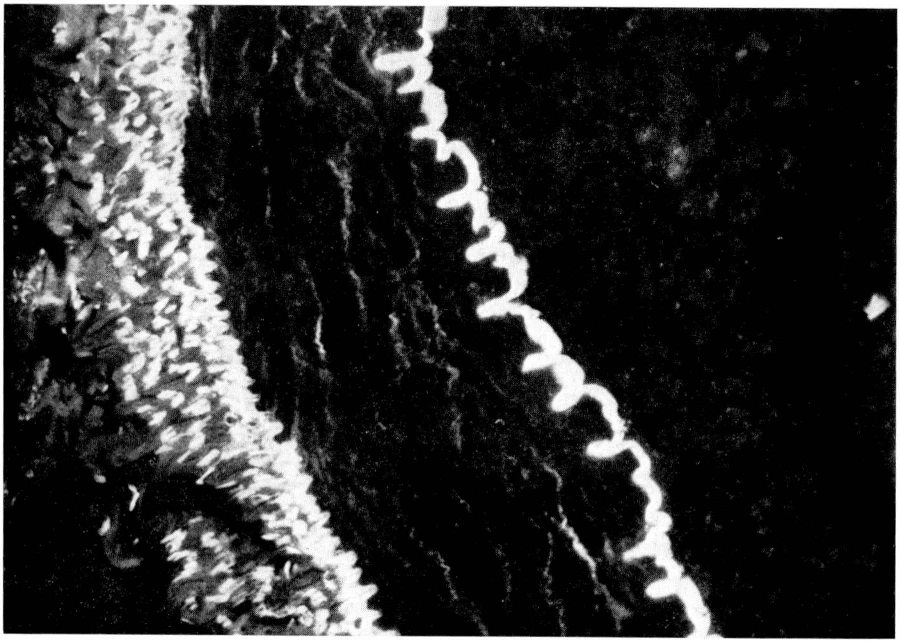

Fig. 5. No noradrenaline fluorescence in the superior mesenteric artery of a progesterone-treated rabbit, fed on a cholesterol-containing diet. × 128.

normal rabbits and the artery of the pyridinolcarbamate-treated rabbits which had the cholesterol-containing diet (Fig. 3). Noradrenaline fluorescence was also seen in the media of the artery of cholesterol-fed rabbits treated with estrogen (Fig. 4). Noradrenaline fluorescence was never observed in the media of the artery of cholesterol-fed rabbits treated with progesterone (Fig. 5).

Aorta

No definite results were obtained from the noradrenaline fluorescence of the aorta of the cholesterol-fed rabbits treated with pyridinolcarbamate, estrogen and progesterone. This needs further investigation.

DISCUSSION

Noradrenaline fluorescence of the artery represents the adrenergic nerve of the artery (Mohri et al., 1969; Tsunekawa et al., 1967). Histological and histochemical studies (Numano et al., 1971) indicate marked degenerative changes of the vascular wall in the cholesterol-fed rabbit. Therefore, the adrenergic nervous system of the vascular wall is assumed also to be affected by cholesterol feeding. Our results show that pyridinolcarbamate prevents the decrease in noradrenaline fluorescence in the vascular wall. Therefore, pyridinolcarbamate has perhaps a preventive effect on the degeneration of the adrenergic nerve of the vascular wall in the cholesterol-fed rabbit. The reason for the preventive effect on nerve degeneration by pyridinolcarbamate and the mechanism of noradrenaline increase by pyridinolcarbamate have not yet been completely clarified.

The antidegenerative effect on adrenergic nerve could possibly be a factor in the anti-atheromatous effect of pyridinolcarbamate. The data from noradrenaline chemical assay of the vascular wall by Hidaka (*This Volume*, p. 145) support these histochemical results. It is well known that estrogen is assumed to protect against atherosclerosis, but its mechanism is not yet clear. The increase in the collagen content in the vascular wall by the administration of estrogen has possibly an important role in the antiatherosclerotic effect and the antidegenerative effect of the adrenergic nerve of the vascular wall. Decrease in the noradrenaline content of the vascular wall by the administration of progesterone corresponds with the histologically extensive degenerative changes in the vascular wall caused by progesterone.

SUMMARY

Noradrenaline fluorescence of the superior mesenteric artery of the rabbit is clearly decreased by cholesterol diet. No significant noradrenaline fluorescence was observed in the media of the superior mesenteric artery of the cholesterol-fed rabbits. Decrease in the noradrenaline fluorescence of the artery by cholesterol diet was markedly inhibited by the administration of pyridinolcarbamate or estrogen, but promoted by administration of progesterone. The anti-decreasing effect of noradrenaline by the administration of pyridinolcarbamate is presumably one of the mechanisms for its antiatherosclerotic effect.

REFERENCES

FUJIWARA, M. (1967): Fluorescence histochemistry of catecholamine and serotonin. *Saisin-igaku, 22*, 10.

MOHRI, K., TSUNEKAWA, K. et al. (1969): Histochemical demonstration of adrenergic fibers in the smooth muscle layer of media of arteries supplying abdominal organs. *Arch. jap. Chir., 38/1*, 236.

NUMANO, F., SHIMAMOTO, T. et al. (1971): Comparative studies on the preventive effect of pyridinol-carbamate and estrogen against aortic and coronary atherosclerosis of cholesterol-fed rabbits. *Acta path. jap., 21/2*, 177, 193.

TSUNEKAWA, K., MOHRI, K. et al. (1967): Histochemical demonstration of adrenergic fibers in the smooth muscle layer of media of dorsal pedal artery in dog. *Experientia (Basel), 23*, 842.

INFLUENCE OF MAST CELL DEGRANULATION ON VENULAR PERMEABILITY

MASAHARU TSUCHIYA, MASAYA ODA, YUKIYOSHI KAMISAKA and CHIKARA OHSHIO
Department of Internal Medicine, School of Medicine, Keio University, Tokyo, Japan

At the First International Symposium on Atherogenesis, Thrombogenesis and Pyridinolcarbamate Treatment in 1969, the authors (Tsuchiya et al., 1969*a*) presented the cinematographic observation of intravascular platelet aggregation following mechanical injuries to the endothelium of mesenteric microvessels by micropuncture and the preventive effect of pyridinolcarbamate on platelet aggregation when injected intravenously in a dose of 5 mg/kg rat body weight preceding the mechanical injuries. At the International Microcirculation Conference in Aalborg in 1970, it was reported by the authors (Oda et al., 1971) that pyridinolcarbamate can improve microcirculatory disorders. In fact, pyridinolcarbamate suppressed vascular permeability, formation of emboli, swelling and degranulation of platelets, and plasminogen activation during the process of thrombus formation.

The present study is designed to demonstrate the role of mast cells in increased vascular permeability and the preventive effect of pyridinolcarbamate on mast cell degranulation.

MATERIALS AND METHODS

Cholera toxin was used to induce an increase in vascular permeability and degranulation of mast cells. This toxin was obtained from the filtrate of strain 569 B and has a potency of about 10,000–50,000 blueing doses. One blueing dose (BD) is the minimal amount of the toxin which produces an end-point reaction (10 × 10 mm) in Menkin's method. The material used in this experiment was previously dialysed against Ringer's solution.

For the observation of the in vivo vascular responses in the mesentery, male rats of the Wistar strain weighing about 200 g were used. The rat, anesthesized by intraperitoneal injection of 2 mg/kg body weight thiopental sodium, was placed in the supine position on a board. After shaving the skin, a midline incision was made in the neck and the abdomen. A vinyl canule was inserted into the left jugular vein, the mesentery was exposed on a glass slide and observed under a phase-contrast microscope. During observation a part of the ileum of the animal was pulled out of the peritoneal cavity and kept humid by covering with pieces of cotton soaked in Ringer's solution containing 1 % gelatin in a chamber maintained at 38 °C.

3 min after the intravenous administration of the toxin, 4 % pontamine sky-blue 6B was injected into the jugular vein. For the morphological observation of extravascular mast cells following application of the cholera toxin, the rat mesentery was promptly fixed with 99.5 % alcohol and stained with toluidine blue according to the method of Villavicencio and De Takats (1963) as shown in Table I. This method is a reasonable technique to calculate mast cell degranulation. In a 1 mm^2 area of the rat mesentery, about 70 normal mast cells were found around a venule of about 50 μ in caliber in the untreated animal (Fig. 1*). The cytoplasmic granules of the mast cells contain many vasoactive substances (Selye, 1965; Smith, 1963).

For the closer observation of the individual granule, it is better to utilize Bloom's technique (1965) in which the materials were also embedded in epoxy resin. Sections 1 μ thick of repre-

* Figures 1–8, see p. 156 a-d

TABLE I

Mast cell staining method (rat mesentery)
(Villavicencio and De Takats, 1963)

Ether anesthesia
ǀ
Laparotomy
ǀ
Spread the mesentery on the slide
ǀ
Free mesenteric attachment
ǀ
Fix in absolute alcohol for 7 hours
ǀ
Rinse with water
ǀ
Stain for 15 sec with 0.1% toluidine blue
ǀ
Rinse for 2 sec with 95% alcohol
ǀ
Clear through xylene for 5 hours

sentative venules were stained with 1% methylene blue at pH 10.0 or 4% toluidine blue at pH 10.9 (Figs. 2 and 3).

The effect of pyridinolcarbamate on mast cell degranulation induced by cholera toxin was compared with the effect of other drugs known to be antagonistic to the toxin and provoking an increase in vascular permeability. Prednisolone 1 mg/kg, chlorpromazine 5 mg/kg, ethacrynic acid 50 mg/kg, cycloheximide 5 mg/kg, leupeptin 50 mg/kg, and pyridinolcarbamate 3 mg/kg were respectively given intravenously 3 min prior to cholera toxin injection. Furthermore, it was investigated whether or not the protective effect of pyridinolcarbamate was directly on the mast cells. Pyridinolcarbamate (3 mg/kg) was given intravenously 3 min prior to the intravenous administration of compound 48/80 in a dose of 2 mg/kg. 3 min after the injection of compound 48/80 morphological observation of the mast cells was carried out. In each experimental group 5 rats of Wistar strain weighing 200 g were used.

RESULTS

1. Cholera toxin given intravenously is able to induce increase in vascular permeability. The phenomenon is just the same as that induced by intravenous injection of histamine (0.1 mg/kg) or serotonin (0.01 mg/kg). 3 min after intravenous injection of 0.5 ml of cholera toxin, pontamine sky-blue started to leak out of the venule. The maximal intensity of the dye was observed 10 min after the injection of the toxin. It should be stressed that the extravasation of the dye takes place first along the venules and not along the arterioles (Figs. 4, 5 and 6).
2. Previous administration of the above-mentioned drugs prevents the increase in the vascular permeability induced by cholera toxin.
3. When the toxin is intravenously injected, extravascular mast cells found in the connective tissue become significantly degranulated (Table II) and the released granules migrate towards the blood vessel (Figs. 7 and 8). These findings suggest that histamine and serotonin contained in these granules appear to contribute, from outside the vessels, to the increase in vascular permeability.

TABLE II

Degranulation of mast cells induced by cholera toxin (rat mesentery)

Treatment	No. of mast cells		Statistical evaluation (χ^2-test)
	Counted*	Degranulated*	
Non-treated	72	8 (11 %)	—
Cholera toxin** (i.v.)	77	46 (59 %)	Significant ($p < 0.001$)

* No. of mast cells per 1 mm² was counted 3 min after treatment.
** 500 BD of toxin 569B was given.

TABLE III

Degranulation of mast cells by cholera toxin and inhibitory effect of some drugs (intravenous injection of toxin)*

Pretreatment (i.v.) Drug Dose	No. of mast cells (per mm²)		Statistical evaluation (χ^2-test)
	Counted	Degranulated	
(Toxin alone)	77	46 (59 %)	—
Ethacrynic acid (50 mg/kg)	86	10 (11 %)	$p < 0.001$
Cycloheximide (25 mg/kg)	57	25 (43 %)	$p < 0.01$
Chlorpromazine (5 mg/kg)	77	14 (18 %)	$p < 0.001$
Leupeptins (50 mg/kg)	87	12 (13 %)	$p < 0.001$
Pyridinolcarbamate (3 mg/kg)	69	8 (11 %)	$p < 0.001$
Prednisolone (5 mg/kg)	70	3 (4 %)	$p < 0.001$

* 500 BD of toxin 569B was injected intravenously, 3 min after pretreatment. 3 min later, the tissue was fixed for mast cell counts.

TABLE IV

Degranulation of mast cells (rat mesentery)

Treatment		No. mast cells (per mm²)		Statistical evaluation (χ^2-test)
		Counted	Degranulated	
Non-treated		72	8 (11 %)	—
Histamine (0.1 mg/kg i.v.)	3 min	64	4 (6 %)	$p > 0.05$
	6 min	98	22 (22 %)	$p > 0.05$
	10 min	53	36 (67 %)	$p < 0.001$
Compound 48/80 (2 mg/kg i.v.)	3 min	62	58 (99 %)	$p < 0.001$
	6 min	67	67 (100 %)	$p < 0.001$
	10 min	67	60 (98 %)	$p < 0.001$

4. The drugs, which have been reported to counteract the increasing action of the toxin in increasing permeability, suppress significantly thede granulation of the mast cells (Table III).

5. Compound 48/80, which is a histamine-releasing factor, degranulates 99 % of the mast cells in 3 min, whereas histamine degranulates only 6 %. However, under in vivo observation, histamine can induce extravasation of the dye from the vessels more markedly after 3 min and extravasation of the dye reaches a maximum in 10 min, at which time degranulation of the mast cells reaches 67 %. Compound 48/80 hardly induces extravasation of the dye after 6 min but degranulation of mast cells had already taken place in 3 min (Table IV).

6. When the animals were pretreated with pyridinolcarbamate, extravasation of the dye was well suppressed both in histamine treated and compound 48/80 treated groups. Pyridinolcarbamate exerted a very strong inhibitory effect on mast cell degranulation (Table V).

TABLE V

Effect of pyridinolcarbamate on mast cells (rat mesentery)

Treatment	No. of mast cells (per mm^2)		Statistical evaluation (χ^2-test)
	Counted	Degranulated	
Non-treated	72	8 (11 %)	—
Compound 48/80 (0.1 mg/kg i.v.) (3 min)	62	58 (99 %)	$p < 0.001$
Pyridinolcarbamate and compound 48/80 (3 min)	66	17 (25 %)	$p > 0.05$

COMMENT

The method of in vivo observation of the microcirculatory system of the rat mesentery established by Chambers and Zweifach (1944) provides a useful tool not only for the study of rheology but also of intravascular components, vascular permeability and extravascular factors. By this method any blood vessels studied by the researcher are easily damaged by a microtrauma and the lesion can be fixed with osmic acid for electron-microscopic study of the processes of bleeding, hemostasis and thrombogenesis. The endothelial layer of the vessels with increased permeability is further investigated with intravenous administration of ferritin or Thorotrast.

The mast cell is one of the extravascular factors including collagen, reticulin and elastin which appear to be of importance in relation to vascular permeability. In this regard, the mesentery is frequently used for experiments to study the relationships between pathophysiological changes in the vessels and perivascular mast cell morphology.

While investigating the importance of vascular permeability in the pathogenesis of cholera diarrhea, it was found that cholera toxin increased the permeability of the venules and degranulated the perivascular mast cells (Tsuchiya et al., 1972). The effects of pyridinolcarbamate have been tested on toxin-induced vascular permeability and mast cell degranulation.

Prednisolone and chlorpromazine have been known to behave as antagonists to the effects of bradykinin, histamine and serotonin (Tsuchiya et al., 1967, 1969*b*). Ethacrynic acid was reported to have a therapeutic effect on experimental cholera in a canine model (Carpenter et al., 1969), and cycloheximide was also reported to prevent cholera toxin induced fluid production by the small bowel as well as edema in the foot pad model (Serebro et al., 1969).

Leupeptin is a new protease inhibitor which has been isolated from an actinomycete by Aoyagi et al. (1969). Leupeptin strongly inhibits proteolytic activities of plasmin, trypsin and papain but not that of chymotrypsin. It also inhibits thrombokinase and coagulation of human or rabbit blood and weakly inhibits the esterase activity of plasmin and trypsin. Oral administration of leupeptin suppresses edema induced by carrageenin in rats. It is very interesting that such various kinds of drugs show antagonistic effects to cholera toxin. However, the specific activity of these drugs responsible for their counteraction against the cholera toxin has not yet been determined. It is also still uncertain whether suppression of the increase in vascular permeability by these drugs results from prevention of functional changes in the endothelium or from inhibition of mast cell degranulation. If pyridinolcarbamate directly affects the mast cell, it seems necessary to know whether the effect of compound 48/80 (a polymer of *N*-methylhomoanisylamine and formaldehyde) will be inhibited by pyridinolcarbamate. This is because the degranulation of the mast cell is induced by the primary effect of compound 48/80, whereas histamine has a secondary effect on the cells.

The results obtained in this paper also indicate that compound 48/80 first degranulates the mast cell. After discharge, these granules could then play an important role in increasing the vascular permeability, particularly of the venules. On the other hand, histamine primarily affects the endothelial cells of the venules resulting in increase in vascular permeability and secondarily induces the degranulation of the mast cells through the leakage of plasma factors from the blood vessel. It was shown that pyridinolcarbamate exerts a direct effect not only on the endothelial cell but also on the mast cell.

CONCLUSION

The importance of mast cell degranulation for the increase in vascular permeability and the preventive effect of pyridinolcarbamate on these phenomena were reported.

Studies of the effects of pyridinolcarbamate upon the microcirculation yielded lots of interesting findings as shown in Figure 9. Namely, this drug would simultaneously affect the blood stream, the microvessels themselves and the perivascular components.

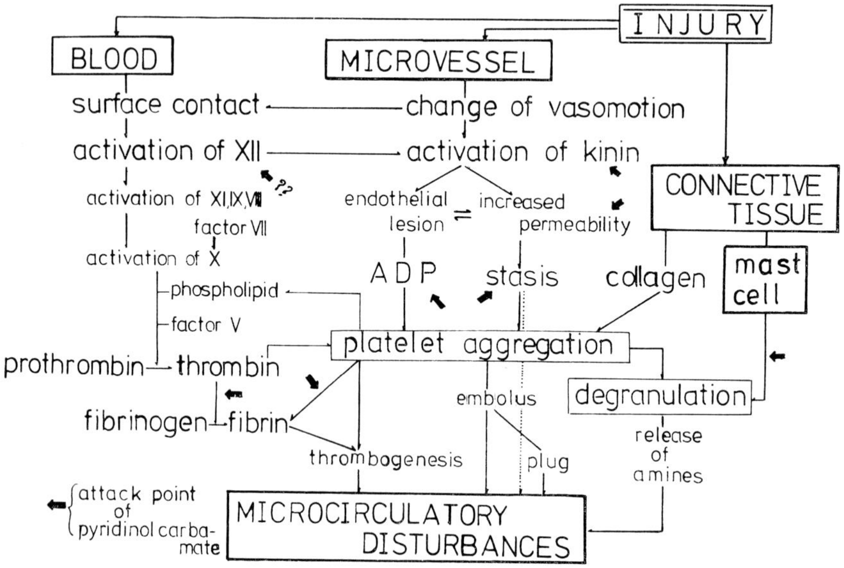

Fig. 9.

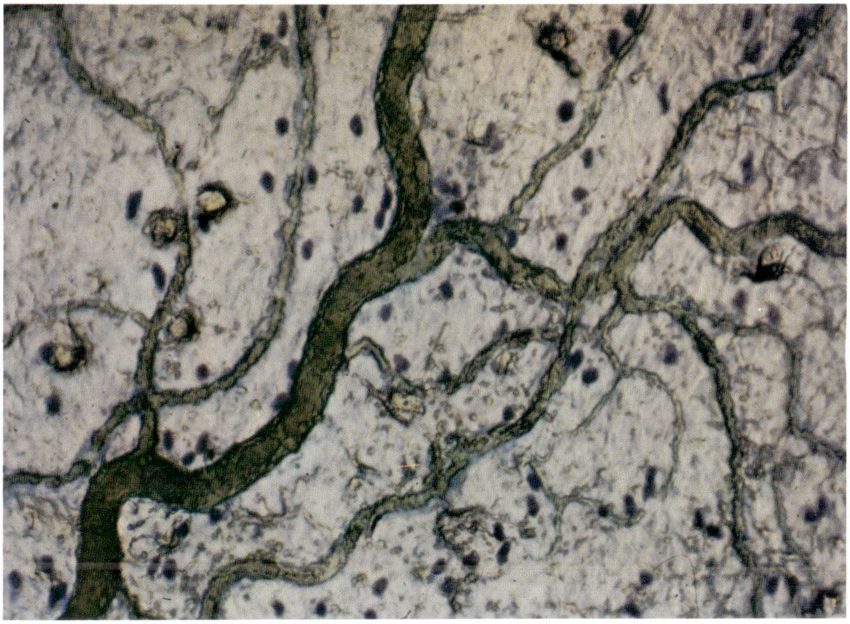

Fig. 1. Normal mast cell distribution in rat mesentery, stained with toluidine blue after fixation with absolute alcohol. x 100.

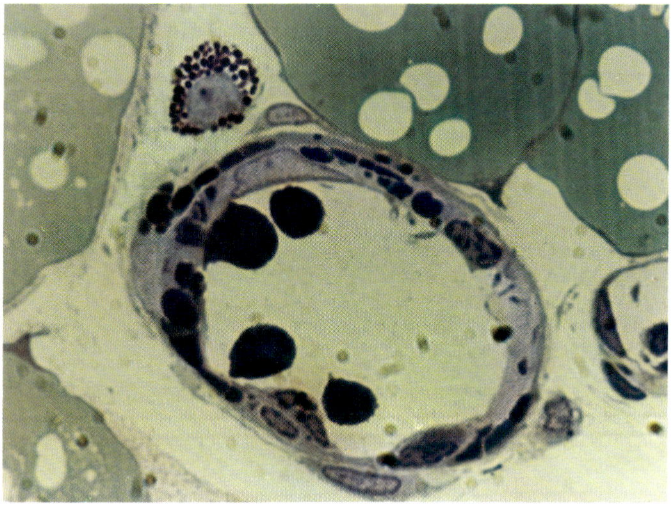

Fig. 2. Normal mast cell around a venule of rat mesentery, stained with toluidine blue after fixation in osmium tetroxide. x 100.

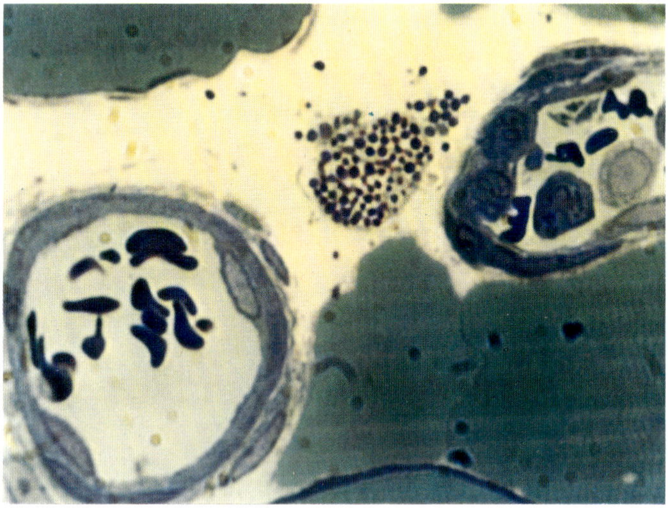

Fig. 3. Degranulated mast cell. x 1000.

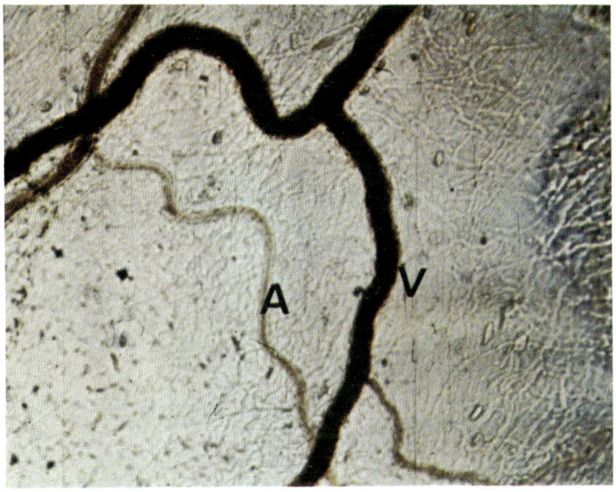

Fig. 4. Microcirculatory bed of rat mesentery before intravenous injection of cholera toxin.

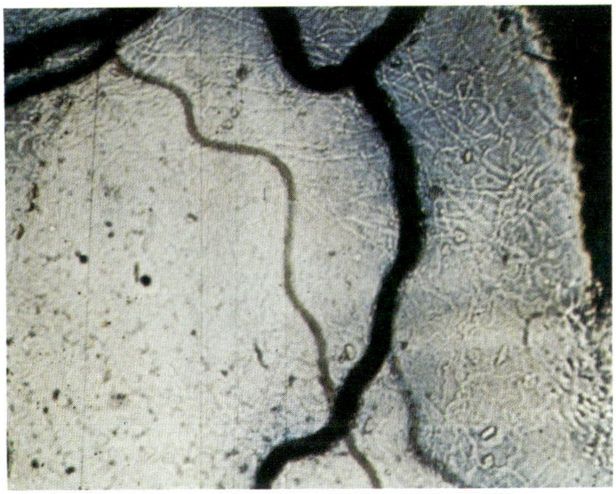

Fig. 5. Three minutes later.

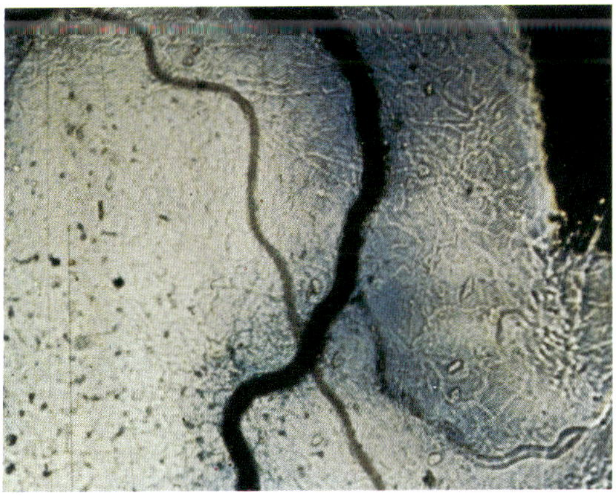

Fig. 6. Ten minutes later.

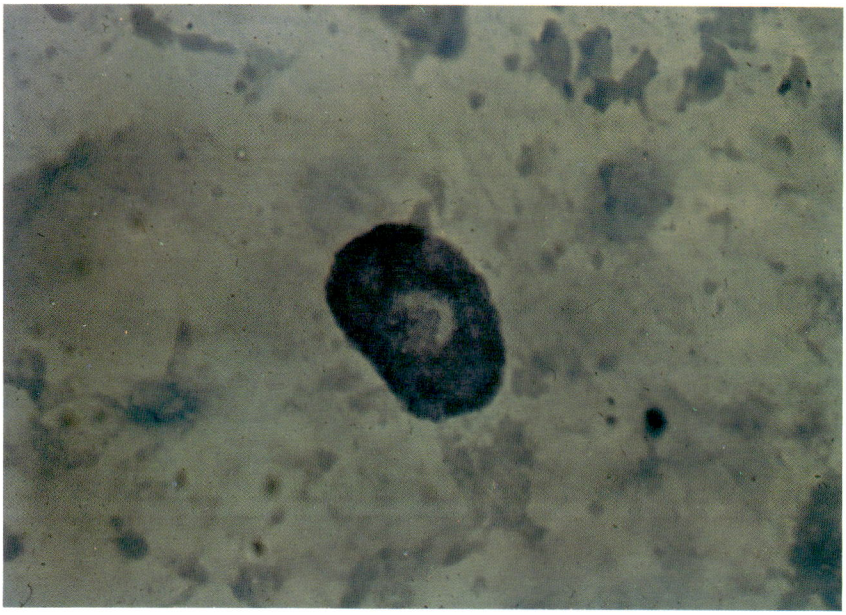

Fig. 7. Normal appearance of mast cell. x 1200.

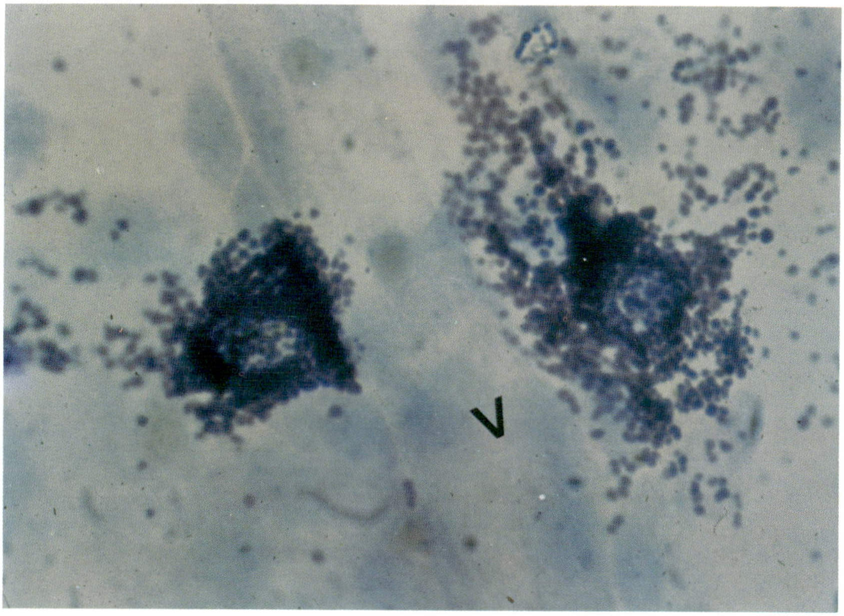

Fig. 8. Degranulation of mast cells. V= small venule. x 1300.

REFERENCES

AOYAGI, T., MIYATA, S., NANBO, M., KOJIMA, F., MATSUZAKI, M., ISHIZUKA, M., TAKEUCHI, T. and UMEZAWA, H. (1969): Biological activities of leupeptins. *J. Antibiot. (Tokyo)*, *22*, 558.

BLOOM, G. D. (1965): Structural and biochemical characteristics of mast cells in the inflammatory process. In: *The Inflammatory Process*, pp. 355–383. Academic Press, New York–London.

CARPENTER, C. C. J., CURLIN, G. T. and GREENOUGH, W. B. (1969): Response of canine Thirty-Vella jejunal loops to cholera endotoxin and its modification by ethacrynic acid. *J. infect. Dis.*, 120, 332.

CHAMBERS, R. and ZWEIFACH, B. W. (1944): Topography and function of the mesenteric circulation. *Amer. J. Anat.*, *75*, 173.

ODA, M., TSUCHIYA, M., SHISHIDO, T., KAMISAKA, Y. and YOSHIMATSU, H. (1971): Effect of pyridinolcarbamate on the thrombogenesis following vascular damage. In: *Proceedings, VI European Conference on Microcirculation, Aalborg 1970*, pp. 387–393. Editors: J. Ditzel and D. H. Lewis. S. Karger, Basel.

SELYE, H. (1965): *The Mast Cells*. Butterworths, Washington, D.C.

SEREBRO, H. A., IBER, F. L., YARDLEY, J. H. and HENDRIX, T. R. (1969): Inhibition of cholera toxin action in the rabbit by cycloheximide. *Gastroenterology*, *56*, 506.

SMITH, D. E. (1963): The tissue mast cell. *Int. Rev. Cytol.*, *14*, 327.

TSUCHIYA, M., FUZISHIRO, Y. and SHISHIDO, T. (1969*a*): Observation vitale de la thrombogenèse. In: *Atherogenesis. Proceedings, I International Symposium on Atherogenesis, Thrombogenesis and Pyridinolcarbamate Treatment, Tokyo 1969*, pp. 145–150. Editors: T. Shimamoto and F. Numano. ICS 201, Excerpta Medica, Amsterdam.

TSUCHIYA, M., KAMISAKA, Y., OHASHI, M. and SHIMADA, T. (1972): Effect of cholera toxin on the microcirculatory bed and the mast cells in the rat's mesentery. *Biochim. Biol. sper.*, *11*, in press.

TSUCHIYA, M., KIRYU, Y., YASUDA, M. and SHISHIDO, T. (1967): Effects of several hormones on the microcirculation. In: *Acta, VII Internationalis Angiologorum Congressus*, pp. 912–914. Cientifico-Medico Swets and Zeitlinger, Amsterdam.

TSUCHIYA, M., SHISHIDO, T. and FUJISHIRO, Y. (1969*b*): Vital observation of the vascular responses to some chemical mediators in the microcirculatory system. In: *Increased Permeability*, pp. 89–99. Editors: T. Shighei and M. Katori. Japan Medical Association and Japan Arteriosclerosis Research Foundation, Tokyo.

VILLAVICENCIO, J. L. and DE TAKATS, G. (1963): Mast cell activity under various forms of stress. *Surgery*, *44*, 312.

DISCUSSION

Dr. MORI: We performed a different type of experiment on stomach ulcer and mast cell degranulation. Administration of adrenaline produces the basic effects of stress. In your experiment, mast cell degranulation is inhibited by administration of adrenaline. Is that correct?

Dr. TSUCHIYA: We did not perform experiments with adrenaline.

Dr. MORI: I also examined in my experiments the histamine and serotonin content. In the stomach wall these are increased.

Dr. TSUCHIYA: But we were unable to measure the amount of serotonin in the tissue. In my experience of the microcirculation, intravenous injection of histamine induces increase in vascular permeability. Previous injection of pyridinolcarbamate completely inhibits this phenomenon. I believe pyridinolcarbamate suppresses the histamine effect on the vessel wall.

Dr. NUMANO: Do you find a significant difference in the number of degranulated mast cells between the control and pyridinolcarbamate-treated groups?

Dr. TSUCHIYA: The difference is not so great. In the normal Wistar strain rat the number of mast cells is 60–70 per mm^2 around the venule. If we count the avascular area, the number becomes different.

Dr. NUMANO: You found 58 mast cells in the control groups, and in the case of pyridinolcarbamate only 17. I feel there is some difference between both groups, don't you?

Dr. TSUCHIYA: Yes, but I do not know the reason for this difference. The number of mast cells in the mesentery is affected by stress. We must take account of cage conditions, season and room temperature.

Dr. AUSTIN: Dr. Tsuchiya, you mentioned that serotonin increased the vascular permeability, and that pyridinolcarbamate blocked this. What concentration of serotonin increased the permeability, and what concentration of pyridinolcarbamate blocked it?

Dr. TSUCHIYA: I did not measure the serotonin content in the blood. I gave serotonin to provoke the vascular permeability increase in the microcirculatory bed of rat mesentery.

Dr. AUSTIN: In what concentration did you give it?

Dr. TSUCHIYA: We injected it intravenously in a dose of 0.01 mg/kg rat body weight. That is a very high dose.

Dr. AUSTIN: And the pyridinolcarbamate?

Dr. TSUCHIYA: Pyridinolcarbamate in a dose of 5 mg/kg body weight was injected intravenously.

EFFECTS OF PYRIDINOLCARBAMATE ON THE α-ACTIVITY OF RABBIT BLADDER DETRUSOR MUSCLE*

DAVID L. KREULEN, GORDON F. ANDERSON and RAYMOND L. HENRY

School of Medicine, Wayne State University, Detroit, Mich., U.S.A.

I presented work here at the First Symposium in 1969 on the effect of pyridinolcarbamate (PDC) on the mechanisms of hemostasis. At that time, I indicated that PDC must be functioning on vascular smooth muscle membranes perhaps by blocking α-adrenergic activity. We knew at that time of the finding in 1965 by Murase et al. that PDC inhibited contractions of rat uterus muscle induced by bradykinin. We also knew about Odakura's finding (1965) that PDC prevented decreases in adhesive platelet counts by the catecholamine, adrenaline. Armed with the information published by Born in 1967 that epinephrine or norepinephrine induces platelet aggregation by stimulation of α-receptors since their effects could be inhibited by phentolamine (an α-adrenergic blocking agent), we could make a logical assumption that PDC likely functioned as an α-adrenergic blocking agent in hemostasis. Finally, Mizukawa and Azuma reported in 1969 that PDC potentiated the hypotensive effects of isoxuprine, a stimulant of adrenergic β-receptors.

We decided to test further the hypothesis that PDC exhibits α-adrenergic blocking activity. For this purpose, we utilized classical pharmacological techniques employing smooth muscle strips under carefully controlled conditions. In addition, we studied the effects of PDC on blood flow and blood pressure in unanesthetized trained dogs. I wish to present our data on this experimentation.

The urinary bladder contains both α- and β-adrenergic receptors. Numerous studies by others have shown that the bladder base and trigone contain mostly α-excitatory adrenergic receptors while the tissue from the fundus or dome (detrusor muscle) contains both α-excitatory and β-inhibitory adrenergic receptors. Paton and Rang (1966), De Sy (1970), and Anderson et al. (1971) found that the predominant response of the rabbit detrusor muscle to catecholamine administration is *inhibition* of the frequency of spontaneous contractions and relaxation. In addition, electrophysiological techniques show inhibition to be the prevailing response. Shigei et al. (1965), Evardson and Setekliev (1966), and Rohner et al. (1971) all produced excitatory responses to catecholamines using β-adrenergic blocking agents. It is well established, then, that bladder detrusor muscle contains distinct and separable α-excitatory and β-inhibitory receptors.

We have obtained evidence that PDC inhibits the α-activity of rabbit bladder detrusor muscle and thereby allows the relaxation (the β-inhibitory response) by catecholamines to be potentiated or magnified.

METHODS AND RESULTS

Paired strips of detrusor muscle 1–1.5 cm long and 0.25–0.5 cm wide were placed in our isolated organ tissue apparatus and signals from force transducers were amplified and re-

* Supported in part by the Michigan Heart Association and the National Defense Education Act, Title IV Fellowship to D. L. Kreulen.

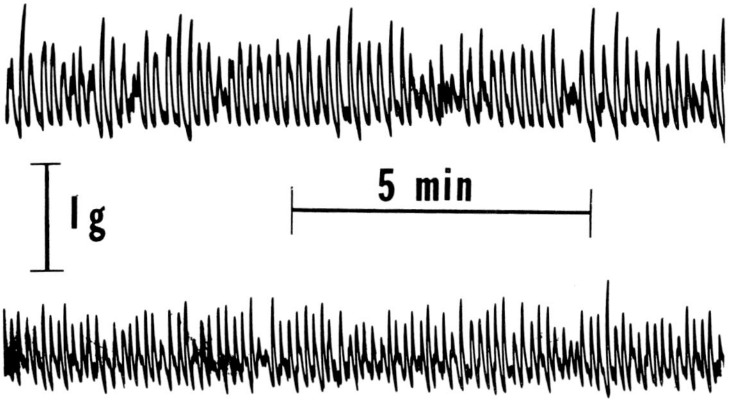

Fig. 1. Spontaneous rhythmic contractions of isolated rabbit detrusor muscle: Tracing demonstrates typical contractile activity of detrusor strips in vitro.

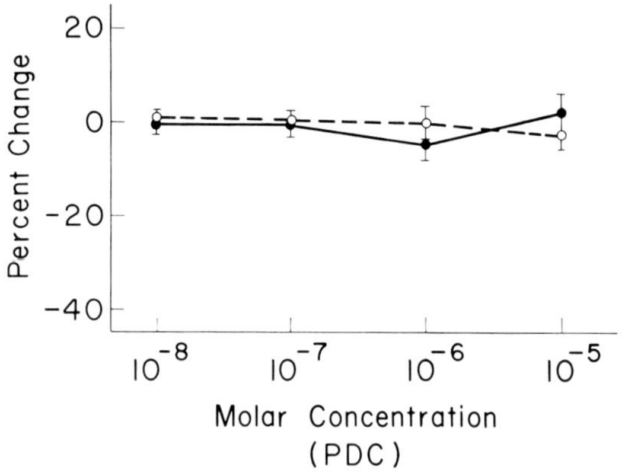

Fig. 2. Changes in detrusor strip motility with pyridinolcarbamate (PDC).
•——• frequency; o– – –o force.

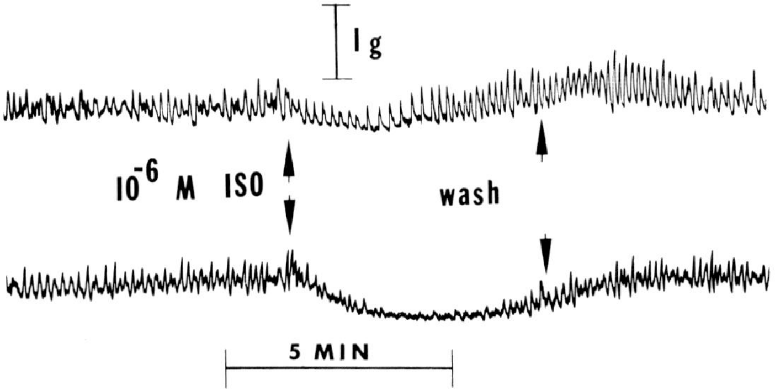

Fig. 3. Administration of 10^{-6} M isoproterenol (ISO) tracing of the pretreated detrusor strip with 10^{-5} M pyridinolcarbamate shows greater depression of spontaneous frequency and tension in the upper untreated case.

corded (Fig. 1). The tracing at the top is the control in Figure 1 and the next few figures, while the bottom tracing is from the paired muscle strip treated in 1×10^{-8} to 1×10^{-5} molar concentrations of PDC.

PDC alone did not affect either the force or the frequency of contractions, i.e. without challenging the muscle with catecholamines (Fig. 2).

Isoproterenol at 10^{-6} M inhibited both the rate and force of contractions and this β-activity is enhanced by PDC (Fig. 3, bottom tracing) because the α-activity had been eliminated. In lower concentrations (10^{-8} M) isoproterenol actually stimulated the muscle be-

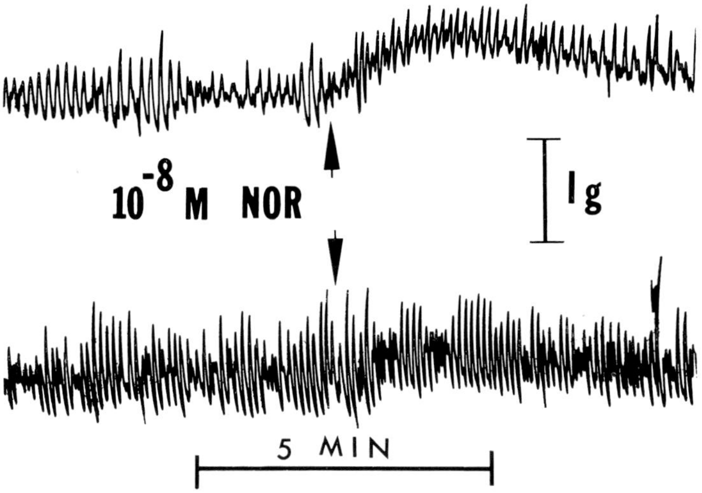

Fig. 4. Administration of 10^{-8} M norepinephrine (NOR): The untreated detrusor strip (upper) shows an increase in force of contractions while the pyridinolcarbamate pretreated strip (lower) shows little or no change from control.

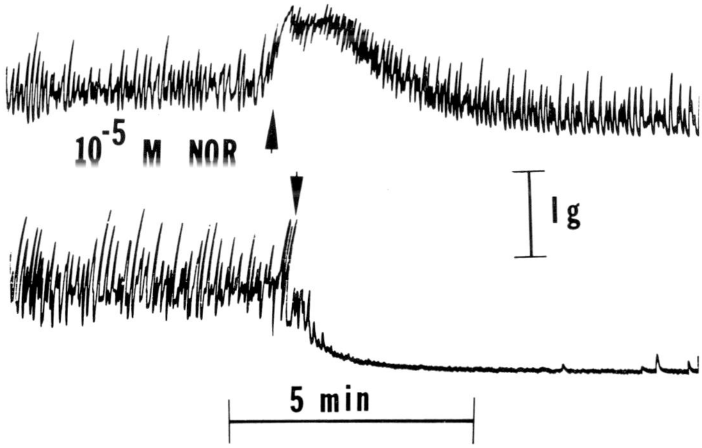

Fig. 5. Administration of 10^{-5} M norepinephrine (NOR): Spontaneous contractile activity of the pyridinolcarbamate pretreated strip (lower) was completely inhibited by norepinephrine while the untreated strip (upper) was stimulated. Pyridinolcarbamate blocked the excitatory action of norepinephrine.

cause the β-activity was diluted out at very low concentrations while the α-excitatory activity remained. Once again PDC eliminated this α-activity.

We see a similar response with norepinephrine in Figure 4. At low concentrations the α-excitatory activity is eliminated by PDC, while at higher concentrations of norepinephrine the α-excitatory activity is blocked and the β-inhibitory activity is allowed to express itself to the fullest degree (Fig. 5).

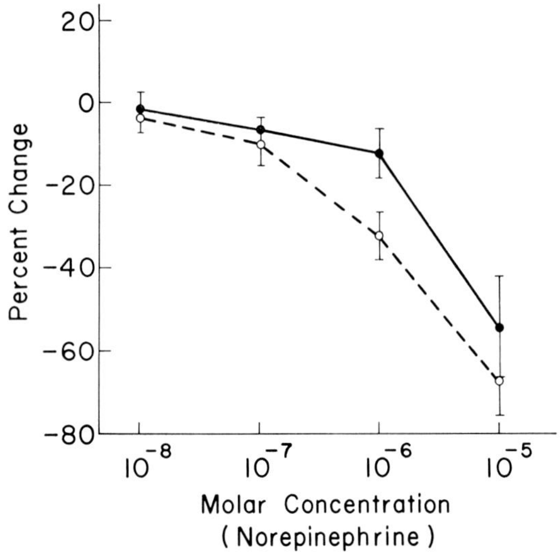

Fig. 6. Changes in detrusor strip spontaneous force with norepinephrine. •——• norepinephrine; ○- - -○ pyridinolcarbamate 10^{-5} M and norepinephrine.

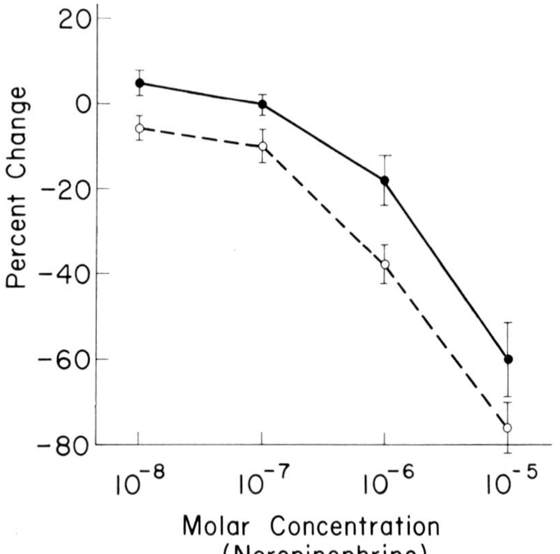

Fig. 7. Changes in detrusor strip spontaneous frequency with norepinephrine. •——• norepinephrine; ○- - -○ pyridinolcarbamate 10^{-5} M and norepinephrine.

Changes induced by PDC were statistically significant in shifting the dose-response curve to the left. Varying molar concentrations of PDC from 10^{-4} to 10^{-7} were equally potent in α-blocking activity. At concentrations as low as 10^{-9} M no blocking activity was exhibited. In Figure 6 we see the enhancement of β-activity on the force of contractions by PDC treatment. One can conclude that the difference between these curves represents α-excitatory activity.

Similarly, the frequencies of contractions were further reduced in the presence of PDC over wide variations of concentrations of norepinephrine (Fig. 7).

Similar results are seen when one uses epinephrine as the stimulating catecholamine. One example of the experimental results is given in Figure 8. Note the enhancement of depressor activity.

I would like now to turn to experiments on unanesthetized trained dogs. These experiments are preliminary but interesting.

Dogs were equipped with blood flow probes and pressure transducers under surgical anesthesia, allowed to recover, and trained to remain quiet while measurements were made during challenges by epinephrine before and after injections of PDC.

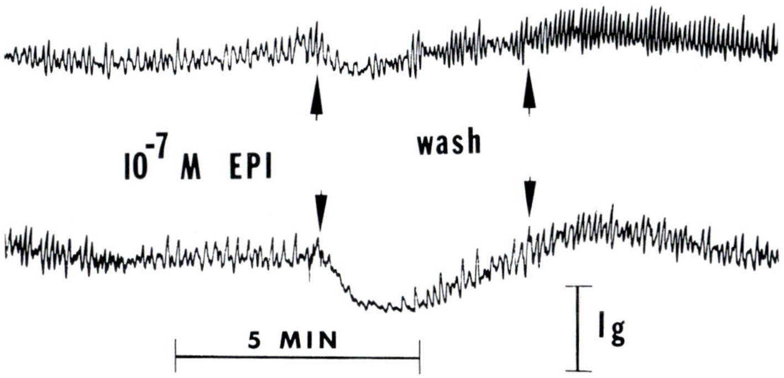

Fig. 8. Administration of 10^{-7} M epinephrine (EPI): The strip pretreated with pyridinolcarbamate (lower) shows greater inhibition of spontaneous frequency and tension of contraction as mediated by epinephrine than the untreated strip (upper tracing).

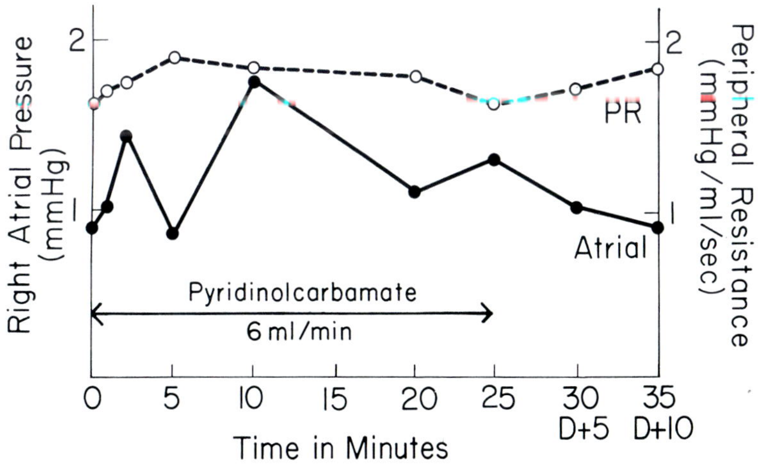

Fig. 9. Effect of Anginin (7.14 mg/kg i.v.) on right atrial pressure and peripheral resistance.

Anginin alone did not alter right atrial pressure or peripheral resistance in these acute studies (Fig. 9). Arterial pressure did not change significantly, although a suggestion of a drop in pressure was noted following the end of infusion of the total dose of PDC (Fig. 10), while aortic blood flow showed a mild increase even in the face of the reduced blood pressure (Fig. 11).

When the dogs were challenged with epinephrine 10 and 20 min after the injection of PDC, the typical 60 sec rise in systolic and diastolic arterial pressure was squashed (Fig. 12).

Cardiac output and aortic blood flow were impressively increased by challenges of epinephrine in the presence of PDC (Fig. 13), while right atrial pressure was at first precipitously dropped and then increased, indicating an improvement in venous return to the heart (Fig. 14).

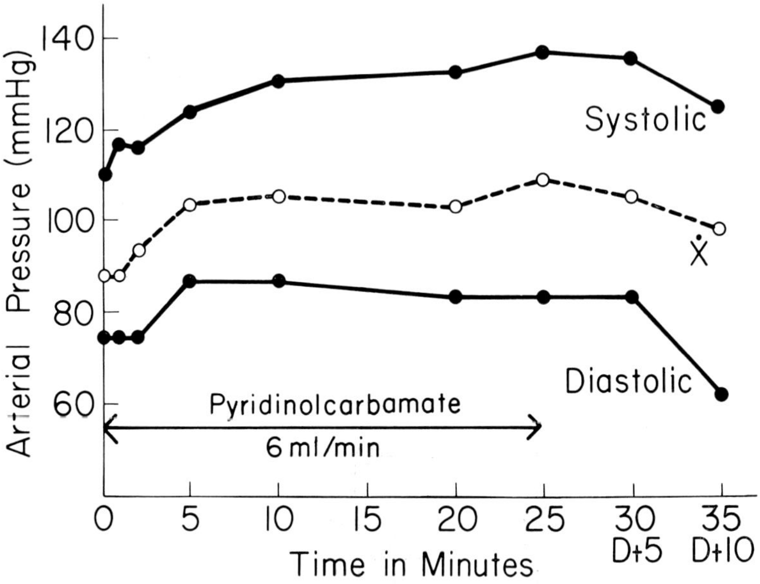

Fig. 10. Effect of Anginin (7.14 mg/kg i.v.) on arterial pressure.

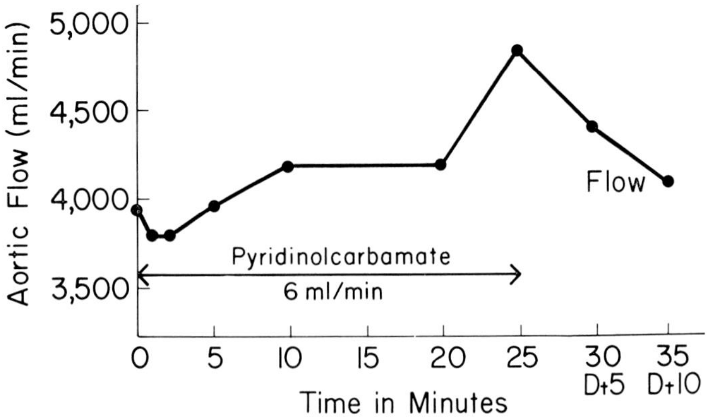

Fig. 11. Effect of Anginin (7.14 mg/kg i.v.) on aortic blood flow.

Taken all together, we feel that PDC in these acute studies was acting to block the vascular constricting activity of epinephrine (its α-excitatory activity), thus allowing better venous return and better aortic blood flow in the presence of reduced blood pressure, a condition likely meaning better tissue blood perfusion. These, of course, were not long-term studies, but may have relevance to benefits possible from PDC under conditions of stress where adrenergic catecholamines are released. An example might be the reduction or elimination of anginal pain by PDC during the Master's two-step test reported by Yamasaki et al. in the *American Heart Journal* in May 1970.

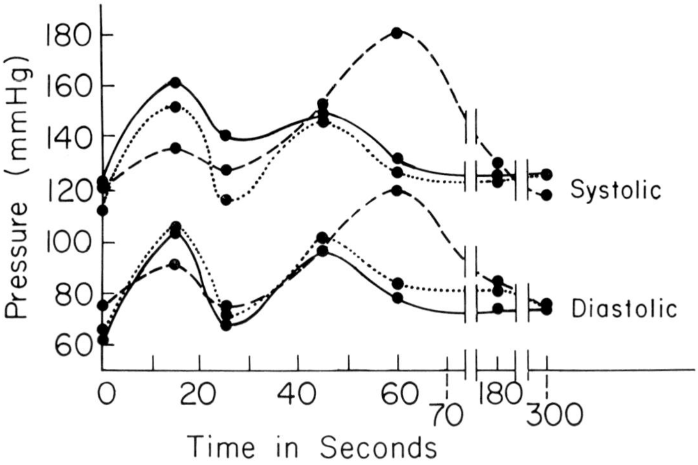

Fig. 12. Blood pressures induced by epinephrine before and after Anginin. ---- control; —— 1st challenge (D + 10); ···· 2nd challenge (D + 20).

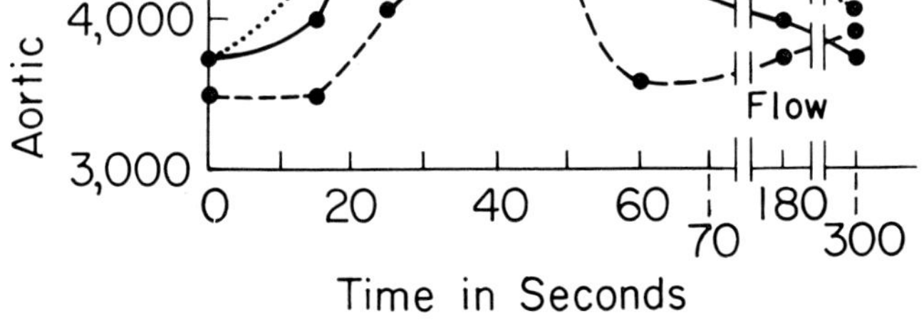

Fig. 13. Epinephrine-induced blood flow before and after Anginin. ---- control; —— 1st challenge (D + 10); ···· 2nd challenge (D + 20).

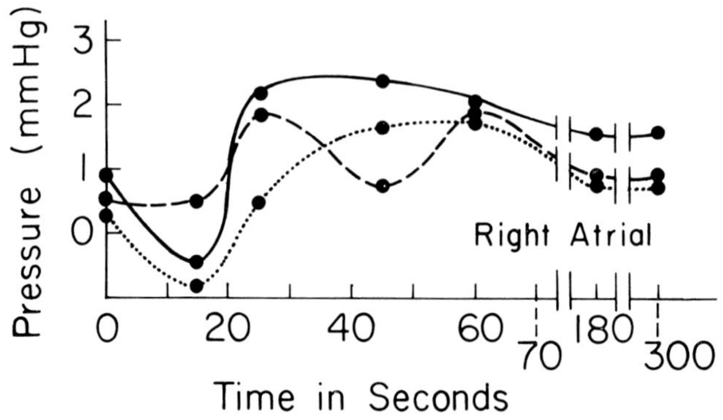

Fig. 14. Right atrial pressure induced by epinephrine before and after Anginin. ---- control; —— 1st challenge (D + 10); ···· 2nd challenge (D + 20).

REFERENCES

ANDERSON, G. F., PIERCE, J. M., FREDERICKS, C. M., ATKINSON, S. M. and GOELLNER, P. (1971): A pharmacologic evaluation of the adrenergic receptors of the rabbit detrusor muscle. *Int. Arch. Pharmacodyn.*, *191*, 220.

BORN, G. V. R. (1967): Possible mechanisms of platelet aggregation by ADP and of its inhibition. *Thrombos. Diathes. haemorrh. (Stuttg.)*, *Suppl. 26*, 173.

DE SY, W. (1970): Receptor responses in isolated smooth muscle of the urinary bladder. *Int. Arch. Pharmacodyn.*, *186*, 188.

EVARDSON, P. and SETEKLIEV, J. (1968): Distribution of adrenergic receptors in the urinary bladder of cats, rabbits, and guinea pigs. *Acta pharmacol. (Kbh.)*, *26*, 437.

MIZUKAWA, T. and AZUMA, I. (1969): Effects of pyridinolcarbamate (Anginin) on intraocular pressure and aqueous humor dynamics. In: *Atherogenesis. Proceedings, I International Symposium on Atherogenesis, Thrombogenesis and Pyridinolcarbamate Treatment, Tokyo 1969*, pp. 295–302. Editors: T. Shimamoto and F. Numano. ICS 201, Excerpta Medica, Amsterdam.

MURASE, H., YAGISHITA, M., SHIMAMOTO, T. and YAMAZAKI, H. (1965): Action of pyridinolcarbamate on isolated rat uterus preparation. *Ochanomizu med. J.*, *13/3*, 313.

ODAKURA, T. (1965): Preventive effect of pyridinolcarbamate against decrease of adhesive platelet count by adrenaline and animal fat in man. *Ochanomizu med. J.*, *13/3*, 309.

PATON, W. D. M. and RANG, H. P. (1966): A kinetic approach to the mechanism of drug action. *Advanc. Drug Res.*, *3*, 57.

ROHNER, T. J., PAEXER, D. M., WEIN, A. J. and SCHOENBERG, H. W. (1971): Contractile responses of dog bladder neck muscle to adrenergic drugs. *J. Urol. (Baltimore)*, *105*, 657.

SHIGEI, T., SAKUMA, A., NISHIWAKI, T. and KATO, H. (1965): Action of pyridinolcarbamate on the heart and coronary vessels of dogs. *Ochanomizu med. J.*, *13/3*, 314.

YAMASAKI, H., SANO, T., ODAKURA, T., TAKEUCHI, K. and SHIMAMOTO, T. (1970): Electrocardiographic and hematological changes by exercise test in coronary patients and pyridinolcarbamate pretreatment. A double-blind crossover trial. *Amer. Heart J.*, *79*, 640.

DISCUSSION

UNIDENTIFIED SPEAKER: How was the Anginin administered, and in what vehicle?

Dr. HENRY: The Anginin was dissolved in physiological saline and injected intravenously.

Dr. BERKOWITZ: We, in some of our studies, when trying to solubilize Anginin, find we have to dissolve it in acid. It does not, in fact, and the studies we presented were all done in suspension. As I commented this morning, there is, I think, a very clear species difference in the effects of Anginin because there is no question in the rat of there being an adrenergic blocking effect. The effect of noradrenaline on blood pressure or the effect of tyrosine, which releases more adrenaline, are not affected, so again we have a species difference. But our results do carry weight and we do focus on the possibility of an adrenergic response somewhere in the effect.

Dr. HENRY: We did not find it a problem to dissolve the Anginin in our physiological electrolyte solution and I have the constituents of that solution if you would like to see it.

Dr. KIPSHIDZE: How long do you have high blood pressure after Anginin?

Dr. HENRY: These were very acute studies, and they were following the challenging doses of adrenaline. We only went to 20 min after the injection, because we were only doing a 10- and 20-min response and relating this to control experiments that we know in these trained dogs. You probably know that these are very expensive and difficult experiments because it takes weeks to train a dog to lie still. We want him to have his normal reflex mechanisms intact and are only timing them for 10 or 20 min during these doses. We do not know the answer for a longer-term response.

Dr. SPECTOR: I wonder if you have looked at ions, namely does Anginin modify calcium? Could you not take some non-specific stimulant on this system itself?

Dr. HENRY: This is a question we are also asking in terms of the isolated muscle strips. Just last week we did some strips, and we found, using Furchgott's system, that 1×10^{-7} M noradrenaline should give at least 50% contraction or more. In our system, I think we had close to that, and in the presence of Anginin, in addition to the noradrenaline, we had to go to 1×10^{-4} M to get the same kind of response as in the control, so that the time factor is of concern as well. These experiments will have to be extended to wash-out procedures etc.

EXPERIMENTAL STUDIES ON METASTASIS FORMATION, WITH SPECIAL REFERENCE TO THE MECHANISM OF CANCER CELL LODGEMENT IN THE MICROCIRCULATION

HARUO SATO and MAROH SUZUKI
Cancer Research Laboratory, Research Institute for Tuberculosis, Leprosy and Cancer, Tohoku University, Sendai, Japan

INTRODUCTION

Experimental studies have been designed to clarify the causes of cancer metastasis by using various strains of transplantable tumors of rats and mice, e.g. Yoshida sarcoma and the ascites hepatomas of rats (Sato, 1964, 1967). Based on the findings on the dynamic behavior of tumor cells in the circulating blood, the mechanism of the lodging of tumor cells, which is an important process in hematogenous metastasis of cancer, was investigated and correlated with disturbances of the microcirculation system. Embolism, passage and adhesion of tumor cells could be observed and recorded in the microcirculation using cinephotography. Tumor cells which embolized to the arterioles or the entrance of the capillaries passed through the narrow capillary lumen by changing shape within a few hours. Then some of them adhered to the walls of venules. It was noted that the disturbance caused by the embolism of tumor cells in the microcirculation could induce events which led to the adhesion of tumor cells to the wall of venules following tumor cell passage through the capillaries. Carrying out some basic experiments to search for a way to prevent metastasis formation, we studied the role of pyridinolcarbamate on the inhibition of metastasis formation and the results are described in this report.

MATERIALS AND METHODS

Several strains of transplantable tumors of rats and mice, mainly ascites tumors, have been used in our series of experiments. Tumor cells grow in the ascites fluid when transplanted into the peritoneal cavity. Tumor cells growing in ascites fluid are either of a free, single-cell type or island-forming type, which is individually characteristic of each strain of tumor. Some examples are shown in Figures 1–4. We are now using more than 80 strains of these transplantable tumors. Each tumor strain has individual characteristics either morphologically or biochemically. Thus, the ascitic picture, chromosome patterns, transplantability, survival, enzymatic patterns, drug sensitivity and metastasis formation have been examined and shown to have features characteristic for each strain (Yoshida and Sato, 1964).

Employing these tumors, a series of model experiments on metastasis has been carried out in our laboratory. The animals used for the experiments in this report are Donryu rats, weighing about 100–120 g.

RESULTS AND DISCUSSION

In talking about metastasis, the term 'metastasis' describes a focus (or foci) such as enlarged tumor nodule(s) in lymph nodes or shadow(s) on an X-ray picture of the chest. Such metastatic lesions are the terminal products of metastatic cancer cells, no matter how small they are. The metastasis begins by the liberation of a cancer cell or cells from the primary site where the cancer developed. The liberated cancer cells migrate in the tissue. Then the cells will get into either lymph vessels or blood vessels, i.e. intravasation will occur. These cells will migrate in the lymph or blood stream in the vessels. Arriving at the distant organs or tissues, some of the cancer cells may lodge. Following this stage, there will be proliferation of cancer cells which we can then recognize as a metastatic focus. In thinking about the procedures of metastasis formation, it should be noted that the procedures are phenomena at the cellular level.

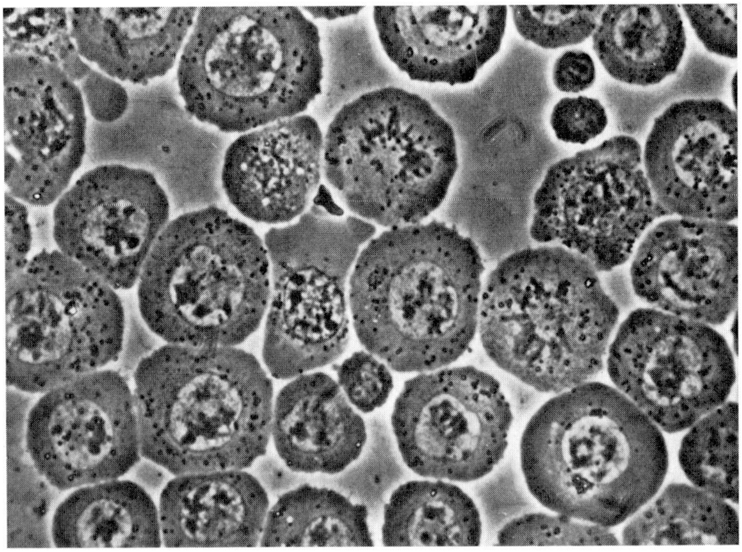

*Fig. 1.** Ascitic feature of AH66F (free-cell type).

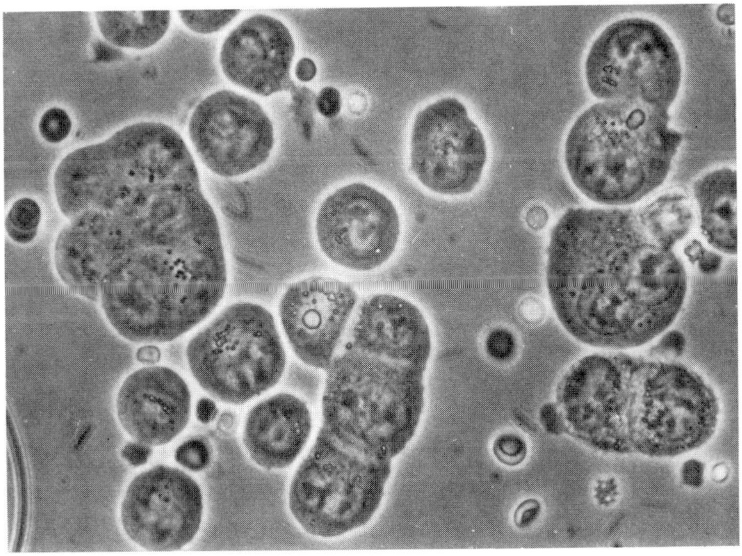

Fig. 2. Ascitic feature of AH66 (mixed type of free cells and small cell complexes).

**Figs. 1–4.* Ascitic picture of the ascites hepatomas of rat. Photographed under phase-contrast microscope.

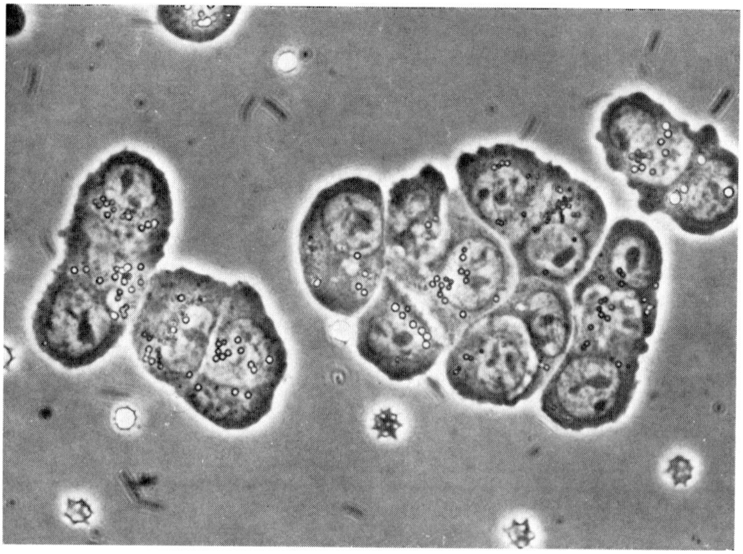

Fig. 3. Ascitic picture of AH7974 (small island type).

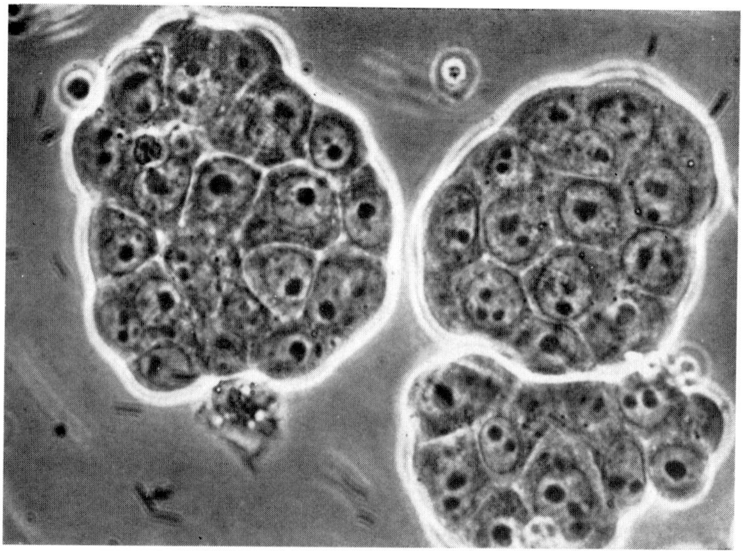

Fig. 4. Ascitic picture of AH601 (large island type).

We have been studying these phenomena by analysing the procedures of metastasis formation. In this paper, some of the findings are related to the mechanism of lodging of cancer cells in blood-borne metastasis.

Dynamic behavior of cancer cells in the circulating blood

During investigation of the mechanism of metastasis formation the dynamic behavior of tumor cells in the circulating blood was examined and recorded on cine film. Observation

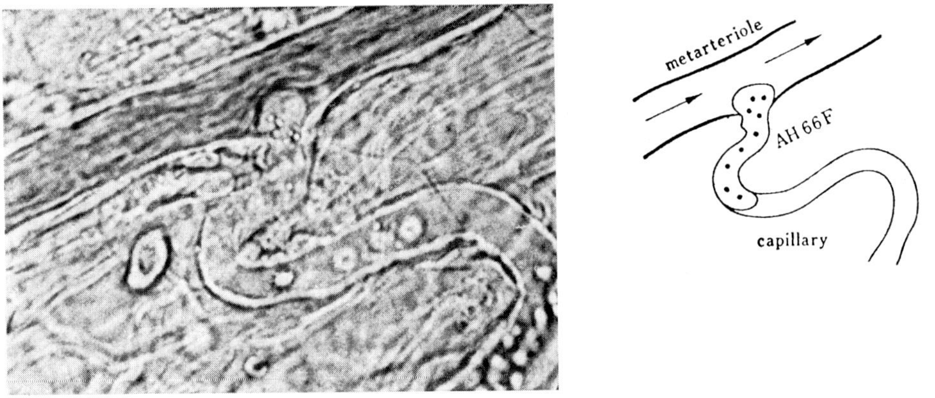

*Fig. 5.** One cancer cell of AH66F (a strain of ascites hepatoma of rat) is embolizing at the entrance to a capillary of the mesentery of rat. The blood stream is flowing in the arteriole, while no flow is seen in the capillary.

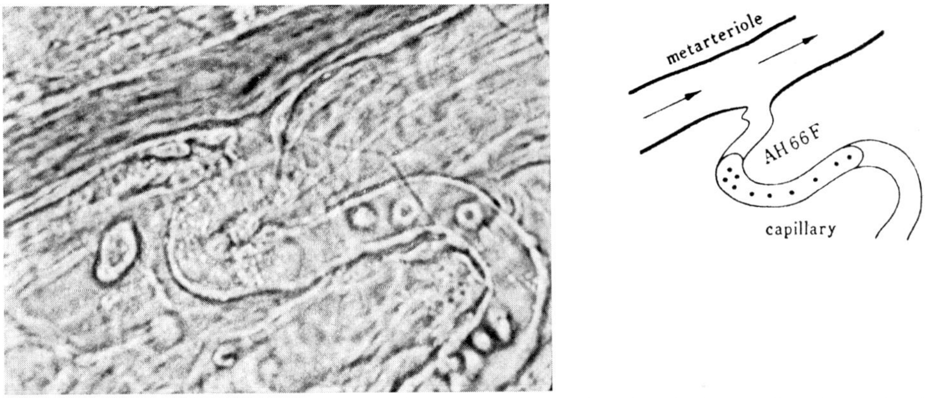

Fig. 6. The embolic cell is forcing its way into the capillary, changing its shape. There is no blood flow yet in the capillary. Fine, bright granules seen in the cell are glycogen granules, which are a characteristic marker of this tumor cell strain.

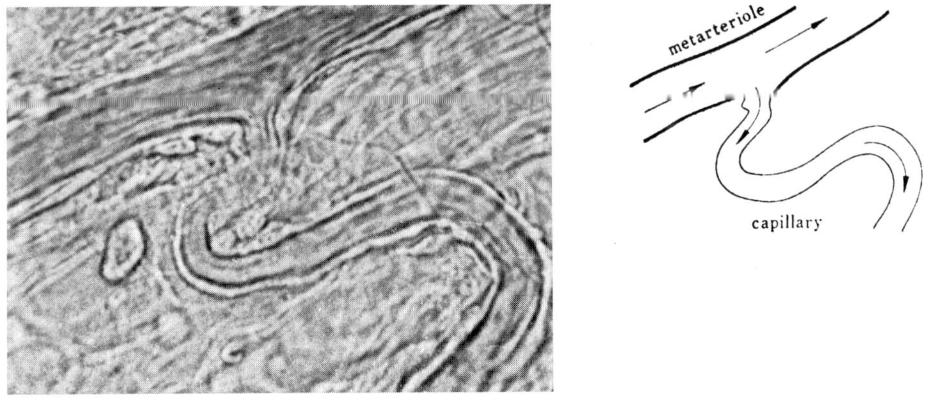

Fig. 7. When the cell passed through the capillary, recovery of blood flow was seen immediately.

**Figs. 5–11.* Embolism, passage, lodging and growth of cancer cells in the microcirculation. All pictures were taken from 16 mm cinemicrographs.

was carried out using the mesentery of living animals (rats) under anesthesia. The mesentery was spread on a warmed glass slide under a microscope. The cinematographic pictures were mainly taken at a camera speed of 24 frames per second. Sometimes a high-speed camera (500 frames per second) was used.

According to the anatomical description of the microcirculation by Chambers and Zweifach (1944), the blood flow streams from the arterioles to venules through either thoroughfare channels or true capillaries or sometimes arteriovenous anastomoses. In the normal condition of the microcirculation, a certain number of tumor cells inoculated into the aorta through the carotid artery reach the peripheral area of circulation of the mesentery within a few seconds after inoculation.

When a cell (or cells) is embolized, sudden changes in the blood stream were seen in the area such as arrest of the stream, backflow etc. (which will be described in detail below). The site of embolism is usually at the entrance of a capillary in the free-cell type of tumor such as AH66F and Yoshida sarcoma or in the large arterioles in the island-type of tumor cells such as AH601 and AH7974. Tumor cells, once embolized, passed through the vessels, changing their shapes (Figs. 5–7). In general, the island type of tumor cells took a longer time to pass

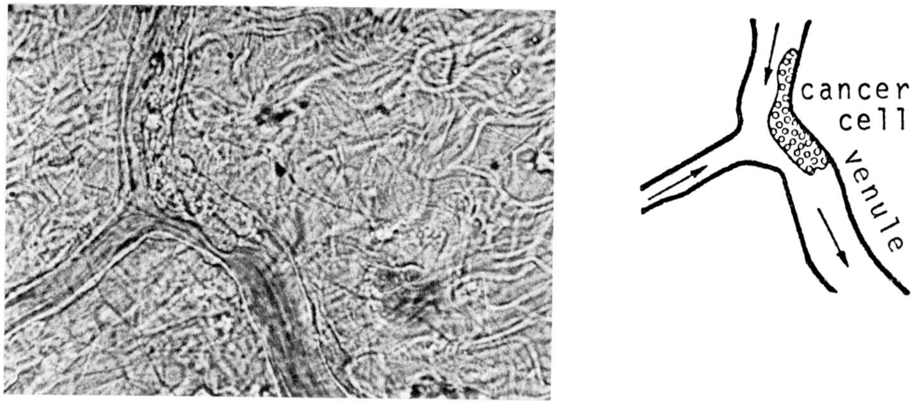

Fig. 8. Adhesion of cancer cell (AH601, a strain of ascites hepatoma of rat) to the wall of a venule of the mesentery of rat. The cell, coming through the thoroughfare channel (left), lodged at the junction of the venule and adhered to the vessel wall.

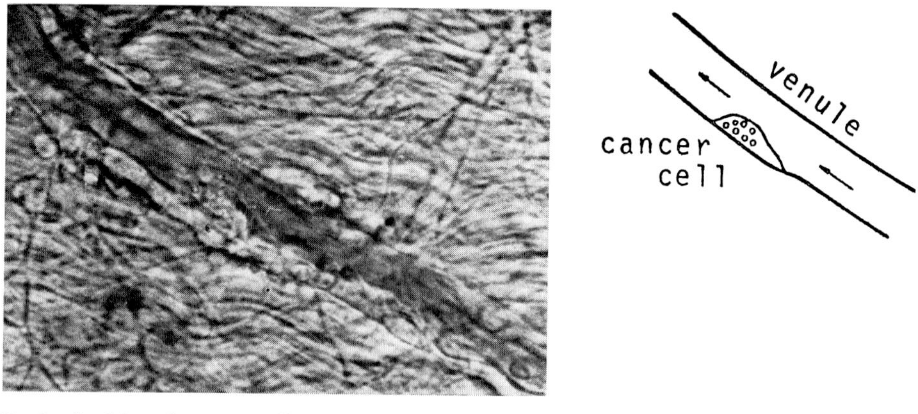

Fig. 9. Lodging of a cancer cell (AH601) on the wall of a venule. After passing through the capillary following the embolism, the cell adhered to the vessel wall. Some pathological features in the microcirculation had been observed, caused by the embolism of tumor cells.

through than the free-cell type. Immediate recovery of the blood flow followed the passing of tumor cells into the venous system. This happened in some cases in which it took more than 2 hours for tumor cells to pass completely through.

Adhesion of tumor cells to the wall of venules

Many tumor cells which passed through and entered the venous system were carried away in the blood stream. However, there were some cells which adhered to the inner walls of either postcapillaries or venules. These cells adhered to, or moved very slowly on, the wall even when the local blood stream recovered to almost normal (Figs. 8 and 9).

Site of initial growth

It was particularly noted that the site of the earliest growth of tumor cells was observed in the area of postcapillaries and venules, not in the blood vessels but outside the vessels (Figs. 10 and 11). These findings were observed 15–30 hours after tumor cell inoculation into the blood stream. Features of mitotic division were also observed in some cases. It was assumed that the adhering tumor cells might have extravasated through the wall of blood vessels as seen in the case of leukocytes.

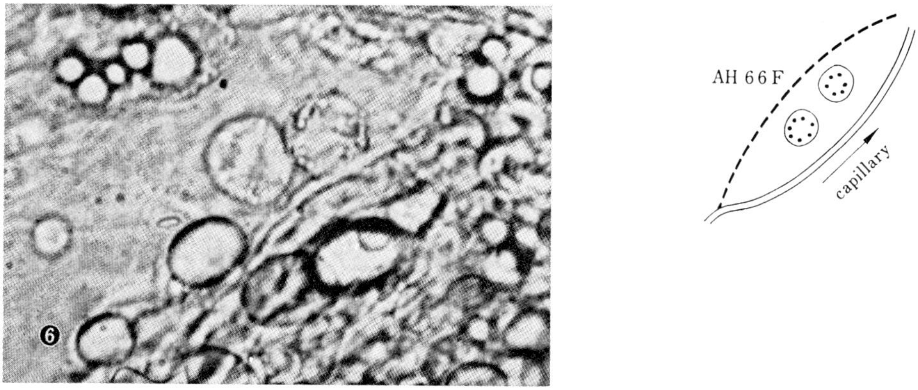

Fig. 10. Early stage of tumor cell growth. Two AH66F cells are seen outside a postcapillary. The cells have many glycogen granules. 48 hours after transplantation.

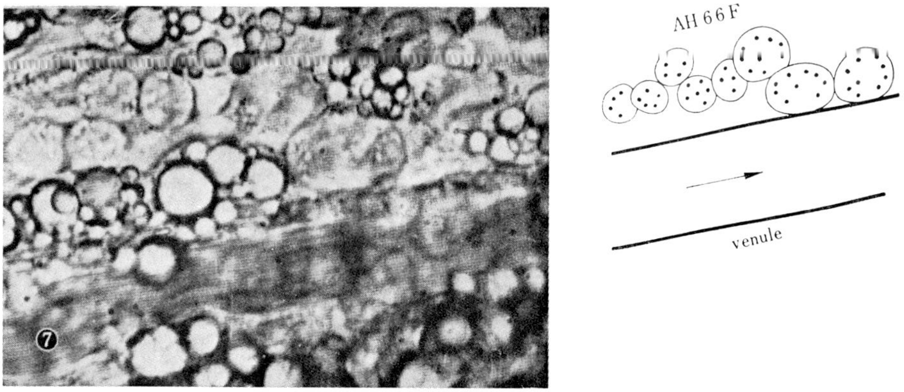

Fig. 11. Growth of tumor cells (AH66F) is seen outside a venule. 8 cells (7 in this picture) were observed; 3 on the right appear to be in mitosis. 60 hours after transplantation into the blood.

Disturbances in the microcirculation

A notable finding seen in the area of microcirculation, when tumor cells embolized at an entrance to a thoroughfare channel, is the abnormal blood flow. For example, sludging, slowing down, backflow or complete arrest of the blood stream, and plasma skimming are observed. When these changes are seen, adhesion of tumor cells seemed to occur to the wall of venules or postcapillaries. Also observed were adhesion of leukocytes and emigration through the wall of venules. Sometimes diapedesis of red cells and thrombus formation were observed in the venules. These findings resemble those found in inflammation.

On the other hand, tumor cells circulating in the systemic circulation were observed even 3 to several days after transplantation. This finding was seen particularly in cases of the free-cell type of tumor such as AH66F or Yoshida sarcoma. Tumor cells pass through a capillary smoothly without staying at the site of embolism for a long time. In such cases adhesion to the venous wall does not occur. In one case of Yoshida sarcoma circulating in the blood 3 tumor cells were observed passing through a capillary within about 1 sec. This was recorded by a high-speed camera. Such a short period of embolism causes little disturbance to the microcirculation and no adhesion is initiated.

Induction of metastasis

To study the correlation between disturbances in the microcirculation and adhesion of tumor cells a series of model experiments on brain metastasis was designed as follows. The tumor cells used are those of AH66F, the free-cell type of tumor. When a certain number of the cells were inoculated into the carotid artery, this strain of tumor does not form metastases in the cerebrum or does so only infrequently because the cells could easily pass through the blood vessels of the cerebrum. (This was confirmed by another series of experiments.) These cells were inoculated into the carotid artery together with some dead cells which were first boiled, fixed with formalin solution and washed. The dead cells are too hard to pass through the capillary because they lose their plasticity together with their viability. The embolism of the dead cells caused severe disturbances in the microcirculation which enhanced the lodgement of the inoculated living tumor cells. The results are shown in Table I. Increased metastasis is induced in the cerebrum and brainstem where no metastases were formed just by giving the living cells.

TABLE I

Experimental induction and inhibition of brain metastasis in rats

Treatment	Site of growth			
	Cerebrum	Brainstem	Cerebellum	Choroid plexus
AH66F (5×10^6)	0/11	0/11	0/11	7/11
AH66F (5×10^5) + dead cells (5×10^5)	7/7	1/7	0/7	6/7
AH66F + dead cells + pyridinolcarbamate*	4/10	0/10	0/10	9/10

* 20 mg/kg i.p.

The tumor cells of AH66F (free-cell type) do not form metastatic lesions in brain parenchyma following introduction into the carotid artery. However, frequent metastases can be induced in the cerebrum by giving dead cells (heat-killed and fixed with formalin) together with the living cells. In this experimental system, metastasis formation can be inhibited in the animals treated by the administration of pyridinolcarbamate.

Permeability of blood vessels by the embolism

As a sign of endothelial injury when the disturbances had occurred in the microcirculation, increased permeability is observed. For example, when pontamine blue dye was injected into the tail vein of rats, permeability was seen to be increased markedly in the area of the mesentery where the tumor cells inoculated into the aorta through the carotid artery had embolized, compared with non-treated animals.

In the next experiment, increased permeability was examined in the lungs of rats in which tumor cells (AH7974, island type), inoculated into the tail vein, had embolized. As seen in Figure 12, marked increase in the permeability was observed in the embolized lungs of

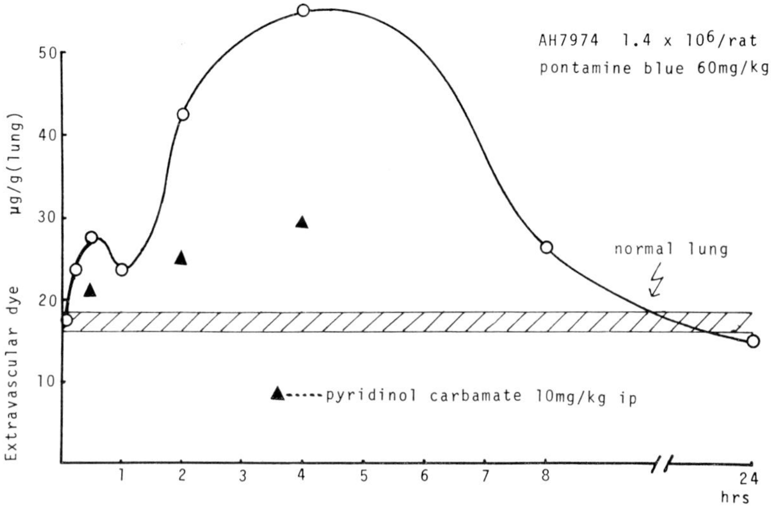

Fig. 12. Increased permeability of dye (pontamine blue) in the lung following the embolism of tumor cells.

The tumor cells of AH7974 (a strain of ascites hepatoma of rat) were inoculated into the tail vein of rats, together with the dye injection. The amount of dye was measured in the lung tissue. The hatched area indicates the value in normal lungs of untreated rats. Increased permeability was maximal at 4 hours after embolism. Administration of pyridinolcarbamate inhibited the permeability markedly.

animals in which 1.4×10^6 tumor cells of AH7974 were inoculated into the tail vein. The maximum increase was observed 4 hours after the time when the cells had embolized. When larger numbers of tumor cells such as 10^7 were inoculated, a greater increase in permeability was found. When the free-cell type of tumor such as Yoshida sarcoma was used, the increase in permeability was rather less.

Based on these findings, it does not seem to be unreasonable to assume that the disturbances in the microcirculation system (abnormality in blood flow and endothelial injury) are related to the mechanism of lodging of cancer cells.

Inhibition of metastasis by pyridinolcarbamate

Understanding the mechanism of the lodging of cancer cells as described above, the following experiments can be designed to study the effect of pyridinolcarbamate, expecting the improvement of disturbances in the microcirculation which have been reported by Shimamoto and Tsuchiya. Thus a marked inhibition of dye permeability was observed as shown in Figure 12. If the increased permeability is the sign which indicates the grade of disturbances in the microcirculation, pyridinolcarbamate, which has the effect of improving disturbances of the microcirculation, could affect those which were initiated by the embolism of tumor cells. Several experiments were carried out to see whether the administration of pyridinolcarbamate could inhibit metastasis formation using various experimental systems. In one of these, the brain metastasis system was used as seen in Table I. Metastasis formation was less (markedly so) in animals treated with pyridinolcarbamate. An adequate dose of pyridinolcarbamate was 10 mg/kg/day, although various doses have been tested.

SUMMARY

It is obvious that cancer metastasis is one of the biggest hazards which interfere with the complete cure of cancer patients. We have to conquer metastasis before we can conquer cancer.

In order to work out the problems of metastasis, we still have a long way to go. However, it is noted that the procedures in metastasis formation could be analysed at the cellular level. Thus, new approaches to find a way to inhibit or prevent metastasis could be developed.

The use of pyridinolcarbamate, for example, seems to be reasonable when the drug is administered to prevent the lodging of cancer cells by improving the disturbances in the microcirculation caused by the embolism or some other (non-specific) agent.

REFERENCES

CHAMBERS, R. and ZWEIFACH, B. W. (1944): Topography and function of the mesenteric capillary circulation. *Amer. J. Anat., 75*, 173.

SATO, H. (1964): Cancer metastasis and ascites tumors. *Nat. Cancer Inst. Monogr., 16*, 241.

SATO, H. (1967): Cancer metastasis, from pathological studies on ascites tumors. *Trans. Soc. Path. Jap., 56*, 9.

YOSHIDA, T. and SATO, H. (Eds.) (1964): Ascites tumors – Yoshida sarcoma and ascites hepatoma(s). *Nat. Cancer Inst. Monogr., 16*.

DISCUSSION

Dr. HENRY: I believe Dr. Sumner Wood of Johns Hopkins University and Dr William Knisely, when he was in Lexington, showed that the aggregation of platelets and white cells around tumor cells enhanced metastasis, and when they reduced the aggregation of the cells by drugs such as heparin or dextrans, it reduced metastasis. In view of the effect of pyridinolcarbamate on reducing the secondary phase of platelet aggregation, I would like to know if it was common for you to find aggregation of platelets on cancer cells in the metastasis.

Dr. SATO: I think that it is a big problem whether or not the blood coagulation system is related to metastasis formation. I think the blood coagulation system could be related partly to the lodging of tumor cells. But in our observations, particularly the in vivo observations, the tumor cells passed through the capillary and adhered to the wall of the venules and in many cases we could not see any blood coagulation at this stage. At a later stage, blood coagulation could be seen, and examples were shown in the cine pictures, so the coagulation of the blood might play a role in fixing the tumor cells where they lodge. However, I do not know whether the coagulation effect is primarily related to the lodging of the tumor cells or not. This problem should be studied more in future.

ENHANCEMENT OF ADP-INDUCED PLATELET AGGREGATION BY ADRENALINE AND CHOLESTEROL IN VIVO AND ITS PREVENTION

HIROH YAMAZAKI, TADAHIRO SANO, ITSURO KOBAYASHI, TAKEO TAKAHASHI and TAKIO SHIMAMOTO

Institute for Cardiovascular Diseases, School of Medicine, Tokyo Medical and Dental University, Yushima, Tokyo, Japan

The importance of adrenaline and cholesterol in atherogenesis and thrombogenesis is well recognized. Previously we have reported that the intravenous injection of a small amount of adrenaline induced an immediate and transient decrease in the adhesive platelet count and an abrupt but transient shortening of the one-stage prothrombin time in rabbits (Shimamoto et al., 1960) and man (Yamazaki et al., 1971). These results suggest the appearance of a thrombogenic tendency induced by adrenaline and that aggregability of platelets may change under such circumstances. We therefore tried to examine changes in aggregability of platelets induced by adenosine diphosphate (ADP) before and after an intravenous injection of adrenaline using the optical density method of Born (1962) and O'Brien (1962). Meanwhile we found that such a thrombogenic tendency induced by adrenaline was prevented by a β-adrenergic but not by an α-adrenergic blocking agent (Yamazaki et al., 1971). The phenomenon was also prevented by pyridinolcarbamate which prevents the edematous changes in the arterial wall induced by adrenaline and is known to have an antithrombotic effect (Shimamoto et al., 1966*a*, *b*). Aspirin has been known to inhibit platelet aggregation induced by ADP and adrenaline in vitro (O'Brien, 1968). According to these results, we examined the effect of pretreatment with the above drugs on changes in platelet aggregation and tried to clarify the mechanism of the thrombogenic tendency induced by adrenaline in vivo. Single-dose treatment with cholesterol also induced an immediate and transient decrease in adhesive platelet count with enhancement of blood coagulability and the change was inhibited by pyridinolcarbamate pretreatment (Shimamoto et al., 1966*b*). Thus we also examined the effect of cholesterol on ADP-induced platelet aggregation and its prevention by pyridinolcarbamate.

MATERIALS AND METHODS

1. Effect of adrenaline on ADP-induced platelet aggregation in vivo

90 male rabbits weighing 1.8–2.9 kg were used. They were divided into 9 groups of 10 rabbits. The rabbits in Groups 1 to 5 were given a gelatin capsule containing 10 mg/kg starch powder; 3 hours after the oral administration Group 1 was injected intravenously with 0.5 ml of physiological saline; 0.1, 1 and 10 μg/kg adrenaline in 0.5 ml saline was injected into Groups 2, 3 and 4, respectively, and 1 μg/kg L-noradrenaline into Group 5. The rabbits in the other 4 groups were given orally 10 mg/kg phenoxybenzamine, propranolol, aspirin and pyridinolcarbamate respectively and then injected with 1 μg/kg adrenaline 3 hours later.

Before the intravenous injection, the rabbits were given an intraperitoneal injection of 1.2 g/kg urethane and then secured in a supine position under light anesthesia. Both carotid arteries were exposed and a polyethylene tube was inserted into the carotid artery to collect 9 ml of blood into a siliconized test tube containing 1 ml of 3.8% sodium citrate solution. The artery was clamped by a forceps and then the intravenous injection was given into the marginal ear vein; 5 min after the injection, 9 ml of blood was collected from the arterial catheter after removal of the forceps. The initial 1 ml was discarded. The artery was ligated and 30 min after the injection, blood was collected from the other carotid artery in the same manner.

Immediately after collection, the blood was centrifuged at 100×*g* for 30 min at room temperature and about 4 ml of citrated platelet-rich plasma (CPRP) was obtained as supernatant. Within 2 hours after the collection of CPRP, the platelets suspended in the CPRP were examined for their aggregability produced by ADP. Since cooling increases the tendency of platelets to aggregate (Zucker, 1961), CPRP was kept at room temperature during the experiment. To detect the degree of platelet aggregation by ADP, a photoelectric system was used as described by Born (1962) and O'Brien (1962). A platelet aggregation meter (Model 169, Evans Electroselenium Ltd., Halstead, Essex, United Kingdom) was used. A polyethylene tube, 45×10 mm, was filled with 1 ml of CPRP and inserted into the photoelectric system and thermostatically warmed to 37 °C for 90 sec before testing. To determine ADP-induced platelet aggregation, 0.1 ml of dilute ADP was added to the CPRP with an Ostwald pipette. After recording the aggregation, the CPRP was centrifuged at 1,000×*g* for 30 min to obtain platelet-free plasma (PFP). Then the optical density (OD) of the PFP was obtained and used as a standard for the changes in the OD of the CPRP (Yamazaki et al., 1970*a*). A horizontal line was drawn from each starting point of the aggregation curve and it was defined as the baseline. The degree of platelet aggregation was calculated as follows:

$$\frac{\text{maximum deflection of OD of CPRP measured from baseline}}{\text{OD of PFP measured from baseline}} \times 100\%$$

2. Effect of cholesterol on ADP-induced platelet aggregation in vivo

66 male rabbits weighing 2.1–3.1 kg were used. They were divided into 3 groups of 22 rabbits. Group 1 was treated orally with 30 ml of water and then with 1 g/kg starch powder dispersed in 30 ml of water. Group 2 was treated with 30 ml of water and then with 1 g/kg cholesterol dispersed in 30 ml of water. Group 3 was treated with 10 mg/kg pyridinolcarbamate dispersed in 30 ml of water, then with 1 g/kg cholesterol dispersed in 30 ml of water. The 2nd administration followed the 1st administration (starch or cholesterol) 3 hours later. For the oral administration a gastric tube was inserted into the stomach of each rabbit through a specially prepared mouthpiece.

Just before the 1st administration, 3 hours after the 1st administration, i.e. just before the 2nd administration, and 3 hours after the 2nd administration, 4.5 ml of blood was taken from the central ear artery by means of a polyethylene disposable syringe containing 0.5 ml of 3.8% sodium citrate solution. Immediately after the collection of blood it was centrifuged at 100×*g* for 30 min to collect CPRP. After removal of CPRP from the specimen, the residual blood was recentrifuged at 1,000×*g* for 30 min to obtain PFP. To detect the degree of platelet aggregation by ADP a photoelectric system and a new microscopic method were used as follows:

a. Optical density method (Born, 1962; O'Brien, 1962): A platelet aggregation meter (Model 300, Chrono-Log Corp., Broomall, Pa., U.S.A.) was used. A polyethylene tube, 50×7 mm, was filled with 0.4 ml of CPRP and inserted into the photoelectric system and thermostatically warmed at 37 °C. CPRP was stirred continuously by a Teflon-coated magnetic rotor revolving at the bottom of the cell. After 90 sec, 0.04 ml of dilute ADP was added to the CPRP by means of a micropipette (H. E. Pederson, Denmark). The degree of ADP-induced platelet aggregation was calculated as in the case of adrenaline.

b. Estimation of platelet sensitivity to ADP aggregation by a new microscopic method (Sano et al., 1971): Using CPRP collected from 10 rabbits of each group, platelet aggregability by ADP was determined by a new microscopic method which measures the minimum concentration of serial doubling dilutions of ADP which induces platelet aggregation. All procedures were carried out at room temperature. The details of the method employed have been described previously. The minimum concentration of doubly diluted ADP (2^{-n} mg/ml) required to induce platelet aggregation was found by mixing and stirring the ADP solution with the same volume of CPRP and observing aggregation microscopically. The absolute value of the exponent of the minimum ADP concentration required to induce aggregation was taken as the value of platelet sensitivity. For example, when the end-point was 2^{-13} mg/ml, the sensitivity was expressed as '13'.

Estimation of plasma cholesterol level: An aliquot of PFP was used for cholesterol level estimation by Zak-Henly's method (Zak, 1957; Henly, 1957).

3. Effect of adrenaline on ADP-induced platelet aggregation in vitro

Using 30 samples of rabbit CPRP, the effect on ADP-induced platelet aggregation of adrenaline was examined in vitro. Adrenaline or L-noradrenaline in a dose of 0.01, 0.1, 1, 10 or 100 μg/ml was added to CPRP which was incubated at 37 °C for 30 sec. Then ADP to a final concentration of 10^{-5} or 3×10^{-6} molar was added and the change in OD measured. The same CPRP was incubated at 37 °C for 30 sec with 1/10 volume of saline as a control and its aggregability by ADP was measured. The degree of platelet aggregation induced by ADP with and without the addition of catecholamines was compared.

4. Preventive effect of pyridinolcarbamate on platelet aggregation induced by ADP or adrenaline in vitro

The hypothesis that pyridinolcarbamate inhibits platelet aggregation in vitro was tested. For this purpose 97 samples of CPRP collected from human subjects were incubated at 37 °C for 90 sec with 1/10 volume of saline or the same amount of saline containing 300 μg/ml pyridinolcarbamate. ADP or adrenaline was then added to a final concentration of 3×10^{-6} molar or 1 μg/ml respectively. Platelet aggregation curves induced by ADP or adrenaline were observed by a platelet aggregation meter (Model 300, Chrono-Log) with or without pyridinolcarbamate pretreatment.

DRUGS

The drugs used in this experiment were as follows: adrenaline (Sankyo Pharmacological Co., Ltd., Japan), L-noradrenaline (Levophed, Winthrop Laboratories, USA), cholesterol (L'Industrie Biologique, France), starch powder (the Japan pharmacopoeia), phenoxybenzamine (Dibenzyline, Smith Kline and French Laboratories, USA), propranolol (Inderal, ICI Ltd., England), aspirin (the Japan pharmacopoeia), and pyridinolcarbamate (Anginin, Banyu Pharmacological Co., Ltd., Japan). The disodium salt of adenosine 5′-diphosphate (Sigma Chemical Co., Ltd., USA) was used for the test. Stock ADP was deep-frozen at a concentration of 10^{-2} molar and pH of the solution was adjusted to 7.4 with Tris buffer (Born and Hume, 1967). The working solution of ADP for the test was prepared by dilution with distilled concentrations of 10^{-4}, 3×10^{-5} molar, respectively. Thus the final concentrations of ADP in the CPRP were 10^{-5}, 3×10^{-6} and 10^{-6} molar, respectively.

RESULTS

1. Effect of adrenaline on ADP-induced platelet aggregation in vivo

Before the intravenous injections, there was little difference in the degree of platelet aggregation induced by ADP between the 5 groups of rabbits pretreated with starch powder (Table I). The mean levels were 44.3–49.9% with 10^{-5} molar, 37.8–39.5% with 3×10^{-6} molar, and 24.4–27.9% with 10^{-6} molar ADP. The standard errors were 2.8–7.8% at 10^{-5} molar, 3.1–8.4% at 3×10^{-6} molar, and 4.8–7.5% at 10^{-6} molar ADP. The coefficients of variance were 5.7–17.6% at 10^{-5} molar, 8.2–21.4% at 3×10^{-6} molar, and 19.7–26.9% at

TABLE I

Changes in degree of ADP-induced platelet aggregation (10 cases each)

Intravenous injection		Before injection (mean ± SE) (%)	Percent of values before injection (mean ± SE)	
			5 min	30 min
Induced by 10^{-5} molar ADP final concentration				
Saline	0.5 ml	47.4 ± 4.3	109.2 ± 6.5	103.6 ± 7.6
Adrenaline	0.1 μg/ml	49.9 ± 3.6	96.6 ± 2.1	98.3 ± 3.2
	1 μg/ml	44.3 ± 7.8	115.1 ± 4.9**	111.5 ± 8.0
	10 μg/ml	49.4 ± 2.8	101.7 ± 2.9	93.5 ± 2.5
Noradrenaline	1 μg/ml	47.4 ± 7.2	107.2 ± 5.5	99.1 ± 5.7
Induced by 3×10^{-6} molar ADP final concentration				
Saline	0.5 ml	39.0 ± 3.2	109.7 ± 4.8	109.8 ± 9.3
Adrenaline	0.1 μg/ml	37.9 ± 3.1	97.7 ± 3.6	107.4 ± 3.1
	1 μg/ml	39.5 ± 7.1	121.8 ± 7.8**	117.9 ± 9.0
	10 μg/ml	37.8 ± 4.2	103.9 ± 4.2	94.6 ± 2.3
Noradrenaline	1 μg/ml	39.2 ± 8.4	110.3 ± 5.4	104.5 ± 6.7
Induced by 10^{-6} molar ADP final concentration				
Saline	0.5 ml	27.2 ± 6.2	107.9 ± 7.7	110.4 ± 7.9
Adrenaline	0.1 μg/ml	24.4 ± 5.4	95.9 ± 6.4	98.9 ± 6.0
	1 μg/ml	24.4 ± 4.8	129.4 ± 12.8*	126.6 ± 12.2
	10 μg/ml	27.3 ± 4.9	106.1 ± 7.4	92.0 ± 6.1
Noradrenaline	1 μg/ml	27.9 ± 7.5	106.9 ± 5.4	96.5 ± 12.5

** $P<0.01$, * $P<0.05$ (compared with value before injection).

10^{-6} molar ADP. There was a tendency for the responses induced by higher concentrations of ADP to show smaller variation. In the above 5 groups, the degree of platelet aggregation by ADP increased significantly 5 min after intravenous injection of 1 μg/kg adrenaline, when the degree of platelet aggregation increased to 115.1±4.9% (mean±SE) with 10^{-5} molar, 121.8±7.8% with 3×10^{-6} molar, and 129.4±12.8% with 10^{-6} molar ADP compared to the preinjection values. The difference was statistically significant in each group at the 1–5% level. 30 min after the injection, the statistically significant enhancement was not observed, although the mean value was higher than that before the injection. The enhancement of platelet aggregation was not observed in the groups of 10 rabbits injected with saline or 1 μg/kg noradrenaline (Table I, Fig. 1).

For the analysis of these results, the degree of platelet aggregation and the dose of ADP were compared in each of the values measured before and 5 and 30 min after the injections, respectively. The correlation between them is shown in Table II. The number in parenthesis shows the correlation coefficient. A positive correlation was observed, although the correlation coefficients were not high. The slopes of each dose-response curve before and 5 min after the injections were almost the same. A statistically significant difference ($P<0.05$) in the degree of platelet aggregation was observed between both the preinjection level and 5 min after the injection of 1 μg/kg adrenaline.

The enhancement of ADP-induced platelet aggregation was observed only in the group injected with 1 μg/kg adrenaline. In the group injected with 0.1 or 10 μg/kg adrenaline, there was no statistically significant difference in ADP-induced platelet aggregation after the injection. 5 min after 0.1 μg/kg adrenaline, the degree of aggregation was 96.6±2.1% with

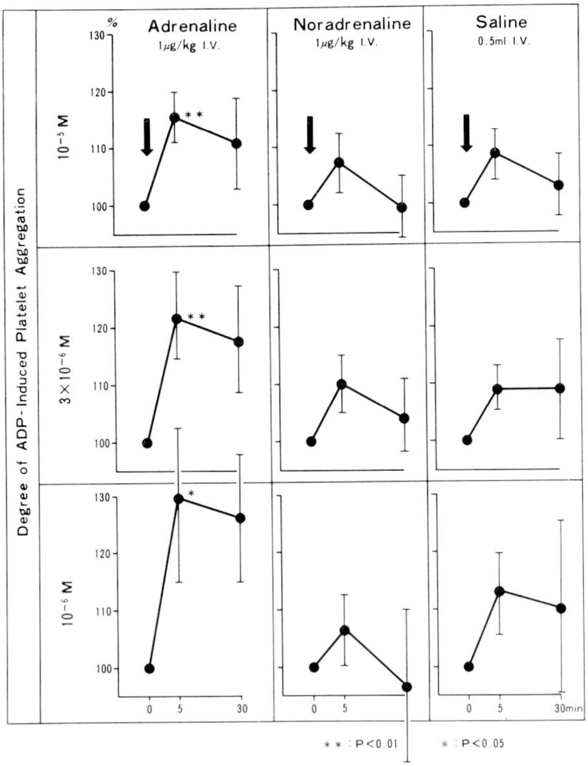

Fig. 1. Changes in ADP platelet aggregation induced by catecholamine in vivo (10 rabbits in each group). Enhancement of ADP-induced platelet aggregation was observed 5 min after i.v. injection of 1 μg/kg adrenaline with statistical significance ($P<0.01 \sim 5$). The enhancement was observed after addition of 10^{-5}, 3×10^{-6} and 10^{-6} molar ADP final concentration. It was not observed after i.v. injection of 1 μg/kg noradrenaline or 0.5 ml saline.

TABLE II

Relationship between degree of platelet aggregation (y) and dose of ADP (x)

Intravenous injection	Before	5 min	30 min
Saline 0.5 ml	$y=25.29+2.08x$ (0.66)	$y=28.97+2.07x$ (0.58)	$y=33.27+1.42x$ (0.31)
Adrenaline 1 μg/kg	$y=28.56+1.85x$ (0.43)	$y=36.17^{*}+1.67x$ (0.38)	$y=35.95+1.61x$ (0.31)
Noradrenaline 1 μg/kg	$y=25.01+1.89x$ (0.45)	$y=28.76+1.88x$ (0.42)	$y=25.07+1.92x$ (0.37)

Number in parenthesis shows correlation coefficient (r).
* $P<0.05$ (compared with value before injection).

10^{-5} molar, 97.7±3.6% with 3×10^{-6} molar, and 95.9±6.4% with 10^{-6} molar ADP compared to the preinjection values. 5 min after 10 μg/kg adrenaline, the degree of aggregation was 101.7±2.9% with 10^{-5} molar, 103.9±4.2% with 3×10^{-6} molar, and 106.1±7.4% with 10^{-6} molar of ADP compared to the preinjection values (Table I).

Next, we examined the preventive effect of oral administration with 10 mg/kg each of α- and β-adrenergic blockade, aspirin and pyridinolcarbamate against the enhancement in-

TABLE III

Prevention of the enhancement of ADP-induced platelet aggregation (10 cases each) by i.v. injection of adrenaline (1 μg/kg)

Pretreatment (p.o. 3 hours before)		Before injection (mean ± SE) (%)	Percent of values before injection (mean ± SE)	
			5 min	30 min
Induced by 10^{-5} molar ADP final concentration				
None		44.3 ± 7.8	115.1 ± 4.9*	111.5 ± 8.0
Phenoxybenzamine	10 mg/kg	34.2 ± 2.9	106.7 ± 7.3	99.2 ± 9.9
Propranolol	10 mg/kg	47.2 ± 3.0	103.0 ± 5.5	97.4 ± 3.8
Aspirin	10 mg/kg	51.1 ± 3.4	106.2 ± 3.2	91.3 ± 5.9
Pyridinolcarbamate	10 mg/kg	50.6 ± 6.2	96.9 ± 5.8	105.4 ± 4.2
Induced by 3×10^{-6} molar ADP final concentration				
None		39.5 ± 7.1	121.8 ± 7.8*	117.9 ± 9.0
Phenoxybenzamine	10 mg/kg	27.3 ± 3.2	101.6 ± 8.7	96.8 ± 8.6
Propranolol	10 mg/kg	35.9 ± 3.5	107.6 ± 6.3	111.5 ± 5.9
Aspirin	10 mg/kg	41.6 ± 3.4	100.5 ± 4.4	93.0 ± 5.7
Pyridinolcarbamate	10 mg/kg	37.7 ± 4.3	105.1 ± 4.9	112.3 ± 7.3

* $P < 0.01$ (compared with value before injection).

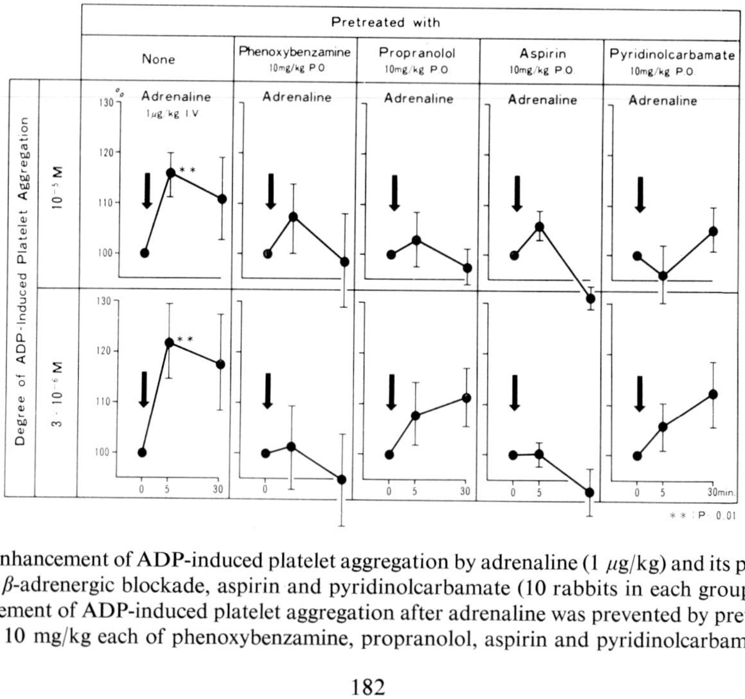

Fig. 2. Enhancement of ADP-induced platelet aggregation by adrenaline (1 μg/kg) and its prevention by α- and β-adrenergic blockade, aspirin and pyridinolcarbamate (10 rabbits in each group). Enhancement of ADP-induced platelet aggregation after adrenaline was prevented by pretreatment with 10 mg/kg each of phenoxybenzamine, propranolol, aspirin and pyridinolcarbamate.

TABLE IV

Degree of ADP-induced platelet aggregation measured by the optical density method (12 cases each)

Group	Treatment	Degree of aggregation (mean ± SE) Concentration of ADP			Correlation coefficient	Regression line
		10^{-5}M	3×10^{-6}M	10^{-6}M		
1	Before water	72.6 ± 1.5	65.5 ± 1.8	54.7 ± 2.3%	0.70	$y = 56.21 + 1.75x$
	Before starch	71.1 ± 1.4	64.9 ± 1.7	54.9 ± 2.5%	0.67	$y = 56.34 + 1.57x$
	After starch	72.2 ± 1.2	65.2 ± 1.5	55.0 ± 2.2%	0.72	$y = 56.55 + 1.65x$
2	Before water	71.8 ± 1.1	65.1 ± 1.6	53.9 ± 2.3%	0.71	$y = 56.00 + 1.68x$
	Before cholesterol	71.4 ± 1.0	64.9 ± 1.5	54.0 ± 2.6%	0.69	$y = 56.08 + 1.63x$
	After cholesterol	75.5 ± 0.8*	70.0 ± 0.8*	58.8 ± 2.1*%	0.74	$y = 61.21 + 1.53x$
3	Before pyridinol-carbamate	73.9 ± 1.3	66.0 ± 2.4	54.3 ± 4.6%	0.68	$y = 56.96 + 1.76x$
	Before cholesterol	73.7 ± 1.8	66.4 ± 3.0	53.8 ± 4.4%	0.63	$y = 57.38 + 1.70x$
	After cholesterol	72.6 ± 1.2	65.1 ± 2.5	54.8 ± 3.9%	0.70	$y = 56.76 + 1.64x$

* $P < 0.05$ (compared with value before cholesterol).

duced by the injection of 1 μg/kg adrenaline. Because the levels of platelet aggregation by 10^{-6} molar ADP were variable and the relationship between dose and response did not show a significant correlation, we used 10^{-5} and 3×10^{-6} molar ADP for the preventive experiment. Before the injection of adrenaline, there was a decrease in degree of platelet aggregation in 10 rabbits pretreated with 10 mg/kg phenoxybenzamine. As shown in Table III, the degree of aggregation by 10^{-5} molar ADP was 34.2±2.9% (mean±SE) in the phenoxybenzamine-pretreated group, while it was 44.3–51.1% in the other pretreated groups. The degree with 3×10^{-6} molar ADP was 27.3±3.2% in the phenoxybenzamine group and 35.9–41.6% in the other groups. However, there was no statistical significance in the difference. None of the pretreated groups with 10 mg/kg phenoxybenzamine, propranolol, aspirin or pyridinolcarbamate showed statistically significant enhancement of ADP platelet aggregation after the injection of adrenaline (Table III, Fig. 2). 5 min after the injection, these values were 96.9–106.7% with 10^{-5} molar and 100.5–107.6% with 3×10^{-6} molar ADP compared with the preinjection values. 30 min after the injection no significant difference was observed also.

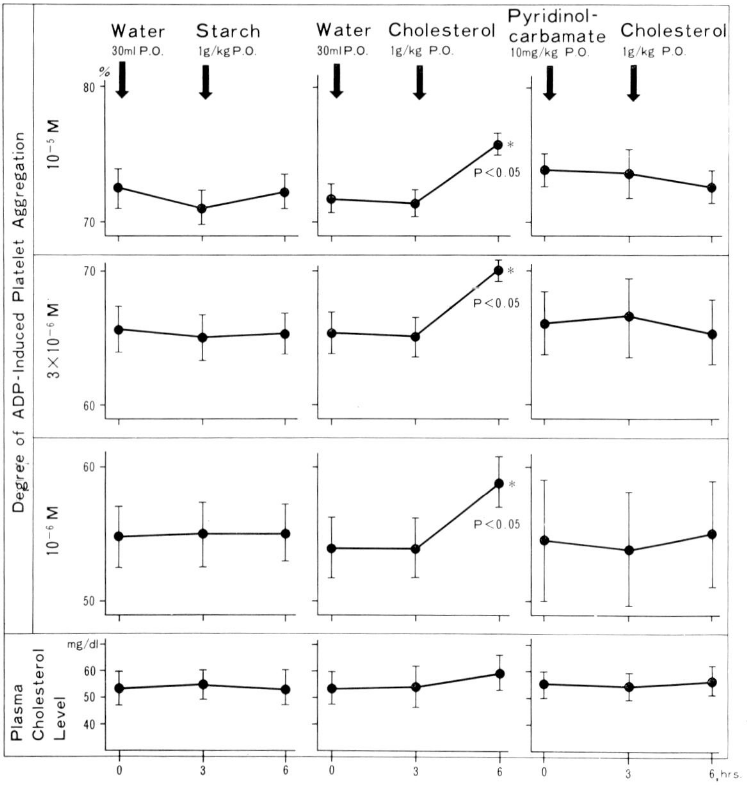

Fig. 3. Enhancement of ADP-induced platelet aggregation by cholesterol intake and its prevention by pyridinolcarbamate in rabbits.

Enhancement of ADP-induced platelet aggregation was observed 3 hours after oral administration of 1 g/kg cholesterol with statistical significance ($P<0.05$). The enhancement was observed after addition of 10^{-5}, 3×10^{-6} and 10^{-6} molar ADP final concentrations. It was not observed after administration of 1 g/kg starch powder. Enhancement after cholesterol was prevented with 10 mg/kg pyridinolcarbamate. Plasma cholesterol levels did not change significantly after any procedure as shown in the lowest column.

2. Effect of cholesterol on ADP-induced platelet aggregation in vivo

a. Degree of platelet aggregation measured by the optical density method No significant difference was observed in the value of the degree of ADP-induced platelet aggregation among 3 groups of 12 rabbits before pretreatment with water or pyridinolcarbamate at any of the 3 concentrations of ADP (Table IV). The mean values were 71.8–73.9% at 10^{-5} molar, 65.1–66.0% at 3×10^{-6} molar, and 53.9–54.7% at 10^{-6} molar ADP. The standard errors were 1.1–1.5% at 10^{-5} molar, 1.6–2.4% at 3×10^{-6} molar, and 2.3–4.6% at 10^{-6} molar ADP. The coefficients of variance were 1.5–2.1% at 10^{-5} molar, 2.5–3.6% at 3×10^{-6} molar, and 4.2–8.5% at 10^{-6} molar ADP. There was a tendency for the responses induced by higher concentrations of ADP to show smaller variations. In the above 3 groups, the degree of platelet aggregation induced by ADP did not change 3 hours after any pretreatment and increased only 3 hours after the oral administration of 1 g/kg cholesterol in 12 rabbits pretreated with water (Fig. 3). At that time, the intensity of platelet aggregation increased to 106.0±2.4% at 10^{-5} molar, 108.5±2.6% at 3×10^{-6} molar and 110.2±3.7% at 10^{-6} molar ADP compared with the value before the cholesterol administration. These values were statistically significant ($P<0.05$) compared with the respective value before the administration. The enhancement was not observed in platelets from 12 rabbits 3 hours after oral administration of 1 g/kg starch powder. Also it was not observed in platelets which were collected from 12 rabbits pretreated with 10 mg/kg pyridinolcarbamate, 3 hours after the oral administration of 1 g/kg cholesterol.

For the analysis of these results, the degree of platelet aggregation and the dose of ADP were compared. In all cases, a statistically significant positive correlation was found between the ADP concentration and the degree of ADP-induced platelet aggregation ($P<0.01$) (Table IV). y is the degree of aggregation and x the concentration of ADP. The correlation coefficients were 0.63–0.74 and the regression lines were almost the same, except in the case obtained 3 hours after cholesterol from water-pretreated rabbits. Here, both regression lines obtained before and after cholesterol administration were compared with a parallel line assay. The slopes of both were parallel ($P<0.01$).

At the same time, the plasma cholesterol levels were examined and statistically significant changes were not observed in any of the 3 groups (Table V, Fig. 3).

b. Sensitivity of platelets to ADP aggregation measured by the microscopic method Before pretreatment, platelets were aggregated in all cases by 2^{-9} to 2^{-12} diluted ADP solution (Fig. 4). Almost all of them were aggregated by 2^{-10} diluted ADP solution. The averages

TABLE V

Changes in plasma cholesterol level (12 cases each)

	Control		
Before (mean ± SE) mg/dl	Pretreatment	3 hr after pretreatment	3 hr after starch 1 g/kg p.o.
51.1 ± 2.0	Water	52.0 ± 1.8	50.1 ± 2.7
	Cholesterol administration		
Before (mean ± SE) mg/dl	Pretreatment	3 hr after pretreatment	3 hr after cholesterol 1 g/kg p.o.
53.4 ± 7.0	Water	56.7 ± 8.4	58.9 ± 7.1
55.1 ± 4.2	Pyridinolcarbamate	54.0 ± 6.1	56.5 ± 5.6

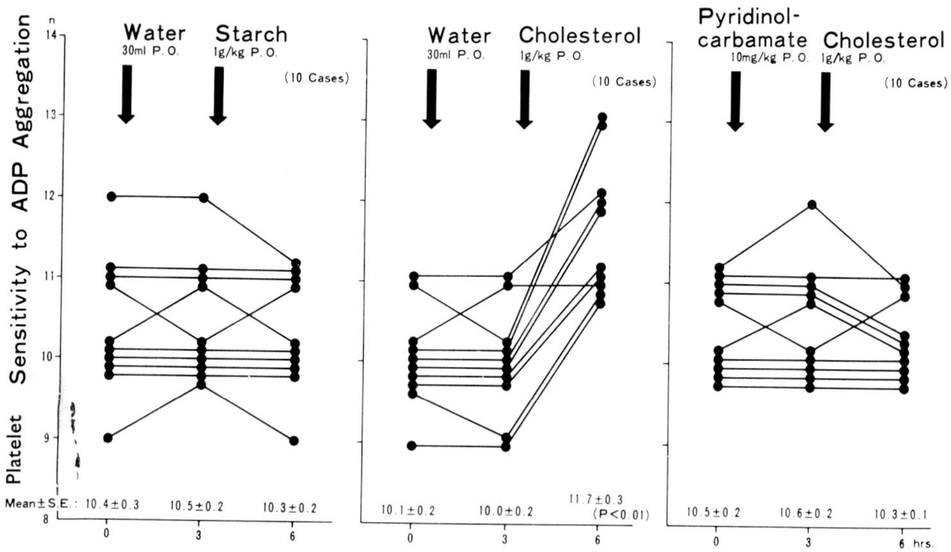

Fig. 4. Enhancement of platelet sensitivity to ADP aggregation induced by cholesterol and its prevention by pyridinolcarbamate in rabbits.

Platelets in CPRP collected from rabbits after 1 g/kg cholesterol were aggregated by $\frac{1}{2}$–$\frac{1}{8}$ diluted ADP solution compared with that collected before the cholesterol in 9 of all 10 cases as shown in the middle column. Enhancement prevented by pyridinolcarbamate pretreatment is shown on the right, the control on the left.

TABLE VI

Platelet sensitivity to aggregation induced by doubly diluted ADP (10 cases each)

Group	Treatment	Platelet sensitivity to ADP aggregation (mean ± SE)
1	Before water	10.4 ± 0.3
	Before starch	10.5 ± 0.2
	After starch	10.3 ± 0.2
2	Before water	10.1 ± 0.2
	Before cholesterol	10.0 ± 0.2
	After cholesterol	11.7 ± 0.3*
3	Before pyridinol-carbamate	10.5 ± 0.2
	Before cholesterol	10.6 ± 0.2
	After cholesterol	10.3 ± 0.1

* P < 0.01 (compared with value before cholesterol).

and standard errors of exponents in each group were 10.4±0.3, 10.1±0.2 and 10.5±0.2 (Table VI). In the 3 groups, the minimum concentration of ADP to aggregate platelets did not change 3 hours after any pretreatment. On the other hand, platelets in CPRP collected from rabbits pretreated with water and tested 3 hours after the administration of 1 g/kg cholesterol were aggregated by $\frac{1}{2}$–$\frac{1}{8}$ diluted ADP solution compared with that collected before administration in 9 of 10 cases (Fig. 4). The minimum effective dose of ADP decreased to $\frac{1}{8}$ in 2, to $\frac{1}{4}$ in 4, and to $\frac{1}{2}$ in 3 cases. In 1 case, the minimum effective dose of ADP did not change. The average exponent increase of 11.7±0.3 was statistically significant ($P<0.01$) compared with that before cholesterol which was 10.0±0.2 (Table VI). The change was not observed in platelets collected from 10 rabbits 3 hours after oral administration of 1 g/kg starch powder. Also, it was not observed in platelets collected from 10 rabbits pretreated with 10 mg/kg pyridinolcarbamate, 3 hours after the oral administration of 1 g/kg cholesterol.

3. Effect of adrenaline on ADP-induced platelet aggregation in vitro

Besides the above experiment, in which the effect of adrenaline was examined on ADP-induced platelet aggregation in vivo, we examined whether an enhancement of ADP platelet aggregation by adrenaline or noradrenaline is present in vitro. Out of 30 CPRP from rabbits, slight platelet aggregation occurred in 9 cases and in the other 21 cases no aggregation was observed during 90 sec after the addition of 0.01–100 μg/ml adrenaline or noradrenaline. The levels of aggregation in the former 9 CPRP were 5–15%. However, after incubation at 37 °C for 30 sec with 0.01, 0.1, 1, 10 or 100 μg/ml adrenaline or noradrenaline in vitro, the degree of platelet aggregation induced by 10^{-5} or 3×10^{-6} molar ADP in any CPRP was almost the same as that without adrenaline or noradrenaline (Fig. 5).

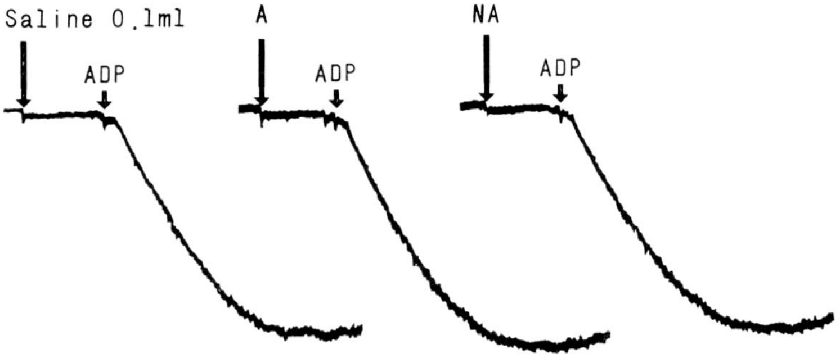

Fig. 5. Rabbit platelet aggregation by ADP (3×10^{-6} molar) was not enhanced by preincubation with adrenaline (0.1 μg/ml) (A) or noradrenaline (0.1 μg/ml) (NA) in vitro.

4. Preventive effect of pyridinolcarbamate on platelet aggregation induced by ADP or adrenaline in vitro

Figure 6 shows aggregation curves induced by 3×10^{-6} molar ADP added to CPRP, which was incubated with saline or 300 μg/ml pyridinolcarbamate at 37 °C for 200 sec. Both primary and secondary platelet aggregation were inhibited by pyridinolcarbamate. Figure 7 shows aggregation curves induced by 1 μg/ml adrenaline. Both primary and secondary aggregation were again inhibited by pyridinolcarbamate. A summary of the in vitro experiments is shown in Table VII. In human platelet aggregation by 3×10^{-6} molar ADP, 86 of 97 samples of CPRP showed a primary aggregation curve. After incubation with 300 μg/ml pyridinolcarbamate in vitro, 57 of the 86 samples showed a smaller response than when incubated with saline. The degree of primary aggregation decreased to 6.7±1.4% of the control value. In secondary

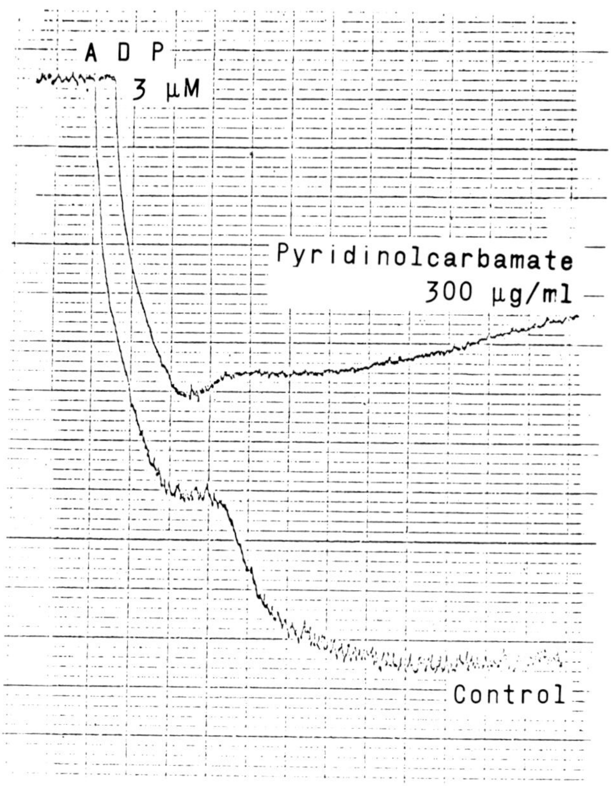

Fig. 6. Platelet aggregation curves induced by 3×10^{-6} molar ADP. Both primary and secondary platelet aggregation were inhibited by 300 μg/ml pyridinolcarbamate in vitro.

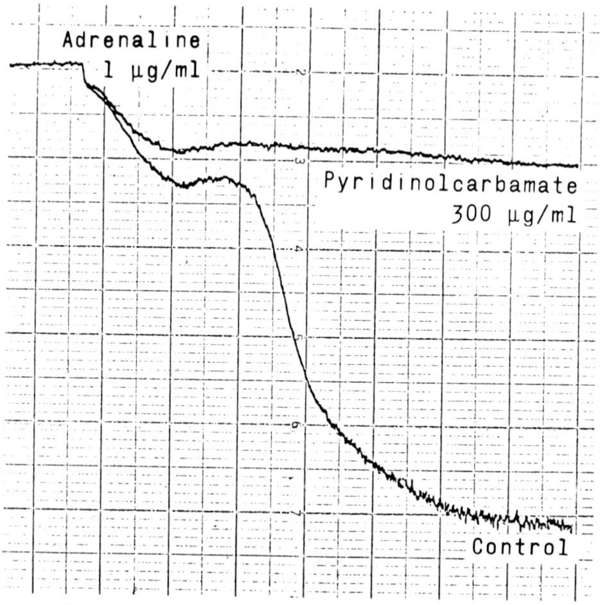

Fig. 7. Platelet aggregation curves induced by 1 μg/ml adrenaline. Both primary and secondary platelet aggregation were inhibited by 300 μg/ml pyridinolcarbamate.

TABLE VII

Inhibition of human platelet aggregation by pyridinolcarbomate (300 μg/ml) in vitro

	Aggregation	Inhibited/total	Inhibition ratio
ADP (3×10^{-6}M)	Primary	57/86 cases	$6.7\pm1.4\%$*
	Secondary	88/97 cases	$33.4\pm2.8\%$*
Adrenaline (1 μg/ml)	Primary	20/27 cases	$12.0\pm2.7\%$*
	Secondary	30/33 cases	$35.2\pm4.8\%$*

* $P<0.01$

aggregation 88 of 97 samples of CPRP were inhibited by pyridinolcarbamate. The inhibition ratio was $33.4\pm2.8\%$. As regards primary aggregation by 1 μg/ml adrenaline, 20 of 27 samples of CPRP were inhibited by pyridinolcarbamate with an inhibition ratio of $12.0\pm2.7\%$. Secondary aggregation was inhibited by pyridinolcarbamate in 30 of 33 samples with an inhibition ratio of $35.2\pm4.8\%$. The inhibition of primary aggregation by adrenaline was stronger than that by ADP, while both primary and secondary aggregation were similarly inhibited by pyridinolcarbamate. This suggests that pyridinolcarbamate may inhibit release of intrinsic ADP from platelets.

DISCUSSION

It has been found (Mitchell and Sharp, 1964) that adrenaline enhances human platelet aggregation by ADP when adrenaline is added to CPRP in vitro. However, the enhancement of ADP-induced platelet aggregation by adrenaline in vivo has not been clarified, except in a report by Sano and Yokoyama (1971). They found that ADP-induced platelet aggregation was enhanced 5 min after an intravenous injection of 1 μg/kg adrenaline in rabbits, using a new microscopic method which measures the minimum concentration of serial doubling dilutions of ADP to induce platelet aggregation. Using the optical density method, we have found enhancement of platelet aggregation by the addition of ADP to CPRP collected from rabbits which were injected with 1 μg/kg adrenaline intravenously 5 min before the collection. We have already reported that a direct relationship between ADP concentration and the maximum optical density of CPRP collected from humans could be observed. There was apparently a dose dependency between ADP and the degree of platelet aggregation, especially using 10^{-6} to 10^{-5} molar ADP (Yamazaki et al., 1970*a*). A similar correlation was found also in the present experiments using rabbit platelets. As shown in Table II, the same relationship between degree of platelet aggregation and dose of ADP was observed in each group. Moreover, before and after the intravenous injection of 1 μg/kg adrenaline, the slopes of the dose-response curves were almost the same while the intensity of response increased after adrenaline ($P<0.05$). This correlation was found in human platelet aggregation by ADP before and after Master's 2-step test in coronary patients (Yamazaki et al., 1970*a*).

To clarify the mechanism of the enhancement by adrenaline, we examined the preventive effect of α- and β-adrenergic blocking agents. Because the intensities of platelet aggregation by 10^{-6} molar ADP were variable, we used 10^{-5} and 3×10^{-6} molar ADP for the preventive experiment and found a preventive effect of oral administration of 10 mg/kg phenoxybenzamine or propranolol against the enhancement of ADP-induced platelet aggregation by the intravenous injection of 1 μg/kg adrenaline. Mills and Roberts (1967) found a preventive effect of propranolol against human platelet aggregation induced by adrenaline in vitro. Bygdeman and Johnsen (1969) confirmed this and found more potent prevention by phenoxybenzamine in vitro. They concluded that the prevention was not due to inhibition of uptake of catecholamine by receptor blockade and that uptake of catecholamine was not a necessary step in catecholamine-mediated platelet aggregation. Sinakos and Caen (1967) reported that rabbit platelets were not aggregated by adrenaline, but that platelet aggregation induced by ADP was enhanced after preincubation with 1 μg/ml of adrenaline in vitro. However, we could not observe this enhancement by adrenaline in vitro. So the enhancement of ADP-induced platelet aggregation after the intravenous injection of adrenaline may not be due to the simple presence of adrenaline in the circulating blood of the rabbit. The enhancement was not observed on intravenous injection of noradrenaline in vivo, which enhanced human platelet aggregation in vitro (Bygdeman and Johnsen, 1969). It was not observed after the injection of 0.1 or 10 μg/kg adrenaline in these authors' experiments.

Recently we reported that an intravenous injection of 0.1 or 1 μg/kg adrenaline induced a decrease in adhesive platelet count and an enhancement of blood coagulability which may be related to thrombogenesis (Shimamoto et al., 1960; Yamazaki et al., 1971). These changes were not observed after a large amount of adrenaline (Shimamoto et al., 1960). Also, we found that the above hematological changes were prevented by β-adrenergic but not by α-adrenergic blocking agents (Yamazaki et al., 1971). On the other hand, the enhancement of ADP-induced platelet aggregation by adrenaline was prevented by both α- and β-blocking agents. Although a larger amount of adrenergic blockade (10 mg/kg) was used and a large amount of phenoxybenzamine may inhibit β-adrenergic receptors in the present experiment, we could not find a clear-cut explanation to clarify the discrepancy. However, there was a difference between phenoxybenzamine and propranolol pretreatment in the pattern of prevention against the enhancement. In the rabbits pretreated with phenoxybenzamine, there was a decrease in the intensity of aggregation by ADP before the injection of adrenaline as compared with that of the other rabbits. This decrease was not found in rabbits pretreated with propranolol. Pretreatment with phenoxybenzamine may directly influence the sensitivity of platelets to ADP.

It is known that aspirin inhibits platelet aggregation induced by ADP or adrenaline (O'Brien, 1968) and that its mechanism may be related to the acetylation of proteins by aspirin (Pinckard et al., 1968; Al-Mondhiry et al., 1969). On the other hand, an intravenous injection of a small amount of adrenaline induced the edematous arterial reaction, which is always accompanied by adhesion of platelets to endothelial surfaces with a decrease in the circulating adhesive platelet count and enhancement of blood coagulability (Shimamoto, 1963). These changes were prevented by aspirin (Shimamoto et al., 1966*b*), β-adrenergic blocking agents (Yamazaki et al., 1971) and pyridinolcarbamate (Shimamoto et al., 1966*a*,*b*; Yamazaki et al., 1971). These substances prevented the appearance of the enhancement of ADP-induced platelet aggregation by adrenaline in vivo as shown in the present paper. The preventive effect of pyridinolcarbamate has already been reported by Sano and Yokoyama (1971) using their microscopic method. These results suggest that the mechanism of the enhancement of ADP-induced platelet aggregation by adrenaline may be partially related to an interaction between platelets and vessel walls which showed edematous changes induced by adrenaline.

Recently the authors have reported (Yamazaki et al., 1970*b*) a decrease in adhesive platelet count with a concomitant enhancement of blood coagulability in coronary arteriosclerotic patients after Master's exercise test. At the same time, the enhancement of ADP-induced platelet aggregation by Master's test was observed (Yamazaki et al., 1970*a*). These changes were similar to those induced by a small amount of adrenaline and may be related to thrombogenesis as described before (Yamazaki et al., 1971). It suggests that the appearance of ischemic changes induced by exercise may be partially due to adrenaline in circulating blood. The hematological changes induced by exercise or adrenaline were similarly prevented by pyridinolcarbamate pretreatment. In this respect, the results presented in this paper may also suggest the clinical usefulness of these compounds as a new type antithrombotic and anti-anginal agent.

The same situation was observed in cases administered cholesterol orally. The authors have reported (Shimamoto et al., 1966*b*) that the oral administration of cholesterol or fatty meal induced an immediate and transient decrease in the adhesive platelet count with an enhancement of blood coagulability. At that time the aggregability of platelets was enhanced as reported in the present paper. The samples in the cholesterol experiment showed higher platelet aggregability by ADP and smaller variations than those in the adrenaline experiment. The discrepancy may be due to differences in the collection of blood samples and the instrument used to measure the aggregability. Table IV shows the relationship between degree of platelet aggregation and dose of ADP which was also observed in the case of cholesterol. In the water-pretreated group, the slopes of the dose-response curves were almost the same before and after cholesterol, while the degree of response increased after cholesterol.

The enhancement of ADP-induced platelet aggregation by cholesterol was observed also by a new microscopic method which measures the minimum concentration of a doubly diluted series of ADP solutions to aggregate platelets (Sano et al., 1971). This method can measure platelet sensitivity to aggregation by ADP with good reproducibility. Although this method can be carried out with a small amount of CPRP (1 drop), there is another beneficial point in that it is not affected by changes in the turbidity of CPRP and the circulating platelet count. Using this method, we confirmed the enhancement of ADP-induced platelet aggregability after cholesterol administration. The percentage change at 3 hours after cholesterol intake was 117.0% of the value before the cholesterol by the microscopic method, whereas by the optical density method the values were 106.0 ± 2.4, 108.5 ± 2.6 and 110.2 ± 3.7% of the value before the cholesterol at 10^{-5}, 3×10^{-6} and 10^{-6} molar ADP, respectively. The confidence level of the significant increase against the value before challenge was at the 1% level by the microscopic method and at the 5% level by the optical density method at any of the 3 concentrations of ADP. The enhancement of ADP-induced platelet aggregation by cholesterol intake was prevented by pyridinolcarbamate pretreatment also. The prevention was clearly observed by both the methods employed.

In considering the preventive mechanism of pyridinolcarbamate on the above hematological changes, we wondered whether pyridinolcarbamate inhibits platelet aggregation by ADP in vitro. Didisheim et al. (1970) reported a preventive effect of this drug against ADP-induced platelet aggregation in vitro. We have also found such prevention by pyridinolcarbamate in a dose of 300 μg/ml in vitro. It inhibited both primary and secondary aggregation by ADP or adrenaline. However, the inhibitory effect was not complete and the inhibition was observed in about 80% of cases. The inhibitory effect was stronger against secondary aggregation (inhibition ratio 33–35%) than against primary aggregation (inhibition ratio 6–12%). It suggests that pyridinolcarbamate may inhibit release of intrinsic ADP from platelets. However, this inhibitory effect in vitro was not enough to explain the inhibition of the enhancement of ADP-induced aggregation after adrenaline, exercise and cholesterol in vivo. The enhancement of platelet aggregability by cholesterol intake was not accompanied by a significant rise in the serum cholesterol level. The relationship between the plasma cholesterol level and the aggregability of platelets by ADP was not obvious. However, Shimamoto (1963) has observed sticking of platelets to endothelial surfaces after administration of cholesterol without a significant rise in the serum cholesterol level. Such a change was prevented by pyridinolcarbamate. According to these experimental results, it is concluded that the enhancement of ADP-induced platelet aggregation after cholesterol administration may be partially related to an interaction between platelets and the blood vessel wall as in the case of adrenaline.

SUMMARY

The authors report a transient decrease in adhesive platelet count and an enhancement of blood coagulability after administration of a small amount of adrenaline (0.1 ~ 1 μg/kg i.v.) or fatty meal including cholesterol in man and rabbit. These changes appear to be related to thrombogenesis and were prevented by pyridinolcarbamate which showed a preventive effect on the appearance of edematous changes in the arterial wall induced by adrenaline or cholesterol. In similar circumstances, the sensitivity of platelets to their aggregation induced by ADP was studied by an optical density (OD) method and by a microscopic method. The degree of platelet aggregation induced by ADP in the OD method was obtained as a percentage of maximum deflection of OD against OD of platelet-free plasma. The latter method measures the minimum concentration of a doubly diluted ADP (2^{-n} mg/kg) solution to induce platelet aggregation. Platelet sensitivity to ADP aggregation was expressed by the absolute value of end-point concentration, i.e. 'n'.

5 min after the i.v. injection of 1 μg/kg adrenaline in 10 rabbits, the intensity of platelet aggregation increased to 115.1$\pm$4.9% (mean$\pm$SE) at 10^{-5} molar, 121.8$\pm$7.8% at 3×10^{-6} molar, and 129.4$\pm$12.8% at 10^{-6} molar ADP of the value before the injection. The difference was statistically significant ($P<0.01 \sim 0.05$). The above change was not observed in each group of 10 rabbits injected with saline, 1 μg/kg L-noradrenaline or 0.1 and 10 μg/kg adrenaline. It was prevented by oral administration of 10 mg/kg phenoxybenzamine, propranolol, aspirin or pyridinolcarbamate 3 hours before the challenge. In 10 rabbits given 1 g/kg cholesterol orally, the degree of platelet aggregation increased to 106.0$\pm$2.4% at 10^{-5} molar, 108.5$\pm$2.6% at 3×10^{-6} molar, and 110.2$\pm$3.7% at 10^{-6} molar ADP, although the plasma cholesterol level did not change. The difference was significant ($P < 0.01 \sim 0.05$). It was also prevented by pyridinolcarbamate pretreatment. Results obtained by the new microscopic method confirmed these results.

To analyse the preventive mechanism of pyridinolcarbamate, the effect of pyridinolcarbamate on platelet aggregation by ADP or adrenaline in vitro was also studied. In 88 of 97 samples of citrated platelet-rich plasma (CPRP) collected from human subjects, platelet aggregation by 3×10^{-6} molar ADP was inhibited by the addition of 300 μg/ml pyridinolcarbamate in vitro. In 30 of 33 CPRP, platelet aggregation by 1 μg/ml adrenaline was inhibited by 300 μg/ml pyridinolcarbamate in vitro. The inhibitory effect in vitro was not enough to explain the inhibition of the enhancement of ADP-induced platelet aggregation after adrenaline or cholesterol in vivo. An important interaction between blood vessel wall and platelets is therefore suggested to clarify the above phenomena in vivo.

REFERENCES

AL-MONDHIRY, H., MARCUS, A. and SPAET, T. H. (1969): Acetylation of human platelets by aspirin. *Fed. Proc., 28*, 576.

BORN, G. V. R. (1962): Quantitative investigations into aggregation of blood platelets. *J. Physiol. (Lond.)*, 162, 67.

BORN, G. V. R. and HUME, M. (1967): Effects of the numbers and sizes of platelet aggregates on the optical density of plasma. *Nature (Lond.), 215*, 1027.

BYGDEMAN, S. and JOHNSEN, Ø. (1969): Studies on the effect of adrenergic blocking drugs on catecholamine-induced platelet aggregation and uptake of noradrenaline and 5-hydroxytryptamine. *Acta physiol. scand., 75*, 129.

DIDISHEIM, P., STURM, R. E. and OWEN JR, C. A. (1970): Experiments on thrombosis and its prevention. Paper presented at: Sherbrooke Symposium on Blood Coagulation, Sherbrooke, Quebec, 1970.

HENLY, A. A. (1957): The determination of serum cholesterol. *Analyst, 82*, 286.

MILLS, D. C. B. and ROBERTS, G. C. K. (1967): Effects of adrenaline on human blood platelets. *J. Physiol. (Lond.), 193*, 443.

MITCHELL, J. R. A. and SHARP, A. A. (1964): Platelet clumping in vitro. *Brit. J. Haematol., 10*, 78.

O'BRIEN, J. R. (1962): Platelet aggregation. II. Some results from a new method of study. *J. clin. Path., 15*, 452.

O'BRIEN, J. R. (1968): Effects of salicylates on human platelets. *Lancet, 1*, 779.

PINCKARD, R. N., HAWKINS, D. and FARR, R. S. (1968): In vitro acetylation of plasma proteins, enzymes and DNA by aspirin. *Nature (Lond.), 219*, 68.

SANO, T., BOXER, M. G. J., BOXER, L. A. and YOKOYAMA, M. (1971): Platelet sensitivity to aggrega-

tion in normal and diseased groups – a method for assessment of platelet aggregability. *Thrombos. Diathes. haemorrh. (Stuttg.)*, *25*, 524.
SANO, T. and YOKOYAMA, M. (1971): Effect of pyridinolcarbamate on platelet aggregation. *Amer. J. med. Sci.*, *262*, 205.
SHIMAMOTO, T. (1963): The relationship of edematous reaction in arteries to atherosclerosis and thrombosis. *J. Atheroscler. Res.*, *3*, 87.
SHIMAMOTO, T., MAEZAWA, H., YAMAZAKI, H., ATSUMI, T., FUJITA, T., ISHIOKA, T. and SUNAGA, T. (1966*a*): Pyridinolcarbamate, a bradykinin antagonist in veins. *Amer. Heart J.*, *71*, 297.
SHIMAMOTO, T., MAEZAWA, H., YAMAZAKI, H., ISHIOKA, T., SUNAGA, T. and FUJITA, T. (1966*b*): Edematous arterial reaction and its relationship to atherosclerosis and thrombosis. *Meth. Achiev. exp. Path.*, *1*, 337.
SHIMAMOTO, T., YAMAZAKI, H., INOUE, M., FUJITA, T., SAGAWA, N., ISHIOKA, T. and SUNAGA, T. (1960): Effect of adrenaline and noradrenaline on 'silicone-like property' of blood vessels. *Proc. Jap. Acad.*, *36*, 234.
SINAKOS, Z. and CAEN, J. P. (1967): Platelet aggregation in mammalians (human, rat, rabbit, guinea-pig, horse, dog) – a comparative study. *Thrombos. Diathes. haemorrh. (Stuttg.)*, *17*, 99.
YAMAZAKI, H., KOBAYASHI, I. and SHIMAMOTO, T. (1970*a*): Enhancement of ADP-induced platelet aggregation by exercise test in coronary patients and its prevention by pyridinolcarbamate. *Thrombos. Diathes. haemorrh. (Stuttg.)*, *24*, 438.
YAMAZAKI, H., SANO, T., ODAKURA, T., TAKEUCHI, K., MATSUMURA, T., HOSAKI, S. and SHIMAMOTO, T. (1971): Appearance of thrombogenic tendency induced by adrenaline and its prevention by β-adrenergic blocking agent, nialamide and pyridinolcarbamate. *Thrombos. Diathes. haemorrh. (Stuttg.)*, *26*, 251.
YAMAZAKI, H., SANO, T., ODAKURA, T., TAKEUCHI, K. and SHIMAMOTO, T. (1970*b*): Electrocardiographic and hematological changes by exercise test in coronary patients and pyridinolcarbamate pretreatment. A double-blind crossover trial. *Amer. Heart J.*, *79*, 640.
ZAK, B. (1957): Simple rapid microtechnic for serum total cholesterol. *Amer. J. clin. Path.*, *27*, 583.
ZUCKER, M. B. (1961): In: *Blood Platelet*, p. 141. Editors: S. A. Johnson, R. W. Monto, J. W. Rebuck and R. C. Horn. Little, Brown and Co., Boston, Mass.

DISCUSSION

Dr. TERRY: I do not think there will be any doubt that the effects of pyridinolcarbamate on platelets are extremely important. However, we ran into 2 problems which I assume a number of others have also encountered and perhaps discussing it may perhaps help others too.

The first problem was that we were unable to identify patients according to severity of disease by the response in the platelet test we used. We use the Salzmann procedure. If I use the terms 'normal' and 'abnormal' these are obviously only very relative terms. We found abnormal responses in untreated patients or normal responses regardless of the severity of the disease. Following treatments with the drug, because we did not know whether it was the pyridinolcarbamate or the placebo, we found responses practically unchanged. Again we could not relate it to any clinical manifestation or laboratory procedure. We can add that subsequently a number of people in the field who were using other substances had run into the very same problem. Any suggestions will be more than welcome.

Dr. KRITCHEVSKY: Dr. Yamazaki, did you measure the release of any of the platelet constituents such as platelet Factors 3 or 4 or ADP, and, if so, is this inhibited by pyridinolcarbamate as you suggested might be possible?

Dr. YAMAZAKI: In answer to your question, I have not measured the release of ADP or Factors 3 and 4 from platelets.

Dr. COLMAN: I have 2 comments and a question. First, in the adrenaline enhancement experiments I think you used 3×10^{-6} molar ADP. I suggest that if you drop your concentration a bit, you will have enhancement because other people have done this experiment.

In the effect of pyridinolcarbamate and, for that matter, pyridinolcarbamate on platelets, in order to get inhibition of platelet aggregation one must use 300 μg/ml. But at the blood levels which one achieves in man, 24–25 μg/ml have absolutely no effect on aggregation. So one has to be concerned with what the mechanism is. Is it metabolic? Is it local concentration or are we not using the right test to measure the effect?

The question concerns the time. You always express this as a percentage both here and also in your article on thrombosis. I would be interested to know the number of seconds shortening you actually got because on most prothrombin curves between 195% there is a $\frac{1}{2}$ sec difference.

Dr. YAMAZAKI: I said in my report that the inhibitory effect of pyridinolcarbamate in vitro was not enough to explain the inhibition of the enhancement of ADP-induced aggregation in vivo. The interaction between the blood constituents and the blood vessels may be important. The third question was the prothrombin time?

Dr. COLMAN: Yes. Could you give an example of the number of seconds shortening that you see? You give percentages but I would like to know what you are measuring – 1 sec, 5 sec, or $\frac{1}{2}$ sec?

Dr. YAMAZAKI: We used the standard method. However, I forget the correct value. I am sorry.

Dr. SHKHVATSABAYA: Could you tell me at what time of day you would measure the aggregation, because normally during the day this parameter is changed?

Dr. YAMAZAKI: We only measure the changes in aggregability of platelets before and after some kind of stress, e.g. intravenous injection of adrenaline, so I cannot know the absolute value of platelet aggregability. But I think you had better hear from Dr. Cotton.

Dr. DIDISHEIM: I would like to make one other comment regarding the platelet function tests which Dr. Colman and Dr. Terry raised. I think it is a very crucial one. Some reports recently – one by Dr Jenkin from Denver, and another from Seattle by Dr. Harker – indicate that the present survival by the chromium-51 method is perhaps the most sensitive test of platelet function that we know. In these 2 centers, when the platelets of patients with cardiac diseases were studied, all other tests including platelet aggregation by Born's method and platelet adhesiveness by the Salzmann method and a number of others were completely normal. The only test which showed abnormality was platelet survival, and it could be corrected instantly by treatment with various ADP agents. I think it would be very useful to repeat these experiments with the ADP agent pyridinolcarbamate in patients with coronary disease and other vascular diseases.

EFFECT OF PYRIDINOLCARBAMATE ON PLATELET AGGREGATION IN VITRO AND ADP-INDUCED CHANGES IN VIVO: COMPARATIVE EFFECTS OF AMP AND ATP*

PAUL DIDISHEIM and ITSURO KOBAYASHI
Department of Laboratory Medicine, Mayo Clinic, Rochester, Minn., U.S.A.

Platelets play an essential role in the early stages of thrombogenesis in arteries and probably in veins as well (Sherry et al., 1969). This fact may explain why agents such as heparin and dicumarol, which prevent fibrin formation but do not inhibit platelet functions, are not always effective antithrombotic agents. The limitations of these anticoagulants are particularly evident in the prevention of thrombosis in systemic arteries and arterioles, where platelets play a particularly prominent role.

For these reasons, it is desirable to find agents which will safely inhibit the participation of platelets in thrombosis in man. Aspirin, dipyridamole, and sulfinpyrazone may eventually be found satisfactory for this purpose (Didisheim, 1969; Evans et al., 1968; Mustard et al., 1967). The following is a report on in vitro and in vivo studies with pyridinolcarbamate. The studies suggest that this agent may have a place in antithrombotic therapy.

METHODS AND MATERIALS

Platelet aggregation was studied by the turbidimetric method of Born (1962). Pyridinolcarbamate (Banyu) was dissolved in 0.9% NaCl. Adenosine nucleotides (Sigma) were obtained as their sodium salts and were dissolved in 15.4 mM tris buffer, pH 7.4 and stored frozen in small aliquots until use. Collagen was a saline extract of rat tail tendon, stored as above. Epinephrine and thrombin were from Parke Davis and were prepared immediately before use. Inhibition of platelet aggregation was calculated from the relative heights of the control and pyridinolcarbamate light transmission curves above baseline at the times specified. Pyridinolcarbamate or 0.9% NaCl was incubated with platelet-rich plasma at 37°C with continuous mixing before the aggregating agent was added.

Male 400–600 g rats were anesthetized with pentobarbital. A polyethylene tracheotomy tube was inserted. Arterial pressure was continually recorded via a femoral artery cannula and transducer. A femoral vein and carotid artery were cannulated for injection of agents and collection of blood, respectively. Heparin, 100 U/kg, was injected to prevent clotting in the cannulas during the experiment. Platelets were counted on a Coulter Model B counter. Blood gases were measured on an IL 112 blood gas analyzer. Electrocardiograms and respirations were recorded on a Grass Model III D 6 channel electroencephalograph. Respirations were sensed by a temperature-sensitive transducer attached to the tracheotomy tube. Nucleotides were injected intravenously within one second's time.

RESULTS

Pyridinolcarbamate inhibited platelet aggregation when induced by ADP, tendon extract, or epinephrine, but not by thrombin (Tables I, II).

Intravenous injection of ADP caused an immediate drop in platelet count. The amount of drop was related to the dose of ADP injected (Fig. 1). Prior administration of pyridinol-

* This work was supported, in part, by grants from USPHS, NIH (NS-06663) and from the Japan Arteriosclerosis Research Foundation.

TABLE I

Platelet aggregation.
Inhibition by pyridinolcarbamate

Agent	Final concentration	% Inhibition by pyridinolcarbamate	
		200 μg/ml	300 μg/ml
ADP	10 μM	4	11
	3	3	21*
	1	2	35*
	0.3	11	37*
Tendon extract	2.3 mg/ml	8	14*
(collagen)	1.5	22*	27*
	0.8	42*	58*
	0.4	70*	80*
Thrombin	0.5 NIH U/ml	10	10
	0.3	15	−4

* $P < 0.01$; for all other values, $P > 0.05$.

TABLE II

Platelet aggregation by epinephrine.
Inhibition by pyridinolcarbamate

Epinephrine	% Inhibition by pyridinolcarbamate			
	200 μg/ml		300 μg/ml	
	at 3 min	at 7 min	at 3 min	at 7 min
50 μM	28	35	46	58
5 μM	25	37	40	52

For all data, $P < 0.01$.

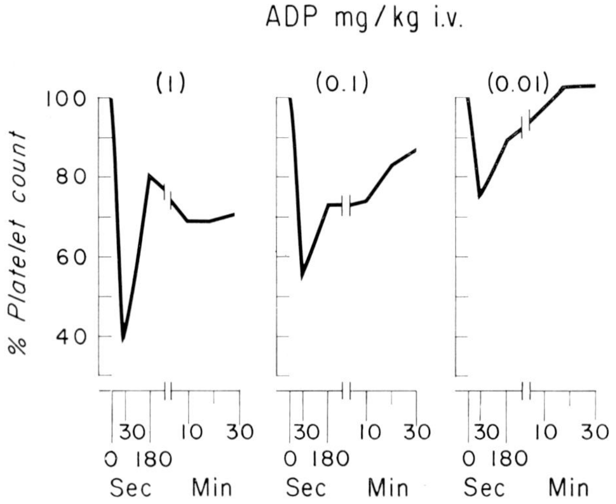

Fig. 1. Effects of injecting various doses of ADP intravenously on the platelet count in the rat.

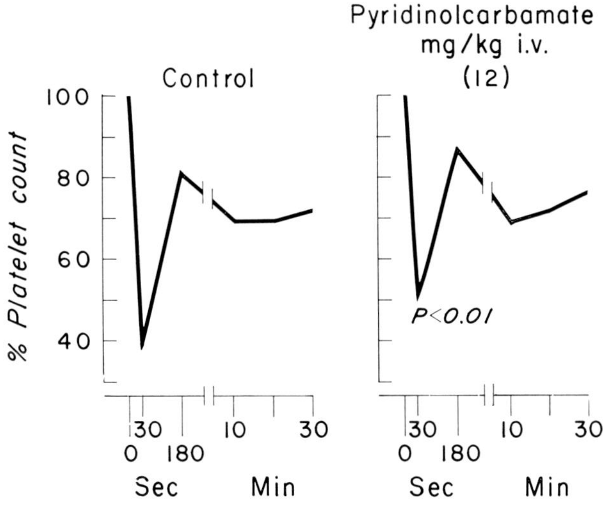

Fig. 2. Effect of prior pyridinolcarbamate infusion on the thrombocytopenia induced by intravenous injection of ADP, 1 mg/kg.

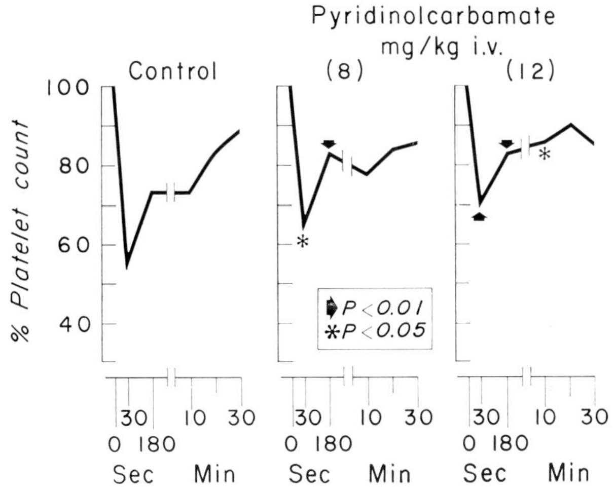

Fig. 3. Same as Fig. 2 except that ADP dose was 0.1 mg/kg.

carbamate reduced the amount of platelet drop (Figs. 2 and 3). ADP also had various respiratory effects including shallow respirations, slow respiration, or respiratory arrest. These effects were usually of short duration, were related to the dose of ADP administered, and were reduced by prior administration of pyridinolcarbamate (Table III). In addition, the injection of ADP was followed by a drop in carotid arterial Po_2 (Table IV) and in heart rate (Table V) as well as in the appearance of flutter-fibrillation (Table VI) and variable A–V block (Fig. 4). These changes were all related to the dosage of ADP administered, and all values returned to near normal within 3 min or less. In each case, the severity of the abnormality was reduced by prior administration of pyridinolcarbamate.

In contrast to ADP, intravenous injection of AMP or ATP had much slighter effects on platelet count (Fig. 5), respiration (Table VII), arterial Po_2 (Table VIII), heart rate (Table IX), or heart rhythm (Table X).

TABLE III

ADP-induced respiratory changes.
Effect of pyridinolcarbamate (PDC)

PDC	ADP	Resp./min (time after ADP)			Respiratory arrest	
(mg/kg i.v.)		Before	0–40 sec	3 min	No. rats	Sec
0†	1	62	31	61	10/10	13
12	1	59	49*	58	9/9	7*
0†	0.1	59	49	50	12/13	9
8	0.1	67	64*	73*	6/11*	4**
12	0.1	67	65*	65*	4/10*	5**

† 0.9 % NaCl.
* For difference between groups, $P < 0.01$.
** For difference between groups, $P < 0.05$.

TABLE IV

ADP-induced changes in arterial Po_2.
Effect of pyridinolcarbamate (PDC)

No. rats	PDC	ADP	% Po_2 change (time after ADP)	
	(mg/kg i.v.)		30 sec	3 min
10	0†	1	−24	+2
9	12	1	− 1*	0
13	0†	0.1	−18	−4
11	8	0.1	−14	0
10	12	0.1	+ 4**	+7

† 0.9 % NaCl.
* For difference between groups, $P < 0.01$.
** For difference between groups, $P < 0.05$.

TABLE V

ADP-induced changes in heart rate.
Effect of pyridinolcarbamate (PDC)

No. rats	PDC	ADP	Beats/min (time after ADP)		
	(mg/kg i.v.)		Before	0–40 sec	3 min
10	0†	1	296	100	274
9	12	1	297	156**	260
13	0†	0.1	338	202	248
11	8	0.1	344	265	298
10	12	0.1	360	293*	325*

† 0.9 % NaCl.
* For difference between groups, $P < 0.01$.
** For difference between groups, $P < 0.05$.

TABLE VI

ADP-induced arrhythmia.
Effect of pyridinolcarbamate (PDC)

PDC (mg/kg i.v.)	ADP (mg/kg i.v.)	Flutter-fibrillation (no. rats)	Duration of arrhythmia (sec)
0†	1	6/10	36
12	1	2/9	23*
0†	0.1	0/13	14
8	0.1	0/11	8**
12	0.1	0/10	4*

† 0.9 % NaCl.
* For difference between groups, $P < 0.01$.
** For difference between groups, $P < 0.05$.

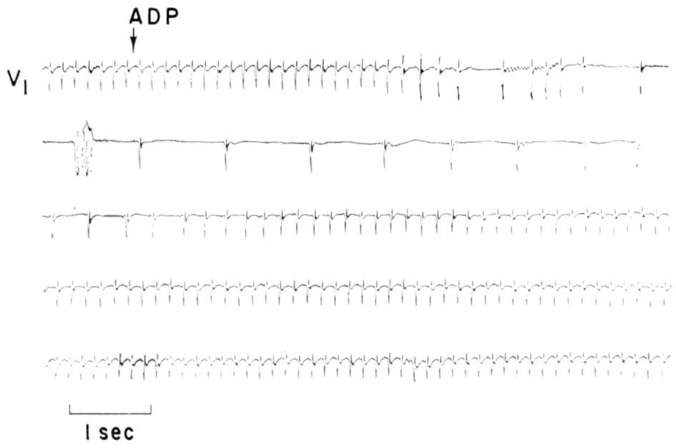

Fig. 4. Effect of intravenous injection of ADP, 0.1 mg/kg, on the electrocardiogram in the rat.

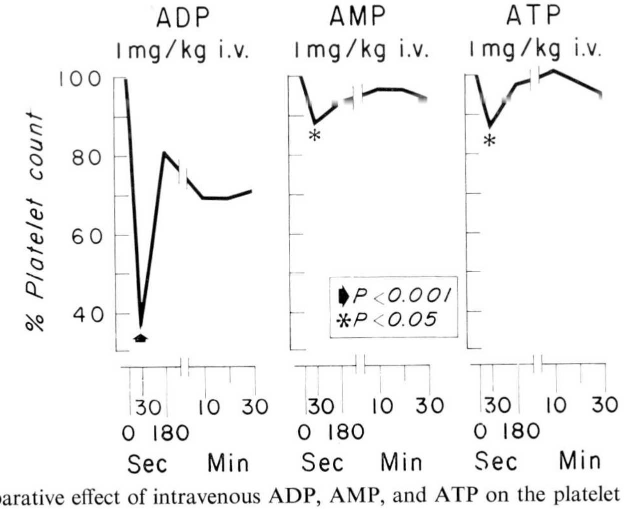

Fig. 5. Comparative effect of intravenous ADP, AMP, and ATP on the platelet count in the rat.

TABLE VII

Nucleotide-induced respiratory changes

Nucleotide (1 mg/kg i.v.)	Resp./min (time after nucleotide)			Respiratory arrest	
	Before	0–40 sec	3 min	No. rats	Sec
ADP	62	31	61	10/10	13
AMP	67	72*	75	2/12*	3
ATP	74	88*	74	1/8*	6

* For differences from ADP group, $P < 0.01$.

TABLE VIII

Nucleotide-induced changes in arterial Po_2

No. rats	Nucleotide (1 mg/kg i.v.)	% Po_2 change (time after injection)	
		30 sec	3 min
10	ADP	−24	+2
12	AMP	− 4*	+4
8	ATP	− 4*	+1

* For differences from ADP group, $P < 0.01$.

TABLE IX

Nucleotide-induced changes in heart rate

No. rats	Nucleotide (1 mg/kg i.v.)	Beats/min		
		Before injection	After injection	
			0–40 sec	3 min
10	ADP	296	100	274
12	AMP	347	245*	347
8	ATP	399	285*	383

* For differences from ADP group, $P < 0.01$.

TABLE X

Nucleotide-induced arrhythmia

Nucleotide (1 mg/kg i.v.)	Flutter-fibrillation (no. rats)	Duration of arrhythmia (sec)
ADP	6/10	36
AMP	0/12*	11*
ATP	0/8*	12*

* For differences from ADP group, $P < 0.01$.

DISCUSSION

Previous studies from this laboratory have demonstrated the inhibition of platelet aggregation by pyridinolcarbamate (Didisheim et al., 1971). The present studies indicate that intravenous pyridinolcarbamate inhibits the effects of intravenous ADP. This suggests that most, if not all, of the changes noted following injection of ADP are related to platelet aggregation in vivo.

The mechanism of respiratory changes following ADP injection is not clear, but the inhibition of these changes by pyridinolcarbamate suggests that they are caused by platelet aggregates in the pulmonary microcirculation. The respiratory changes, along with the platelet aggregates in small pulmonary vessels, combine to produce a ventilation-perfusion defect which would explain the arterial desaturation observed.

The bradycardia, flutter-fibrillation, and A–V block observed following intravenous ADP injection, and the inhibition of these changes by pyridinolcarbamate, suggest that these changes too are in large part caused by multiple platelet aggregates, in this case lodging in vessels which nourish the A–V conduction system and nearby tissue. It is postulated that some of the injected ADP crosses the pulmonary microcirculatory bed before it is metabolized, and that it then causes aggregation of platelets which enter the coronary microcirculation.

These observations are supported by others (Yamazaki et al., 1970*a*, *b*), showing that pyridinolcarbamate prevents certain electrocardiographic and hematologic changes induced by exercise in patients with coronary artery disease. Together they support the concept that pyridinolcarbamate may have a beneficial effect in the prevention and treatment of thromboembolic disorders, particularly involving small systemic arteries, including coronary artery disease.

There is a parallel between the degree of platelet drop and the severity of the changes (respiration, arterial Po_2, heart rate, arrhythmia) induced by ADP, AMP and ATP. These findings confirm and extend previous studies (Jørgensen et al., 1967) and support the concept that the effects observed are largely due to the formation of platelet aggregates in the pulmonary and myocardial microcirculations.

SUMMARY

Intravenous injection of ADP in rats causes numerous transient effects. These include a drop in platelet count, shallow or slow respirations or apnea, a fall in arterial Po_2, bradycardia, flutter-fibrillation, and A–V block.

These effects are partly or completely prevented by prior infusion of pyridinolcarbamate. AMP and ATP cause some of the same effects but to a lesser degree. There is a parallel between the degree of platelet drop and the severity of the other effects following injection of the 3 nucleotides.

These observations support the concept that most, if not all, of the effects observed following ADP injection are due to the formation of platelet aggregates in the pulmonary and myocardial microcirculations.

ACKNOWLEDGEMENT

Miss Marfina R. Briones and Mr. William L. Donovan gave valuable technical assistance.

REFERENCES

BORN, G. V. R. (1962): Quantitative investigations into the aggregation of blood platelets. *J. Physiol. (Lond.)*, *162*, 67.

DIDISHEIM, P. (1969): Inhibition by dipyridamole of arterial thrombosis in rats. *Thrombos. Diathes. haemorrh. (Stuttg.)*, *20*, 257.

DIDISHEIM, P., STURM, R. E. and OWEN JR, C. A. (1971): Experiments on thrombosis and its prevention. *Thrombos. Diathes. haemorrh. (Stuttg.)*, *Suppl. 46*, 177.

EVANS, G., PACKHAM, M. A., NISHIZAWA, E. E., MUSTARD, J. F. and MURPHY, E. A. (1968): The effect of acetyl salicylic acid on platelet function. *J. exp. Med.*, *128*, 877.

JØRGENSEN, L., ROWSELL, H. C., HOVIG, T., GLYNN, M. F. and MUSTARD, J. F. (1967): Adenosine diphosphate-induced platelet aggregation and myocardial infarction in swine. *Lab. Invest.*, *17*, 616.

MUSTARD, J. F., ROWSELL, H. C., SMYTHE, H. A., SENJI, A. and MURPHY, E. A. (1967): The effect of sulfinpyrazone on platelet economy and thrombus formation in rabbits. *Blood*, *29*, 859.

SHERRY, S., BRINKHOUS, K. M., GENTON, E. and STENGLE, J. M. (Eds.) (1969): *Thrombosis*. National Academy of Sciences, Washington, D.C.

YAMAZAKI, H., KOBAYASHI, I. and SHIMAMOTO, T. (1970*a*): Enhancement of ADP-induced platelet aggregation by exercise test in coronary patients and its prevention by pyridinolcarbamate. *Thrombos. Diathes. haemorrh. (Stuttg.)*, *24*, 438.

YAMAZAKI, H., SANO, T., ODAKURA, T., TAKEUCHI, K. and SHIMAMOTO, T. (1970*b*): Electrocardiographic and hematologic changes by exercise test in coronary patients and pyridinolcarbamate pretreatment – a double blind crossover trial. *Amer. Heart J.*, *79*, 640.

DISCUSSION

Dr. TERRY: How important would you consider the release of vasoactive substances during aggregation and the effect on the microcirculation?

Dr. DIDISHEIM: We know that serotonin, adrenaline, and noradrenaline are released from the platelets as part of the general release reaction, and it could well be that pyridinolcarbamate acts upon these as well.

Dr. BERKOWITZ: You mentioned that there is a number of other drugs which blocked platelet aggregation in addition to pyridinolcarbamate. When one gives aspirin in a dose which would block platelet aggregation with ADP, would you then block the respiratory changes that you saw? Is the effect specific to pyridinolcarbamate?

Dr. DIDISHEIM: No, not particularly. We have done some studies with aspirin and we find an effect rather similar to that with pyridinolcarbamate.

Dr. BERKOWITZ: On the platelet aggregation or on blocking the respiratory effects as well?

Dr. DIDISHEIM: In both systems: in vitro in inhibiting the second phase of platelet aggregation, as has also been shown by a number of others, and in vivo as well.

Dr. BERKOWITZ: What were the respiratory effects?

Dr. DIDISHEIM: It partly inhibits the respiratory effects of ADP in a manner rather similar to pyridinolcarbamate.

Dr. BERKOWITZ: The other point is one in the pharmacodynamics of AMP and ATP which you are giving along with the ADP. I wonder how long they last in the blood relative to the ADP. For example, do they stay in the blood as long, so that the effects in fact would be comparable, or do they disappear slower or perhaps faster?

Dr. DIDISHEIM: They all disappear very rapidly, being metabolized by enzymes in the blood, and their effect following the cessation of continuous infusion disappears within minutes.

Dr. CONSTANTINIDES: Dr. Didisheim, when you inject ADP intravenously, you have first this dramatic drop within 30 sec down to 40% or so, indicating aggregation produced by ADP, and within almost 30 or 40 sec it goes back; it is half-way to recovery. That is too fast for the bone marrow to get the signal to start pouring out new platelets; it must indicate dispersal. Is this an indication that the effect of ADP is very short-lived? Has it to be there all the time to keep them aggregated?

Dr. DIDISHEIM: Yes, I agree with you. Continuous infusion of ADP can cause a sustained reduction in the platelet count, whereas one dose injection will cause just this brief one. I agree with you — this brevity argues for rapid disaggregation of circulating platelets rather than production of new ones.

Dr. CONSTANTINIDES: What blood levels of ADP do you think are achieved in the blood following intravenous injection? And if you have any information on this, has anybody measured the blood levels of ADP in cases of cardiac arrhythmias to see if one ever gets such an accumulation of ADP-like compounds systemically, in vivo, in the diffused blood? I can quite believe that you would have a high concentration locally in a microenvironment. But in whole blood, what levels of ADP are required to cause such an aggregation, and do they ever occur normally?

Dr. DIDISHEIM: We can, of course, easily calculate what the initial level is, after injection of 1 or 0.1 or 0.01 mg/kg as we did, and we also know that these nucleotides are rapidly metabolized after injection. There is also evidence that adenosine levels in the coronary circulation may have something to do with coronary flow control, so that adenosine levels have been measured in the hearts of animals and perhaps patients.

Dr. CONSTANTINIDES: And have they been found increased in cardiac arrhythmias?

Dr. DIDISHEIM: I do not have any information about that. What we plan to do in the future is to lower the doses of ADP that we inject to the level which causes very minimal change, which would perhaps approximate the physiological levels.

Dr. AUSTIN: Platelets contain ADP. Is the level of ADP in the platelet such that, when the platelets were degranulated, this might achieve a high local concentration starting the aggregation?

Dr. DIDISHEIM: The only evidence we have about that is from some other studies that I have not reported here, which involved the injection of collagen extract intravenously. This causes all of the same changes, except that they occur later. I presume that what happens is that the collagen infusion causes intravascular release of ADP from the circulating platelets. This is known to take roughly 20–30 sec. This is, in fact, the delay that we observed in animals that were injected with collagen. We interpret this to indicate that the platelets are induced to release their own ADP; this in turn causes thrombocytopenia, reduced arterial Po_2, increased central venous pressure, which I did not indicate but which also occurs after ADP or collagen injection, and ECG abnormalities as well.

Dr. YAMAZAKI: Is there any difference in mechanism between pyridinolcarbamate and aspirin?

Dr. DIDISHEIM: I am aware of the studies which suggest the mechanism whereby aspirin works. I think that may not be the entire story about the mechanism of action of aspirin. A few conflicting data have been reported recently which are hard to explain by that mechanism. It is one thing to demonstrate that aspirin acetylates platelets, but I am not sure that this is the mechanism whereby platelets are inhibited from aggregating. The conflicting data relate to the dose-response effect of aspirin. It is hard for me to understand why doubling doses of aspirin would increase the inhibitory effect against the platelet aggregation, and yet that is what some people are finding. There is a dose-response relationship between the amount given to animals or man and the effect on aggregation. This in fact goes against the popular concept of 'an aspirin a day will keep thrombosis away'.

FUNCTIONAL CHANGES DURING PHARMACOLOGICAL MODIFICATION OF HYPERACUTE RENAL ALLOGRAFT REJECTION

ROBERT W. COLMAN* and GEORGE J. BUSCH

Deparment of Medicine, Massachusetts General Hospital, Peter Bent Brigham Hospital and Harvard Medical School, Boston, Mass., U.S.A.

Although this investigation deals with thrombosis rather than atherosclerosis, the relationship between these 2 pathological processes is probably very close since each may complicate the other.

Renal transplantation has become an accepted clinical procedure for the treatment of chronic renal failure. However, unfortunately a certain number of grafted kidneys fail immediately after implantation. This phenomenon, which usually occurs in recipients presensitized by blood transfusion, is termed 'hyperacute rejection'. Although the underlying mechanism is probably immune, 3 processes which are secondary to immunological injury are in fact responsible for the immediate graft failure. This triad consists of intravascular coagulation, platelet aggregation, and vasoconstriction. On the other hand, from experience with human patients, activation of 2 other systems in the blood, the fibrinolytic and kallikrein systems, may frequently play a protective role and may be favorable for graft survival.

The aim of this study is to define the functional and morphological correlates of experimental hyperacute allograft rejection and to evaluate the pharmacological modification of this model with intra-arterial heparin and pyridinolcarbamate (PDC). Macaca monkeys were chosen since the kinetics of the coagulation, kallikrein, fibrinolytic and complement systems are very close to those in man. The model of hyperacute renal allograft rejection is most suitable for looking at graft rejection in general, since it represents the most intense form of human reaction and also provides measurable functional and morphological changes within rather short periods of time.

Four groups of monkeys were studied. In the untreated group the graft is rejected in 2 min or shortly thereafter, at which point renal venous flow ceases. Hence, in these animals one can get only a very limited amount of data. A second set of monkeys was pretreated with heparin, 2 mg/kg, and was used to assess its effect. These animals were in turn contrasted with a 3rd group who, in addition to the pretreatment, received continuous heparin intra-arterially during the entire time that the graft was in place. The heparin was perfused at the rate of 0.3 mg/kg/hr. In a 4th experimental set, the effects of inhibition of platelet aggregation as well as suppression of the inflammatory reaction was investigated, using PDC. The drug was administered at levels of 15 mg/kg 3 hours prior to the graft vascularization.

Paired monkeys were used which were specifically presensitized to one another by exchange skin grafting. Lymphocytotoxic antibody levels which correlate with graft rejection were in the range of 1 : 4 to 1 : 512 in all animals. Kidney allografts were then performed from one animal to another and the graft was anastomosed to an indwelling Schribner arteriovenous shunt. Both renal arterial and renal venous samples were obtained prior to the anastomosis and at intervals up to 180 min following graft anastomosis. These samples were then analyzed for coagulation Factors II, VIII, X and XII by standard one-stage assays. Plasminogen was measured by a caseinolytic technique after streptokinase activation. Fibrinogen degradation products (FDP) were measured with the staphylococcal clumping test; kallikreinogen and

* Dr. Colman is the recipient of Career Development Award No. HL–48075 (USPHS [NIH]).

kallikrein inhibitor were measured by an esterolytic technique. The 3rd component of complement was measured by radial immunodiffusion.

In addition, renal biopsies were obtained at 5–240 min post-transplantation and were studied using light- and electron-microscopic and immunofluorescent techniques. These findings will be discussed in the companion paper.

Even prior to renal transplantation, certain changes were noted. For example, rejection of skin grafts themselves was associated with moderate changes in coagulation factors, fibrinolytic parameters or complement components. Insertion of the A-V shunt is accompanied by a rather sharp rise in fibrin degradation products with titers ranging from 1:16 to 1:512, possibly due to surface activation via Hageman factor. All results except the split products were expressed in terms of percent of control values for each animal, obtained just prior to anastomosis but after formation of the shunt.

In the untreated group, rejection of the graft occurs within minutes of its revascularization. Usually only a 2-min sample is obtained from these grafts because venous flow ceases so promptly. In these animals, paradoxically, no functional changes were observed in the coagulation, kallikrein, complement and fibrinolytic systems. The cortical vasoconstriction and thrombosis proceed so rapidly that cortical blood flow through injured areas rapidly subsides. Thus the renal venous blood flow drains unaffected areas and does not reflect any alteration that might be present in plasma proteolytic enzyme systems. However, pretreatment with heparin allows collection of venous samples up to 180 min. It is interesting that, although the renal venous flow continued in the animals that were on heparin, the grafts appeared virtually identical to the untreated controls. This group of monkeys pretreated with heparin and essentially a second control group will be contrasted with the intra-arterial continuous heparin as well as the PDC groups.

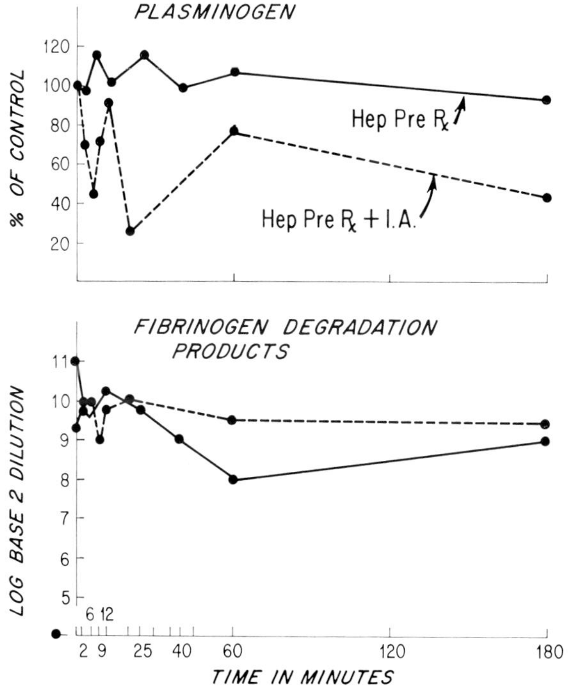

Fig. 1. The fibrinolytic system. Heparin pretreatment ●—●; heparin pretreatment followed by intra-arterial heparin ●---●. Each value is the mean of several animals in the group.

Figure 1 displays the fibrinolytic parameters. The immediate rise in fibrinogen degradation products (FDP) occurred even before the graft is anastomosed and after creation of the arteriovenous shunt. The levels of FDP are so high that subsequently few changes are observed. However, the fibrinolytic system does seem to be activated by the allograft rejection, since although the heparin-pretreated sample essentially shows no change, in contrast, the animals who received intra-arterial heparin throughout the procedure show a gradual fall of plasminogen levels to 40-50% of the original values. This observation indicates that the fibrinolytic system can be activated by mechanisms other than thrombin in vivo and this may allow dissolution of fibrin deposits. Failure to observe any change in the plasminogen in the group pretreated with heparin again suggests that the blood is not draining from the injured portions of the renal cortex.

No significant changes were observed in the levels of the 3rd component of complement in the group pretreated with systemic heparin. In contrast, the animals receiving continuous intra-arterial heparin showed a fall in C_3 to about 60% of control values by the first 25 min. This observation indicates activation of the complement system either by antibody-antigen reaction or by Hageman factor in the fluid phase.

Moderate arteriovenous differences were observed in the measurements of prothrombin and Factor X shown. However, the more significant changes occurred in the renal venous samples (Fig. 2) in both groups. Both Factors II and X in the intra-arterial heparin group

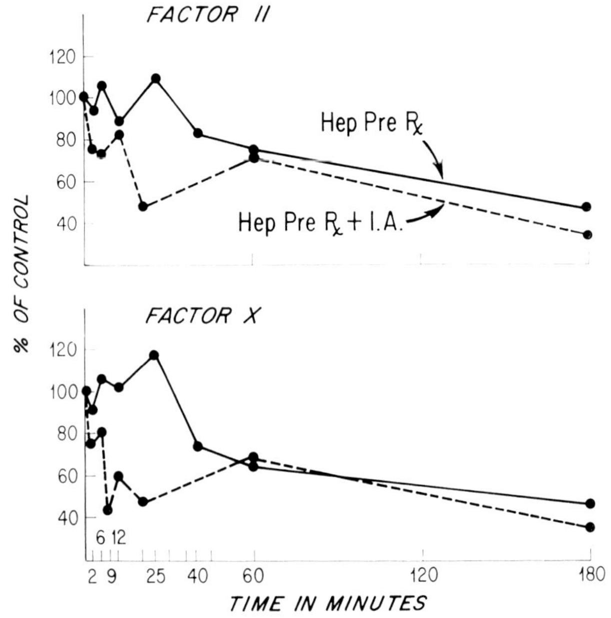

Fig. 2. The coagulation system. For explanation, see legend of Fig. 1.

show a significant decline within the first 60 min compared to the pretreatment group. Thereafter, the 2 groups become very similar. This indicates that, although heparin can block fibrin deposition, it does not interfere completely with the formation of thrombin or of the production of Factor Xa with the respective depletion of its precursors Factor II and Factor X.

The changes of Factor VIII are surprising in their amplitude. In Figure 3 are displayed venous and arterial levels in the animals that received heparin only as a pretreatment.

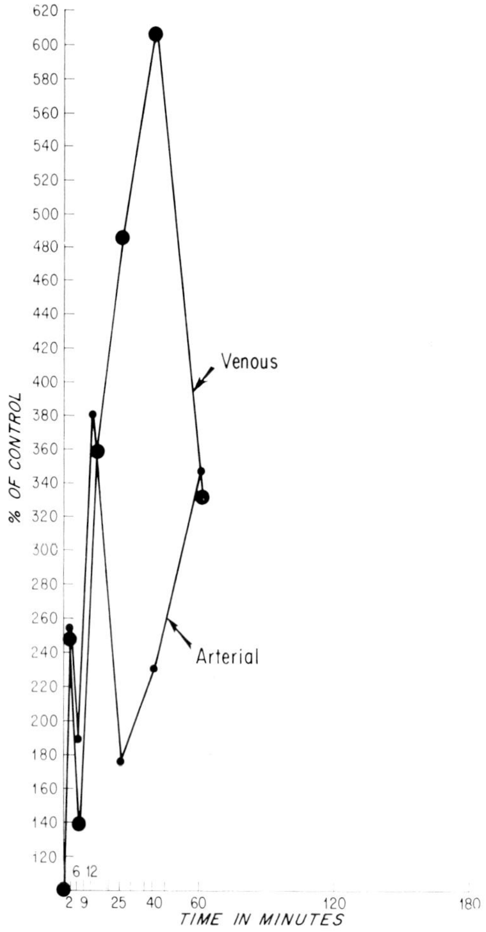

Fig. 3. Factor VIII. Heparin pretreatment. Renal venous ●—● and renal arterial •—• levels are shown.

Enormous A-V differences occur with a marked increase in Factor VIII up to 600% of the control levels followed by a decline. A number of possibilities exist to explain these results. First, an increase in Factor VIII has been noted in stress and these kinds of levels in people who exercise or receive epinephrine may occasionally be seen. However, this would hardly account for the A-V differences observed in these kidneys. The second possibility is that the kidney is thought to be one site of production of Factor VIII. Perfusion of kidneys has yielded net amounts of Factor VIII, and Factor VIII has been isolated from kidney homogenates. The kidney, in the face of extensive injury, may react as does the liver, which is known to release large amounts of Factor VIII. A more attractive possibility is that Factor VIII remains at the same concentration but is converted to a much more active form by thrombin. The consequence of this would be an increase in activity and then a decay due to existence of an unstable form. This has been shown in vitro by a number of workers and may very well operate in this case in vivo. This latter hypothesis gains some credence from Figure 4. In monkeys given heparin intra-arterially, although there were still some increases in Factor VIII, the levels are very much lower and the A-V differences are much less impres-

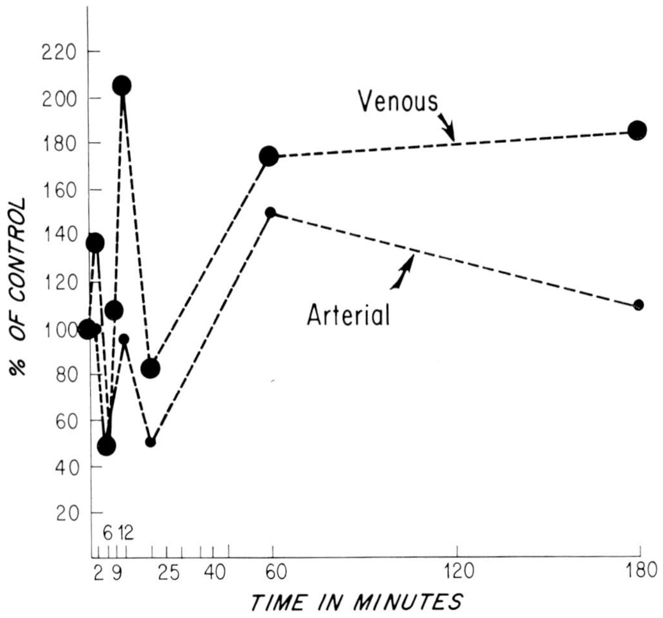

Fig. 4. Factor VIII. Heparin pretreatment followed by intra-arterial heparin. ●----● indicates renal venous effluent values; •----• indicates values from renal arterial blood.

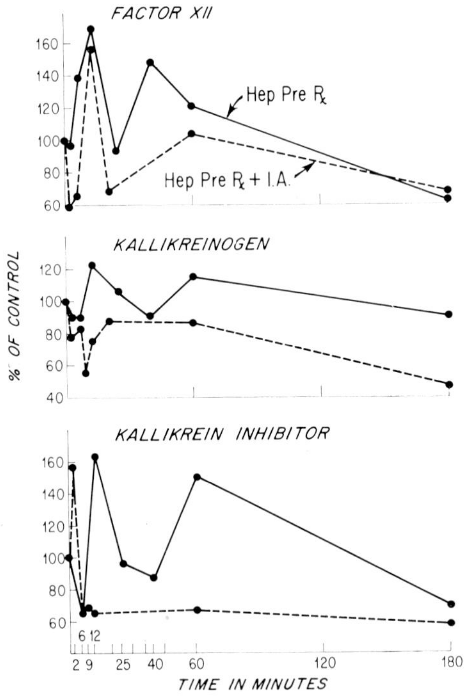

Fig. 5. Kallikrein system. For explanation, see legend of Fig. 1.

sive. This effect of heparin suggests that it may be partially blocking the thrombin activation of Factor VIII in these cases.

Since bradykinin is the most potent vasodilator in mammalian organisms, kallikrein, which is responsible for its release, is of primary concern. The kallikrein system is definitely activated in hyperacute renal allograft rejection and this can be seen very well in the animals who received the intra-arterial heparin (Fig. 5). Kallikreinogen concentration decreases progressively until termination of the experiment when it is less than 50% of the original levels. This represents the decrease of a precursor converted to the active enzyme. The parallel fall in kallikrein inhibitor indicates that free kallikrein is combining with its naturally occurring inhibitor to form a complex which has either inhibitor or kallikrein activity. This activation of the kallikrein system does not occur to any appreciable extent in animals pretreated only with heparin and which are not receiving heparin during the course of the rejection. These phenomena apparently are mediated in part through Factor XII. If samples are obtained very early in the course of rejection, Factor XII rises and then declines. This finding suggests that this protein may be activated and then cleared by a hepatocellular mechanism or by combining with the major kallikrein inhibitor which is identical to the Cl esterase inhibitor. The kallikrein system may be very important in the graft survival because the more kallikrein released, the greater the ability of the organism to antagonize the extensive vasoconstriction that occurs in the untreated animals. This vasoconstriction, probably mediated through the sympathetic system, may itself cause the graft to fail. Experimental results by McKay, using another animal model, showed that large amounts of epinephrine alone can produce extensive renal damage. The activation of the kallikrein system is probably a defense mechanism which increased renal blood flow in the affected areas. Figure 6 shows the changes in the formed elements (white cell and platelet counts)

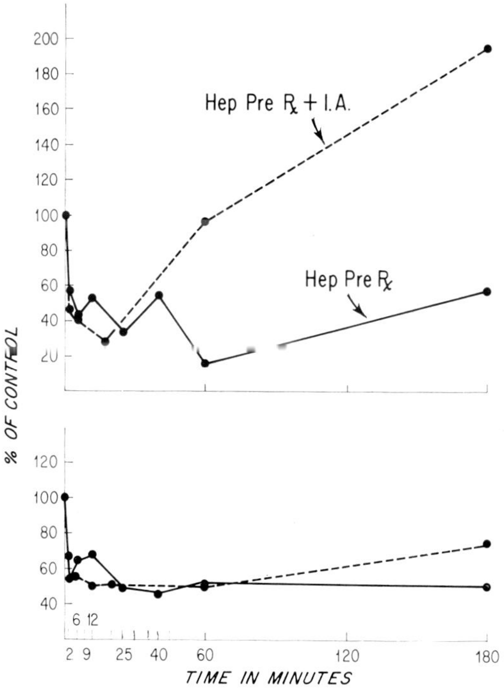

Fig. 6. Cellular response. Upper graph records white blood cell count, lower graph, platelet count. Groups same as in Fig. 1.

of these animals. In both groups, an initial drop occurs within the first few minutes, due to sequestration of platelets and white cells within the graft. Blockage of fibrin deposition by intra-arterial heparin appears to be associated with subsequent release of white cells from the graft. This reversal does not seem to be as marked for platelets.

The functional changes are closely mirrored in the morphological observations presented in the companion paper. In animals which are treated with heparin both before and after the procedure, there is still extensive white cell accumulation but intravascular thrombosis and fibrin deposition is inhibited. In contrast, in untreated animals and animals which are merely pretreated with heparin, intrarenal thrombosis is a prominent feature.

Since white cells and presumably platelets are still present in the graft, it seemed appropriate to try to prevent graft rejection with an inhibitor of white cell and platelet function. We chose to study a group of monkeys treated orally with 15 mg/kg of PDC 3 hours prior to the anastomosis of the donor kidney to the circulation of the presensitized host. Figure 7

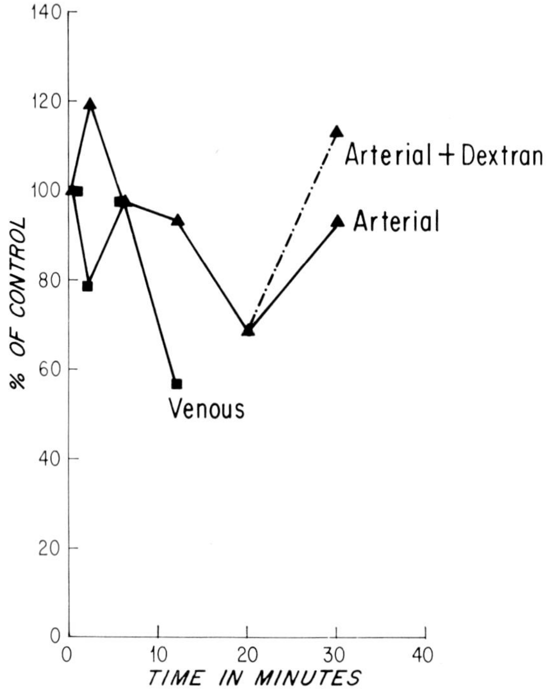

Fig. 7. White blood cell count. Pyridinolcarbamate pretreatment. Renal venous ■—■ and renal arterial levels ▲—▲ are recorded. ▲–·▲ indicates values of 1 animal using 50% dextran.

illustrates the arterial and venous white cell counts. The white blood cell count drops in the venous samples below arterial levels, indicating a net increase of white cells in the graft. All of the experimental points represent 3–5 animals. In one animal we were able to do an additional experiment which was to give a dextran infusion to the animal at a time when the white cell count had decreased. Following the dextran, there was a rise in the white cell count as if the white cells were being released from the graft. This result could be a direct effect of dextran on the white cells or simply an effect of volume expansion.

This phenomenon is seen much more dramatically with the platelets (Fig. 8). Here, when we gave the dextran, the platelet counts increased markedly. Again, one sees the same initial

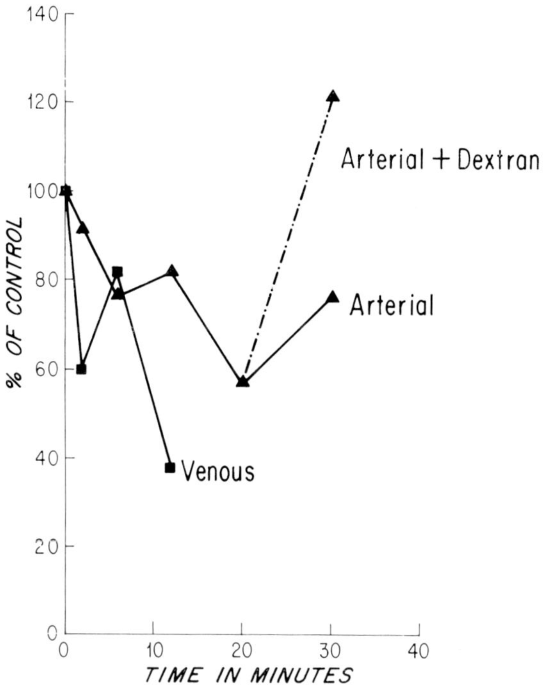

Fig. 8. Platelets. Pyridinolcarbamate pretreatment. Same groups as in Fig. 7.

fall with the significant A-V difference across the graft in platelets. The mechanism of this reversal of the sequestration is probably due to the ability of PDC to block the secondary wave of platelet aggregation which is part of the irreversible platelet reaction. In the presence of PDC platelets are able to disaggregate and allow the possibility of being flushed from the graft.

The coagulation results in the animals receiving PDC (Fig. 9) are strikingly like the intra-arterial heparin group. However, there is no heparin in this system, only PDC. The same degree of activation of Factors II and X occurs as previously seen with heparin alone. The fact that we can see these changes occurring indicates that blood is flowing from the cortical areas, which in the untreated or low-dose heparin animals we were never able to sample. The parallel with intra-arterial heparin continues with Factor VIII (Fig. 10). The enormous rise of Factor VIII that was seen in the animals given only pre-systemic heparin suggested thrombin activation. The increase in Factor VIII observed in the animals treated with PDC is a much more moderate one and quite similar to the effects of the intra-arterial heparin alone. When one examines the histology of the graft, only occasional thrombosis and very little white cell accumulation are apparent. The lesions in the graft in the PDC-treated animals are indeed much less than in any of the other 3 groups, and yet despite that, the graft eventually failed. In Figure 11 the kallikrein system is again examined – this time in the PDC-treated animals. Again, we see activation of Factor XII and a decrease in kallikreinogen, indicating that kallikreinogen is being converted to kallikrein. Quite surprisingly, there is no significant decline and, in fact, an actual rise in the kallikrein inhibitor occurs. This is exactly the finding one might observe if PDC is a kallikrein inhibitor, as has been suggested. As kallikrein is formed, there is another inhibitor, PDC, that competes with the natural inhibitor, so that it is no longer depleted. If kallikrein were inhibited by PDC, there would be no bradykinin available to promote the essential vasodilation that must occur if the graft is to have a chance to

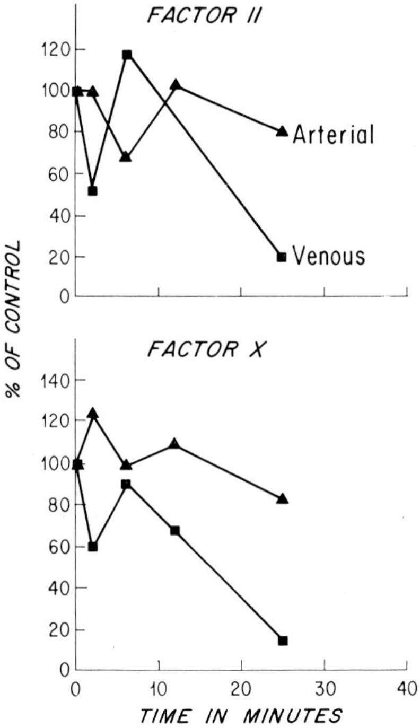

Fig. 9. Coagulation system. Pyridinolcarbamate pretreatment. Same groups as in Fig. 7.

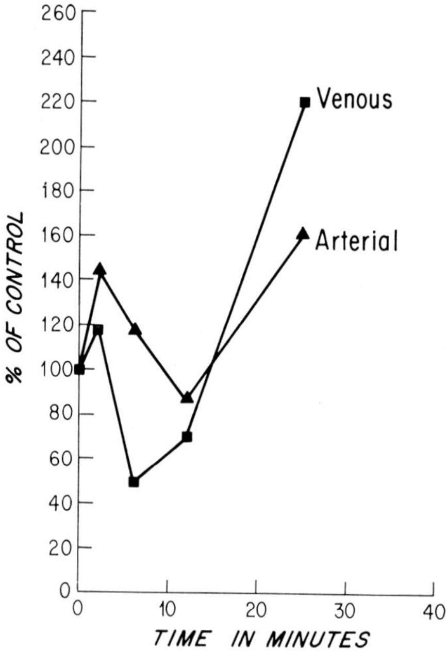

Fig. 10. Factor VIII. Pyridinolcarbamate pretreatment. Same groups as in Fig. 7.

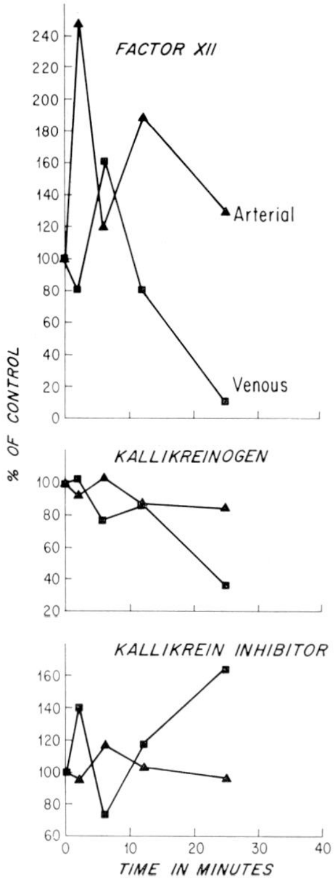

Fig. 11. Kallikrein system. Pyridinolcarbamate pretreatment. Same groups as in Fig. 7.

survive. If the protective effect of the kallikrein system is blocked, the unopposed catecholamine-mediated vasoconstriction may cause graft rejection. This observation will then explain rejection without thrombosis or platelets and white cell aggregates. The mechanism by which PDC prevents fibrin deposition is not clear. The ability to block platelet and white cell function probably explains its ability to inhibit cellular sequestration. These findings suggest that if PDC could be combined with an adrenergic blocking agent, it would have the potential to prevent hyperacute renal allograft rejection. Such a regime, as well as combined PDC and heparin therapy, is currently being evaluated.

For discussion see page 221.

THE PATHOGENESIS OF HYPERACUTE RENAL ALLOGRAFT REJECTION: MORPHOLOGIC CHANGES DURING PHARMACOLOGIC MODIFICATIONS IN THE PRIMATE

G. J. BUSCH and R. W. COLMAN

Department of Pathology, Peter Bent Brigham Hospital and Department of Medicine, Massachusetts General Hospital, Boston, Mass., U.S.A.

There are two primary mechanisms by which a kidney or any other organ transplanted between members of the same species may be rejected. The first is a cell-mediated, or delayed hypersensitivity, form of rejection involving thymus-derived lymphocytes; the second is a circulating antibody mediated, or humoral, rejection with the bone marrow derived lymphocyte as the recognition and effector system.

Humoral rejection, manifest as hyperacute or slowly progressive, has become one of the most important clinical problems in human renal allotransplantation today. Most of the 200 kidney transplant centers around the world are now accumulating ever increasing numbers of patients who have become sensitized to histocompatibility antigens not shared with their prospective donors.

To date, 24 human lymphocyte histocompatibility (HL-A) antigens have been identified. Of these, 10 reside at the HL-A sublocus, and 14 reside at the 4 sublocus; these two subloci are closely contained on a single chromosome. The normal haplotype consists of one such antigen at each respective sublocus. Therefore, the simple Mendelian, non-independent segregation is such that in a family having 5 offspring, 2 might be expected to be HL-A identical, whereas when donors are sought from the general population, the chance of donor-recipient HL-A identity is only 1:100,000.

Thus, most transplant situations involve some degree of histoincompatibility, and many potential recipients may have had a prior encounter with the foreign HL-A antigen(s) either during the course of multiple whole blood transfusions or multiparity, and have developed an immunity against the foreign antigens. Presensitization may be recognized by a cross-match test using recipient serum and donor lymphocytes. A positive test predicts an immediate graft failure rate of 80%.

In the event that a presensitized recipient is inadvertently transplanted with an incompatible donor kidney, hyperacute rejection ensues. Upon revascularization, the kidney becomes immediately cyanotic, mottled, flaccid and renal venous flow ceases.

Figure 1 is a schematic representation of the pathogenetic mechanism of humoral renal allograft rejection. The first stage in this cycle is the binding of specific antibody, formed against the donor's foreign HL-A antigens, with those antigens present on the plasma membranes of the graft endothelial and vascular smooth muscle cells. This reaction is mediated by serum complement, with release of chemotactic factors (e.g. C_{5-6-7}), initiating plasma membrane injury. On the endothelial side of this cycle, the injured endothelial cells contract and often undergo necrosis, thus exposing vascular basement membranes. This injury is followed by adhesion, clumping and degranulation of platelets, local activation of the coagulation system, mural thrombosis and vasoconstriction. At this point a very delicate interplay begins to take place. If the thrombosis is severe, with vascular occlusion, the graft becomes ischemic and undergoes cortical necrosis. In the event that thrombosis is not occlusive, or that the fibrinolytic system can lyse thrombi as they form, there is intramuralization of the thrombotic debris, with subsequent organization and re-endothelialization. These

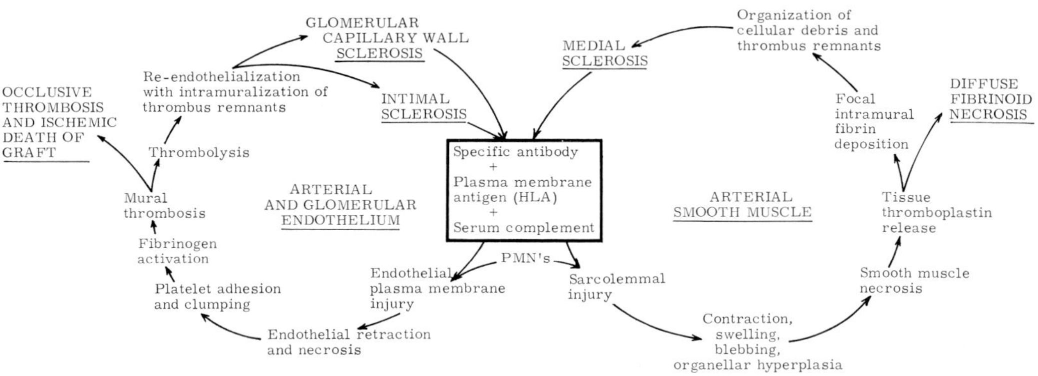

Fig. 1. Pathogenetic mechanism of humoral rejection in renal allografts. Reproduced from *Medicine* (*50*, 1971) by courtesy of Williams and Wilkins Co., Baltimore, Md.

endothelial lesions are similar in glomerular and peritubular capillaries, and in arteries. These alterations result in sclerosis of the endothelial side or intima of vessel walls and narrowing of the lumen. This cycle of injury may be repetitive, depending on the persistence of anti-HL-A antibody levels. On the arterial side of the cycle, in the media, the same antigen-antibody complement-mediated reaction takes place with direct injury to the sarcolemmal plasma membranes, and results in contraction, swelling, blebbing, organellar hyperplasia, smooth muscle cell necrosis, and release of thromboplastins. If this injury is extensive, as is seen with higher antibody titers, diffuse fibrinoid necrosis of smooth muscle occurs and the graft fails. When this reaction is local, the foci of injury undergo repair and the result is one of organization and focal medial sclerosis.

In man, a hyperacutely rejecting kidney becomes immediately cyanotic and flaccid, and shows a marked reduction in renal venous blood flow. The initial histologic features are focal aggregation of red blood cells in dilated peritubular and glomerular capillaries. Shortly thereafter these injured areas also show microthrombi, increased numbers of PMN's, and evidence of endothelial cell injury, namely pyknosis, cellular retraction and nuclear debris. As rejection proceeds, increasingly larger areas of renal cortex are involved, increasing numbers of PMN's are present, capillary thrombosis becomes occlusive and areas of denuded capillary basement membrane are readily evident. These changes may all be seen on a 1-hour biopsy, which may also show necrosis of hilar arterioles in glomeruli and similar endothelial cell injury in small cortical arteries. By 3 hours, focal fibrinoid necrosis and thrombosis may be present in cortical arteries. These lesions progress to extensive endothelial cell destruction, vascular necrosis, occlusive luminal thrombosis and cortical necrosis. The pattern is one of diffuse vascular destruction in the absence of interstitial mononuclear cell infiltration.

Immunofluorescence studies show initial binding of host immunoglobulins G and M, as well as B_1C/B_1A, along portions of the vascular endothelial surface, and by 3 hours to sarcolemmal plasma membranes, with more diffuse staining of some smooth muscle cells. The observation of such immunoglobulin deposits in the media of arteries at any time within the initial 2 months is associated with an immediate poor prognosis for the graft. Similarly, immunofluorescent stains for fibrinogen show extensive deposits within the media of arteries, along vascular basement membranes, and in many areas as dense, occlusive thrombi within dilated peritubular and glomerular capillaries, and in arteries. Proteinaceous material within tubular lumina also stains brilliantly for fibrinogen.

Electron microscopy confirms the light-microscopic findings and further illustrates the extensive endothelial injury with retraction of pyknotic cells away from adjacent cells and underlying basement membrane, while other endothelial cells show prominent blebbing, swelling and lysis. Granulated as well as degranulated platelets and neutrophiles and formed fibrin strands are often but not invariably present in areas of endothelial cell injury. Figures 2 and 3 are representative electron micrographs obtained from a portion of a hyperacutely rejected human kidney allograft, removed 3 hours after transplantation.

Slowly progressive humoral rejection occurs in many kidney grafts over a period of months

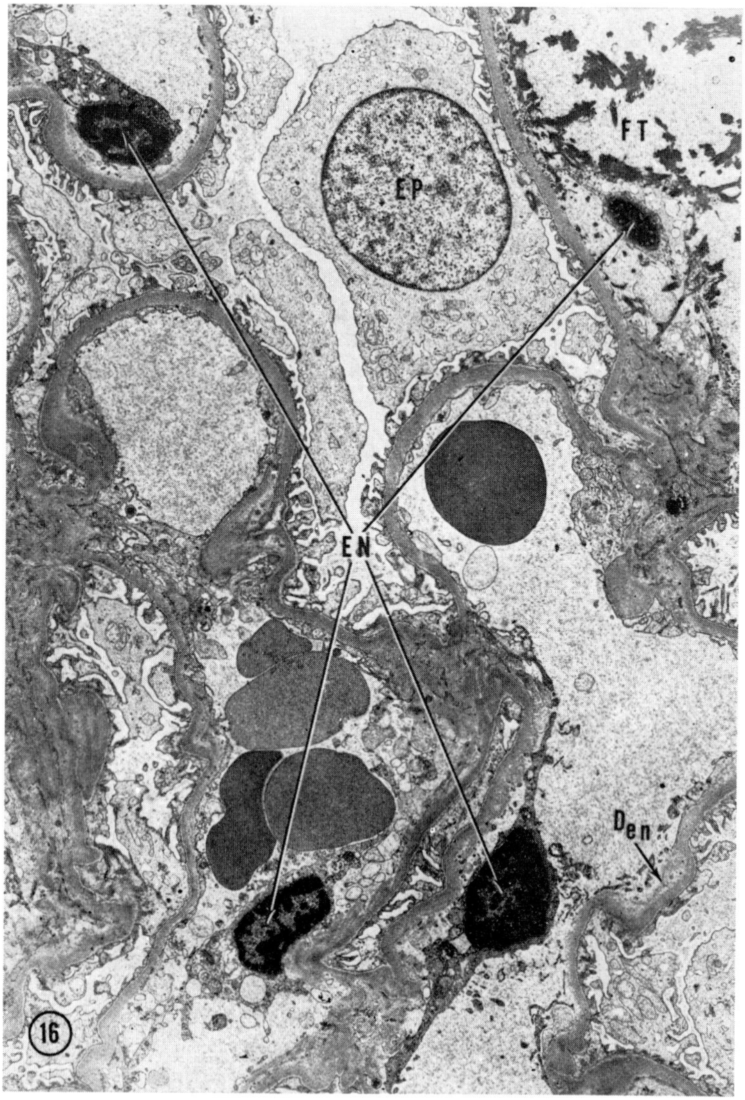

Fig. 2. Biopsy of a hyperacutely rejected human kidney graft at 3 hours. A glomerulus shows endothelial cells with pyknotic nuclei (EN), while their cytoplasm shows increased density, is discontinuous and retracted from underlying basement membrane exposing it to capillary lumen. Focally, electron-lucent amorphous deposits lie against the endothelial surface of the basement membrane. Fibrin strands (upper right) extend into the subendothelial space through discontinuities in endothelial cell cytoplasm. EP = epithelium, FT = fibrin thrombus, D_{en} = deposit, subendothelial. × 5,500 (reduced 30 %). Reproduced from *Medicine* (*50*, 1971) by courtesy of Williams and Wilkins Co., Baltimore, Md.

to years post-transplantation. These lesions appear as focal necrosis of small groups of smooth muscle cells in the walls of scattered cortical arteries, associated with immunofluorescent deposits of IgG, IgM, B_1C/B_1A and fibrinogen in areas of injury. In other areas the media of arteries show areas of patchy fibrosis as evidence of prior injury. Most striking, however, are the changes in the endothelial lining and intima, where there are initial foci of endothelial cell injury and destruction, usually associated with small clumps of aggregated and adherent platelets, marginated PMN's, and fibrin strands. These foci also show positive

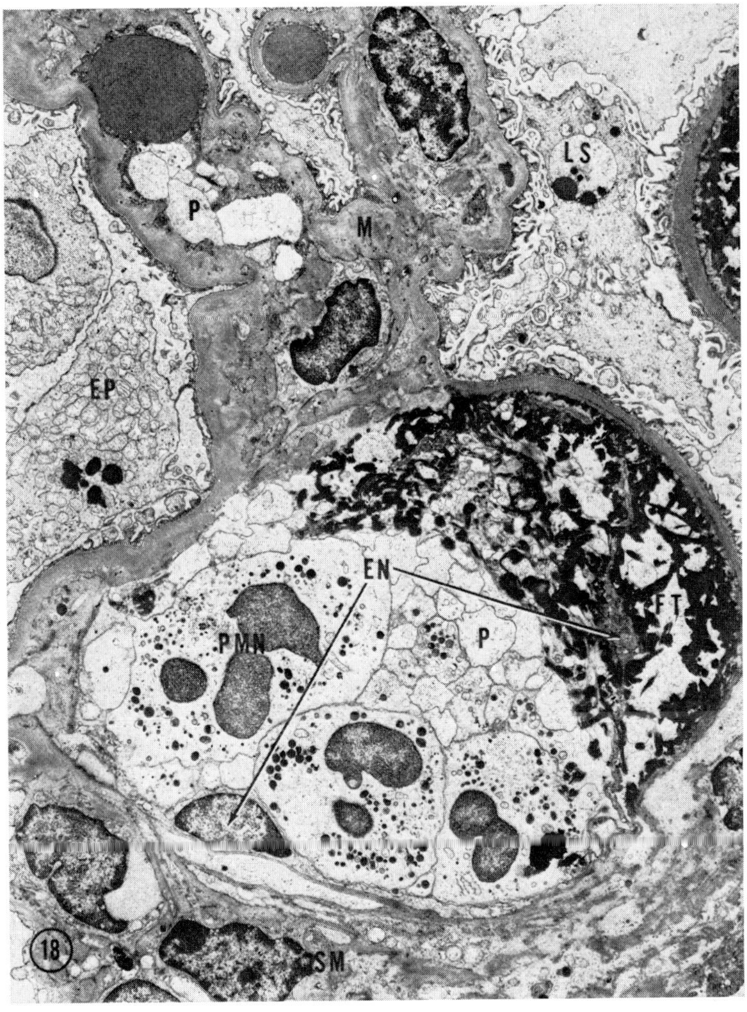

Fig. 3. Vascular pole of glomerulus from same biopsy as in Fig. 2. Smooth muscle (SM) is at lower left. A laminated fibrin, platelet and PMN thrombus fills the capillary lumen. The endothelial cell cytoplasm is reflected from the basement membrane in the region of fibrin deposition and fibrin is deposited between endothelium and basement membrane. Elsewhere the endothelium appears intact. Most platelets are degranulated. More distal capillary lumens (top) show retraction of endothelium, platelet degranulation and aggregation (top left). There is moderate fusion of epithelial cell foot processes. EP = epithelium, FT = fibrin thrombus, LS = liposome, M = mesangium, P = platelet, PMN = polymorphonuclear leukocyte. × 4,800 (reduced 30 %). Reproduced from *Medicine* (*50*, 1971) by courtesy of Williams and Wilkins Co., Baltimore, Md.

immunofluorescence as outlined above. Soon thereafter, layers of lipid-laden macrophages accumulate along the denuded arterial basement membranes, fibromyocytes migrate through the altered internal elastica and organization of the altered intima occurs, followed by re-endothelialization. The process is repetitive, resulting in dense fibro-obliterative lesions in most cortical arteries and gradual ischemic atrophy of the graft over a period of months to years. These lesions show a marked similarity to the atherosclerotic process, but are most likely due to repetitive immune injury to the endothelium, and illustrate a final common pathway for vascular repair.

Our prior experiments in various animal model systems showed that the time of onset and histologic lesions of hyperacute renal allograft rejection seen in the primate (Macaca monkeys) most closely resembled our observations during similar rejections in man. The purpose of this experiment was twofold: (1) an attempt to abrogate the secondary thrombotic injury and thus permit graft survival, and (2) to dissect the sequence of vascular injury. Our observations were confined to a period ranging from 5 minutes to 3 hours post-transplantation.

Kidneys placed in untreated control animals failed with cessation of renal venous blood flow within the initial 5 min, and biopsies showed extensive endothelial cell injury and fibrin-platelet thrombosis in capillaries as described above. These changes are illustrated in an electron micrograph obtained from a 5 min biopsy of one of these grafts (Fig. 4).

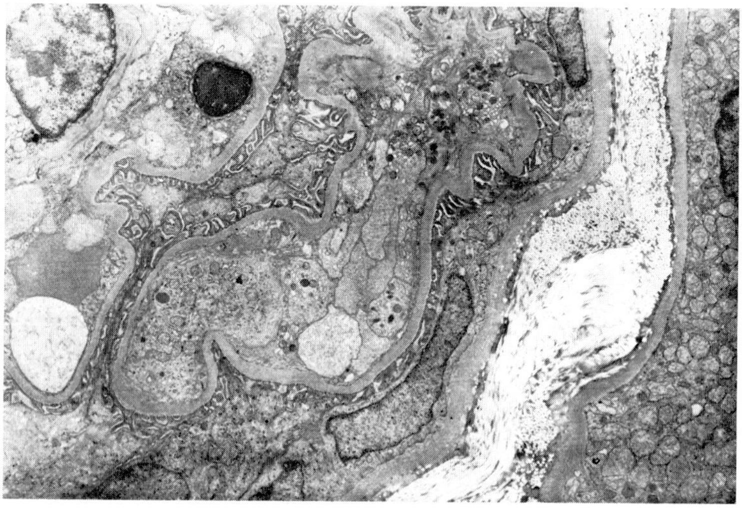

Fig. 4. Biopsy of an untreated, hyperacutely rejected primate graft at 5 min post-transplantation (lymphocytotoxic titer 1:512). A glomerulus shows moderate focal folding of the capillary basement membrane. Capillary lumina are occluded by granulated and degranulated platelets and trapped RBC's. Endothelium shows multifocal discontinuity, nuclear pyknosis and cytoplasmic swelling. Fibrin strands are inconspicuous in this field. × 5,500 (reduced 50%).

Systemic pretreatment with heparin (2 mg/kg, i.v.) revealed similar endothelial cell injury, but the onset and progression of intravascular thrombosis were delayed. However, at the time of graft failure (average cessation of renal venous flow was 93 min), the degree of vascular injury and thrombosis was indistinguishable from that seen in control grafts.

The addition of constant intrarenal arterial perfusion with heparin (1 mg/3 kg/hr) to systemic heparin pretreatment prolonged renal venous flow to an average of 105 min. Early biopsies obtained at 10 and 30 min showed endothelial injury similar to that seen in prior groups; however, intravascular thrombosis was markedly reduced, the numbers of PMN's within vessels were markedly increased and the extent of cortical vascular injury appeared

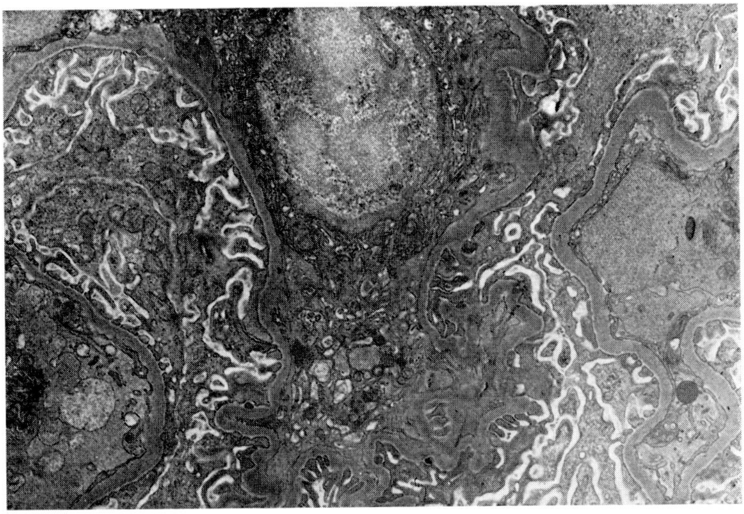

Fig. 5. Biopsy of an intrarenal arterial heparin perfused graft at 60 min post-transplantation (lymphocytotoxic titer 1:512). A capillary loop (center) shows severe contraction of a portion of the basement membrane, collapse of endothelium and many degranulated platelets. The endothelial cell nucleus appears markedly swollen. Capillary at the right shows discontinuity of endothelium with cytoplasmic projections, while on the left, a capillary also shows cytoplasmic vacuolization and intraluminal degranulated platelets and debris. × 5,500 (reduced 50%).

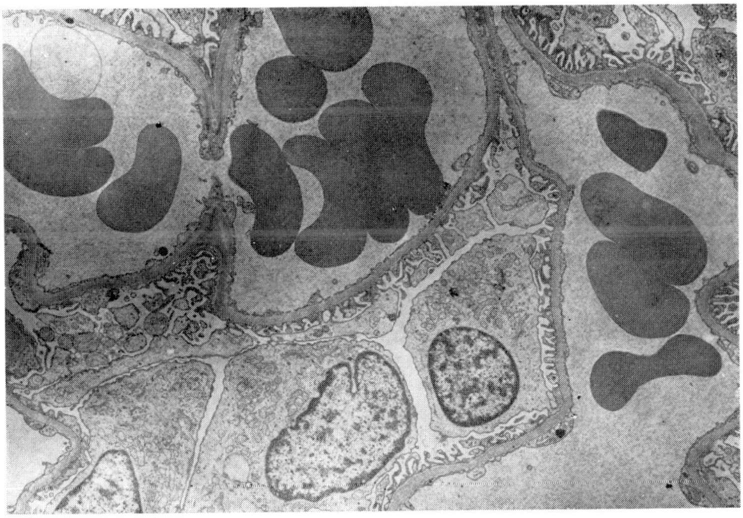

Fig. 6. Biopsy of a pyridinolcarbamate-treated graft at 50 min (lymphocytotoxic titer 1:32). A glomerulus shows RBC stasis, but capillary lumina are otherwise patent. The capillary endothelial lining shows minimal alterations. Only occasional platelets (some degranulated) were noted. × 5,500 (reduced 50%).

more diffuse. Subsequent biopsies showed a diminution in the number of PMN's within these grafts, a finding which correlated with the progressive net increase of PMN's in the venous effluent. Although the degree of intravascular thrombosis gradually increased, at the times of graft failure it was not as prominent as seen in the prior groups. Of interest in this group was the finding of prominent glomerular basement membrane folding. The changes observed are illustrated in Figure 5.

Animals pretreated with pyridinolcarbamate (150 mg, p.o., at −3 hours) had cessation of renal venous flow from their grafts at an average of 43 min. However, biopsies showed a remarkable preservation of the renal cortex with a marked reduction in intravascular thrombosis, few PMN's within vessels, and only scattered vascular endothelial pyknosis, when compared to the prior groups. However, cortical arteries appeared constricted with prominent folding of the elastic lamina and smooth muscle cell nuclei. This relative paucity of morphologic findings was most apparent in grafts from recipient animals which had lower lymphocytotoxic titers (e.g. 1:32), whereas these titers are regularly associated with immediate graft failure and the histologic changes described earlier in this report. Figure 6 is a representative electron micrograph and illustrates the more normal appearance of a pyridinolcarbamate-treated graft.

Thus, this experimental primate system duplicated both the morphologic lesions and the changes in coagulation, fibrinolytic and kinin systems that we have previously reported to occur during hyperacute rejection in man. With this model we hope to be able to dissect further the morphological and biochemical changes as they may occur and investigate the role of pharmacologic agents for the prevention of hyperacute rejection in man. The ultimate objective is to be able to transplant those patients who are known to be presensitized. Agents shown to be effective in abrogating the immediate and profound injury just illustrated will almost certainly be effective in preventing the more slowly progressive form of humoral rejection.

For discussion see page 221.

DISCUSSION

Dr. Henry: Dr. Colman, I wonder if you have considered an inhibitor of Factor VIII? Factor VIII assay measures activity and not concentration. Dr. Mammen showed that he could find an inhibitor which could be removed by ether and probably is a lipid-type inhibitor. Heparin may be functioning through such a system.

Dr. Colman: I think this is a possibility one has to consider. However, Factor VIII also fails to rise with pyridinolcarbamate in the absence of heparin, which does not support the postulate that heparin is a co-factor for the inhibitor. The inhibitor would also have to be transient, appearing and disappearing as Factor VIII varies. I think that one can always postulate an inhibitor, but that more likely other mechanisms are involved. Although as yet unproven, thrombin activation of Factor VIII or the release of Factor VIII from the kidney itself as a function of damage to the kidney seems more likely. The former is established in vitro and the latter is seen with liver injury in hepatitis and carbon tetrachloride poisoning.

Dr. Constantinides: Dr. Busch, do you think it possible that the glomerular basement membrane contraction may have been caused by contraction of the podocytes induced by serotonin? Podocytes can theoretically contract and could have microfilaments, but I do not know whether Dr. Becker has identified any actomyosin in them. What do you think about this possibility?

Dr. Busch: There are several possibilities; podocyte contraction is one of them. If one believes that mesangial cells also have contractile properties, particularly in response to a stimulus such as serotonin, this would be a most attractive possibility and would correlate very nicely with the contraction, and prominent folding of elastica, that we see in cortical arterial walls. I suppose other possibilities include the dense platelet aggregation with retraction so that there may be retraction of the basement membrane rather than contraction by surrounding structures. The third possibility is just collapse. I do not know which of these mechanisms are actually involved in producing this change.

Dr. Terry: Dr. Colman, you mentioned the use of dextran, did you use dextran 30?

Dr. Colman: No, this was dextran 70, the clinical dextran.

I would like to emphasize that this was one preliminary experiment. We do not know whether this effect was merely due to the volume expansion. We think we should pursue this observation further with suitable controls, e.g. albumin vs dextran. Of course, we all know that dextran may have specific effects on platelets and high molecular weight dextrans precipitate fibrinogen.

Dr. Busch: I would like to comment on this particular point. The animal which responded to dextran, interestingly, had persistent renal venous flow: in other words, it was perfusing the renal cortex and dextran was certainly able to get into this kidney. It has been shown that by diluting hyperimmune serum, and thus a reduction in antibody titer, one can get a return of adequate blood flow and lessen the severity of rejection. We tried the same experiment in another animal where the venous flow had already ceased, and saw no effect.

Dr. Redisch: Did you say it was without use of pyridinolcarbamate?

Dr. Busch: With pyridinolcarbamate.

Dr. Austin: What does aspirin or steroid glucocorticoids do in this system?

Dr. Colman: We have not tried aspirin or steroids on our experimental model as yet. However, Dr. Busch has previously studied aspirin in dogs.

Dr. Busch: Our study of aspirin was in a series of hypersensitized dogs; one group was treated with heparin and another with aspirin. Canines have a very active fibrinolytic system and heparin worked well in that species. As long as heparin infusion into the renal artery was maintained, there was no evidence for rejection, but once heparin infusion was stopped for 24 hours the kidneys rejected hyperacutely. Aspirin seemed only to delay in time the rapidity of hyperacute rejection.

Dr. Colman: I would like to make one further comment. The reason we used monkeys is the crucial importance of species differences. Anyone who has worked in the area of thrombosis knows that rabbits and dogs are extremely different. The Shwartzman phenomenon can be easily induced in rabbits, whereas in the dog it is impossible to produce this reaction. Therefore, we tried to get as close to the human system as possible. In addition, we have investigated the kallikrein system in the rabbit and the dog and they are quite different from man. Therefore, I think only limited information can be drawn from work in rabbits, in particular, since these animals are not very similar to humans.

NEPHROPATHY IN SPONTANEOUSLY DIABETIC MICE AND ITS POSSIBLE PREVENTION BY PYRIDINOLCARBAMATE (PDC)*

RAFAEL A. CAMERINI-DAVALOS, THEODORE EHRENREICH, DHANOO PATEL** and WERNER OPPERMANN

Diabetes Center, New York Medical College, New York, N.Y., U.S.A.

Nakamura (1962) was the first investigator to report on the diabetic syndrome in the Japanese strain of KK mice, considering it as human-type maturity-onset diabetes. Our group (Oppermann et al., 1968*a*) and Iwatsuka et al. (1970) described later the metabolic disturbance of KK mice as chemical diabetes, since they show mainly impaired tolerance to glucose, but no glycosuria or hyperglycemia in the fed state. In 1970 (Camerini-Davalos et al., 1970), it was described in more detail that the impairment in tolerance to glucose is age-related, since the highest blood glucose values were found in the 2–6 month old KK mice. In the same study, maximal serum immunoreactive insulin (IRI) values were determined in them at 9–12 months of age.

As preliminary data, microaneurysms of the retina and gangrene of the posterior extremities were reported in these animals. Diabetic-like glomerular lesions were first described by us in this strain of mice in 1968 (Oppermann et al., 1968*b*). The ultrastructure of these renal lesions was presented in another report (Ehrenreich et al., 1971).

In the present study, the progression of the diabetic-like glomerulosclerosis in the KK colony will be discussed. The severity and the relation to factors such as age, weight and degree of glucose dysmetabolism will be reviewed. In an attempt to delay, prevent or ameliorate the development of diabetic glomerulopathy, KK mice were treated with pyridinolcarbamate (PDC).

MATERIAL AND METHODS

We received the stock of our KK mice colony 6 years ago from Smith, Kline and French Laboratories, which received them directly from Nakamura in Japan. The mice were kept under constant laboratory conditions and fed an 11% fat-containing regular mouse chow diet (Old Guilford). Primarily, brothers and sisters were mated at 2–6 months of age, and their genetic background was individually documented. The animals have now been bred in our laboratory over 17 generations. As controls, Swiss Albino mice (S_1) were kept under the same laboratory conditions. Similarly to the KK mice, 2–4 animals were kept in a cage in the same room with automatic light control, and they were given the same type of food. Breeding of this strain of Swiss Albino mice (brother/sister/cousin) has been carried out over the past 5 years for 11 generations.

The mice were weighed every week. After an 8-hour fast, the oral glucose tolerance test (OGTT) was performed by forced feeding of 0.1 mg/10 g body weight of a 30% glucose solution. Blood samples for glucose and insulin were obtained from the orbital plexus of the animal at 0, 30, 60, and 120 min, and the blood glucose was determined by Hoffmann's ferricyanide method in the Technicon autoanalyzer. Blood for insulin was collected in plain micro-blood-collecting tubes (Natelson No. A-2939, 150 × 1.5 mm ID) and centrifuged at 3000 rpm for 30 min after 30 min refrigeration. The serum, separated by breaking the micro-

* Supported by the Japanese Arteriosclerosis Research Foundation and N.I.H. Grant No. AM13343.

** N.I.H. Trainee.

tube, was collected in micro-plastic tubes and stored at 4 °C until assayed. IRI was measured by our micromodification of the double antibody technique (Oppermann et al., 1969). The Uristix paper strip was used for the determination of glucose and proteins in the urine. Blood urea nitrogen was measured by the micromethod of Beale and Croft (1961). Triglycerides were determined by the method of Van Handel and Zilversmit (1957). The eyes were examined for microaneurysms of the retina by the trypsin digestion or by a silver nitrate perfusion technique (Kaczurowsky, 1969; Kuwabara and Cogan, 1960).

Metabolic and histological findings in untreated and treated KK and control mice will be reported.

PDC was given to the treatment groups by forced feeding and started at 2 months of age. It was given daily (7 days a week) in the 2 different doses of either 50 or 250 mg/kg of body weight. The medication was suspended in saline with 5% Acacia in the volume of 0.1 ml/10 g body weight. The control animals received plain saline with 5% Acacia.

Metabolic and structural studies were carried out in the KK and control mice at 1, 2, 4, 6, 9, 12, 15 and 18 months of age. A certain number of animals was sacrificed in each age group. Complete autopsies were performed on a few animals. The kidneys were removed from all the KK and control mice for light-microscopic studies. They were bisected and fixed in 10% neutral formalin. After paraffin embedding, sections were cut at 3–4 μ and stained with hematoxylin and eosin (H and E), periodic acid Schiff (PAS) and chromotrope silver methenamine (SCM). A representative number of kidneys from animals of each age group was studied in addition by electron microscopy. The histological and metabolic evaluations were performed according to number in a completely blind fashion.

RESULTS

The findings for the untreated animals are based on studies of 130 KK and 64 Swiss Albino mice (S_1) in equal age and sex distribution. Gangrene of the posterior extremities has been found (Fig. 1) so far in KK mice. Histological examination revealed extensive gangrenous tissue with muscle and bone involvement. The arteries and arterioles were thick-walled; no visible occlusions were present.

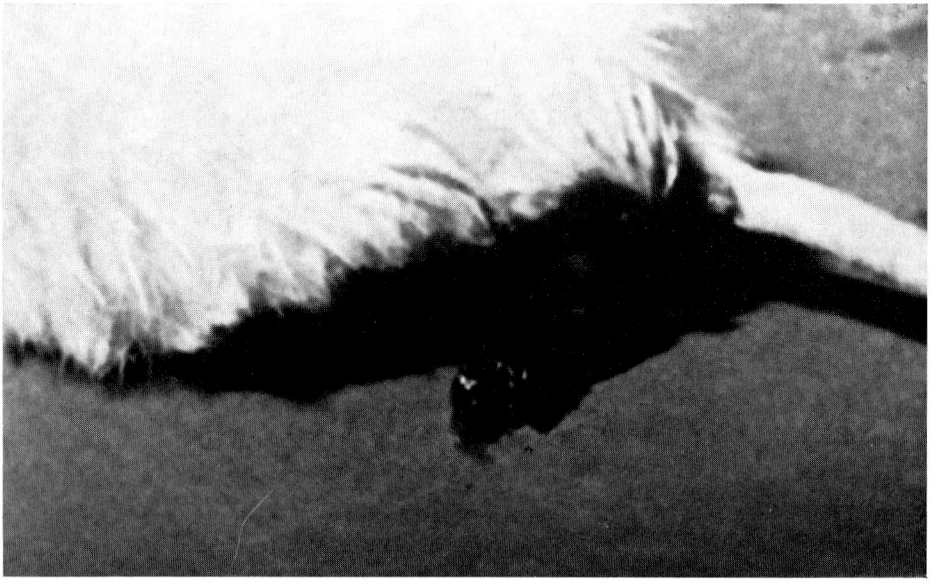

Fig. 1. Wet gangrene in a 6-month-old KK mouse.

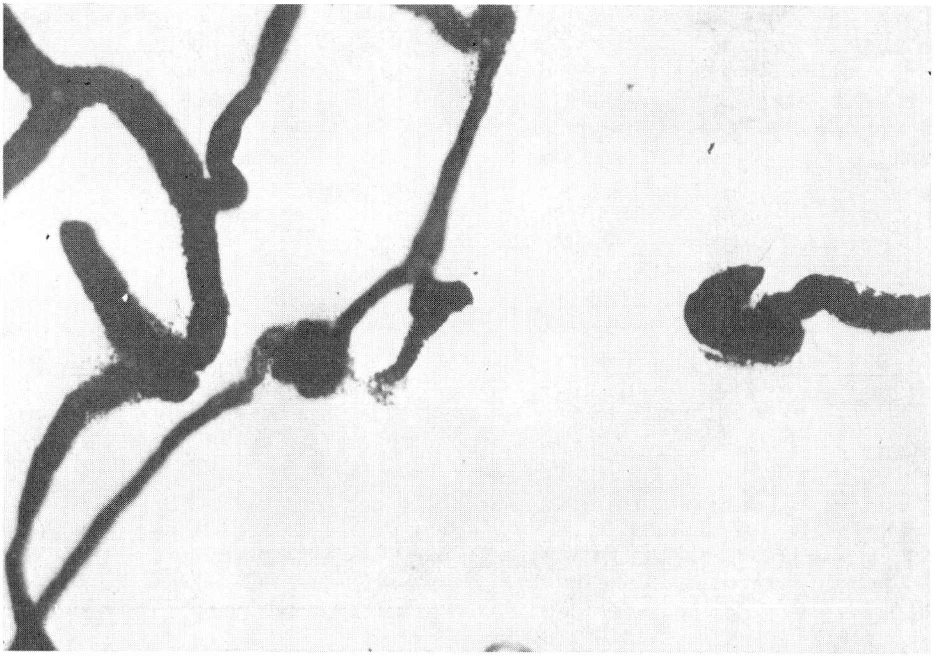

Fig. 2. Microaneurysms of the retina in a 12-month-old KK mouse (silver staining technique).

As preliminary data, microaneurysms of the retina were demonstrable on 7 KK mice (Fig. 2).

The histological evaluation of the kidneys revealed that, among the KK mice studied at various age groups, 77% showed significant glomerulopathy. A less advanced type of such glomerular lesions was found in only 28% of the control mice (S_1) (Fig. 3).

The glomerular abnormalities are present in different degrees. An increase in mesangial

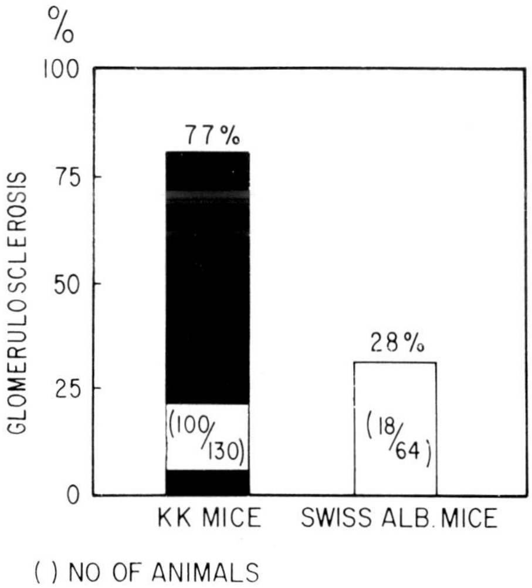

Fig. 3. Incidence of significant glomerulosclerosis in KK and Swiss Albino mice (S_1) of both sexes and all age groups (1–18 months).

matrix and cells is noted in the younger animals (2–6 months, Fig. 4). These changes progress with age. Older animals (9–16 months) show significant mesangial widening and changes resulting in a diffuse and nodular-type sclerosis (Fig. 5). The nodular lesions are more frequently located near the hilus, and they consist of mesangial matrix and cells; they are rarely acellular. So-called 'exudative' lesions are conspicuous in the older age group and absent in younger animals (Fig. 6). Segmental thickening of capillary walls and basement membrane is noted, frequently in association with exudative-like or nodular lesions. The glomerular lesions have many points in common with human diabetic nephropathy: the genesis of the nodular lesions, the presence of exudative-like lesions, the segmental thickening of the basement membrane and the relatively early glomerulosclerosis. Our studies of the ultrastructure of these renal lesions confirmed the light-microscopy findings (Ehrenreich et al., 1971).

In Figure 7 the incidence of significant glomerular lesions among the KK and control mice of both sexes is plotted according to age groups. The significantly higher incidence of renal lesions at 2 months, and the relatively steeper increase thereafter among the KK versus the control mice is apparent on this graph. We may conclude from these data that the diabetic syndrome in the KK mice is not only associated with a higher incidence of glomerulosclerosis, already at a young age, but that it furthermore accelerates the development of kidney pathology.

Figure 8 summarizes the incidence of severe glomerulopathy in the KK mice in relation to various factors. It is interesting to note that the incidence of the severe form of glomerulosclerosis rises significantly during the same age period of 9–12 months in which the KK mice have reached their highest weight and show maximal serum IRI levels. Tolerance to oral glucose is already markedly less impaired at this period.

The mean serum triglyceride levels in 28 KK mice were 91 mg% versus 60 mg% in 25 matched Swiss Albino control mice. No correlations between these data and the incidence of

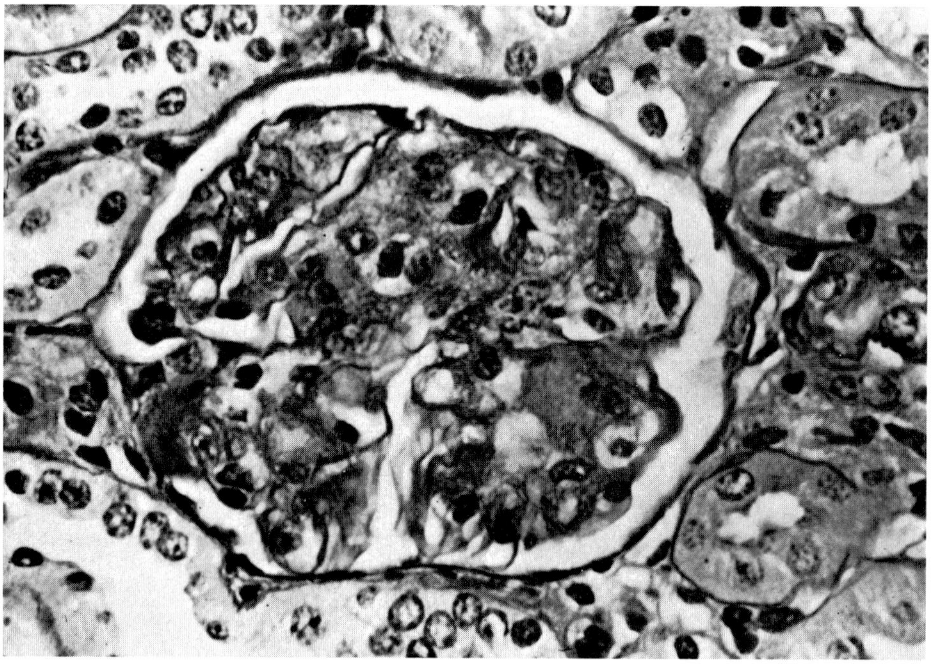

Fig. 4. Marked diffuse increase of mesangial matrix and cells with obliteration and compression of capillaries. PAS stain; × 640; 13-month-old animal.

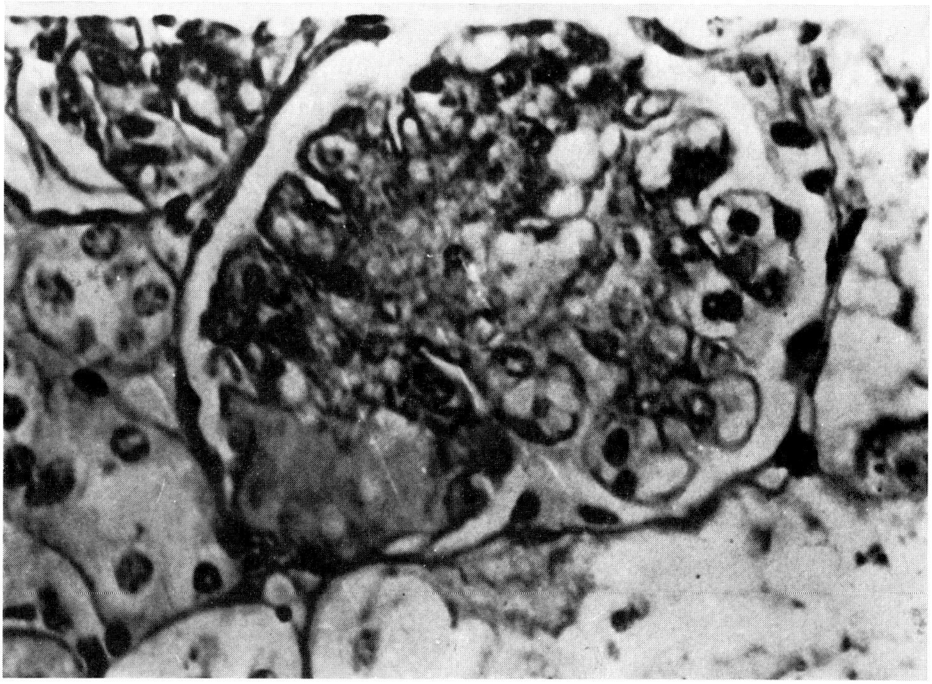

Fig. 5. Nodular-type sclerosis in one part of the glomerulus. Diffuse glomerulosclerosis, mesangial widening and moderate segmental thickening of capillary walls in other parts. PAS stain; ×600; 9-month-old animal.

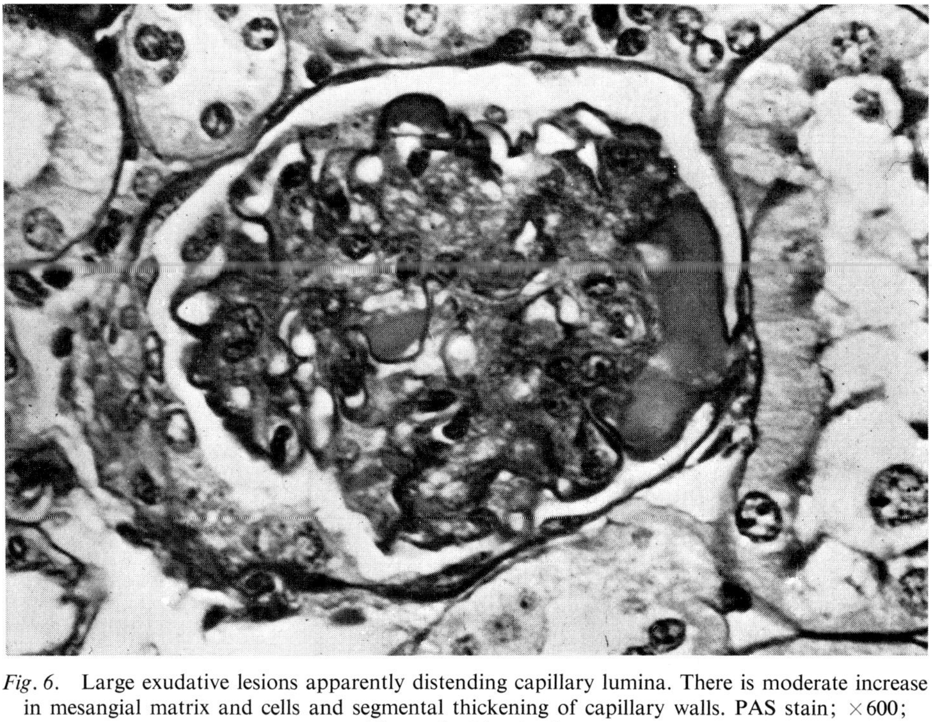

Fig. 6. Large exudative lesions apparently distending capillary lumina. There is moderate increase in mesangial matrix and cells and segmental thickening of capillary walls. PAS stain; ×600; 15-month-old animal.

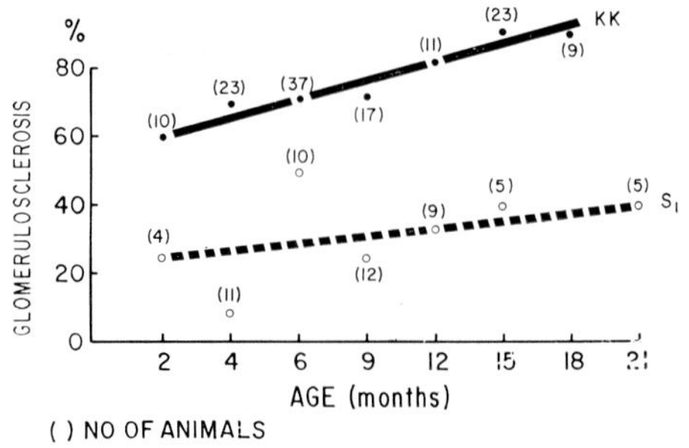

Fig. 7. Frequency of age-related glomerulosclerosis in KK and Swiss Albino (S_1) mice.

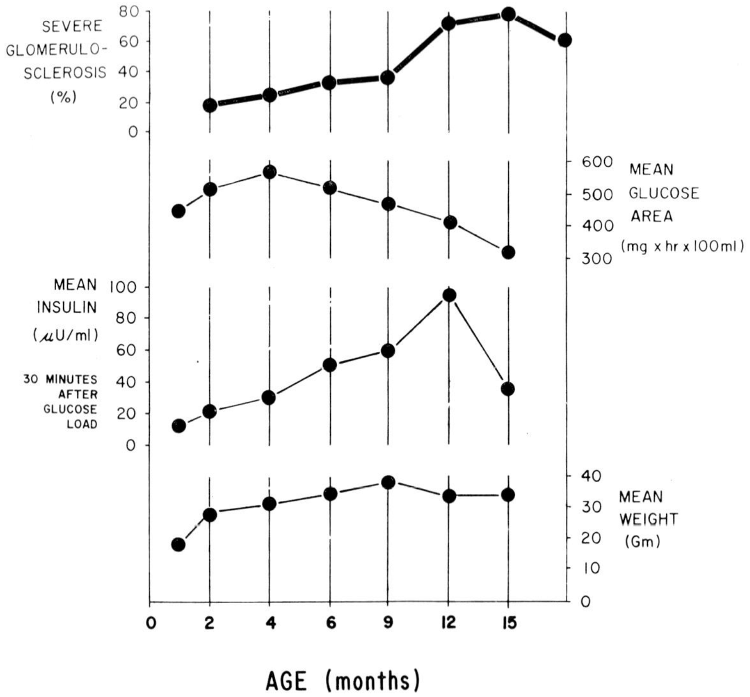

Fig. 8. Severe glomerulosclerosis in KK mice related to various factors.

glomerulopathy could be noted. The average blood urea nitrogen (BUN) level ranges, for KK and control mice, between 15 and 35 mg%. Marked BUN elevations up to 150 mg% can be occasionally observed in older KK mice with more advanced glomerular lesions. More than 1+ proteinuria was in most instances seen in KK mice with severe glomerulopathy.

RESULTS OF TREATMENT

94 KK and 70 Swiss Albino mice (S_1) in equal sex and age distribution were treated either with plain saline or with PDC in doses of 50 or 250 mg/kg body weight.

Figure 9 demonstrates that there is no significant difference in the occurrence of glomerulosclerosis between the groups of S_1 control mice treated with plain saline or Anginin (50 and

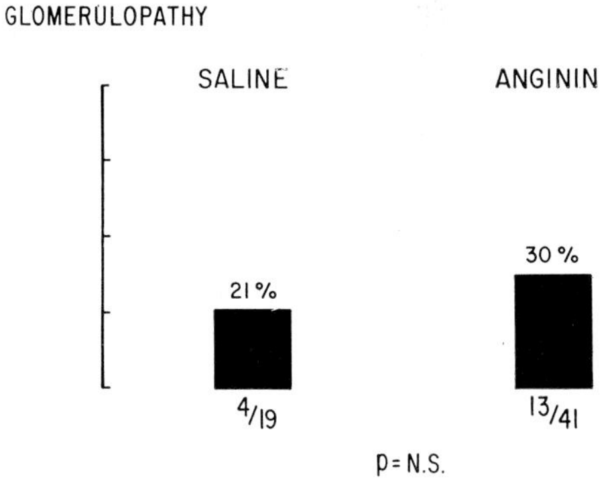

Fig. 9. Incidence of glomerulopathy in Swiss Albino mice (S1) treated with saline versus treatment with Anginin (50 or 250 mg/kg).

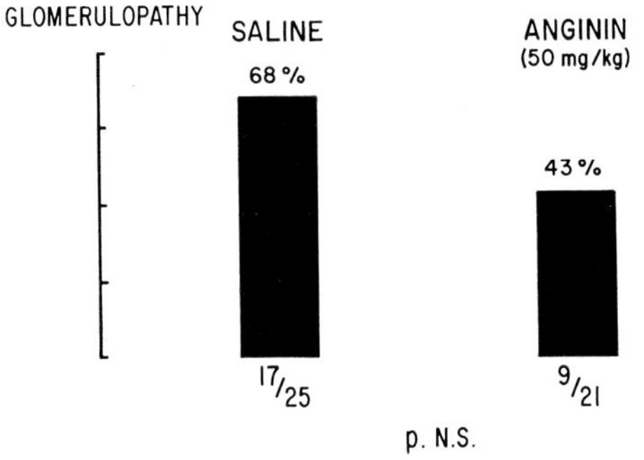

Fig. 10. Incidence of glomerulopathy in KK mice treated with saline versus treatment with Anginin (50 mg/kg).

250 mg/kg). The incidence of glomerulopathy in the untreated Swiss Albino mice lies also in the same range (Fig. 3).

Similar to the findings in the control animals, no significant difference in the incidence of glomerular lesions was found between the groups of KK mice 'treated' with plain saline or untreated.

When the KK mice were, however, medicated with 50 mg/kg of PDC daily, 25 % fewer animals showed glomerulopathy (43 % versus 68 %, Fig. 10).

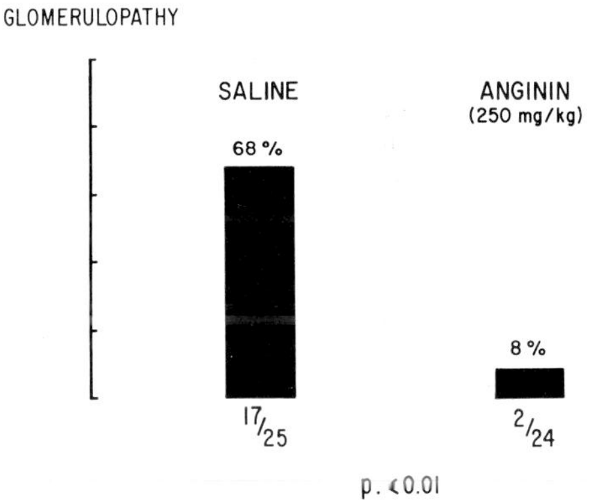

Fig. 11. Incidence of glomerulopathy in KK mice treated with saline versus treatment with Anginin (250 mg/kg).

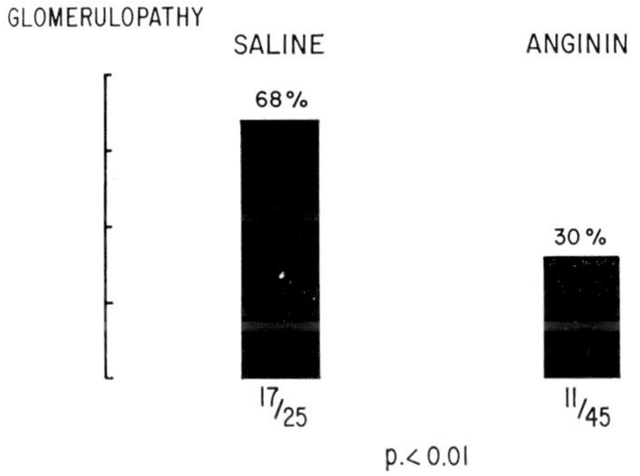

Fig. 12. Incidence of glomerulopathy in KK mice treated with saline versus treatment with Anginin (50 or 250 mg/kg).

This decrease of glomerular lesions became very striking for the group of KK mice treated with 250 mg/kg of PDC every day (8 % versus 68 %, Fig. 11).

For 2 of the treatment groups of KK mice which received 50 and 250 mg/kg of PDC daily, 38 % less glomerulopathy was found in comparison to the untreated diabetic animals (30 % versus 68 %, Fig. 12).

DISCUSSION

It could be demonstrated by light- and confirmed by electron-microscopic studies that there is a high incidence of 'diabetic' glomerulopathy in the Japanese strain of KK mice (Figs.

4, 5, 6). Evidence for the occurrence of wet gangrene of the posterior extremities and for the presence of retinal microaneurysms suggests that vasculopathy may also be present in organs other than the kidney of this strain of animals (Camerini-Davalos et al., 1970; Figs. 1, 2).

Since the tolerance to oral glucose is significantly impaired in these mice in comparison to control animals over the life period of at least 6 months from 2 to 9 months of age, the vasculopathy can be considered as part of the genetically determined diabetic syndrome in the KK mice.

According to the observations of our group (Fig. 7) and more recently of Like et al. (1972), mild glomerulosclerosis can be seen in normal control mice. But the glomerular lesions in the KK mice are more advanced and significantly more frequent at the early age of 2 months.

The question arises whether the duration of the diabetic syndrome is responsible for the development of the severe type of glomerulopathy. Or can one or several 'environmental' factors such as hyperglycemia, hyperinsulinism or weight gain be regarded as the main cause of this phenomenon?

The now generally accepted importance of duration of the disease for the development of advanced diabetic vasculopathy in humans can clearly be demonstrated for the KK mice (Fig. 7). The aging process can also be found as an accelerating factor for vascular disease in the control mice but to a much lesser extent.

The fact that the age period with the highest degree of intolerance to glucose precedes the evolution of severe glomerulopathy by half a year (Fig. 8) does not exclude impaired tolerance to glucose as an important factor in the development of severe glomerular lesions.

The steep increase in the incidence of glomerulopathy occurs in an age period when the KK mice have reached their highest weight. This observation, as well as the higher incidence of glomerular lesions in KK mice with obesity induced genetically or by dietary means (Iwatsuka, 1973), suggests weight as an important accelerating factor for the development of glomerulopathy.

No significant difference in the incidence of glomerulopathy could be found among the KK and control mice between non-treated and saline-treated groups (Figs. 3, 9, 10). It could, however, be demonstrated that the daily oral treatment of Anginin prevents the development of glomerulopathy in the KK mice (Fig. 12). The protective effect of this drug appears to be dose-related since a significantly lower incidence of glomerulopathy was found among the KK mice treated with 250 mg/kg (Fig. 11) versus those treated with only 50 mg/kg of Anginin daily (Fig. 10).

It is emphasized here that we are very concerned and hesitant at presenting these striking data on the preventive effect of PDC in the development of diabetic-like nephropathy, which are also surprising to us. But we feel justified and even obliged to do so for the following reasons:

1. The correlative studies are performed in a blind fashion.
2. The numbers of animals in each group are large enough to allow tentative conclusions.
3. KK and control mice are carefully age-matched.
4. No significant differences in weight are found between the animal groups without and with treatment of PDC.

The mechanisms by which PDC may prevent diabetic-like vasculopathy in the KK mice are not clear to us at the present time. Studies of blood sugar and serum insulin levels in treated and untreated mice give no conclusive data. It appears suggestive, however, that the early initiation of therapy at 2 months may play an important role in the preventive effect.

REFERENCES

BEALE, R. N. and CROFT, D. (1961): A sensitive method for the colorimetric determination of urea. *J. clin. Path., 14*, 418.

CAMERINI-DAVALOS, R. A., OPPERMANN, W., MITTL, R. and EHRENREICH, T. (1970): Studies on the KK mouse. *Diabetologia, 6*, 324.

EHRENREICH, T., SUZUKI, Y., CHURG, J., OPPERMANN, W. and CAMERINI-DAVALOS, R. A. (1971): Ultrastructure of glomerular lesions in KK mice with glucose dysmetabolism. *Amer. J. Path.*, *62*, 55A.

IWATSUKA, H. (1973): In: *Vascular and Neurological Changes in Early Diabetes*, p. 305. Editors: R. A. Camerini-Davalos and M. S. Coke. Academic Press, New York, N.Y.

KACZUROWSKY, M. S., Wills Eye Hospital, Philadelphia, Pa. (1969): Personal communication.

KUWABARA, T. and COGAN, D. G. (1960): Studies of retinal vascular pattern. I. Normal architecture. *Arch. Ophthal.*, *64*, 904.

LIKE, A. A., LEVINE, R. L., POFFINBARGER, P. L. and CHICK, W. L. (1972): Studies in the diabetic mutant mouse. VI. Evolution of glomerular lesions and associated proteinuria. *Amer. J. Path.*, *66*, 193.

NAKAMURA, M. (1962): A diabetic strain of the mouse. *Proc. Jap. Acad.*, *38*, 348.

OPPERMANN, W., MEHTALIA, S. D., SODERO, E., COLE, H. S. and CAMERINI-DAVALOS, R. A. (1969): A sensitive micromethod for the simultaneous insulin and growth hormone determination by double antibody precipitation. *Clin. Biochem.*, *2*, 341.

OPPERMANN, W., PENHOS, J. C. and CAMERINI-DAVALOS, R. A. (1968*a*): Genetic carbohydrate dysmetabolism. *Bull. N.Y. Acad. Med.*, *44*, 1135.

OPPERMANN, W., TRESER, G., EHRENREICH, T., LANGE, K., CAMERINI-DAVALOS, R. A. and LEVINE, R. (1968*b*): Specific glomerular lesions in a genetically diabetic mouse. *Clin. Res.*, *16*, 347.

VAN HANDEL, E. and ZILVERSMIT, D. B. (1957): Micromethod for the direct determination of serum triglycerides. *J. Lab. clin. Med.*, *50*, 152.

DISCUSSION

Dr. SPECTOR: Have you ever administered a 'concomitant' with pyridinolcarbamate, such as a protein inhibitor, because you are implying that pyridinolcarbamate is perhaps stimulating the enzymes and synthesis of the transferase system?

Dr. CAMERINI-DAVALOS: On the contrary, we believe that pyridinolcarbamate may delay the enzyme activity.

Dr. SPECTOR: If you give puromycin or actinomycin, you might reverse this.

Dr. CAMERINI-DAVALOS: We have not tried this.

Dr. COTTON: Did you observe any increase in liver weight in the diabetic rats?

Dr. CAMERINI-DAVALOS: I do not think so. To be absolutely sure, let me ask Dr. Oppermann.

Dr. OPPERMANN: We have done several complete autopsies but did not find any significant change.

Dr. DIDISHEIM: I find these studies of great interest in view of their possible relation to the report last year by Dr. Jameson, of the Red Cross Laboratories, Washington. I believe Dr. Jameson and his colleagues reported that aspirin inhibits glucosyltransferase and he postulated that this is the mechanism by which aspirin inhibits adherence of platelets to collagen, so that this is a very analogous situation. He postulated that aspirin inhibits the transfer of glucose from the platelet membrane to collagen which is the bond between platelets and collagen. It could very well be that pyridinolcarbamate has a similar action and thereby inhibits adherence of platelets to a basement membrane which is a type of collagen. That glucosyltransferase is increased in the blood and particularly in platelets will give us an avenue of research in the future.

II

CLINICAL STUDIES ON THE TREATMENT OF ATHEROSCLEROSIS AND THROMBOSIS

CLINICAL, METABOLIC, AND PERMEABILITY STUDIES WITH PYRIDINOLCARBAMATE

JAMES H. AUSTIN, JOHN SHEPPARD, THOMAS WISELY, MARIE LAFRANCE, JOACHIM GERLOFF and WILLIAM REPPERT

Division of Neurology, University of Colorado Medical Center, Denver, Colo., U.S.A.

INTRODUCTION

We have long been interested in two mechanisms: (1) those by which lipid is deposited and (2) those by which membrane permeability is increased in disease. The present report summarizes certain clinical and experimental findings using pyridinolcarbamate (PDC; Anginin).

CLINICAL STUDIES

Studies in hypertrophic neuritis

Mr. J.D. is a 71-year-old man with a known diagnosis of hypertrophic interstitial neuritis (Austin, 1956). He was first admitted to the Colorado General Hospital on 4/19/71 with a chief complaint of progressive weakness in his legs and hands. He had no symptoms until 3 years before admission when he noted the gradual onset of paraesthesias, pains and weak ness in his hands and feet. By early 1969 he had slight foot drop. In March, 1971 he was hospitalized elsewhere. Lumbar puncture showed a slightly xanthochromic fluid with a total protein of 780 mg/100 ml. Right median nerve conduction time was 10 m/sec, right ulnar nerve conduction time 27 m/sec. Conduction time could not be measured in the common peroneal nerve. A left sural nerve biopsy showed hypertrophic interstitial polyneuropathy. He had no previous symptoms consistent with syphilis and had no prior episode of polyneuropathy.

Neurological examination revealed 2 mm pupils. They did not react to light but did react well to accommodation. There was bifacial lower motor neurone weakness, moderate in degree. He had a marked weakness of the extremities more evident distally than proximally. There was bilateral minimal atrophy. He had a bilateral foot drop. Deep tendon reflexes were 2 + in the upper extremities, 1 + at the knee and absent at the ankle. Plantar responses were bilaterally flexor. He had a high steppage gait. There was a fading glove and stocking loss to light touch and pinprick. Position sense was absent in the toes and intact in the upper extremities.

The ulnar, peroneal and greater auricular nerves were $1\frac{1}{2}$–2 times enlarged. They were firm, not nodular, not tender.

Lumbar puncture showed normal pressure and slightly xanthochromic fluid on both occasions. There were no cells. The protein on 2 occasions was 1,235 and 985 mg/100 ml. Serological tests for syphilis were negative.

A lumbar puncture performed 24 hours after the injection of homologous fibrinogen intravenously showed no radioactivity in the spinal fluid. This was interpreted to mean that no large fibrinogen molecules were leaking into the subarachnoid space.

Baseline motor status and sensory status evaluations were made independently both by two neurologists and by physiotherapy. Baseline movies were obtained of his gait and other functions. Baseline nerve conduction measurements were obtained. He started out on pyridinolcarbamate (PDC) placebos, 500 mg, 3 times a day.

He was readmitted for the second time on June 8, 1971. At this time he had been on PDC itself for 4 weeks (since May 6). Serial tests of nerve conduction velocities showed essentially no change. Lumbar puncture revealed an opening pressure of 160 and a total protein of 1,700 mg/100 ml. Again the fluid was slightly xanthochromic. The dosage of PDC was increased to 750 mg t.i.d. After 2 days on this dosage he developed nausea, vomiting and abdominal bloating. The PDC was reduced to 625 mg t.i.d. which the patient tolerated without discomfort. Lumbar puncture showed a total protein of 1,400 mg/100 ml.

Clinical impression This study was begun to test whether or not PDC would change the abnormally increased permeability (manifested by increased CSF protein) in hypertrophic neuritis. Over the period of 2 months, there was no consistent evidence that PDC, in dosages up to 625 mg t.i.d., altered the patient's course, motor or sensory deficit, nerve conduction, or CSF protein in comparison with the placebo. Follow-up, off therapy one year later (May, 1972), indicated that his condition continued to deteriorate slowly.

Studies in multiple sclerosis

Mrs. J. T., a 30-year-old woman, first noted blurring of vision in both eyes in January, 1971. In February she noted mild dizziness and unsteadiness. During early March she noted numbness, tingling and weakness of both feet and lower legs. Lumbar puncture revealed a protein of 35 mg/100 ml; 12.2% of this was gamma globulin.

On examination later in March, 1971 mental status was normal. She had a moderate left central scotoma with slight pallor of the disc and a small right central scotoma. The jaw jerk was brisk. There was a slight right upper motor neurone facial weakness. Cerebellar functions were considered normal except for slight finger to nose tremor. Her gait was unsteady with a slightly wide base. There was marked decrease in position sense and vibration sense of both feet. Pinprick was decreased on the left to the level of the iliac crest. There was slight weakness of the right deltoid and right external rotators with questionable weakness in the right hip flexors. Deep tendon reflexes were hyperactive throughout. There was a right reflex preponderance, right extensor plantar response and a flexor plantar response on the left. Abdominal reflexes were absent. On March 29, 1971 she was started on PDC, but only in a dosage of 250 mg $\times$ 3 per day instead of 500 mg $\times$ 3 per day.

By discharge on April 5, there was no essential change. Laboratory studies included blood, SGOT, alkaline phosphatase and LDH, which were all within normal limits.

Re-examination on April 12 showed minimal improvement and some improvement in use of her legs. Vibration sense had returned in both ankles.

On April 26, in association with the onset of the menses she noted marked worsening in vision. Re-examination of the visual fields documented an increase in the central scotoma especially on the left. There was increased weakness in both legs. There were new symptoms referable to the right arm — numbness and hypalgesia involving the C_5 through C_7 dermatomes. This coincided with a relative depression of the right biceps and right brachioradialis reflexes. Other findings were as before. At this point, appreciating that she was only on PDC 250 mg per day, her dosage was increased to 500 mg 3 times a day for the first time.

By May 3, 1971 visual field changes and leg strength had improved. The sensory loss in the right arm and the reflex reduction had both returned to their previous levels. Her reflexes were now 2 + and symmetrical in both arms. Re-examination on May 17 showed continued improvement. Arm strength was symmetrical, as were her reflexes. Spasticity was still marked in the legs, greater on the right. Vibration and position senses were preserved and pinprick appreciation was not altered on the left.

Re-examination on August 16 showed definite spasticity in both legs, more on the right. Vibration sense was absent below the knees bilaterally. Tandem gait was minimally impaired. The plantar response was still extensor on the right and flexor on the left. Blood counts and

SGOT were within normal limits. On August 16 she noted rather severe nausea, reduced PDC from 6 to 4 tablets per day, and added Compazine. One day later numbness returned in her legs for one day. This was associated with clumsiness in her legs. She gradually returned to a dosage of 500 mg PDC 3 times per day. On September 27, re-examination showed leg strength definitely improved over that recorded previously. She was able to feel vibration sense with maximal stimulation of the ankles. Her vision was somewhat improved.

On September 10, 1971 she was switched from PDC to placebos, 6 per day.

Re-examination on October 29 revealed continued mild improvement in right hip flexor strength, reduction in ankle clonus and bilateral flexor plantar responses. There was no alteration in pinprick.

The patient was again seen on December 11, 1971. She was still on placebos. For $1\frac{1}{2}$ months she had noted increasing general fatiguability and worsening of balance. Re-examination revealed some return of spasticity in the legs, more on the right. Vibration sense was absent below the hip on the right and the knee on the left, a worsening from the previous examination. Position sense was relatively intact bilaterally. The right plantar response was again extensor. The findings were interpreted as a reaccentuation of old symptoms rather than appearance of discrete new plaques.

On January 10, 1972 she complained of increasing symptoms of stiffness, weakness and clumsiness of gait. She noted numbness below the hips, vague and mild in degree. Re-examination revealed slight weakness of the left arm. Vibration sense was absent below the hips. Position sense was mildly impaired at the toes. Both plantar responses were extensor. Spasticity had increased bilaterally, the gait was both spastic and ataxic. Pinprick and touch were preserved.

Re-examination on January 29 showed an accentuation of all previous symptoms and signs without any single new clearcut sign being present. This occurred in the setting of her menses. On this day the placebo was discontinued. PDC itself was reinstituted, 500 mg $\times$ 3 per day.

Her symptoms continued to progress over the next 2 weeks. The findings then included intense weakness in both legs, greater on the right, intense spasticity in the legs, greater on the right, a vague sensory level to pinprick from T_6 down on the left, some slight diminution to pinprick over the right lower extremity below the knee, loss of vibration and position sense below the costal margins. Her gait was spastic; deep tendon reflexes were hyperactive in the legs and the right arm. Plantar responses were bilaterally extensor.

PDC did not appear to be effective in checking her symptoms in the dosage and time employed. Accordingly, she was begun on ACTH gel, 80 units per day intramuscularly. Within 4 days she showed signs of improvement, particularly an increase in leg strength and a decrease in spasticity. On discharge, there was no longer any alteration of pinprick. Position sense had improved markedly, although vibration sensation was only minimally improved. The sustained knee and ankle clonus previously present was no longer observed. PDC was discontinued at the end of the 10-day period of ACTH gel therapy. Over the next $2\frac{1}{2}$ months her course gradually stabilized, off therapy of all kinds, and she has had no further progression of symptoms.

Clinical impression This study was begun to test whether or not PDC might obviously decrease a local increase in permeability in a patient with multiple sclerosis to a degree such that a clinical effect might be apparent. Previous studies by Lykke et al. (1967) have raised the possibility that PDC might favorably influence the course of disease by such a mechanism.

Evaluation of therapy is difficult in a disease which spontaneously exacerbates and remits. This patient's symptoms and signs, observed over a 1-year period, worsened both on placebos and on PDC. Moreover, she has improved both on placebos and PDC. At the termination of therapy ACTH gel appeared to be effective in mobilizing her at a time when PDC had been given for 2 weeks without benefit. An interesting component of her illness was a diffuse progression in signs and symptoms in association with the menses. No single plaque could be discretely identified which appeared or disappeared during the period of observation. Thus, the study does not clearly indicate whether or not PDC, in appropriate dosage, might affect one isolated plaque, in part because multiple lesions were present.

One other woman, patient A. L., with definite multiple sclerosis, has been maintained on placebo for the past 7 months. No new symptoms have occurred thus far.

Other comments PDC was very well tolerated by both patients. The highest dosage well tolerated was 625 mg 3 times per day. A dosage of 750 mg 3 times per day produced nausea and vomiting. Multiple routine hematological, enzymic, and chemical studies showed no adverse affects due to PDC at any time.

Studies of platelet aggregation and of platelet counts

In a preliminary study, the effect of PDC was compared with that of placebo and aspirin in 3 subjects. They were all healthy young men in the 20's, were on no other medications, did not imbibe alcohol and were subject to no unusual stresses during the period of this study. Samples were drawn at the same time each day.

PDC (500 mg $\times$ 3 per day) produced no definite change in platelet count which could be differentiated from that of aspirin (600 mg $\times$ 3 per day) (Fig. 1). Platelet counts were higher after PDC and aspirin were withdrawn. However, the known variability in platelet counts precludes further conclusions on this point. (Note that the counts varied before either drug or placebo was started.)

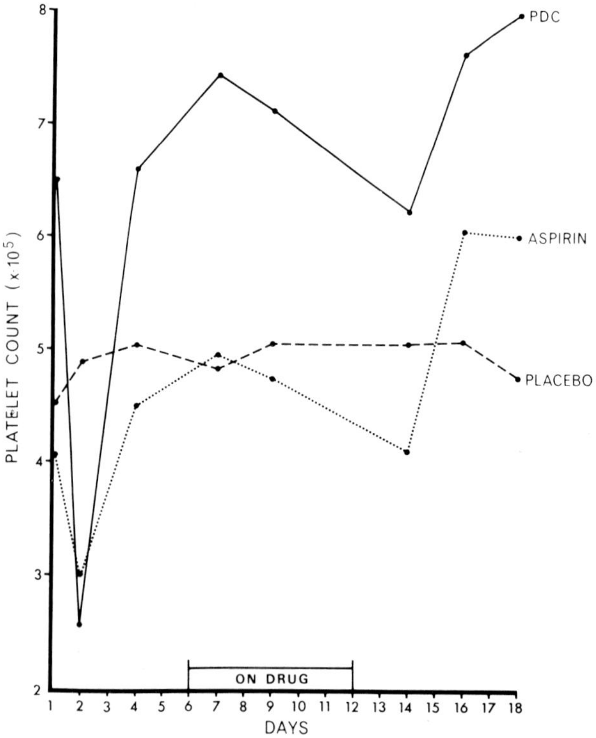

Fig. 1. Platelet counts. The effect of PDC cannot be distinguished from that of aspirin. Note the variability of the platelet count.

Platelet aggregation was studied in the same 3 subjects identified in Figure 1. In this experiment (Fig. 2) we studied the effect of PDC on collagen-induced platelet aggregation. The responses to 60 or 10 μl of collagen solution were examined. The response to PDC could not be distinguished from that to the placebo. The platelet aggregation of the subject placed on aspirin was sufficiently variable both before and after the drug to preclude further comment.

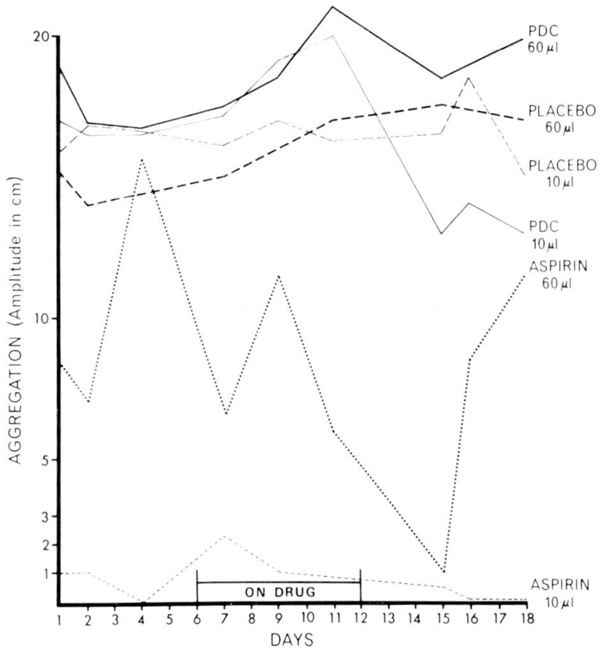

Fig. 2. Platelet aggregation. No definite effect of the various medications on platelet aggregation was demonstrated in this experiment.

STUDIES OF LIPID METABOLISM

A turnover disorder of lipids occurs in atherosclerosis. It was considered of interest to test the effect of PDC both on lipid anabolism and catabolism. The 2 key substrates selected were triglycerides and cholesterol esters. The results of these studies are summarized in Table I. Over the dosage range tested, there was no evidence that PDC affected lipid metabolism, or adenylcyclase metabolism. The morphology of cultured cells was not affected.

PERMEABILITY STUDIES

In vivo permeability

Evans blue, an azo-binding dye, accumulates focally in several discrete areas of the aorta 24 hours after it is injected intravenously. The intimal-medial surface shows more contrast than does the adventitial side. This evidence, corroborating that of other investigators (Klynstra and Bottcher, 1970; McGill et al., 1967; Somer and Schwartz, 1971), suggests that certain regions of the aorta differ in their permeability. When the living rabbit is also given radiolabeled cholesterol, the areas of increased dye accumulation and of radiolabeled uptake were found in general to coincide.

TABLE I

Effect of PDC on lipid metabolism and adenylcyclase activity

PDC concentration added in vitro	System studied	Tissue studied	Result
3×10^{-4} M	Hydrolysis of ^{14}C-palmitate from labeled triglyceride	Rabbit iris	No change
10^{-2} M through 10^{-8} M	Hydrolysis of ^{14}C-palmitate from labeled triglyceride	Rabbit iris and rabbit ear skin	No change
3×10^{-4} M	Hydrolysis of ^{14}C-palmitate from labeled cholesterol palmitate	Rabbit iris	No change
10^{-2} M through 10^{-8} M	Hydrolysis of ^{14}C-palmitate from labeled cholesterol palmitate	Rabbit iris and rabbit ear skin	No change
3×10^{-4} M 3×10^{-4} M	Incorporation of ^{14}C-palmityl CoA into triglyceride	Rabbit iris and rabbit ear skin	No change
10^{-2} M through 10^{-8} M 5×10^{-5} M	Adenylcyclase*	Cultured mouse fibroblasts (3T3)	No change
PDC administered in vivo	**System studied**	**Tissue studied**	**Result**
PDC given in vivo for 120 days in dosage of 30 mg/kg/day (n = 6)	Hydrolysis of ^{14}C-palmitate from labeled triglyceride and labeled cholesterol. Incorporation of ^{14}C-palmitate CoA into triglyceride or cholesterol palmitate	Rabbit iris and rabbit ear skin	No change from saline controls

* From Krishna et al. (1968).

In vitro permeability

How much of this increased permeability reflects hemodynamic factors present within the arterial system of living animals? To answer this question, we wished to see if the same kinds of regions of 'high permeability' were also present in aortas excised from the rabbit, incubated in a nutrient medium, and later exposed in vitro to Evans blue or to radiolabeled cholesterol. It turned out that the uptake of dye and of radiolabeled cholesterol also tended to coincide under these in vitro conditions. The possibility that PDC would affect this differential permeability pattern was then tested.

The data reported herein are to be viewed as exploratory and preliminary, because permeability to Evans blue appears to differ even among littermates, because the isotope system tested itself gives somewhat variable results, and because the numbers of animals studied are still quite small.

In *all* cases in this report it was the thoracic aorta *caudal* to the arch which was selected for study. The contour of this portion of the aorta was most uniform and free of bends. Moreover, it would appear to be theoretically less subject to mechanical hemodynamic stress both in vivo and perhaps agonally.

Methods and techniques for studying in vitro permeability of the thoracic aorta

The in vitro permeability studies of rabbit aortas were carried out as follows. Adult male rabbits (white, New Zealand strain, 1.5–2.5 kg) were fed a normal diet ad lib. The rabbits were either littermates or were carefully matched for age and weight. The rabbit was sacrificed by decapitation, and the thoracic aorta was carefully dissected out using sterile instruments. The pericardial end of the aorta was held gently and the remainder was removed by careful caudal dissection. The aorta caudal to the left subclavian artery and proximal to the superior mesenteric was used. The aorta was immediately placed in 100 ml of isotonic saline solution and gently rinsed to remove blood. It was then incubated at 37 °C with gentle agitation. The incubation periods varied from 2–4 hours as noted. When the aortas were preincubated there was no Evans blue present.

The incubation mixture contained: (1) 50 ml of Dulbecco's modified Eagle medium supplemented with 10% calf serum, 0.5 mM glutamine and 1% penicillin-streptomycin and the pH was adjusted to 7.3 with 1 M HCl. (2) 0.5 ml of Evans blue dye (2%) in isotonic saline (large volumes were autoclaved and aged for 2 weeks before using). (3) Radiolabeled cholesterol (^{3}H-chol-7α). After sonication, this was added in certain experiments (100 μCi in 100 μl of 95% ethanol were added for each 50 ml of medium). (4) Cholesterol palmitate-1-^{14}C was added in certain other experiments. (250 μCi were suspended by sonication in 1.0 ml of 95% ethanol at room temperature. This suspension was then added to 100 ml medium at 37 °C. The mixture was then shaken by hand and then centrifuged for 15 min at 15,000 $\times$ *g*. The supernatant was counted (2.2 $\times$ 10^6 counts/min/ml). No Evans blue was added.) (5) ^{3}H-leucine 50 μCi in 0.5 ml phosphate buffered saline was added on one occasion.

After incubation the stained aorta was thoroughly washed in isotonic saline and was then cut longitudinally. The cut margins were pinned down in a pan filled with paraffin. The different permeabilities of the aorta are expressed by different degrees of blue staining. These were photographed. Different light- and dark-staining areas were separately dissected out with scalpel, fine scissors, and forceps. The tough adventitial layer, forming a clear plane of cleavage with the rest of the wall of the aorta, was discarded. The tissue was then blotted dry and weighed. The fragments were then cut into small pieces. Comparable weights of the 2 tissues were homogenized in 2 ml chloroform-methanol (2:1, V/V) for 20 sec in a Polytron homogenizer. 10 ml of chloroform-methanol was added to the homogenate, and the lipid was extracted overnight with constant agitation. The filtered lipid extract was then dried with a stream of air, redissolved in 1 ml solvent, and then counted in a scintillation counter. Light and dark areas from a normal rabbit, a saline-injected control rabbit, and a PDC-injected rabbit were then compared with regard to dye and cholesterol uptake. In the chronic injection experiments, the rabbit had his last injection of PDC 15 hours before sacrifice. When, at autopsy, the subcutaneous injection sites of PDC and saline were inspected over the back, the PDC sites showed no unusual scarring, inflammation or discoloration.

The areas of increased dye uptake in the thoracic aorta caudal to the arch corresponded in general with those usually affected by lipid deposits in human and experimental atherosclerosis. The dye was concentrated more in this portion of the aorta irrespective of whether the rabbit was injected 24 hours earlier with Evans blue while alive or whether the aorta was excised and exposed to the dye during incubation in vitro.

Acute, in vitro, experiments on rabbit aorta

In Table II the data from 4 untreated adult rabbits suggest that areas which stain darker with Evans blue also tend to have a greater uptake of ^{3}H-cholesterol and of ^{3}H-leucine. No drug was added in this experiment.

In Table III the data again suggested that there was slightly greater ^{3}H-cholesterol uptake in the dark-staining areas. In this instance, PDC was given chronically, s.c., over the back

TABLE II

Acute, in vitro, experiment. Difference between light and dark areas of rabbit aorta in the uptake of ^{3}H-cholesterol and ^{3}H-leucine

Nature of experiment	Drug given	^{3}H molecules added	Counts in 2 areas of differing permeability	
			Light	Dark
Normal adult rabbit	None	Cholesterol	58	115
Normal adult rabbit	None	Cholesterol	35	178
Normal adult rabbit	None	Cholesterol	310	666
Normal adult rabbit	None	Leucine	81	407

TABLE III

PDC given chronically. Difference between light and dark areas of rabbit aorta when ^{3}H-cholesterol is added post mortem*

Nature of chronic experiment	Drug given in vivo	Counts** in 2 areas of differing permeability	
		Light	Dark
Normal adult rabbits	None	0	0
Injected for 15 months	Saline × 2 per day	0	0
	PDC 45 mg × 2 per day	43	84
Normal adult rabbits	None	43	73
Injected for 15 months	Saline × 2 per day	55	69
	PDC 45 mg × 2 per day	91	104
Normal adult rabbit	Saline × 2 per day	36	55
Injected for 9 months			
Normal adult rabbit	PDC 45 mg × 2 per day	65	89
Injected for 15 months			

* Rabbits were male littermates.

** Counts/min/mg tissue

in a dosage of 45 mg twice a day before the aortas were removed. These chronic PDC injections were associated with an uptake of cholesterol slightly greater than that in controls. In 5 separate rabbits injected with PDC for 16 months (2), 9 months (1), and 6 months (2) the uptake of Evans blue appeared grossly diffusely greater than that of their saline controls ($n = 5$).

During the course of the acute experiments, summarized in Table IV, the aortas were preincubated before staining either in PDC or in media only. The aim of this preincubation step was to give the aorta additional exposure to the drug. The data were less uniform than those found in other subsequent experiments. The fact that control aortas of 3 *different* rabbits varied noticeably in ^{3}H-cholesterol uptake precludes a final assessment of the effects of PDC in different animals under these conditions.

Viewed grossly in separate experiments, the presence of PDC (10^{-3} M) in the incubation medium for 3 hours was associated with slightly greater Evans blue staining in 3 aortas, and with about the same degree of staining in 3 other aortas.

In Table V, a segment of the aorta of one rabbit was exposed to PDC. The uptake of ^{3}H-cholesterol into this portion of the aorta was contrasted with that in the corresponding segment of aorta from another rabbit. When PDC was added to the incubation medium,

TABLE IV

Acute experiment, in vitro, using ^{3}H-cholesterol. Measuring differences between light and dark areas of rabbit aorta

Nature of in vitro experiment	Drug preincubated with entire aorta in vitro for 1 hr		Counts* in 2 areas of differing permeability	
			Light	Dark
Normal adult rabbit aortas	Medium only	4 °C	257	43
	PDC (10^{-3} M)	4 °C	37	39
	PDC (10^{-3} M)	37 °C	30	169
Normal adult rabbit aortas	Medium only	37 °C	506	2967
	Medium only	37 °C	837	538
	PDC (10^{-4} M)	37 °C	429	543
	PDC (10^{-5} M)	37 °C	665	626
	PDC (10^{-6} M)	37 °C	517	613
	PDC (10^{-5} M)	37 °C	1048	615

* Counts/min/mg tissue.
The data are from an early experiment and are presented, as found, even though the figures of 2967 and 1048 in particular do not inspire confidence.

TABLE V

Acute experiment, in vitro, measuring ^{3}H-cholesterol uptake in one segment of aorta

Nature of in vitro experiment	Drug exposed to aorta in vitro for 3 hr at 37 °C	Area of aorta stained	Counts* between first and second intercostal segment
Normal adult rabbit	Medium only	Entire	63
Normal adult rabbit	PDC 10^{-3} M	Entire	65

* Counts/min/mg tissue.

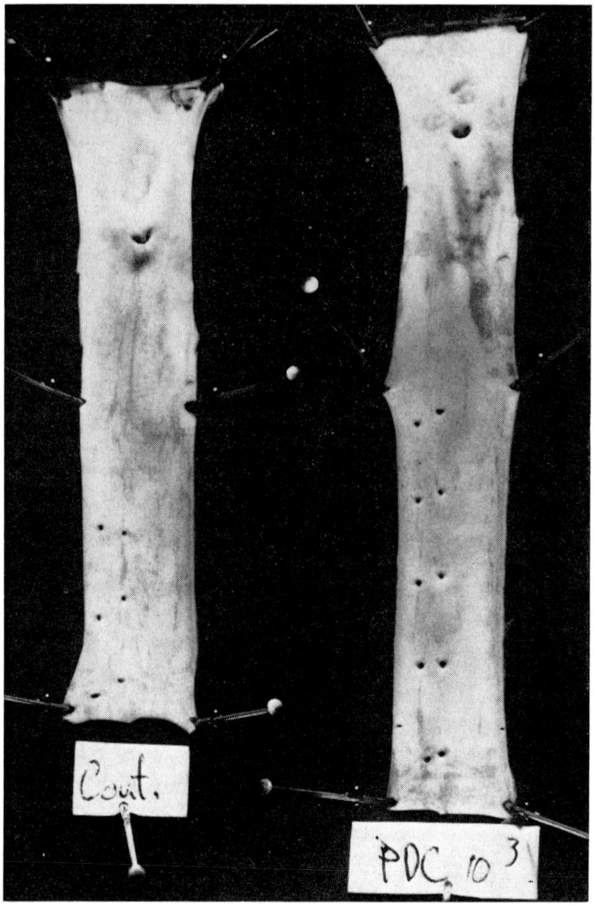

Fig. 3. Rabbit aortas, stained with Evans blue. Rabbits were male littermates 4 months old on a normal diet. Control aorta (cont. at left), was preincubated in medium per se for 1 hour. Evans blue and ^{3}H-cholesterol were then added to the medium, and the aorta was then incubated for 2 more hours. The PDC aorta (PDC 10^{-3}, at right) was preincubated and incubated in medium exactly the same way except that PDC was present. The ^{3}H-cholesterol was extracted as specified from that segment of aorta between the ostia of the first and second intercostal arteries. These counts are indicated in Table V.

TABLE VI

PDC given chronically. Differences in uptake of ^{3}H-cholesterol between rostral and caudal segments of the aorta

Nature of chronic experiment	Drug given in vivo	Counts* in different segments of aorta		Comment
		Rostral	Caudal	
Adult rabbits	Saline × 2 per day	96	129	Saline total counts 360
Injected for 6 months	Saline × 2 per day	78	67	
	PDC 45 mg × 2 per day	92	66	PDC total counts 357
	PDC 45 mg × 2 per day	108	91	

* Counts/min/mg tissue.

there was no difference in the uptake of cholesterol into the small segment of the aorta studied (Fig. 3).

In Table VI, when PDC was injected chronically for 6 months, there was no change in the subsequent uptake of ^{3}H-cholesterol into the *different* aortas tested.

Comparisons *between* animals may be difficult. Therefore, in Tables VII and VIII, each rabbit served as his own control. This method has intrinsic advantages. In Table VII, the uptake of ^{3}H-cholesterol was assessed in the unstained thoracic aorta. The aorta below the arch was divided horizontally into rostral, intermediate, and caudal thirds. Each of these segments was then split into sagittal halves. Thus, the right half was incubated in media only at the same time that the left was incubated in media with PDC. In subsequent segments, the treatment given to the 2 sides was always alternated. Aortas exposed to media only

TABLE VII

Acute experiment, in vitro, measuring ^{3}H-cholesterol uptake in rostral, intermediate, and caudal portions of the aorta

Nature of in vitro experiment	Counts in control half preincubated for 1 hr at 37 °C	Counts in PDC half preincubated in 10^{-3} PDC for 1 hr at 37 °C
Normal adult rabbit	338 (rostral) 185 (intermediate) 366 (caudal)	414 (rostral) 341 (intermediate) 227 (caudal)
Normal adult rabbit	205 (rostral) 182 (intermediate) 272 (caudal)	199 (rostral) 266 (intermediate) 248 (caudal)
Total	1548	1695

TABLE VIII

*Acute experiment, in vitro, measuring cholesterol palmitate-^{14}C. Uptake in rostral, intermediate, and caudal portions of the aorta**

Nature of in vitro experiment	Counts in control half preincubated for 1 hr at 37 °C	Counts in PDC half preincubated in 10^{-3} M PDC for 1 hr at 37 °C
Normal rabbit	283 (rostral) 118 (intermediate) 223 (caudal)	167 (rostral) 342 (intermediate) 299 (caudal)
Normal rabbit	203 (rostral) 89 (intermediate) 117 (caudal)	215 (rostral) 168 (intermediate) 220 (caudal)
Total	1033	1411

* Cholesterol palmitate is poorly soluble when taken from benzene into ethanol. Solvents which might keep it in solution are not appropriate to use when the question of permeability is being studied. Therefore, what little cholesterol palmitate-^{14}C did go *into solution* in the medium was used. To remove that cholesterol palmitate which only remained in suspension, the mixture was centrifuged at $15{,}000 \times g$ as specified, and only the supernatant was used. At the end of the experiment, an aliquot of the lipid which was extracted from the aorta was examined by thin-layer chromatography. 98 % of the ^{14}C lipid was identified as labeled cholesterol palmitate, and 0.5 % as labeled free palmitate.

showed no consistent segment of increased uptake. PDC-treated segments showed no appreciable difference in total uptake of ^{3}H-cholesterol when compared with controls.

In Table VIII the uptake of cholesterol palmitate (^{14}C) was assessed in male littermates. The unstained aorta was again divided into rostral, intermediate and caudal thirds. Each of these segments was split into sagittal halves and treated as specified above. The aortas exposed to media only showed a more rostral segment of increased uptake. In general, the PDC-treated segments tended to have slightly more uptake of cholesterol palmitate-^{14}C than did the corresponding control segments from the same animal.

SUMMARY AND CONCLUSIONS

1. Under the conditions of the experiment the clinical course and abnormal CSF protein permeability in hypertrophic neuritis were not improved by PDC.
2. Under the conditions of the experiment the clinical course of one patient with multiple sclerosis was not obviously influenced by PDC.
3. In a preliminary test, PDC produced no definite change in platelet count which could be differentiated from aspirin. The effect of PDC on collagen-induced platelet aggregation could not be separated from that of the placebo.
4. In the in vitro systems cited, PDC did not appear to affect the metabolism of 2 lipids of interest in atherogenesis. Thus, it did not alter the incorporation of ^{14}C-palmityl CoA into triglyceride, or the hydrolysis of ^{14}C-palmitate from labeled triglyceride or labeled cholesterol palmitate. PDC did not alter the adenylcyclase activity in cultured mouse fibroblasts.
5. In the in vitro studies, there was a tendency for areas of the thoracic aorta which stained more deeply with Evans blue also to show an increased uptake of ^{3}H-cholesterol.
6. The thoracic aortas of animals chronically injected for 15 months with PDC tended to show an increased uptake of Evans blue and of ^{3}H-cholesterol.
7. Aortas removed from rabbits given chronic PDC injections for 6 months showed no consistent effect of this prior PDC on the subsequent uptake of ^{3}H-cholesterol.
8. In acute experiments, in vitro, comparing aortas from different animals, there was no consistent effect of PDC (10^{-3} M) on ^{3}H-cholesterol uptake.
9. In acute experiments, comparing sagittal halves of the same aorta, those portions of the rabbit aorta exposed to PDC (10^{-3} M) showed about the same uptake of ^{3}H-cholesterol as did the corresponding control segments.
10. In acute experiments comparing sagittal halves of the same aorta, those portions of aorta exposed to PDC (10^{-3} M) showed slightly more uptake of cholesterol palmitate than did the corresponding control segments.

ACKNOWLEDGEMENTS

Dr. Robert Scaer kindly referred patient J.T. and participated in the careful serial examinations which were part of her single-blind evaluation. All platelet studies were kindly performed in the Coagulation Laboratory of Dr. Kurt von Kaulla. Dr. Robert Elwell kindly referred patient J.D. for studies. Mrs. Doris Gaskin assisted in the tissue culture experiments, Mr. Richard Cromwell in the chronic injection studies, and Mr. Robert Meyers in the adenylcyclase experiment.

REFERENCES

AUSTIN, J. (1956): Observations on the syndrome of hypertrophic neuritis (the hypertrophic interstitial radiculo-neuropathies). *Medicine (Baltimore)*, *35/3*, 187.

KLYNSTRA, F. and BOTTCHER, C. (1970): Permeability patterns in pig aorta. *Atherosclerosis*, *11*, 451.

KRISHNA, G., WEISS, B. and BRODIE, B. B. (1968): A simple sensitive method for the assay of adenylate cyclase. *J. Pharmacol. exp. Ther.*, *163*, 179.

LYKKE, A., WILLOUGHBY, D. and KOSCHE, E (1967): Thymic permeability factor: Its relationship to lymph-node permeability factor and its antagonism by pyridinol carbamate (Anginin) and other anti-inflammatory agents. *J. Path. Bact.*, *94*, 381.
MCGILL, H., GEER, J. and HOLMAN, R. (1967): Sites of vascular vulnerability in dogs demonstrated by Evans blue. *Arch. Path.*, *64*, 303.
SOMER, J. and SCHWARTZ, C. (1971): Focal ^{3}H-cholesterol uptake in pig aorta. *Atherosclerosis*, *13*, 293.

DISCUSSION

Dr. KRITCHEVSKY: I would like to ask first – you mentioned that you have studied the breakdown of the palmitate in the triglyceride and cholesterol ester. Did this refer to just hydrolysis of the various esters or actual oxidation of the palmitate?

Dr. AUSTIN: No, this is hydrolysis. The work 'breakdown' was used to contrast with 'synthesis' solely in relation to the fatty acid ester linkage.

Dr. KRITCHEVSKY: Because you mentioned the early phases, you know it has been shown that, in the aorta, the cholesterol ester synthesis goes up a week after cholesterol feeding commences before you see any lesion whatsoever, so it may very well be that you are studying an earlier phase of this disease than you thought, because you do not have to wait for the appearance of plaques to get an increase in cholesterol ester synthesis in either the pigeon or the rabbit.

Dr. NELSON: What do you think you were looking at with the Evans blue stained aorta in terms of good old-fashioned light microscopy, utilizing H and E and perhaps Sudan stain? In the areas that were blue or not blue?

Dr. AUSTIN: In these local areas, I think we are probably looking at a diffuse increase in the uptake of Evans blue.

Dr. NELSON: And is this associated with alterations at the light-microscopic level? Or did it look like normal aorta?

Dr. AUSTIN: These aortas in all instances are really grossly normal.

Dr. NELSON: And look normal histologically?

Dr. AUSTIN: Yes, you recall that these animals are on a normal diet. Now, for example, this 2-month-old aorta is a *normal* aorta. The animal has *not* been on a high fat diet; nothing else has been done to these aortas. I am glad you asked the question, because what we have elected to do first is to study a situation in which disease has not been introduced by abnormal feeding or by any other abnormal manipulation. The inference here is that *permeability normally varies from portion to portion of the aorta.* Moreover, these variations in permeability are evident whether you give Evans blue, as I mentioned, either 24 hours before death or if you take the aorta out and then incubate it in Evans blue. Both intravitam and postmortem staining has been used.

Dr. NELSON: Well, would you go so far as to say that the sites of blue darkening, of bluishness then, are the sites at which further atherosclerosis may develop?

Dr. AUSTIN: I would not like to stick my neck out there. It is premature to move, I think, from 'bluishness' to 'anything else-ishness'. However, these studies have been found to hold true by other investigators (Klynstra and Bottcher, 1970) in the pig as well as the rabbit. I think it suffices to say here that permeability does vary in the normal aorta (Klynstra and Bottcher, 1970).

TREATMENT OF CEREBRAL VASCULAR DISEASE WITH PYRIDINOLCARBAMATE

J. G. BERNARD
108, Boulevard Raspail, Paris 6e, France

Our group of 54 patients includes cases of varying severity and of varying duration of impairment of cerebral blood flow. The distribution of the disease among male and female patients and among age groups is shown in Table I.

TABLE I

Distribution of patients according to age

Age group	Male patients	Female patients
40–49	3	
50–59	12	3
60–69	16	
70–79	11	4
80 and above	2	3
Total	44	10

The average duration of treatment was 4½ months. For 24 patients, it lasted 6 months or more. The dosage of the drug varied from 2 to 6 tablets a day, with an average of 4 tablets. As a general rule, the initial dose of 4–6 tablets a day was followed by a maintenance therapy of 3–4 tablets a day, when the effects of the drug became visible.

Our results are given in Tables II and III which show the changes in functional and psychic (or intellectual) symptoms for the 5 main groups of diseases.

Psychometric tests were instituted for 14 patients after treatment for only 30 days. The average values thus found are summed up in Table IV; the slight improvement in performance had no statistical significance.

Electroencephalography was performed on each patient during the course of treatment and at its termination. Marked and permanent improvement was observed in only 10 cases. The ocular fundus was altered in 12 patients only; in 4 of these pyridinolcarbamate therapy brought about an improvement of this condition.

In the case of focal lesions and associated motor disturbances, a prompt recovery was observed in patients treated within 5 days of the first vascular accident. Without control subjects, evaluation of this effect is difficult. On the other hand, therapy instituted for the 5 patients more than a fortnight after the first vascular accident did not seem to have had any effect whatever on motor recovery.

There were also other aspects of vascular damage in our patients: we found that out of 7 cases of coronary arteritis only one was improved. In 5 cases, lower limb Stage II mild arteritis did show improvement. All these disorders were minor and were not the cause which brought our patients to seek medical help.

Our overall results are shown in Table V. It is apparent that the drug operates best when:

TABLE II

Evolution of subjective symptoms under treatment

Class of patients	No. of cases	Headache				Subjective noises				Dizziness				Muscae volitantes			
		No.	++	+	0	No.	++	+	0	No.	++	+	0	No.	++	+	0
Incipient cerebral atherosclerosis	24	12	10	1	1	2	–	1	1	8	6	1	1	11	9	2	–
Marked cerebral atherosclerosis	6	1	–	1	–	–	–	–	–	1	–	1	–	–	–	–	–
Cerebral atherosclerosis with dizziness	10	5	5	–	–	3	–	1	2	10	6	4	–	3	3	–	–
Focalized lesions	10	7	2	5	–	2	–	1	1	1	–	1	–	4	2	1	1
Parkinsonian syndrome	4	–	–	–	–	2	–	–	2	1	–	1	–	1	–	–	1
Total	54	25	17	7	1	9	–	3	6	21	12	8	1	19	14	3	2

TABLE III

Evolution of objective symptoms under treatment

Class of patients	No. of cases	Memory				Intelligence				Reasoning				Affectivity				Depressive state				Disorientation			
		No.	++	+	0	No.	++	+	0	No.	++	+	0	No.	++	+	0	No.	++	+	0	No.	++	+	0
Incipient cerebral atherosclerosis	24	12	2	8	2	16	4	9	3	13	1	9	3	11	1	7	3	17	2	13	2	1	1	–	–
Marked cerebral atherosclerosis	6	6	–	1	5	6	–	–	6	6	–	1	5	6	–	–	6	4	–	1	3	6	–	–	6
Cerebral atherosclerosis with dizziness	10	7	1	3	3	4	1	2	1	1	–	1	–	1	–	1	–	2	1	–	1	0	–	–	–
Focalized lesions	10	2	1	1	–	0	–	–	–	0	–	–	–	1	–	1	–	2	2	-	–	0	–	–	–
Cerebral atherosclerosis with Parkinson's disease	4	1	–	–	1	2	–	1	1	2	–	1	1	4	–	–	4	2	–	1	1	0	–	–	–
Total	54	28	4	13	11	28	5	12	11	22	1	12	9	23	1	9	13	27	5	15	7	7	1	–	6

TABLE IV

Psychometric tests

Test	Before treatment	1 month after beginning of treatment	t
Benton's test	3.67	4.25	1.6
Immediate recollection of digits	4.5	5	1.21
Delayed recollection of words	9.5	10.6	1.44
Crossing-out test	22	22.5	0.5

TABLE V

Results of treatment per class of patients

Class of patients	Results					
	Very good (++)	Good (+)	Limited (±)	No visible effects	Definite failures	Total
Incipient cerebral atherosclerosis	7	8	3	5	1	24
Marked cerebral atherosclerosis				6		6
Cerebral atherosclerosis with dizziness	5	4	1			10
Focalized lesions	1	6	1	1	1	10
Cerebral atherosclerosis with Parkinson's disease				4		4
Total	13	18	5	16	2	54

the impairments are still evolving; patients belong to a younger age group (14 cases of improvement out of 18 patients under 60 years, 17 out of 36 patients over 60 years); the patient is female (7 cases of improvement among 10 women, although, on average, they were among the older patients).

The effects of the drug are stronger on functional symptoms – notably so on dizziness or vertigo – than on intellectual impairment and more marked on the latter than on psychic disorders.

General and biological tolerance of the drug was excellent. Nevertheless, there were among this group a number of instances of gastric intolerance that we tried to alleviate by administering the tablets during meals or by giving a smaller dose. Several patients suffered from diarrhoea which in 2 instances caused the treatment to be stopped.

Thus, on the whole, pyridinolcarbamate has been found to have an effective action: the results have been good or very good in 60% of cases belonging to 'the common run' of medical practice, especially so in patients with recent lesions which showed marked improvement in 70% of the cases. This suggests that the drug should be prescribed at the first symptoms and that it could possibly have a prophylactic action.

TREATMENT OF CHRONIC LOWER LIMB ARTERIOPATHY WITH PYRIDINOLCARBAMATE

J. G. BERNARD
108, Boulevard Raspail, Paris 6e, France

Our study of the treatment of chronic lower limb arteriopathy comprised a group of 45 patients, aged 35–85 years (average, 57 years), who had senile or presenile atheromatous arteritis and a 46th patient with juvenile arteriolitis of Buerger. The average duration of treatment was 6 months. We would like to emphasize that all those patients who, after the first 2 months of treatment, felt that their condition began to improve, attended follow-up clinics regularly. In Table I, the cases are classified according to their severity together with the effect of treatment on the main symptoms observed.

We noticed the following:

A somewhat parallel evolution in the improvement of pulse and the improvement of oscillography.

A very favourable influence on the evolution of the disorder (Stages I, II–III, III–IV), as evidenced by reduced decubitus cramps (13 out of 16 patients) and eschar (4 out of 5). Marked variability of results noted for Stage II (26 patients). At this Stage, the illness has settled in and, for the great majority of cases, diagnosis is usually obvious upon interrogation, as the functional syndrome is so clear. The duration of the evolution of the disease varied greatly. However, in two-thirds of our cases, functional signs had appeared from 6 to 12 months before the first medical examination. None of these patients had received treatment previously. In the other third, disorders had developed long before and had been more or less stabilized by various therapeutic means. In 2 cases, surgical therapy had been previously attempted. Thus, this group is less homogeneous than the former one; although it comprises comparable cases of arteritis, they differ in their previous clinical history.

Overall results are given in Table II.

After completion of this study, we found that results were good in 75% of cases against 6% definite failures. This series of cases, characterized by arteritis at various stages of development, does not enable us to be definite as to the anti-atheromatous effect of pyridinolcarbamate. Nevertheless, we feel we can confirm the previous findings of Shimamoto on 1368 cases which he himself has already supported by several studies of smaller groups of patients observed under rigorous double-blind conditions.

In our opinion, 3 factors support this view:

1. Most important seems to be the varying effect of the drug depending on whether the disorder is progressing or quiescent.

2. The second factor is the almost constant action of the drug on decubitus pains, nocturnal cramps and paraesthesias. This analgesic action on a syndrome notably tenacious and typical of aggravating arteritis can be compared with what the Japanese authors have described as an anti-imflammatory vascular effect of anti-bradykinin type. In fact, it is probable that quinones play an important part in the physiopathology of this type of pain of ischaemic origin.

3. A third argument in favour of this assumption is the occurrence, in 4 cases, of relapses 2 months after interruption of treatment, and their complete recovery 2–3 weeks after resuming treatment. Although less significant than the first 2 arguments, it is an additional reason in favour of this physiopathological theory.

TABLE I

Evolution of symptoms under treatment

Class of patients	No. of observations	Walking perimeter				Decubitus cramps				Arterial oscillations				Pulse				Skin temperature				Eschar			
		No.	+	0	—	No.	+	0	—	No.	+	0	—	No.	+	0	—	No.	+	0	—	No.	+	0	—
Stage I	8	2	2	–	–	0	–	–	–	8	7	1	–	8	6	2	–	8	1	7	–	0	–	–	–
Stage II	26	20	11	7	2	6	4	1	1	26	6	18	2	26	6	18	2	10	1	9	–	0	–	–	–
Stage II–III	4	4	4	–	–	4	4	–	–	4	1	3	–	4	1	3	–	4	1	3	–	1	1	–	–
Stage III–IV	7	6	4	2	–	6	5	1	–	7	1	6	–	7	–	7	–	6	4	2	–	4	3	1	–
Total	45	32	21	9	2	16	13	2	1	45	15	28	2	45	13	30	2	28	7	21	–	5	4	1	0

TABLE II

Results of treatment per class of patients

Class of patients	Results					Total
	Very good (++)	Good (+)	Limited (±)	No visible effect	Definite failure	
Stage I	3	5				8
Stage II	7	8	3	5	3	26
Stage II–III	1	3				4
Stage III–IV	4	2		1		7
Buerger's disease	1					1
Total	16	18	3	6	3	46

Biological tolerance of pyridinolcarbamate was very good although a few cases of digestive side-effects have been noted. Only one caused us to stop the therapy prematurely.

In the present study, we have not attempted to combine pyridinolcarbamate with other drugs, especially of the vasodilator type, as our only purpose was to evaluate the effects of pyridinolcarbamate alone. But it would be relevant to try it in combination with other drugs, so as to associate different physiopathological effects in order to obtain better results in long-term therapy which we deem necessary for this type of disorder.

The view of Shimamoto that pyridinolcarbamate counteracts the 'inflammatory alteration' of arterial walls, which is the evolutive process of atherosclerosis, and thus improves arteritis, agrees with the fact that our best results were obtained with developing forms or in cases where the disease had recently developed.

THE ACTION OF PYRIDINOLCARBAMATE IN THE TREATMENT OF ARTERIAL AND VENOUS ANGIOPATHY: EXPERIMENTAL AND CLINICAL CONTRIBUTIONS

F. PRATESI, C. DEIDDA and A. NUTI

Department of Angiology, Main Regional Hospital of S. Maria Nuova, Florence, Italy

In the study of angiopathies and blood vessel pharmacodynamics, research workers tend to devote their attention principally to the calibre of the 'macrovessels' – the large, medium and small arteries proximal to and the veins distal to the microvessels. In the field of pharmacology attention is concentrated on the calibre of vessels which are largely controlled by nervous regulation. On the other hand, the calibre of the microvessels – meta-arterioles, capillaries, preferential canals, and venules, the calibre of which is mainly regulated by substances produced by the tissues – is much neglected. In our opinion, this particular approach to the subject has contributed to slowing down the progress of knowledge of the pathogenesis of vascular diseases and to hindering the perfection of the appropriate treatment.

In considering the variations in calibre of the microvessels it is necessary to free ourselves of the concept of vasoconstriction and vasodilatation as being the consequence exclusively of the activity of contractile elements. On the contrary, it is necessary also to consider these variations in microvessel calibre as being the expression of variations in the chemical and chemicophysical state of the microvessel wall. They may even be consequent on compression by the surrounding tissues.

As stated below, in a vascular area where circulatory insufficiency exists, it is probable that the behaviour of the microvessels is of fundamental importance in determining the clinical consequences. To study these ideas, my collaborators and I have been and are at present carrying out a series of studies in clinical pharmacology, in order to determine the effect of certain drugs on the behaviour of the microvessels in relation to ischaemia.

For these studies we have employed 2 methods: (1) fluximetry of postischaemic reactive hyperaemia in human limbs with or without arterial obliteration; (2) observation of ultrastructural changes of the microvessels of the cerebral cortex in the rabbit consequent on circulatory insufficiency brought about by ligature of the 2 common carotids.

The drugs which we have used belong principally to the following groups: (1) anti-inflammatory agents, (2) antihistaminics, (3) antiserotoninics, (4) antiadrenergics, and (5) antibradykininics.

In our opinion, the classification of these drugs should not be accepted in too narrow a sense. Obviously no drug has a rigorously specific antagonistic action but is antagonistic to groups of substances which are relatively alike.

The present research has been with a drug belonging to the antibradykinin group, pyridinolcarbamate*.

* Our studies were already in progress when, on 20th March 1972, we received an invitation to take part in this Symposium. In this short period of time, we have not been able to bring them to a conclusion. We limit ourselves, therefore, to presenting certain results in the way of a preliminary communication. On the basis of these we shall plan the direction which we consider useful for our future studies.

POSTISCHAEMIC REACTIVE HYPERAEMIA

Method

In a group of 20 subjects (14 men and 6 women) suffering from atherosclerotic arteriopathy with obliteration of a superficial femoral artery or of an external iliac artery, we calculated the blood flow in: (1) an upper limb free from obliteration; (2) the lower limb with arterial obliteration; (3) the other lower limb without arterial obliteration. We then compressed the limb for 5 min by means of a sphygmomanometer at the base of the limb inflated to a pressure of 20 mm Hg higher than the maximum systemic pressure to arrest the circulation. We then measured the blood flow immediately afterwards at 1, 2, 3, 4, and 5 min intervals following cessation of the ischaemia; 2–3 days later, we repeated the same examination, administering 0.50 g of pyridinolcarbamate orally 1, 2 or 3 hours before examination. The same experiment was also carried out in the upper and lower limb in another group of 8 subjects of equivalent age who suffered no obliterative atherosclerotic arteriopathy. Finally, we checked the behaviour of the blood flow after ischaemia of varying duration, i.e. after ischaemia lasting 1, 3, 5, 10 and 15 min.

For determination of the blood flow, we used the method of Kaindl. As is known, this method is equivalent in conception to the method of venous congestion of Goetz, from which it differs in that it makes use of impedance plethysmography instead of mechanical plethysmography. It is based on measurement of the increase in impedance which takes place in a segment of a limb immediately following the setting-up of a venous stasis, thus allowing the number of ml of blood per 100 ml of tissue to be calculated.

Results

We confirmed the familiar observation that on cessation of ischaemia there is an increase in the blood flow with respect to the values present before the onset of ischaemia. After this increase there is a decrease, which brings the blood flow back to the starting values. During the decrease oscillations may be observed in the value of the flow, so that at certain times this may be measurably lower than the starting values. We were able to observe that, while maintaining these general characteristics, the behaviour of the blood flow may show quantitative variations which differ considerably from subject to subject.

These differences may be attributed to: (1) age, (2) sex, (3) the absence of clinically demonstrable atherosclerosis, (4) the presence of non-obliterative atherosclerosis (limbs without arterial obliteration in subjects with arterial obliteration in other limbs, and (5) the presence of atherosclerotic arterial obliteration.

We do not as yet have sufficient cases to permit us to define precisely the characteristics of the behaviour of the blood stream in postischaemic reactive hyperaemia in relation to each of these parameters.

The administration of pyridinolcarbamate during the hours preceding examination modifies the results of the test. The effect of pyridinolcarbamate on reactive hyperaemia may be summarized in the following manner (Figs. 1–10):

1. It inhibits increased blood flow.
2. This inhibition may not be present in the very early phases of reactive hyperaemia, where it may cause a transient increase in blood flow.
3. This action is particularly evident and repeatable in the second phase of reactive hyperaemia, i.e. in the phase of decreased flow. In other words, pyridinolcarbamate causes a more rapid return to normal of the blood flow. During this phase when the blood flow returns to normal under the action of pyridinolcarbamate, certain periods are frequently observed in which the flow is invariably below starting value.

This effect of pyridinolcarbamate is remarkably constant in its general pattern. However, it shows remarkable quantitative variations from subject to subject. We do not yet possess sufficient cases to enable us to indicate precisely what these differences are in relation to

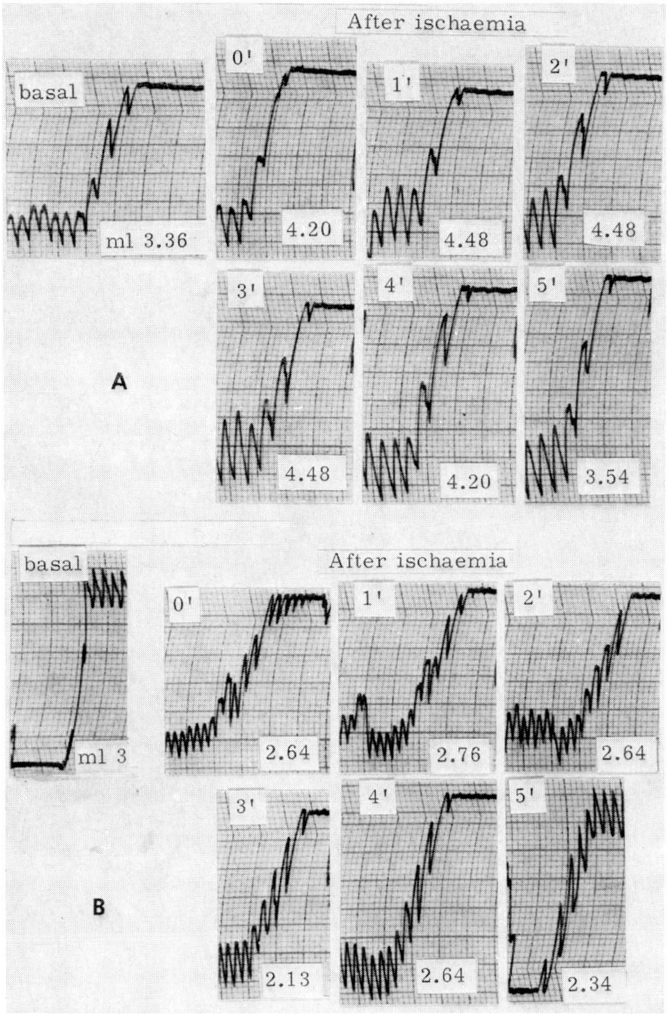

Fig. 1. T.N., aged 63. Reactive hyperaemia. Forearm blood flow in limb without arterial obliteration. A. Before pyridinolcarbamate. B. After pyridinolcarbamate.

single local circulatory conditions. However, we are in possession of sufficient information to provide valid grounds for the hypothesis that there is a parallelism between the clinical picture and the effect of pyridinolcarbamate on reactive hyperaemia, a parallelism which may be of important practical interest.

Comments

In a normal subject the behaviour of fluximetry in reactive hyperaemia is different in relation to the duration of ischaemia (Patterson and Whelan, 1955). More precisely, with an increase in the duration of ischaemia: (1) the increase in the flow becomes greater; (2) the return to starting values takes a longer period of time.

We ourselves have been able to confirm with our own method the findings obtained by Patterson and Whelan.

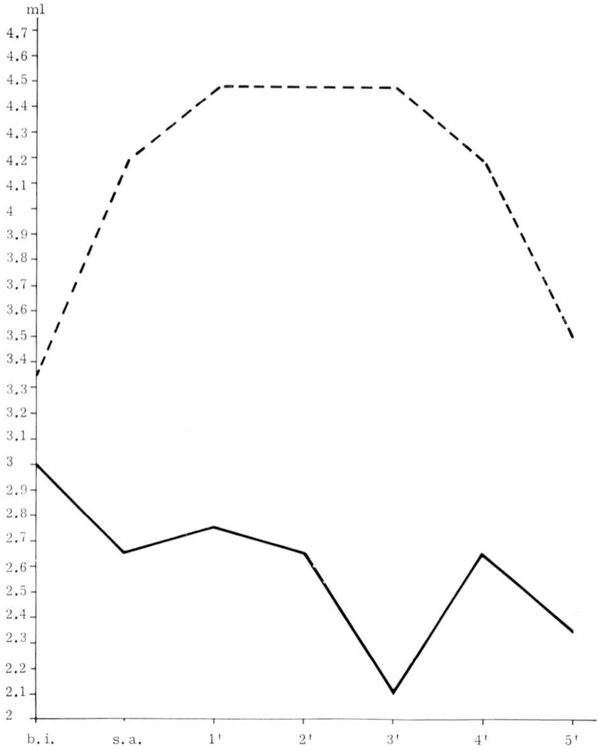

Fig. 2. T.N., aged 63. Forearm blood flow in limb without arterial obliteration. ---- basal; —— after pyridinolcarbamate. ml = blood flow in ml/100 ml tissue/min; b.i. = before ischaemia; s.a. = soon after ischaemia.

Interpretation of the phenomenon of reactive hyperaemia, the study of which was begun by Cohnheim (1882) at the end of the last century, may be summarized schematically in the following manner:

1. If the ischaemia is of very short duration, there is a vasodilatation which is directly due to a diminution in the tone of the smooth muscle fibres consequent on a reduction in pressure. This vasodilatation is in the potential state only as long as ischaemia lasts. With the cessation of ischaemia and therefore with the return of the blood flow into the blood vessels, it manifests itself. After a very brief interval, a vasoconstriction occurs which is due to a sharp increase in blood pressure.

2. If the ischaemia is a little more prolonged, there is a vasodilatation which is due to substances liberated by the tissues during ischaemia. These substances act predominantly on the microvessels distal to the vessels of resistance. The cessation of vasodilatation is due to the removal of these substances brought about by the restoration of the circulation of blood flow after ischaemia.

3. If the ischaemia is still further prolonged, the vasodilatation of the microvessels consequent on the release of the substances by the tissues in a state of ischaemia may be excessive. Under these conditions the return to normal may take much longer. The excessive release of tissue substances probably occurs as a consequence of an initial tissue metabolic breakdown.

4. If the ischaemia is still further prolonged, i.e. if it exceeds a certain limit of time, a micro-

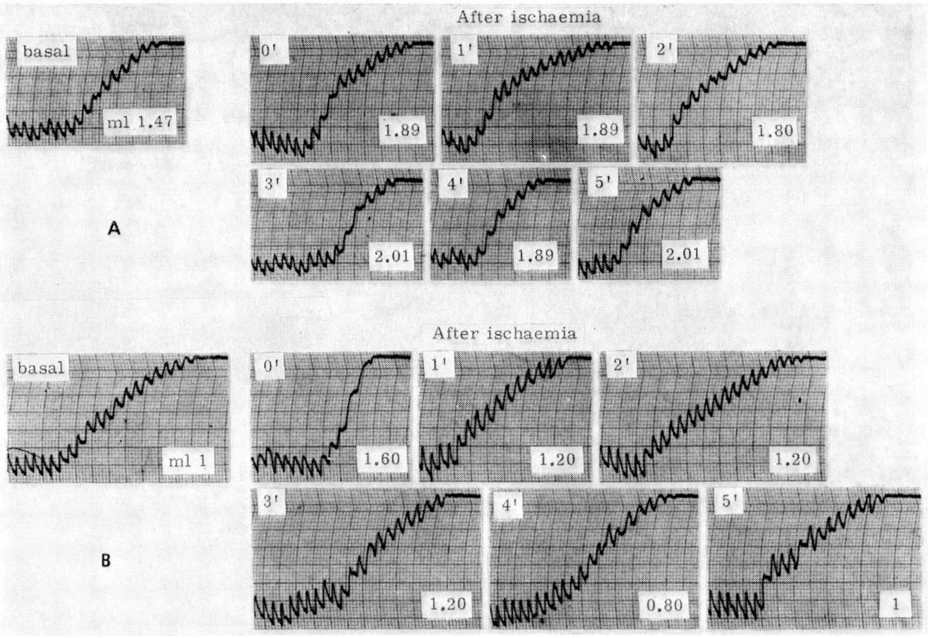

Fig. 3. G.G., aged 58. Reactive hyperaemia. Leg blood flow in limb without arterial obliteration. A. Before pyridinolcarbamate. B. After pyridinolcarbamate.

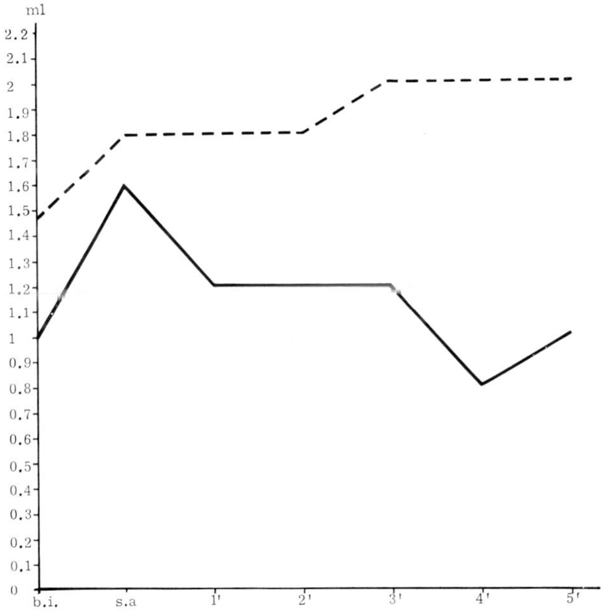

Fig. 4. G.G., aged 58. Leg blood flow in limb without arterial obliteration. ---- basal; —— after pyridinolcarbamate. ml = blood flow in ml/100 ml tissue/min; b.i. = before ischaemia; s.a. = soon after ischaemia.

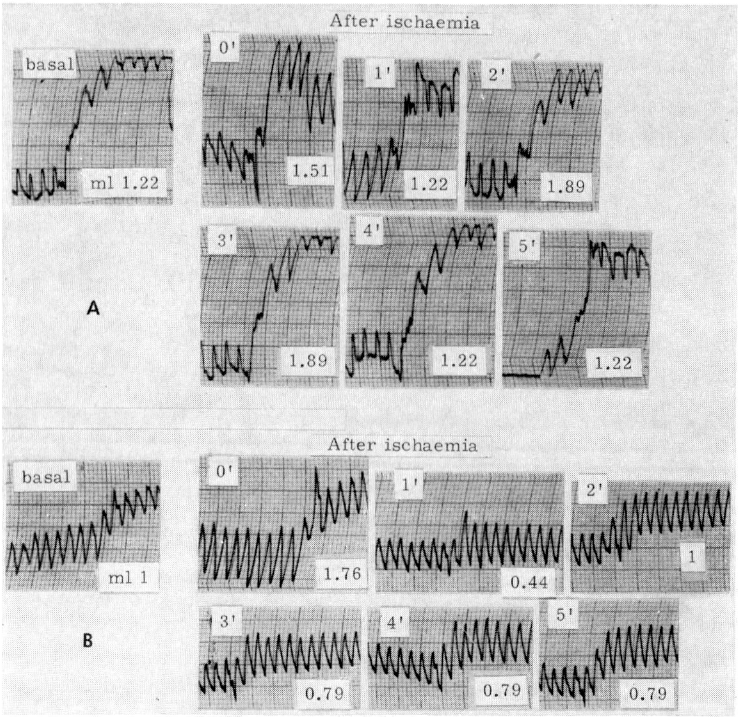

Fig. 5. G.G., aged 58. Reactive hyperaemia. Forearm blood flow in limb without arterial obliteration. A. Before pyridinolcarbamate. B. After pyridinolcarbamate.

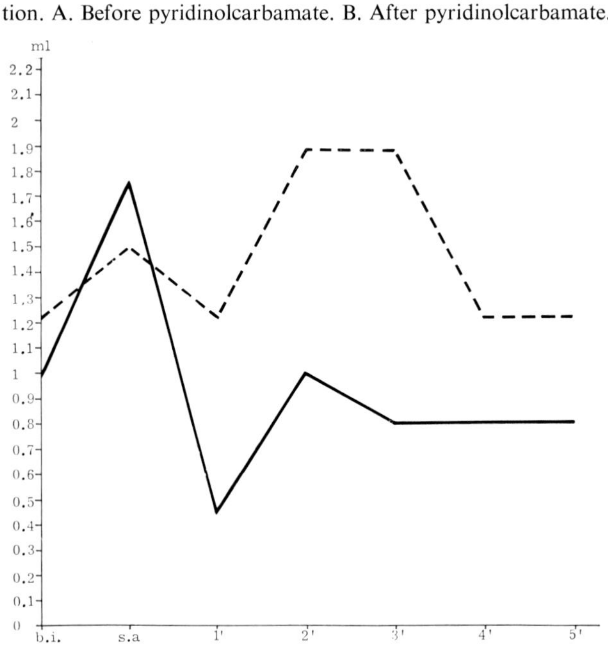

Fig. 6. G.G., aged 58. Forearm blood flow in limb without arterial obliteration. ---- basal; —— after pyridinolcarbamate; ml = blood flow in ml/100 ml tissue/min; b.i. = before ischaemia; s.a. = soon after ischaemia.

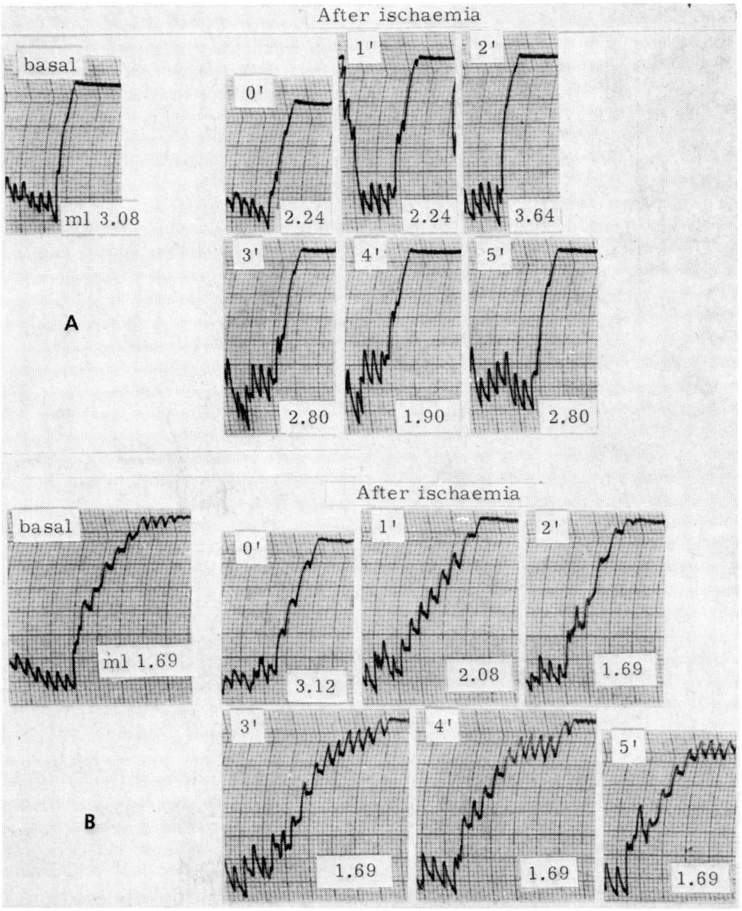

Fig. 7. F.I., aged 54. Reactive hyperaemia. Forearm blood flow in limb without arterial obliteration. A. Before pyridinolcarbamate. B. After pyridinolcarbamate.

vessel dilatation occurs which becomes irreversible. This is due to permanent ischaemic damage of the microvessels. When this microvessel vasodilatation is excessive, there is a disproportion between the inflow of blood and the capacity of the microvessel bed. This disproportion produces stasis of the blood.

It is our opinion that the stasis of blood is more harmful than ischaemia itself as regards the life of the tissues. We base this opinion on numerous tests among which the principal are the following:

1. Clinical evidence. In a limb with circulatory insufficiency due to arterial obliteration, as long as there is clinical evidence of pure ischaemia, i.e. as long as one observes a pallor of the skin, gangrene does not occur. The appearance of cyanosis, which is an expression of microvessel vasodilatation and of disproportion between the inflow of blood and the capacity of the microvessel bed, is a prelude to the onset of gangrene.

2. Experimental evidence. Ligature of the aorta at its origin in an animal causes cerebral lesions which are more easily reversible and therefore less grave than ligature of the aorta accompanied by ligature of the upper vena cava (Hossmann, 1972).

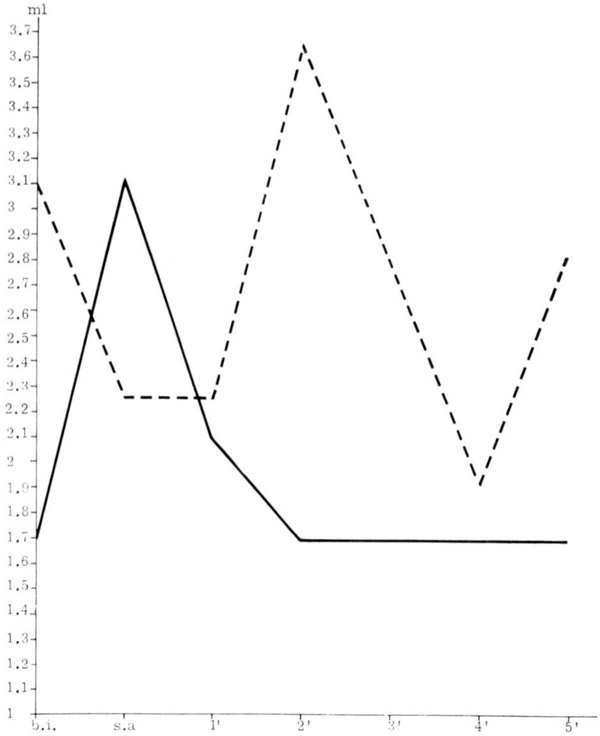

Fig. 8. F.I., aged 54. Forearm blood flow in limb without arterial obliteration. ---- basal; —— after pyridinolcarbamate. ml = blood flow in ml/100 ml tissue/min; b.i. = before ischaemia; s.a. = soon after ischaemia.

The traditional way of studying the pathogenesis of the clinical manifestations of obliterative arterial diseases and of considering their therapy is almost always concentrated on the blood flow and therefore on the calibre of the 'macrovessels' situated proximal to the vessels of resistance. Usually the capacity of the microvessel bed is overlooked. In our opinion, one may validly put forward the hypothesis that an increase in this microvessel capacity with excessive dilatation of the microvessels may be very important in the pathogenesis of tissue damage consequent on circulatory insufficiency due to obliterative arteriopathy.

If this hypothesis is correct, it suggests the use of drugs which antagonize excessive microvessel dilatation in the treatment of obliterative arterial diseases. It is probable that in the sphere of vasodilatatory substances produced by the tissues in ischaemia bradykinin is a major factor. Pyridinolcarbamate, with its antibradykininic action, could act at this level and antagonize the action of a substance such as bradykinin. It is also possible that pyridinolcarbamate may antagonize other microvessel dilatatory substances produced by the tissue during ischaemia.

ULTRASTRUCTURAL CHANGES DUE TO ISCHAEMIA

In order to examine the effect of drugs at the level of the microvessels distal to the vessels of resistance, we carried out a series of studies with the electron microscope. We used several drugs and briefly describe the results obtained with these, because they seem to us better to exemplify the concepts described above.

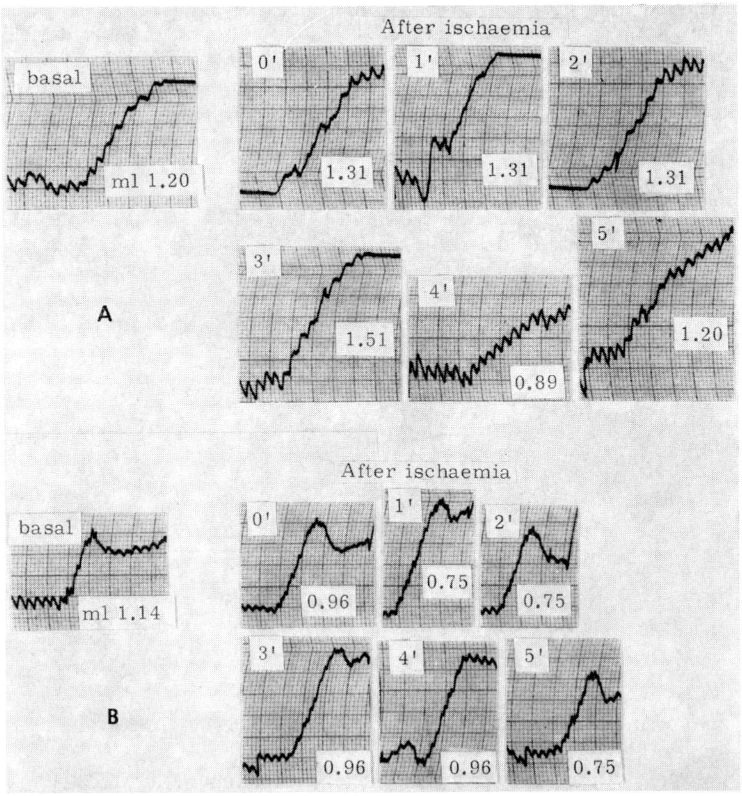

Fig. 9. T.N., aged 63. Reactive hyperaemia. Leg blood flow: iliac artery obliteration. A. Before pyridinolcarbamate. B. After pyridinolcarbamate.

Flavodate disodium (Intercyton) (sodium benzo-γ-pyrone 2-phenyl-5,7-dioxyacetate)

In one batch of rabbits, we ligatured the 2 common carotids. The resulting circulatory insufficiency in the anterior parts of the cerebral hemispheres is well tolerated by the animals, probably because of excellent collateral circulation through the vertebral arteries. After 12 hours the animals were sacrificed and the anterior zones of the cerebral cortex were examined with the electron microscope.

In a second lot of rabbits, we carried out the same experiment after administering parenterally 100 mg of flavodate disodium (Intercyton) per day, for 15 days.

Results. The circulatory insufficiency caused by ligature of the carotids produces on the vessels and surrounding microglia of the cerebral cortex of the rabbit the following changes observable with the electron microscope:

1. The calibre of the vessels is considerably diminished.
2. The surrounding neuroglia appears denser and decidedly less hydrated.
3. The boundaries between the endothelial cells are much more tortuous and thickened, and often show signs of fission proper.
4. Pinocytosis is strongly decreased in the endothelial cells, with diminution or complete absence of fission proper, both towards the surface facing the lumen and on the opposite surface; this diminution appears to be the more accentuated, the more the calibre of the capillaries is reduced.

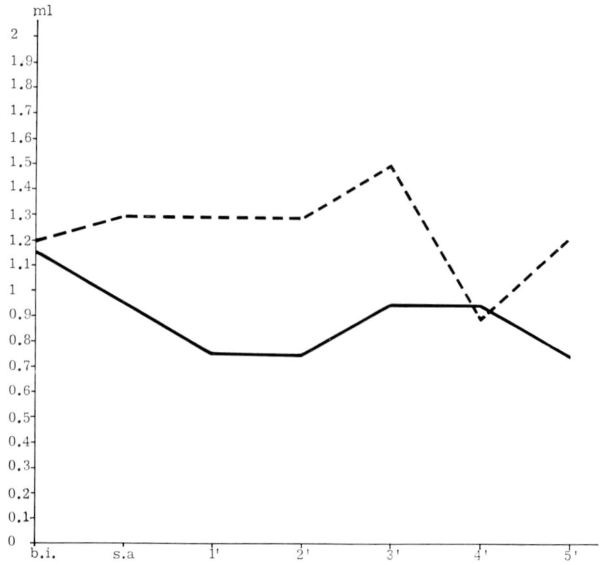

Fig. 10. T.N., aged 63. Leg blood flow: iliac artery obliteration. ---- basal; —— after pyridinol-carbamate. ml = blood flow in ml/100 ml tissue/min; b.i. = before ischaemia; s.a. = soon after ischaemia.

5. The basal membrane appears much thicker and in certain cases shows appearance of fibrillary structures.
6. The lysosomes of the pericytes tend to increase in number and size.
7. The mitochondria tend to present a greater density of their matrix.

In animals treated with flavodate disodium, circulatory insufficiency induced by ligature of the 2 carotids does not produce any significant changes in the vessels and the surrounding neuroglia of the cerebral cortex, i.e. the findings with the electron microscope are identical to those obtained with completely normal control animals of the same weight.

Nicotinic acid

In a third lot of rabbits, we carried out the same examination with the electron microscope, after injecting parenterally into the animal 30 mg of nicotinic acid immediately following ligature of the carotids and 2 hours before sacrificing the animals.

Results. In these animals compared to the controls, the ultrastructural changes produced by circulatory insufficiency as regards the microvessels and the surrounding microglia are as follows:

1. The calibre of the microvessels is even more diminished.
2. The surrounding neuroglia appears even denser and even less hydrated.
3. Pinocytosis is strongly diminished or completely absent, with absence of fission proper on the endothelial surfaces.
4. The basal membrane is even thicker and more opaque.
5. The lysosomes and the mitochondria show signs of greater activity.

Comment

From the ultramicroscopic results described above, it is possible to deduce that: (1) it is possible to modify by pharmacological means changes in the microvessels produced by circulatory insufficiency; (2) the examples considered demonstrate the possibility of influencing in opposite ways microvessel ultrastructural changes due to circulatory insufficiency – flavodate disodium inhibits, and nicotinic acid increases, these ultrastructural alterations; (3) at the present stage of knowledge, we do not know enough to allow us to state which of the 2 types of drugs is the more favourable. In fact we do not know how much of the ultrastructural changes consequent on circulatory insufficiency caused by ligature of the carotids is the expression of tissue damage, and how much is the expression of a useful mechanism of compensation.

Analogous tests are underway with pyridinolcarbamate. We have not, however, had time to complete them. From the preliminary results obtained it seems possible that this method may also be useful in the study of the mechanism of action of pyridinolcarbamate.

CLINICAL INVESTIGATIONS

Running parallel with the experimental investigations reported above, we carried out an investigation into the therapeutic effects of administration of pyridinolcarbamate on subjects suffering from angiopathy of the limbs or the brain. The investigation was carried out on 850 subjects whom we examined and treated in our clinic. These were divided as follows:

1. 462 subjects suffering from atherosclerotic arteriopathy with obliteration localized in the superficial femoral artery, or in the iliac artery of one side, of whom (*a*) 405 showed clinical and instrumental signs of relative circulatory insufficiency of the limb, and (*b*) 57 showed clinical and instrumental signs of absolute circulatory insufficiency.
2. 205 subjects suffering from atherosclerotic cerebral infarct in a non-acute phase.
3. 183 subjects suffering from postphlebitic disease in one or both lower limbs.

In all these subjects, except the group of 57 subjects with complete circulatory insufficiency of the lower limbs, we administered pyridinolcarbamate orally, for 2 months, at a dose of 4 tablets of 0.025 g per day. Pyridinolcarbamate was given in addition to our usual treatment for angiopathic patients. As a control group, we used a group of 400 subjects suffering from the same vascular disease of the limbs or the brain, and in these we used the usual treatment without the addition of pyridinolcarbamate.

To assess the therapeutic effects of pyridinolcarbamate we used the following parameters:

1. For subjects with relative circulatory insufficiency of the lower limbs due to atherosclerotic obliteration of the femoral artery or the iliac artery: the distance walked before onset of intermittent claudication, intensity of pain in intermittent claudication, general assessment of intermittent claudication, and morpho-oscillographic examination.
2. For subjects suffering from cerebral infarct: intensity of paresis or paralysis, mental condition, and general assessment of the course of the disease.
3. For subjects suffering from postphlebitic disease of the lower limbs: intensity of pain, degree of oedema, extent of dermatitis, course taken by ulceration, and general assessment of the course of the disease.

In those subjects suffering from absolute circulatory insufficiency of the limbs due to femoral or iliac atherosclerotic obliteration, treatment with pyridinolcarbamate could not always be carried out over a period of 2 months. Furthermore, pyridinolcarbamate was added to different treatments, according to the urgency of the particular case. In these subjects, any assessment of the therapeutic effect of pyridinolcarbamate is therefore less exact and objective. It was, however, based on the following parameters: pain at rest in a horizontal position, evolution of ulcers and gangrene, and morpho-oscillographic examination.

The therapeutic results are summarized in Tables I–III. From these, one can observe that treatment with pyridinolcarbamate certainly produces in a really very high percentage of cases a regression of the clinical symptomatology of the vascular diseases considered.

TABLE I *Obliterative atherosclerotic arteriopathy of the lower limbs (462 cases)*

	After treatment with pyridinolcarbamate				
	Improved		Unchanged		Deteriorated
	No.	%	No.	%	No. %
1. Subjects with relative circulatory insufficiency (405 cases)					
a. Intermittent claudication					
Distance walked before onset	362	89.4	43	10.6	0
Intensity of pain	368	90.9	37	9.1	0
Time of disappearance of pain	341	84.2	64	15.8	0
General assessment of intermittent claudication	362	89.4	43	10.6	0
b. Morpho-oscillography	222	54.8	183	45.2	0
2. Subjects with absolute circulatory insufficiency (57 cases)					
a. Pain at rest in horizontal position	48	84.2	9	15.8	0
b. Ulcers and/or gangrene	28	49.1	29	50.9	0
c. Morpho-oscillography	32	56.1	25	43.9	0

TABLE II *Cerebral infarct in second stage (205 cases)*

	After treatment with pyridinolcarbamate				
	Improved		Unchanged		Deteriorated
	No.	%	No.	%	No. %
1. Paresis or paralysis	53	25.4	153	74.6	0
2. Mental condition	172	83.9	33	16.1	0
3. General assessment	160	78.1	45	21.9	0

TABLE III *Postphlebitic disease (183 cases)*

	After treatment with pyridinolcarbamate				
	Improved		Unchanged		Deteriorated
	No.	%	No.	%	No. %
1. Pain	161	88.0	22	12	0
2. Oedema	27	14.8	156	85.2	0
3. Dermatitis	148	80.9	35	19.1	0
4. Ulcers	115	62.8	78	37.2	0
5. General assessment	155	84.7	28	15.3	0

Comment

An interpretation of the mechanism by means of which pyridinolcarbamate produces its therapeutic effects in the vascular diseases described above can be attempted only by formulating hypotheses. In formulating these hypotheses, the results which we obtained during our experimental studies may serve some useful purpose. What we have seen of the effect of pyridinolcarbamate on reactive hyperaemia, i.e. on the behaviour of the microvessels in the presence of acute experimental ischaemia, may suggest a hypothesis for interpreting the effects of this drug on the behaviour of the microvessels in relation to the chronic spontaneous ischaemia or stasis of the blood which is due to particular vascular diseases. The hypothesis which we would propose is, firstly, that pyridinolcarbamate acts by improving the way in which the tissues support circulatory insufficiency. Secondly, this improvement comes about by antagonizing certain substances (among which is very probably bradykinin) liberated by the tissues during ischaemia and which may unfavourably influence the microvessels distal to the vessels of resistance. Thirdly, the unfavourable action of these substances consists of an excessive dilatation of the microvessel bed, and, fourthly, after this excessive vasodilatation there follows a disproportion between the inflow of blood into the tissues and the capacity of the microvessel bed. Fifthly, this disproportion causes the stasis of blood, the effect of which on the viability of the tissues is particularly harmful.

Should this hypothesis concerning the mechanism of the therapeutic action of pyridinolcarbamate in clinically manifest arteriosclerotic disease be confirmed by further evidence, it may be possible to hazard a further and even bolder hypothesis. This would deal more closely with the early stages of the pathogenetic mechanism of the atherosclerotic process, i.e. when it is not yet manifest clinically. This further hypothesis, which derives from the ingenious ideas of Shimamoto, may be stated in the following manner:

1. The first stage of the atherosclerotic process consists of a reduction in the blood flow which feeds the wall of the large arteries, both through the endothelium lining the lumen of the vessel and through the vasa vasorum. This reduction in the flow may also be the expression of normal aging of the artery.
2. If the tissues which compose the wall of the artery react well to this circulatory insufficiency, liberating adequate substances (among which is bradykinin), the atherosclerotic process is not set up and one encounters merely the normal aging of the artery.
3. If, on the other hand, the tissues of the wall of the artery do not react in a suitable manner, the atherosclerotic process is set up.
4. In this hypothesis, a drug such as pyridinolcarbamate, which has the capacity of improving the reaction of the tissues in relation to circulatory insufficiency, may really be a drug which acts favourably at a pathogenetic level on arteriosclerosis.

I said at the beginning that this paper is merely a preliminary note concerning a group of research studies which we are at present carrying out. It is chiefly intended, therefore, to pave the way for further research on the subject.

In this preliminary phase, all hypotheses, even the most daring, are justified. Only further pursuance of the experimental investigations to which we propose to devote ourselves in the future can determine whether these are correct and lead to new knowledge on the pathogenesis of arteriosclerosis and the possibilities of prophylaxis and specific treatment.

SUMMARY

By means of fluximetry, the action in man of pyridinolcarbamate was studied on postischaemic reactive hyperaemia in limbs with atherosclerotic arterial obliteration, and in limbs without arterial obliteration.

Further studies were carried out in the rabbit on the action of certain drugs on ultrastructural changes produced in the microvessels of the cerebral cortex by means of ligature of the 2 common carotids.

Finally, an investigation was carried out on the therapeutic effects consequent on treatment with pyridinolcarbamate in a group of 850 subjects suffering from angiopathy of the limbs (obliterative atherosclerotic arteriopathy, atherosclerotic cerebral infarct, and postphlebitic disease).

On the basis of the results obtained, it was possible to advance the hypothesis that one of the principal actions of pyridinolcarbamate consists in improving the way in which the tissues tolerate circulatory insufficiency. The drug might antagonize certain substances which are liberated by the tissues daring ischaemia and which produce excessive dilatation of the microvessel bed.

REFERENCES

HOSSMAN, K. A. (1972): Personal communication.

KAINDL, F., KAUTER-OGRIS, E., POLZER, K., SCHUFRIED, F. and TISO, B. (1967): Indirect quantitative blood flow measurements in the extremities of subjects with unimpaired circulation and patients with arterial obliterating disease. *Angiology*, *18/8*, 528.

PATTERSON, G. C. and WHELAN, R. F. (1955): Reactive hyperaemia in the human forearm. *Clin. Sci.*, *14*, 197.

PRATESI, F., SPINELLI, P., CARAMELLI, L. and TESI, M. (1970): Ultrastructural aspects of cerebral angiological pharmacodynamics. *Folia angiol. (Pisa), 96, 99,* 75.

PYRIDINOLCARBAMATE TREATMENT IN PERIPHERAL OBLITERATIVE ATHEROSCLEROSIS WITH ISCHEMIC SKIN LESIONS AND ITS EVALUATION

F. LUND

Stureby Sjukhus Geriatric Unit, Enskede, Stockholm, Sweden

This study is connected with the one reported in 1969 at the First International Symposium on Atherogenesis, Thrombogenesis and Pyridinolcarbamate Treatment (Lund *et al.*, 1969). The major part of the patient material presented at that time comprised cases of intermittent claudication and only a few cases showed trophic skin lesions. The present investigation on pyridinolcarbamate (Anginin) is restricted to cases of advanced skin ischemia with subsequent trophic skin lesions in a geriatric population.

The fact that spontaneous healing diminishes with age does not justify the claim that even limited ischemic skin lesions in geriatric cases have a very poor prognosis with gradual progressive deterioration. Hence there is a need for a controlled trial or at least an acceptable comparative series. This has been included in our study.

METHODS

The methods used are in principle the same as described by Lund et al. in 1969. They are summarized below.

Photography Cases of advanced skin ischemia with discoloration of the skin, necrotic changes or ischemic ulcerations are very suitable for photographic recording of the course of disease. All patients were repeatedly photographed in color, including close-up pictures of the lesions. The photographic technique was standardized in terms of distance, illumination and other exposure details.

Elevation-dependency tests In both the Anginin and comparative series these tests were performed (cf. also a special paper by Lund et al., *This Volume*, pp. 281–286). The results were recorded by color photography at the beginning of observation for comparison with repeated examinations later on.

Vital capillary microscopy with photography of the microvascular pattern was performed in isolated cases by means of a technique previously described by Fagrell and Lund (1969).

Skin temperature recording (thermocouple) from toes and fingers was carried out regularly before and after vasodilatation as a preparatory procedure before digital pulse plethysmography. In a few cases the skin temperature gradient at various levels from proximal to distal parts of the legs was recorded.

Pulse recording methods Arterial insufficiency of the legs, as diagnosed by clinical pulse palpation and auscultation over the iliac and femoral arteries, was routinely confirmed by:
oscillometry carried out at all levels of the limbs using the Collen's or Comparat oscillometer,
oscillography from the small of the legs by use of the Pulsorette oscillograph, a highly sensitive apparatus, and
digital pulse plethysmography by the method of Lund (1956, 1967). Vasoconstriction obviously influences the amplitude of the digital volume pulse; therefore, in order to abolish vasoconstriction moderate warming of the body by a heating box in combination with oral alcohol intake was used. Smoking before the examination was not permitted.

In evaluation of pulse recording results the amplitude of the deflections should be expressed as relative rather than absolute values. The quotient between the pulse amplitude from the leg and that from the corresponding level of the arm is used. This implies that in digital plethysmography the amplitude of the toe pulse curve is expressed as the ratio to the amplitude of pulse curves from the terminal phalanx of a finger (usually left index). In normal cases this quotient is $\geqslant 0.5$.

As in most cases arterial reconstructive surgery could not be considered as a therapeutic alternative, arteriography was performed only rarely. The location and extension of the obliterative changes were investigated by means of pulse recording methods. The reliability and sensitivity of these indirect methods compared to arteriography have been evaluated in a study by Lund and Hellström (1969).

In some cases the *Doppler ultrasound technique* was used for recording pulsations and distal blood pressure at the small of the leg as compared to that of the arm.

MATERIAL

Type and location of lesions

Both the Anginin and the comparative series comprised patients with one or more distinct lesions limited to the toes, heel, malleolar or other circumscribed areas of the foot or lower leg. In consideration of the latency from commencement of Anginin therapy until a clinically obvious effect could be observed, patients with very extensive necrotic changes and gangrene were excluded from the comparative study. The patients of both series had been considered as unsuitable for arterial reconstructive surgery either because of age, extensive atheromatosis and distal location of the arterial obliterations, or because of other coexistent diseases and poor general condition.

Criteria of ischemic lesions

When deciding upon whether trophic lesions of the foot or leg ulcers are in fact caused by ischemia as a result of arterial insufficiency, it is unsatisfactory to rely exclusively on the presence of intermittent claudication or arteriographically proven arterial stenosis and segmental arterial occlusion as sole criteria. Not infrequently normal resting blood flow is observed in patients with claudication. In both series only patients were included with absent or minimal pulsations in oscillography from the small of the legs, and in toe pulse plethysmography (quotient $\leqslant 0.10$). Some of the patients also had coexistent venous insufficiency following venous thrombosis revealed by history and clinical examination.

Characteristics of comparative series

The comparative group, referred to as controls in the following Tables, is a retrospective series, chosen mainly from material of the last 5 years, during which time our therapeutic principles have shown no essential change, except for the supplementation with Anginin.

Age and sex distribution

This is shown in Table I. Mean age in the control group of 43 patients was 73 years (range 58-89 years) and in the Anginin group of 25 patients, 77 years (range 63-89 years). The proportion of diabetic cases (in this and the following Tables indicated by figures within brackets) was higher among the controls (18 out of 43) than in the Anginin-treated cases (6 out of 25).

Anginin dosage

Patients were given a daily dose of 1.5–1.0 g of Anginin. At the commencement of treatment a gradual increase in dosage up to the standard dose was preferred. If the patients could not tolerate the 1.5 g dose because of side-effects (mainly of the gastrointestinal type) the treatment was continued with a daily dose of 1.0 g in some cases.

Concurrent treatment

In a view of the serious degree of disease the patients in the Anginin group were subjected to other therapeutic measures intended to improve peripheral circulation and tissue nutri-

TABLE I

Age and sex distribution

Age	Control		Anginin	
	♂	♀	♂	♀
85–89	2(2)	1	1(1)	3(1)
80–84	3(1)	4(2)	5	1
75–79	6(2)	1	5(1)	2(1)
70–74	5(1)	4(1)	2	2(1)
65–69	9(5)	1(1)	2(1)	1
60–64	2(1)	1(1)	1	
55–59	3(1)	1		
Σ	30(13)	13(5)	16(3)	9(3)
Total	43(18)		25(6)	

Figures in brackets = diabetics.

tion, or at least to prevent progression of the disease. These measures, e.g. muscular exercise, 'syncardial massage' given by the Vasotron equipment, and oral anticoagulants, were the same as the treatment given to patients in the comparative group.

Other drug therapy, e.g. conventional vasodilators, was not used as a routine and was used less extensively in the Anginin than in the comparative group. Of such drugs, Cyclomandol (Brocades, The Netherlands), Hydergin (Sandoz, Switzerland) and sometimes local treatment with a nitroglycerin cream were preferred, as well as Ido-E (Ferrosan, Sweden), an α-tocopherol compound the effect of which, however, is supposed to differ from that of a vasodilating agent.

Smoking

13 out of 25 of the Anginin patients smoked and of these only 2 were heavy smokers, smoking more than 20 cigarettes per day. Most of the others smoked between 3 and 10 cigarettes per day. Attempts to make the patients stop smoking were not very successful. In no case was smoking completely stopped during the trial, although a few patients (not the 2 heavy smokers) reduced their consumption to some degree.

Observation period

A period of 3 months was chosen as the lowest time limit for evaluation of the course of disease in both series. A few cases receiving Anginin for a period shorter than 3 months are not included in the series. The mean period of Anginin treatment is approximately 17 months. Patients obviously improving or even healing during Anginin treatment continued to take the drug to prevent possible recurrences. This accounts for the comparatively long mean duration of treatment. The shortest treatment period in the series is in fact 5 months (2 cases who deteriorated and in whom further treatment was assumed to be futile).

RESULTS

Course of disease

Control series Table II shows the results in the comparative group without Anginin, with separation into out- and in-patients as well as into cases respectively with and without concurrent anticoagulant therapy. Out of 43 cases, 21 (49%) healed or showed significant improvement. More cases of deterioration were found in the in-patient group. This group represents patients with a more pronounced general or local condition compared with the out-patient group. As mentioned above, the control group included a high proportion of diabetics: 18 cases, out of which 10 deteriorated.

Anginin series Table III illustrates in the same way the course of disease in the Anginin-treated group. Healing or improvement was observed in 18 out of 25 cases (72%). In this series there were 6 diabetics and 2 of these deteriorated. It may be mentioned that the improved cases included 10 smokers (out of 13 in the series), and in fact both of the very heavy smokers.

TABLE II

Controls: Course of disease during observation period

	Improved		Deteriorated		
	Anticoagulants	No anticoagulants	Anticoagulants	No anticoagulants	Σ
Out-patients	8	4(2)	7(5)		19(7)
In-patients	8(5)	1(1)	11(5)	4	24(11)
Total	16(5)	5(3)	18(10)	4	43(18)

Figures in brackets = diabetics.

TABLE III

Anginin: Course of disease during observation period

	Improved		Deteriorated		
	Anticoagulants	No anticoagulants	Anticoagulants	No anticoagulants	Σ
Out-patients	5(2)	3(1)	1		9(3)
In-patients	8(1)	2	6(2)		16(3)
Total	13(3)	5(1)	7(2)		25(6)

Figures in brackets = diabetics.

TABLE IV

Amputations (excluding toes) during observation period

	Total no. of patients	Total no. of patients amputated	Foot	Lower leg	Thigh
Control	43	8	1(1)	7(2)	4(1)
Anginin	25	3		3	

Incidence of amputations in control and Anginin series Frequency and magnitude of major amputations as shown in Table IV reflect to some degree the severity of deterioration. However, it should be emphasized that an amputation, which per se might have been a logical therapeutic measure, was not performed in some cases for one reason or another, e.g. very poor condition of patient because of general deterioration possibly with subsequent death, patient's absolute opposition to mutilating surgery, etc.

In the control series, 8 out of 43 patients were amputated (about 19%). The total number of 12 amputated legs in this group reflects the fact that 4 patients had a bilateral amputation. There were 4 thigh amputations. In the Anginin-treated series, 3 out of 25 patients (12%) had an amputation, none bilaterally. There was no femoral amputation in this group.

Thrombotic episodes during Anginin treatment

Having been for many years an advocate of long-term therapy with oral anticoagulants in advanced cases of peripheral arterial disease, not least in order to prevent complicating venous thrombosis (Lund, 1957; Lund and Tillgren, 1966), I had most patients (17 out of 25)

TABLE V

Anticoagulant therapy

Before and during Anginin therapy	Instituted after thrombotic episode with Anginin
17	3

treated with anticoagulants from the start of Anginin treatment (Table V). In 3 further cases anticoagulant therapy was instituted because of thrombotic episodes occurring during Anginin therapy.

Thrombotic episodes were encountered during Anginin therapy without anticoagulants not only in the series with ischemic skin lesions but also in another series of 30 cases of Type II peripheral atherosclerosis, i.e. only intermittent claudication. With both groups added together (a total of 55 patients) we had 5 cases of venous thrombosis in the leg, which is often a serious complication in cases of arterial insufficiency, and at least 2 cases of arterial thrombosis in the leg. Furthermore, during Anginin treatment without anticoagulants 2 cases of cerebrovascular accident and 3 cases of myocardial infarction occurred. These last observations are mentioned with great reservation as the clinical evidence of a thrombotic occlusion is always difficult to assess in such cases.

Incidence of side-effects

In 6 cases the continuation of Anginin treatment was impossible because of gastrointestinal side-effects. As the treatment was discontinued during the very first weeks and anyhow before 3 months, these cases are, of course, not included in the series of 25 cases presented. This implies that in about 1/5 of the cases (6 out of 31) side-effects were so severe that treatment had to be stopped.

Slight or moderate symptoms of gastritis could sometimes be corrected by antacids or other specific therapy which facilitated continued Anginin therapy. Side-effects presenting as persistent frequent and softer motions or possibly diarrhea were considered to be particularly unfavorable because of the danger of dehydration and subsequent tendency to thrombosis. If these side-effects persisted in spite of a reduction in the daily Anginin dose to 1.0 g, treatment was discontinued.

The cause of discontinued therapy in one of the 6 cases was a gastric hemorrhage in a patient undergoing concurrent anticoagulant therapy. This hemorrhage from an ulcer could be associated with anticoagulant treatment. However, Anginin cannot be excluded as a contributing factor to the bleeding.

Illustrations of individual Anginin cases

In the evaluation of the effect of Anginin, emphasis should be placed on the reported comparative study, and less attention given to illustrations of successful cases. However, it seems appropriate to demonstrate in a visual way the implication of the terms 'healing or significant improvement' as used above, and on this account a few case reports are added to the text (Figs. 1–3, p. 276*a*). At least 2 of the illustrated cases serve as their own controls (see legends of Figs. 1 and 4).

In some other cases Anginin was added after deterioration following a couple of months' treatment with other therapy. A special account of these cases serving as their own controls will not be given here. In the continued study now in progress we try to follow such a protocol. As a matter of fact, we sometimes dare not postpone the institution of Anginin therapy too long because of obvious progression of the ischemic skin lesions.

DISCUSSION

Duration of observation period

An obvious healing tendency of skin lesions was observed in many Anginin cases before the minimum 3 months' period of treatment had passed. However, in evaluation of both Anginin and comparative cases, it seemed advisable to define a sufficiently long observation period, not least with regard to the age of patients and the retarded healing disposition of ischemic skin lesions in these cases. Therefore an observation period of at least 3 months was chosen.

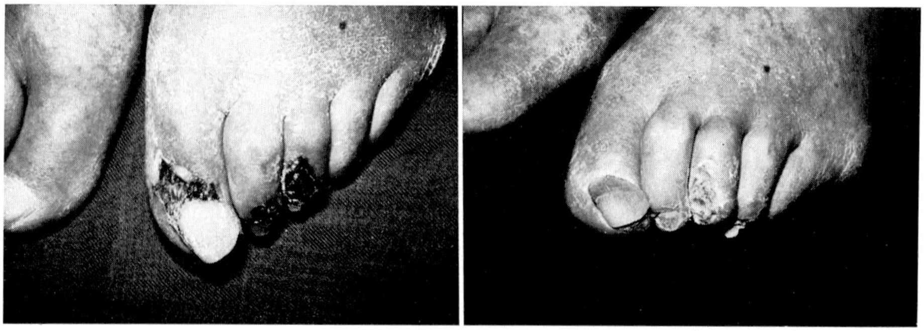

a *b*

Fig. 4a–b. Left foot of 84-year-old man with necrotic toe lesions which had shown progressive tendency in spite of anticoagulant (dicoumarol) and other conservative treatment. Marked improvement after supplementation with Anginin.

Fig. 4a. At commencement of Anginin treatment (in addition to dicoumarol).

Fig. 4b. After 3 months: lesions almost healed.

Vital capillary microscopy showed at commencement of Anginin treatment no capillaries in the skin near to the toe lesions. After Anginin treatment, capillaries were obviously seen in corresponding areas, as could be expected from the clinical signs of improved skin circulation. A similar finding was encountered in another Anginin-treated case of this series, showing clinical improvement (cf. also Fagrell, 1972).

During this period the pattern of ischemic lesions will usually not remain unchanged. As a rule something will occur, either deterioration with aggravated pain and/or progression and extension of the necrotic changes and ulcerations, or improvement revealing itself as relief of pain, demarcation of the necroses, reduced susceptibility to local infection and healing of ulcerations with reduced danger of a necessary major amputation. Unchanged pain and a completely unaltered appearance of the necroses and the ulcerations for a period of 3 months are in fact very rare. Despite this, such an unchanged local pattern of the disease was classified as deterioration in our evaluation.

Evaluation of the results

Considering the spontaneous variations occurring in the course of peripheral atherosclerosis, circumspection is essential when results of new therapeutic measures are evaluated. Undoubtedly the finding that 18 out of 25 Anginin-treated patients showed improvement in their ischemic skin lesions is a surprisingly positive observation, in particular as the patient material is a geriatric one with a mean age of 77 years. Nevertheless we have to ask at least the following 2 questions:

1. Does the course of disease in this series really deviate from the spontaneous course, i.e. are the observed improvements anything else than variations in the spontaneous course? If this first question has an affirmative answer, then the second question follows:

2. Are the observed improvements associated with the Anginin treatment or with other therapeutic measures?

The spontaneous course of obliterative arterial disease of the limbs was studied among others by Bloor (1961) and by Mathiesen et al. (1970*a*, *b*). The latter group was able to report improvement in 67% of 58 cases with ischemic skin lesions. Of course, the presumption was that local infections were treated adequately and that the necessary correction of diabetes was made in such cases. If the patients stopped smoking, the percentage rate of improvement (12 out of the 14 patients) seemed to be further increased.

However, the series reported by Mathiesen et al. represents a more selected group of patients than ours. They excluded not only all patients with extensive necrosis and gangrene who were potential candidates for amputation as in our investigation, but also, and this is important, very old patients and cases suffering from other complicating diseases as well as those patients who died during the period of observation. The authors did not report the mean age of their series. However, out of 58 patients 32 were below 65 years of age and only 26 older, i.e. a much younger group than ours with a mean age of 77 years.

As mentioned above, the evaluation of the Anginin series is undoubtedly complicated by other concurrent therapeutic measures, a fact which cannot be neglected in the discussion of the results. However, those other measures were resorted to before we started our clinical trial with Anginin, and certainly we were not at that time accustomed to encounter in old age improvement in the course of disease in so many cases.

It is important, however, that this conception, which is nothing more than a 'clinical impression', agrees with the results of the retrospective comparative series of patients of the last 5 years in which only those other types of therapy were used. 21 out of 43 cases (49%) improved as compared to 18 out of 25 (72%) in the Anginin series. Undeniably this comparison is not free from criticism, above all that it is not a simultaneously performed comparative study and still less a controlled trial of the double-blind type. For many reasons – ethical, insufficient access to comparable cases and also others which will not be recalled here – such a clinical trial in severe arterial insufficiency with incipient gangrene and danger of amputation did not seem very attractive, although it would represent good science. At any rate, a comparison with a retrospective series stood out as a superior alternative to just a 'clinical impression'. It is possible that the above-mentioned approach with patients serving as their own controls, which is applied in our continued study now running, will be able to give still more conclusive data.

Fig. 1a–c. Left leg (lateral and medial supramalleolar region) of 89-year-old woman, non-diabetic, with combined venous and severe arterial insufficiency. For 20 years she suffered from leg ulcers, originally caused by venous insufficiency. During the past few years obvious deterioration with no healing at all was observed because of progressive arterial insufficiency (toe pulsations almost abolished). Trials with local dermatological measures were futile. Effective compressive therapy of leg ulcers was not tolerated because of unfavorable influence on arterial circulation. After commencement of Anginin therapy there was obvious improvement of leg ulcers.
No concurrent anticoagulant therapy.

Fig. 1a. At commencement of Anginin treatment.

Fig. 1b. After 3 months.

Fig. 1c. After 5 months.

A few months later ulcers were completely healed and patient could be discharged from hospital to return home. Her comment at discharge was: 'Certainly it was about time that my ulcers finally did heal. As they had been more or less open for 20 years I had begun to be a little impatient with them, I must confess!' With some justification this case can be regarded as its own control.

Fig. 2a–c. Right foot of 84-year-old diabetic woman with prenecrotic discoloration of big toe and a necrotic ulceration on its dorsal side. Patient happened to visit our clinic the day before she was due to have an amputation performed at another hospital because of almost unendurable nocturnal pains in the foot. She had Anginin treatment instead of amputation and also initially antibiotics but no anticoagulants. Pain diminished markedly after a few weeks and later disappeared completely.

Fig. 2a. At commencement of Anginin treatment.

Fig. 2b. After 5 months. Obviously improved.

Fig. 2c. After $1\frac{1}{2}$ years. Complete healing.

Patient has been an out-patient all the time and is still very well at home after $2\frac{1}{2}$ years, with her daily Anginin dose reduced from 1.5 to 1.0 g.

Fig. 3a–d. Right foot of 76-year-old diabetic man. Bilateral severe arterial insufficiency (toe pulsations completely abolished). Originally the patient had presented with a necrotic toe lesion of left foot which healed within 4 months after start of Anginin treatment. Then extensive prenecrotic and necrotic changes in right foot due to complicating venous thrombosis occurred during Anginin treatment without anticoagulants. In spite of extremely severe pain the patient declined a femoral amputation recommended at another hospital. He himself elected to continue with Anginin, which was supplemented by dicoumarol. Antibiotics were required for shorter periods.

Fig. 3a. At commencement of observation period.

Fig. 3b. After $\frac{1}{2}$ year of continued Anginin treatment combined with dicoumarol. Pain alleviated. Good demarcation of necrotic toes.

Fig. 3c. After 1 year. 5th toe had sloughed off and been found in bandage. 2nd toe could be removed quite simply by tweezers without any sharp instrument.

Fig. 3d. After $1\frac{1}{2}$ years. Foot deprived of 2 toes but painless and very serviceable for walking.

lat.

med.

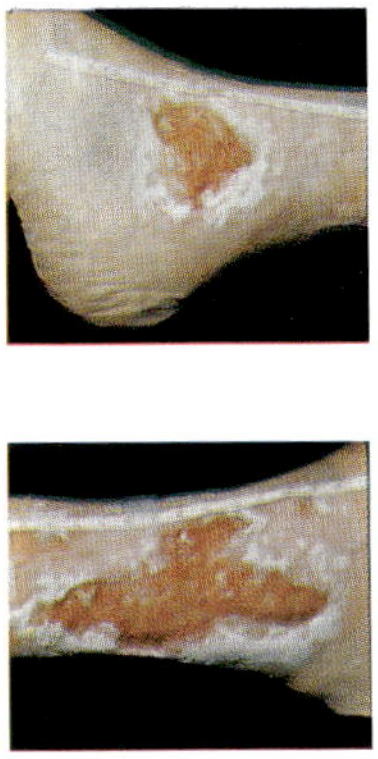

Fig. 1a

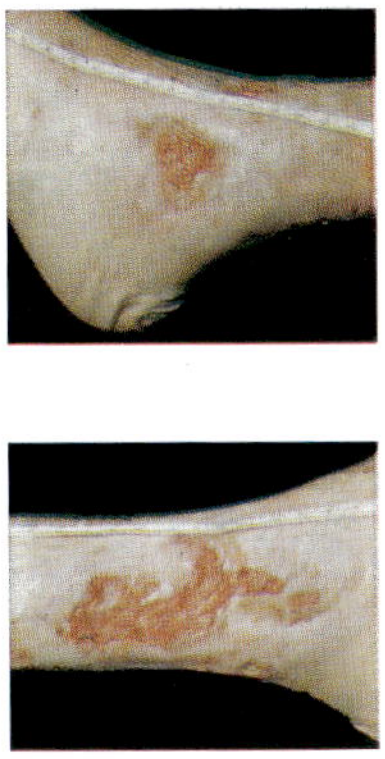

Fig. 1b

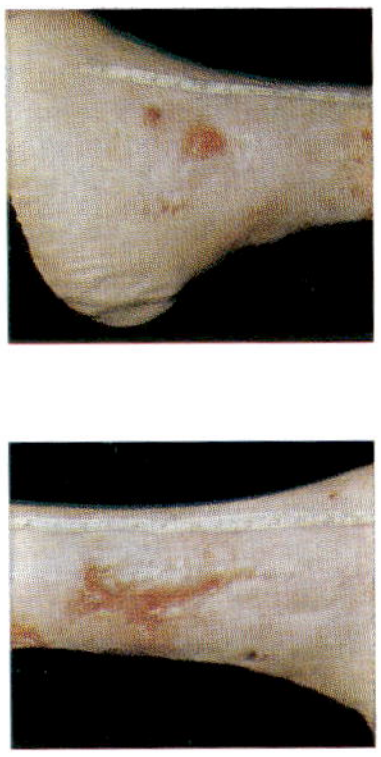

Fig. 1c

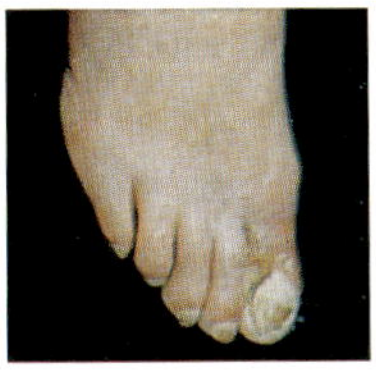

Fig. 2a

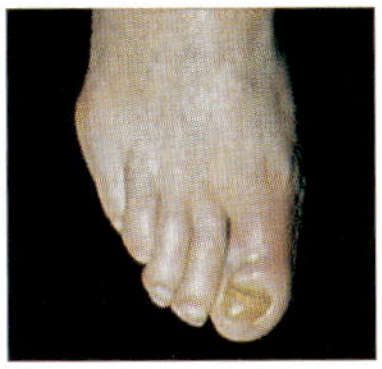

Fig. 2b

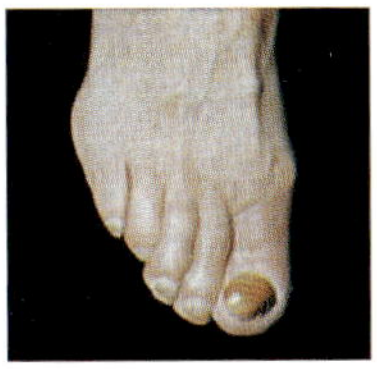

Fig. 2c

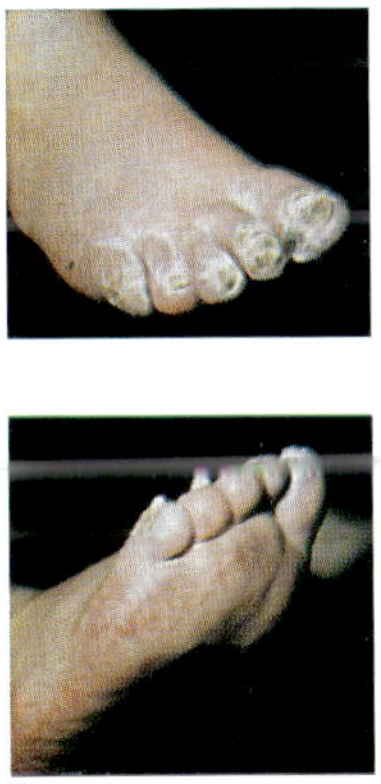

Fig. 3a

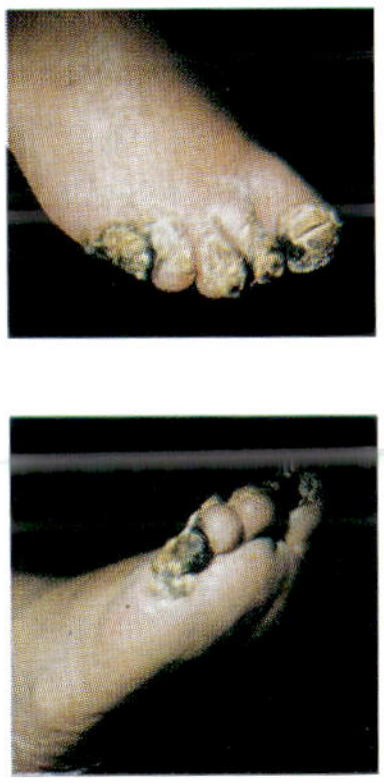

Fig. 3b

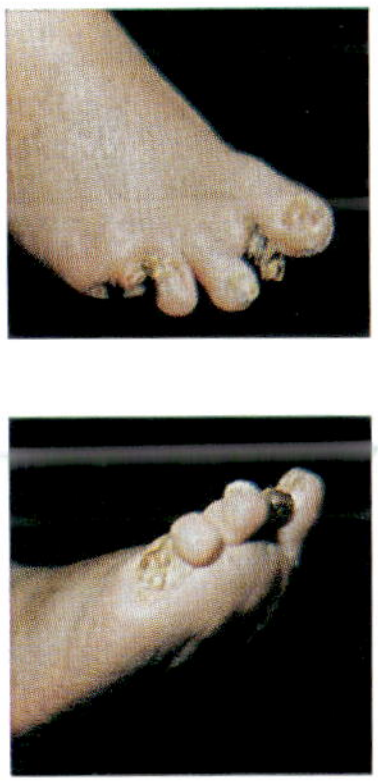

Fig. 3c

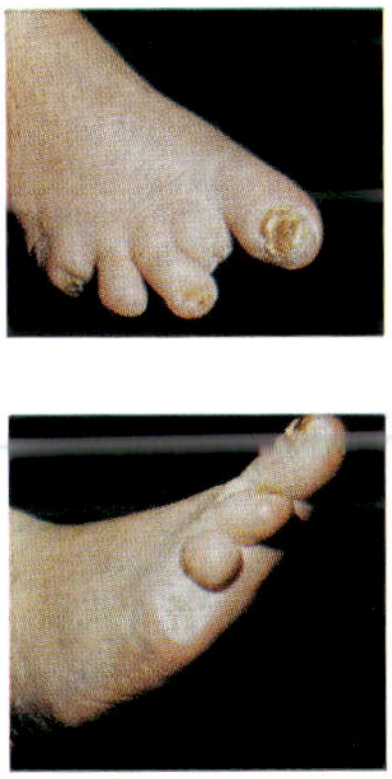

Fig. 3d

Role of smoking

As shown in studies by Silbert and Zazeela (1958), Juergens et al. (1960) and Mathiesen et al. (1970*a*, *b*), smoking plays an important role in the prognosis of obliterative arterial disease of the limbs. These clinical observations agree with the experimental findings of Hess and Frost (1968) and Kjeldsen (1969). Therefore, in evaluation of a supposed clinical effect of a new drug one has to pay due regard to possible changes in smoking habits. The results in our Anginin series cannot be explained on the basis of a change in smoking habits. In no case was smoking stopped completely during the period of observation and only a few of the smokers reduced their moderate consumption to some degree. Further, 10 of the 13 smokers in the series were among the improved cases and in fact both of the very heavy smokers. Of course, these findings do not decrease the great importance of smoking in the prognosis of peripheral atherosclerosis. Possibly the cessation of smoking might have changed the course of disease in the 3 deteriorated smokers, and maybe also among the improved cases in terms of healing time.

In a geriatric clientele, the majority of whom are long-term-care in-patients, it is often very difficult for psychological reasons to have the patient stop or reduce smoking, especially if the consumption is not more than moderate or minimal. Possibly our efforts were not sufficiently energetic in this way. It may be a sort of consolation that we avoided an experimental error by desisting from combining institution of Anginin with interruption of smoking. Some of the non-smokers in the series were ex-smokers who had discontinued long before their participation in the clinical trial with Anginin.

How can a favorable effect of Anginin on ischemic skin lesions be explained?

The positive observations with Anginin could be associated with a microcirculatory action, maybe of the rheological type with an inhibitory effect on agglutination of blood cells. A cellular metabolic influence, possibly combined with changes in the surface electrical charges of the cells, involving also the function and structure of the vascular intima besides the blood cell system, is a conceivable interpretation. An improved nutritional exchange could be the final result, even without primary hemodynamic changes.

The occurrence of thrombotic episodes (venous or arterial), both in the present series and in another Anginin group comprising cases of intermittent claudication, indicates that a marked clinical antithrombotic effect of Anginin cannot be expected in these patient groups. On that account concurrent anticoagulant therapy seems to be justified in cases accessible to such long-term treatment. This view is supported by the study of Hess (1971) who, among 42 arteriographically examined patients treated with Anginin, found 6 cases of further arterial occlusion in spite of treatment, as well as 2 cases of venous thrombosis and 1 cerebrovascular accident.

The capacity of long-term anticoagulant therapy to reduce the incidence of total occlusions in stenosed femoral and popliteal arteries was demonstrated by use of repeated arteriographies (Tillgren et al., 1963; Lund and Tillgren, 1966). In severe arterial insufficiency the purpose of anticoagulant treatment is not least to prevent complicating venous thrombosis.

Preliminary observations in a few patients indicating an effect of Anginin on platelet adhesiveness as determined by use of Hellem's method (mentioned by Lund et al., 1969) could not be confirmed in an extended study (Bygdeman and Lund, *This Volume*, pp.392–393). Our rather negative finding does not exclude, however, that some function or functions of the platelets other than adhesiveness to glass beads may be influenced in vivo by Anginin, e.g. aggregation.

Recanalization of larger arteries of the legs in some claudication patients on Anginin was reported at the Symposium in Tokyo 3 years ago including one case by our own group (Lund et al., 1969). A similar observation was published by Hess (1970), who, however, after observations made in further studies (Hess, 1971) is reluctant to associate the recanalization observed with the treatment. On the whole we had better be cautious in establishing a definite causal connection between an observed increase in the vascular lumen and long-term drug treatment. Spontaneous regression of stenotic changes in limb arteries may sometimes occur (Lund and Hellström, 1969; Schoop, 1971).

Nevertheless, I would say that cases presenting during treatment a reopening of limb arteries totally occluded by thrombosis, not by emboli, may still justify interest as regards a possible drug effect. Hiemeyer (1967) found recanalization in 18% of limb arteries occluded by emboli (17 out of 93 cases) but only in 0.9% of thrombotic arterial occlusion (1 out of 108 cases; this single case was a femoral thrombosis of traumatic origin in a 19-year-old patient).

It might be added that, although Anginin was not able to prevent formation of thrombosis, this fact does not consequently exclude the possibility that it may increase the effectiveness of the endogenous fibrinolytic system's attempt to reopen occluded vessels, provided that rethrombosis does not occur.

Anginin in cases of combined obliterative atherosclerosis and diabetes

The fact that in the Anginin series 2 out of 6 diabetics deteriorated while 10 out of 18 diabetics deteriorated in the comparative series does not, of course, justify any conclusion or supposition, considering the small number of cases. Possibly the findings will direct future interest to a question very interesting in itself, i.e. does Anginin have some particular effect on diabetic microangiopathy? The microvascular involvement in diabetes requires special attention and in presentation of our material the incidence of diabetics has been mentioned in all the Tables.

It might be objected that in comparison between the Anginin and control series the proportionally smaller number of diabetics in the former than in the latter has influenced the total healing results. Certainly, for many years diabetes in combination with obliterative atherosclerosis has been found to aggravate the general prognosis of the vascular disease both in respect of mortality and amputation rate (cf. Silbert and Zazeela, 1958).

However, there are controversial views on the role of diabetes in the prognosis of ischemic skin lesions in peripheral atherosclerosis. It is reasonable that coexistent microangiopathy could cause deteriorated healing conditions. On the other hand, it is well known that, as ischemic skin lesions in diabetics are often infected, a fairly good tendency to heal is shown with appropriate treatment of the infection and correction of the diabetes if required.

CONCLUSIONS

Our results show that the prognosis of limited ischemic skin lesions, even in a geriatric patient population, does not necessarily need to be predominantly poor. Quite frequently satisfactory results can be obtained by active conservative treatment, without pyridinolcarbamate (Anginin). Our findings do, however, indicate that the addition of Anginin extends our therapeutic possibilities and improves healing.

The incidence of thrombotic episodes (venous and arterial) during Anginin therapy as observed in this material, and also in a series of cases suffering from intermittent claudication only, indicates that a marked clinical antithrombotic effect cannot be expected in these patient groups. Concurrent anticoagulant therapy on this account seems to be justified.

The beneficial effect of Anginin is probably associated with a microcirculatory and microvascular action. Recanalizations of larger arteries in a few claudication patients during Anginin treatment have previously been published, one case by our own group. A direct correlation to the treatment cannot, however, be taken for granted as it has been shown that spontaneous regression of stenotic changes in limb arteries does occasionally occur. Cases presenting during treatment a reopening of limb arteries totally occluded by thrombosis (not by emboli) may still justify interest as regards a possible drug effect.

REFERENCES

BLOOR, K. (1961): Natural history of arteriosclerosis of the lower extremities. *Ann. roy. Coll. Surg. Engl.*, *28*, 6.

BYGDEMAN, S. and LUND, F. (1972): Effect of pyridinolcarbamate on ADP-induced platelet adhesiveness. *This Volume*, pp. 392–393.

FAGRELL, B. (1972): Vital capillaroscopy. A clinical method for studying changes in skin microcirculation in patients suffering from vascular disorders of the leg. *Angiology*, *23*, 284.

FAGRELL, B. and LUND, F. (1969): Vital capillary microscopy as a test method for therapeutic procedures in peripheral vascular diseases. In: *Proceedings, International Congress on Clinical Evaluation of Testing Methods of Vasoactive Drug Effects, Rome 1968*, p. 329. Edizione CEPI, Rome.

HESS, H. (1970): Überlegungen zur Physiopathologie obliterierender Angiopathien. II. Zur Pathogenese und Therapie. *Fortschr. Med.*, *88*, 923.

HESS, H. (1971): Paper read at the round table conference on 'Kann die Angininwirkung objektiviert werden?' In: *Verhandlungen, VI Angiologisches Symposium, Kitzbühel 1971*. F. K. Schattauer Verlag, Stuttgart. In press.

HESS, H. and FROST, H. (1968): Rauchen und arterielle Verschlusskrankheiten. *Fortschr. Med.*, *86*, 841.

HIEMEYER, V. (1967): Spontanlyse von arteriellen Verschlüssen. In: *Thrombolytische Therapie. Verhandlungen, IV Symposium der deutschen Gesellschaft für Angiologie, München*, p. 66. Editor: H. Hess. F. K. Schattauer Verlag, Stuttgart.

JUERGENS, J. L., BARKER, M. V. and HINES JR, E. A. (1960): Arteriosclerosis obliterans. Review of 520 cases with special reference to pathogenetic and prognostic factors. *Circulation*, *21*, 188.

KJELDSEN, K. (1969): *Smoking and Atherosclerosis*. Munksgaard, Copenhagen.

LUND, F. (1956): Morphological analysis of the digital volume pulse as a diagnostic method. In: *Comptes Rendus, II Congrès International d'Angéiologie, Fribourg (Suisse) 1955*, p. 223. Editors: L. Laszt, R. Meier and A. Müller. Editions universitaires, Fribourg.

LUND, F. (1957): Arterial thrombosis. *Bibl. cardiol. (Basel)*, *8*, 50.

LUND, F. (1967): Digital plethysmograph for recording of the digital volume pulse. *Scand. J. clin. Lab. Invest., Suppl. 99*, 110.

LUND, F. (1971): Angininbehandlung in Stadium III–IV der Gliedmassenarterienverschlüsse in der Geriatrie. Paper read at the round table conference on 'Kann die Angininwirkung objektiviert werden?' In: *Verhandlungen, VI Angiologisches Symposium, Kitzbühel, 1971*. F. K. Schattauer Verlag, Stuttgart. In press.

LUND, F., ALGOTSSON, A. and LUND, S. (1972): Elevation and dependency tests in peripheral vascular disease. Standardization and increased accuracy by use of modern electronic phototechniques. *This Volume*, pp. 281–286.

LUND, F. and HELLSTRÖM, L. (1969): Evaluation of oscillography and digital volume pulse recording as compared to arteriography in follow-up studies of occlusive arterial disease. With application to long-term nicotinic acid treatment. In: *Proceedings, International Congress on Clinical Evaluation of Testing Methods of Vasoactive Drug Effects, Rome 1968*, p. 199. Edizione CEPI, Rome.

LUND, F., HELLSTRÖM, L. and FRISCH, P. (1969): Pulse recording and arteriography in a long-term study with pyridinolcarbamate. In: *Atherogenesis. Proceedings, I Symposium on Atherogenesis, Thrombogenesis and Pyridinolcarbamate Treatment, Tokyo 1969*, pp. 181–190. Editors: T. Shimamoto and F. Numano. ICS 201, Excerpta Medica, Amsterdam.

LUND, F. and TILLGREN, C. (1966): Anticoagulant therapy in occlusive peripheral arterial disease and its evaluation. In: *Pathogenesis and Treatment of Thromboembolic Diseases, including Coronary, Cerebral and Peripheral Thrombosis. Proceedings, International Symposium, Basel 1965*, p. 385. Editors: F. Koller, F. Duckert and F. Streuli. F. K. Schattauer Verlag, Stuttgart.

MATHIESEN, F. R., ERREBO LARSEN, E. and WULFF, M. (1970*a*): Some factors influencing the spontaneous course of arterial vascular insufficiency. *Acta chir. scand.*, *136*, 303.

MATHIESEN, F. R., ERREBO LARSEN, E. and WULFF, M. (1970*b*): Arterial insufficiency in the legs. I. A clinical statistical analysis. *Acta chir. scand.*, *136*, 477.

SCHOOP, W. (1971): Paper read at the round table conference on 'Kann die Angininwirkung objektiviert werden?' In: *Verhandlungen, VI Angiologisches Symposium, Kitzbühel 1971*. F. K. Schattauer Verlag, Stuttgart. In press.

SILBERT, S. and ZAZEELA, H. (1958): Prognosis in arteriosclerotic peripheral vascular disease. *J. Amer. med. Ass.*, *166*, 1816.

TILLGREN, C., STENSON, S. and LUND, F. (1963): Obliterative arterial disease of the lower limbs studied by means of repeated femoral arteriography. *Acta radiol. (Stockh.)*, *1*, 1161.

DISCUSSION

Dr. PRATESI: In the pictures you have shown there is a lot of local infection in the lesions. How much is this element important in the evolution of the lesions?

Dr. LUND: It is well known that infection is very common in all these lesions. I have shown the Anginin-treated group. If sufficient time had been available, I could have shown pictures from the comparative series. Then you would have found the same signs of infection there – not least in cases of diabetes. Of course, it is very important not only to give Anginin and anticoagulants but also to treat infection effectively.

Dr. JANUSHKEVICHIUS: Dr. Lund, do you allow smoking in patients with peripheral atherosclerosis?

Dr. LUND: This is a very important question which is discussed in the paper to be printed. Most of the smokers were not heavy but were only moderate or minimal smokers. Our attempts to make the patients stop smoking were not very successful. Possibly, our efforts in this way were not sufficiently energetic. In fact, such attempts are often not very easy in geriatric patients of this type. Anyhow, considering the incidence of smokers and non-smokers among the improved and deteriorated cases in our series, I do not think that this factor would be attributed a significant role in the interpretation of our Anginin results.

ELEVATION AND DEPENDENCY TESTS IN PERIPHERAL VASCULAR DISEASE

Standardization and Increased Accuracy by Use of Modern Electronic Phototechniques

F. LUND, A. ALGOTSSON and S. LUND
Stureby Sjukhus Geriatric Unit, Enskede, Stockholm, Sweden

INTRODUCTION

The elevation-dependency test (Ratschow's *Lagerungsprobe*) is based on color variations of the extremities occurring in connection with postural changes. These variations have been well known for many years. In most textbooks (e.g. Wright, 1958; Allen et al., 1972) the tests are advocated as being a simple and important diagnostic aid in obliterative arterial disease. Ratschow (1959) states that these tests constitute the simplest and also the most reliable diagnostic method in circulatory disorders of the limbs. In spite of these strong recommendations the tests have, as judged from the literature, been adopted to a comparatively limited extent in diagnosis and follow-up studies.

In our studies on the effect of therapeutic measures on the course of obliterative arterial disease of the limbs, e.g. in evaluation of pyridinolcarbamate (Anginin), elevation-dependency tests were performed amongst other methods (cf. also Lund et al., 1969). The following procedures were adopted:

1. Skin color of the feet, particularly the soles, in a horizontal position.
2. Occurrence of pathological pallor of the soles and dorsum of the feet after elevation of the legs to 45° for 2 min in combination with active movements at the ankle-joints.
3. Occurrence of pathological cyanotic rubor on the dorsum of the feet after dependency for 3 min, during which period the duration before return of skin color and venous filling was also roughly estimated.

In all cases examined the results were recorded by color photography at the beginning of treatment for comparison with repeated examinations later on.

With time, however, it became increasingly obvious that the elevation-dependency tests were associated with considerable inaccuracy unless they were thoroughly standardized in certain experimental respects, both with regard to the patient examined and the technical set-up. We concluded that the limited use of the tests by other investigators might have been due to lack of standardization and subsequent difficulties in following and interpreting changes in the sequence of events when only ocular observation and infrequent photography were used.

Therefore, we began a methodological study in order to improve the basis for interpretation and to make full use of the positional color changes of the extremities in diagnostic assessment. For this purpose, rapid sequence photography was done by ordinary color photography as well as in some cases with infrared (IR) black-and-white and color film. (N.B. Not to be confused with long-wave infrared, so-called 'passive IR photography' measuring thermal radiation, i.e. thermovision-thermography.)

It ought to be mentioned that, as the study is still in progress, the observations should be regarded as preliminary. The conclusions and recommendations which so far would seem to be justified may be supplemented and possibly modified in some detail after future studies.

These will include a systematic comparison between the results of the elevation-dependency tests and other examination methods.

EQUIPMENT

Photographic equipment

Camera A Nikon F with a Micro Nikkor Auto 55 mm/3.5 lens has been used with manual exposures at short intervals. An electrically driven camera with cassettes for 20–36 exposures would have been preferable; such cameras with cassettes for 250 exposures cannot be used, particularly for IR color film which is available in 20-frame lengths only.

Illumination Two flashes fed by a flash generator of the Pro-1 type (Profoto AB, Scheffersgatan 6–8, Stockholm) supplying 300–600 Wsec to each of the flashes with a repetitive frequency of down to 1 flash per sec (at 300 Wsec) were used to illuminate the feet directly. The recommended lighting angle, i.e. the angle between the lamp-subject and the lens-subject axis, is about 55°, hence 110° between the flashes. Distance from flash to subject was 1.3 m. Black velvet served as background.

Film data and filters Ordinary color photography was performed with Kodachrome II Film, IR black-and-white photography with Kodak High Speed Infrared Film 2481 and a Kodak Wratten Filter No. 87, and IR color photography with Kodak Ektachrome Infrared Aero Film 8443 and a Kodak Wratten Filter No. 12.

Set-up for the elevation test

Moderate elevation This was achieved by the aid of a 'camping-chair' with a cloth seat to support the lower legs.

High elevation The legs of the patient, who was lying on a low couch, were kept in an elevated position by a padded strap adapted to the desired level in a doorway.

Set-up for the dependency test

No special equipment was required except a foot-stool covered with black velvet on which the patient put his feet when sitting at the edge of the examination couch with the legs hanging down immediately after elevation.

PHOTOGRAPHIC PROCEDURES

Elevation test

The development of pathological pallor of the soles of the feet and its regression as sometimes seen after cessation of muscular exercise was photographically recorded at intervals of 10 sec for a period of 3–6 min. As a rule, the elevation test was performed in combination with dorsoplantar foot movements at the ankle joint at frequency of about 1 per sec for the first $1\frac{1}{2}$ min. The time of each photograph was recorded with a stopwatch simultaneously photographed while attached to the background of the black velvet. Up to the present time, only ordinary color film has been used for the recording of the elevation test.

Dependency test

From the start of dependency photographic exposures were made at intervals of 3–5 sec for the first minute and after that at longer intervals until 3–6 min after the start of the experiment. In this way the return of skin color to the dorsum of the feet after elevation pallor and the filling of veins as well as the appearance of typical cyanotic rubor in pathological cases could be recorded and timed by a stopwatch as described above.

IR photography (black-and-white as well as color) was used in some dependency tests in order to study whether the IR procedure was superior for the purpose of recording venous filling time. It was also of interest to find out whether IR color film possibly had any advantage over IR black-and-white film in this respect.

MATERIAL

So far, 9 patients with occlusive obliterative arterial disease of the legs have been examined with this modified technique. In all cases the diagnosis, localization and extent of obliterative changes had been confirmed by routine clinical examination of arterial pulsations, by oscillography at different levels of the legs, toe pulse plethysmography and determination of skin temperature increase as a result of induced vasodilatation. In some cases pulse recording with Doppler ultrasonic equipment as well as ankle blood pressure measurement using the same method was carried out. Four cases had been subjected to arteriography. The sensitivity and reliability of oscillography and toe pulse plethysmography as compared to arteriography have been assessed in previous studies (Lund and Hellström, 1969; Lund et al., 1969).

REMARKS ON STANDARDIZATION

Standardization of photographic details

In comparative studies between different patients and between repeated examinations in the same patient exposure data, such as illumination, distance between light source and object, filters, diaphragm and exposure times, should of course be kept identical. Many other phototechnical details have also to be considered and kept constant, e.g. angle between the 2 flashes and the object, the color of the background used and the walls of the room. An indirect lighting arrangement either with umbrella reflectors in front of the flashes or with the patient inside a white cubicle will reduce the errors of shadowing which is a problem especially in IR photography (cf. Gibson et al., 1965; *Medical Infrared Photography*, 1969). So far, however, we have not used such an arrangement.

Also, the constancy of the film emulsion is very important, dependent among other things on the duration and temperature of storage.

Standardization of vasodilatation

The degree of vasodilatation is of fundamental importance if the test is to be useful for comparative studies. The sensitivity may be increased if the test is performed during vasoconstriction. It is difficult, however, to produce the same degree of vasoconstriction even in the same patient on different occasions and from patient to patient. With the patient in a state of incomplete vasoconstriction the reliability of the test would be reduced.

A state of vasodilatation during the test is obviously preferable. Smoking must be avoided on the day of examination. The patient should not be hungry and should empty the bladder before the test. Vasodilatation is induced by moderate warming of the body with a heating box in combination with oral alcohol, i.e. the same procedure which is used to advantage in toe pulse plethysmography (Lund, 1955, 1967; Lund and Hellström, 1969).

The successive increase in skin temperature of toes and fingers during induction of vasodilatation is recorded. Temperature measurements should also be performed subsequently to confirm that vasodilatation is maintained. A high temperature of the examination room (at least 25°C) is recommended in order to facilitate vasodilatation and counteract cooling of the patient during the tests.

Standardization of the elevation test

Degree of elevation The resistance to the blood flow in the leg can be varied by changing the degree of elevation, i.e. by having the blood make its way more or less uphill. This implies the possibility of grading the severity of the test. In our study 2 different positions of flexion at the hip joints with inclination angles to the horizontal level of (*a*) about 45° and (*b*) about 75° were found to be convenient. A slight flexion in the knees was allowed to avoid overstretching and pain, which may have an unfavorable effect on the circulation. A maximal elevation to 90° from the horizontal level is very often impossible for these reasons. This is particularly true in geriatric patients with pathological changes of the joints and reduced mobility. Sometimes even an elevation of 75° may be difficult to achieve. It is important, however, that in comparative observations of the same patient at different times the degree of elevation should be the same.

Amount of additional exercise By combined elevation and active dorsoplantar (or circular) movements in the ankle joints the test is accentuated and elevation ischemia more easily produced. The exercising muscles require more blood which, in the presence of obliterative arterial disease, will markedly reduce the amount of blood available for the foot. Our routine procedure as mentioned above is to have the patient perform these movements (1 cycle/sec) for the first 1½–2 min after elevation. In comparative studies the amount of additional exercise should be the same in respect of both rhythm and duration of exercise.

Standardization of the dependency test

A very important factor is that the preceding elevation should be standardized and in each case the technique for inducing elevation ischemia of the foot before the dependency test should be the same in comparative observations. If a change in arterial flow has occurred between 2 examinations, for better or for worse, this may influence the intensity and the extension of ischemia during the elevation phase, and consequently also the following dependency test.

The need for rapid sequence photography is more urgent in systematic studies of the dependency test than in the elevation test. In the former test the successive events may occur more rapidly, particularly in normal cases. Here venous filling and return of pink color to the feet may be observed with the naked eye as soon as 5–10 sec after lowering the leg. It ought to be emphasized, however, that the filling of the veins as well as the return of skin color of varying intensity and type is a gradual process when seen in advanced cases of arterial insufficiency. This fact complicates simple ocular inspection. A continuous photographic record of the sequence of events offers a great advantage as the photographs can later be studied thoroughly and in detail.

In pathological cases the gradual venous filling on the dorsum of the feet may last for a minute or more. In fact, venous filling may be retarded longer in some areas than in others due to local circulatory disturbances, and the development of cyanotic rubor may initially occur in patches. For these reasons the photographic recording of the test should be done at short time intervals.

Supplementary infrared (IR) photography of the dependency test For many years it has been well known that superficial veins are better visualized by IR than by ordinary photography. Since IR color film was made available, IR photography has attracted still more interest in medical work (cf. *Medical Infrared Photography*, 1969).

Using IR black-and-white film the venous filling may be recorded somewhat more intensely than by ordinary color film. The latter, however, gives a more 3-dimensional view of the surface. On the other hand, the IR black-and-white technique would seem to be superior in cases where the venous pattern is partially covered by pigmentation or where the surrounding tissue is edematous. If the edema is advanced, even IR photography may be insufficient.

Gibson et al. (1965) dispelled the fallacy that IR black-and-white film would reveal the deoxygenation of venous blood and the blood in minute vessels of the skin. They found that, with IR black-and-white film, arterial blood photographs even more intensely dark than venous blood. This type of film will therefore not be especially useful in studies of the development of pathological cyanotic rubor.

IR color film does distinguish between oxygenated (green-yellow) and deoxygenated blood (red-brown). It would be interesting to study the assessment of the cyanotic component in skin color to see whether more quantitative information can be obtained by the IR color film than by ordinary color film. Certainly veins as well as arteries passing just beneath and visible through the skin will, because of light scattering by the covering tissues, appear bluish not only to the naked eye and on ordinary color film but also on IR color film (Algotsson et al., 1973). This optical error would, however, play a less important role in IR color photography of blood in the very superficial and thin-walled microvessels of the skin.

DISCUSSION OF ERRORS IN THE ELEVATION-DEPENDENCY TESTS

Errors in the elevation test

An *inflammatory* rubor of an area of skin, e.g. in diabetics, does not always exhibit elevation pallor even in the presence of advanced arterial obliterative disease which may cause pronounced pallor in surrounding areas.

In *obstruction of venous outflow* a skin area with reddish or cyanotic discoloration may persist even in the elevated position of the legs.

Discoloration caused by *prenecrosis* and *necrosis* or due to recent or old *petechiae* and *ecchymoses*, with residual *pigmentation*, does not disappear on elevation.

Skin color is dependent particularly on the amount and quality of blood in the subpapillary venous plexus. In *pure microangiopathy* without obliterative macroangiopathy, as occasionally encountered in diabetics, the venules may be filled with blood by a shunt from the arteriolar side through anastomosing channels. At the same time there is deficient blood flow through the capillaries. In such cases the elevation test would not seem capable of revealing the deficiency in capillary blood flow.

Marked edema of the foot contributes to skin pallor even in the horizontal position which becomes still more obvious in elevation. Edema may cause a further reduction of the blood supply in arterial occlusive disease due partly to compression of a low-pressure vascular system and to insufficient exchange of nutrients because of longer distances from capillaries to cells.

Errors in the dependency test

Coexistent venous insufficiency may shorten the latency time of venous filling and return of skin color. This limits to some degree the reliability of the test in assessing arterial insufficiency. In the evaluation of a test the examiner has to observe whether there is a suspicion of superficial or deep venous insufficiency so as to avoid underestimating the degree of involvement of arterial insufficiency.

As mentioned above, *edema* causes both a concealing of the superficial veins and increased skin pallor. Therefore, in the presence of edema the interpretation of a dependency test may become difficult. The errors caused by slight to moderate edema as well as by *pigmentation* hiding the venous pattern and affecting skin color can to some degree be overcome by use of IR photography which not only visualizes the skin surface but penetrates the skin to layers just beneath it.

CONCLUSIONS

From this report on experimental conditions and on errors inherent in the elevation-dependency tests the reader may falsely conclude that these tests are too complicated for routine use. The authors, however, still are of the contrary opinion, that the elevation-dependency tests do represent a very practicable method of examination.

For obvious reasons our systematic study has focussed attention on the errors and limitations of the method in order to delineate its possibilities. It is our intention and hope that the final study will contribute a basis for routine use of the tests not only in the clinico-physiological laboratory but also at the bedside. Certainly a considerably lower number of photographic exposures will be required later than we have found advisable in our study. Presumably it will also be possible to obtain more definite and reliable information of solely visual observation at the bedside when the necessary standardization of experimental conditions is observed and the possibilities, as well as the limitations, of the method are defined.

So far, it is not quite clear in which respects IR photography is superior to ordinary color photography in the evaluation of test results. Our observations indicate that in the dependency test IR photography, whether by use of black-and-white or color film, seems to record venous filling more distinctly in the presence of edema or skin pigmentation. IR color film gives a more 3-dimensional picture of the venous pattern compared to IR black-and-white film.

REFERENCES

Algotsson, A., Lund, F. and Lund, S. (1973): A comparison between infrared black-and-white and infrared color photography of superficial veins and arteries close to the skin. To be published.

Allen, E. V., Barker, N. W. and Hines, E. A. (1972): In: *Peripheral Vascular Diseases., 4th ed.*, pp. 39, 187. Editors: J. F. Fairbairn, J. L. Juergens and J. A. Spittell. W. B. Saunders Co., Philadelphia–London-Toronto.

Gibson, H. L., Buckley, W. R. and Whitmore, K. E. (1965): New vistas in infrared photography for biological surveys. *J. biol. photogr. Ass.*, *33*, 1.

Lund, F. (1955): Morphological analysis of the digital volume pulse as a diagnostic method. In: *Comptes Rendus, II Congrès Internationale d'Angéiologie, Fribourg (Suisse) 1955*. Editors: L. Laszt, R. Meier and A. Müller. Editions universitaires, Fribourg.

Lund, F. (1967): Digital plethysmograph for recording of digital volume pulse. *Scand. J. clin. Lab. Invest.*, *19*, *Suppl. 99*.

Lund, F. and Hellström, L. (1969): Evaluation of some clinico-physiological methods as compared to arteriography in follow-up studies of the long-term effect of vasoactive substances in the course of occlusive arterial disease. In: *Proceedings, International Congress on Clinical Evaluation of Testing Methods of Vasoactive Drug Effects and Indications for Surgical Angiological Therapy, Rome 1968*, p. 199. Edizione C.E.P.I., Rome.

Lund, F., Hellström, L. and Frisch, P. (1969): Pulse recording and arteriography in a long-term study with pyridinolcarbamate. In: *Atherogenesis. Proceedings, I International Symposium on Atherogenesis, Thrombogenesis and Pyridinolcarbamate Treatment, Tokyo 1969*, pp. 181–193. Editors: T. Shimamoto and F. Numano. ICS 201, Excerpta Medica, Amsterdam.

Medical Infrared Photography (1969): Eastman Kodak Company, Rochester, N. Y.

Ratschow, M. (1959): *Angiologie, Pathologie, Klinik und Therapie der peripheren Durchblutungsstörungen*, p. 329. Georg Thieme Verlag, Stuttgart.

Wright, I. S. (1958): *Vascular Diseases in Clinical Practice, 3rd ed.* Year Book Publishers Inc., New York, N.Y.

A STUDY OF THE EFFICACY AND SAFETY OF PYRIDINOLCARBAMATE IN PATIENTS WITH DEMONSTRABLE OCCLUSIVE ARTERIAL DISEASE

W. REDISCH, E. N. TERRY, R. ROUEN and R. H. CLAUSS
Research Clinic, Department of Surgery, New York Medical College, New York, N.Y., U.S.A.

Although the etiology of atherosclerosis is unknown, Shimamoto and his collaborators have conceived a specific mechanism of pathogenesis involving both the vessel wall and cellular elements of the circulating blood. Shimamoto also indicated the importance of the microcirculation in connection with the development of atherosclerotic manifestations and lesions in the vessel wall, pointing in particular to the vasa vasorum and their significance.

This ongoing study, which I am going to present in part, is an attempt to evaluate the effects of pyridinolcarbamate (PC), on 2 aspects of atherosclerosis in man. One is its influence on the course of existing and manifest atherosclerosis, where both improvement in the diseased limb and maintenance of the spared limb should yield information. We are talking about aortic bifurcation branch disease. The other is on the development of atherosclerosis and its possible prevention studied in successfully reconstructed operated individuals, reassessing their arterial condition and comparing patient treatment postoperatively. A sound pharmacological basis has been laid for the effects of PC material and methods on these parameters.

MATERIAL AND METHODS

Table I shows the composition of the study. To date, 47 patients were re-evaluated in the study. These are the details on the 47 patients, who were given a full explanation of aim, purpose and potential risks involved in participating in the study. Their consent was obtained according to American Law.

TABLE I

Distribution of patients

	No.	Age (range)	Weight (range)	Height (range)
All patients	47	63.5 (44–81)	154 (100–220)	5′3″ (4′11″–6′)
Male	30	63 (44–81)	164 (100–220)	5′6″ (5′1″–6′)
Female	17	64 (45–78)	134 (105–185)	5′2″ (4′11″–5′7″)

In addition to clinical history and physical examination, the following parameters were evaluated in all subjects: Blood flow and perfusion (at rest and after exercise), visualization of microvessels, initial angiography, claudication time and distance, using a treadmill, clinical laboratory workup, complete. Subsequent to the initial evaluation but without reference to results of the examinations, a randomization chart was used to assign patients either to the treatment group receiving PC or to a control group receiving identical-looking placebos.

Patients were seen in the Research Clinic at intervals of 4 weeks. Subjective responses and experiences during the treatment period were recorded as were, of course, clinical and laboratory findings. At each visit, patients received prepared packages of medication identified with the patient's special number unknown to the real investigators.

Patients undergoing reconstructive surgery were subjected to the same investigations and to the same randomization assignment to either placebo or active drug group prior to discharge from the hospital. They were seen at 4-week intervals at the Research Clinic like the others.

Angiography and microcirculatory evaluation are being performed again at about a 1-year interval postoperatively or whenever the clinical changes suggest the need for it.

At the completion of this study, which we hope to have in about one more year's time, the results will be analyzed with regard to their biological significance and evaluated statistically. To date, the code has not been broken. The methods used will be briefly described and I want to say that for those who are interested, and there are a few angiologists here who will be interested in it, we will be glad to supply details of our methods.

Angiography was a standard procedure and carried out by the Department of Radiology. The films, however, at evaluation were reviewed by the radiologists and ourselves. In the discussion, Dr. Clauss will go a little bit more into detail on that. For blood flow determinations, plethysmography was chosen as the most direct and accurate method in a form which is practical, namely the Whitney method, and I will spare you all the details and will only tell you that the examinations were performed at a comfortable temperature of 23°C and 55% humidity, of course in the constant temperature room. It is our belief that plethysmography is only possible in the constant temperature room. As far as significance is concerned, we consider that with this method, which uses mercury in a rubber-silastic strain gauge, the theoretical accuracy is $\pm$0.25 ml per 100 g tissue per minute; in other words, we do not consider anything below 1$\pm$0.5 ml a change, either up or down. The perfusion is, of course, calculated in the usual way. It may be of interest to you that the strain gauge is calibrated mechanically by placing it against a mirrored scale, stretching it through 1 ml; thus the known errors in parallax will be avoided. The result in change in voltage is recorded and used in calculating perfusion from the initial plethysmographic curve. Results obtained in our laboratory with both the gauge and air-volume plethysmograph under controlled conditions were of about the same order of magnitude. The advantages of the gauge are known to all those interested in it.

Exercise blood flow

The patients exercised actively by performing dorsal-plantar flexions at a rate of one per second against a hinged spring pedal board. The resistance offered by the spring was 4 lbs. After 2 min, exercise was stopped and perfusion was measured at 5–10 sec, 30 sec, and at 1 min. Subsequently, measurements are made at 1 min intervals until the flow has returned to the previously established resting levels for a period of 10 min.

Capillaroscopy

In brief, 2 things are described: (1) the method used and (2) the outgrowth of that method, which to me means much more than the method itself, namely the quantitation of microvascular findings in man. At the present time, this is still done from photographs taken at about 1/1300th of a second, so we have a fairly good array of pictures to go ahead with. These have been published in *Microvascular Research*, so I do not have to go into more detail here.

Walking test

An electrically driven treadmill with adjustable elevation is used. Speed and angle of inclination of the treadmill are adjusted to individual patients and maintained until absence of a reaction to walking indicates the need to increase workload. Thus only you can judge improvement or deterioration.

RESULTS

This presentation deals only with those patients in whom for one reason or another an end-point has been reached, while the whole study will not have reached its end-point until after 1 more year. Patients were grouped as in Table II.

The first group (surgical patients) consisted of 12 males and 4 females, with an average age of 60.3, ranging from 44 to 73; 5 of the males were diabetics. The somewhat lower mean age of this group compared to that of the total study population reflects probably rather on their being less of a surgical risk than on any difference in the severity of their disease. Changes in the parameters established are shown in Table III. Apart from improvement or deterioration, the absence of either may be unexpected or significant – we do not know. What we are studying at the same time is the natural history of the disease. New lesions were seen in the angiograms of 2 patients. Figures 1–3 show what we mean by our terminology.

TABLE II

Classification of patients

Group	No.	Definition
1	16	'Surgical' repeat angio
2	8	'Medical' no-repeat angio
3	3	'Amputees'
4	12	'Adverse effects'
5	8	'Discontinuation'

TABLE III

Changes in surgical patients

	Improved	Deteriorated	Unchanged	Total
Angiography				
Old	1	4	11	16
New		2	14	16
Collateral	9		7	16
Microcirculation	3	3	10	16
Blood flow				
Rest	6	4	6	16
Exercise	6	6	4	16
Walking test	3	1	12	16
Blood pressure	1		15	16
Heart rate	2		14	16
Pulses				16
Dorsalis pedis	6		10	16
Posterior tibial		1	15	16
Popliteal	1		15	16
Femoral	1		15	16
Venous filling time	1	1	14	16
Clinical impression	3	4	4* 5	16
			7**	
Patient's subjective judgment	5	1	3	16

* 'Good maintenance'
** 'Very satisfactory'

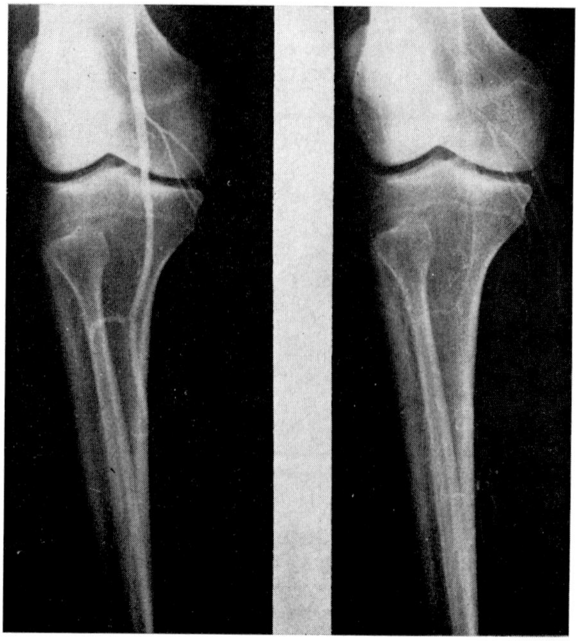

Fig. 1. New lesion. Left, initial angiogram; right, repeat.

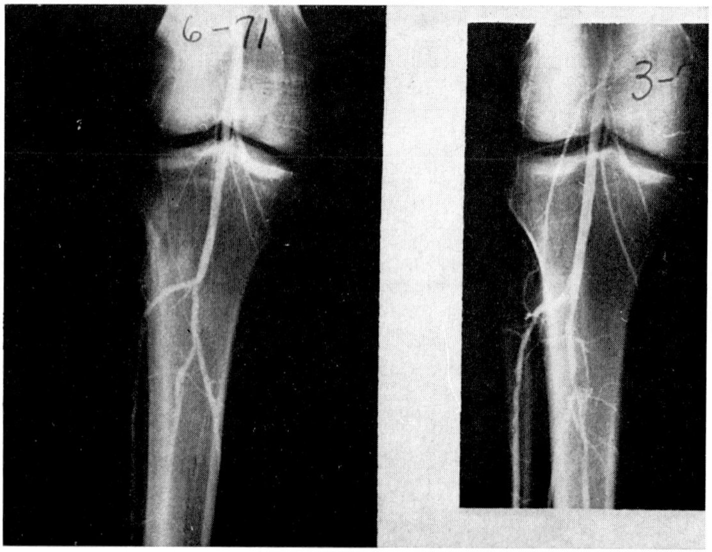

Fig. 2. Development of collateral circulation. Left, initial angiogram; right, repeat.

We speak about a new lesion when the establishment of a block has taken place within the observation period (Fig. 1). We speak about improvement when flow has been obviously improved and a marked further development of collateral circulation (which is very well shown in Figure 2) has been found. And we speak about deterioration of old lesions when this happens (Fig. 3). We know what has happened during the time between 1971 and 1972.

This Table refers to the status prior to their amputation. It would appear that blood flow showed improvement in all of them; walking exercise improved in 1 patient (the non-diabetic); popliteal pulses and femoral pulses deteriorated in 1 patient, respectively. Clinically, and according to his subjective feelings, 1 patient only improved during this study. In both diabetic patients, infection led to gangrene and the need to amputate the involved extremity. In the non-diabetic patient, who had shown pronounced improvement, removal of a toenail followed by infection led to the loss of the extremity.

The 'adverse effects' group totals 12 patients. This number presumably includes patients on

TABLE VI

Adverse effects without challenge

Type of adverse effect	Onset-initiation of R_x
Weakness, sweating	6th day
Dizziness, gastric pain, vomiting	6th day
Weakness, sweating, GI upset, diarrhea	5th day
Intractable diarrhea	1st day
Vomiting	5th month
Pain, right lower chest, liver ↓ 1–2 cm	5th month

Total	Male	Female	Mean age	Concomitant diseases	
6	2	4	68.5	Diabetes	1
			(64–76)	Hypertension	1

active drug as well as patients on placebo. Six patients (Table VI) were not challenged after the occurrence of their adverse effects. It is worthwhile noting that gastrointestinal symptoms are a major feature of their adverse effects. In 3 of the 6, onset was on the 5th or 6th day of treatment. In 1 patient intractable diarrhea occurred on the 1st day of treatment. In the remaining 2 patients adverse effects were noted 5 months after onset of treatment. The patient who had experienced pain in the right lower chest and enlargement of her liver was followed for 4 months after cessation of treatment to ascertain whether or not the effects noted were drug-related. They obviously were not. Mean age in this group was 68.5 years ranging from 64 to 76 years; there were 2 males and 4 females. One suffered from diabetes and 1 from hypertension.

Thanks to the cooperation of 6 patients, we were able to subject these to a challenge following the first occurrence of their adverse effects (Table VII). There were 5 males and 1 female of mean age of 62.5 years, ranging from 52 to 71 years. All their complaints were centered on the gastrointestinal tract. They occurred in 4 patients early in the study; in 2 they occurred on the 60th and 85th day, respectively. The challenge brought about recurrence of their adverse effects, around day 5–7 in 3 of them and began on the 2nd day in one. The 2nd and 3rd rechallenge brought about occurrence of their symptoms on day 6. It is not implied that all the adverse effects noted on the above list are drug-related. As a matter of fact, we believe that gastrointestinal symptoms may be drug-related. However, only challenge with the drug can justify such an assumption. It is interesting to note that in the majority of patients the onset of their adverse effects lies around days 4–6, and is not necessarily dose-related. During the challenge we tried to reduce the dose, but diarrhea or gastrointestinal symptoms occurred nevertheless. They all received initially 2 g/day of pyridinolcarbamate. This is a dose corresponding to an average patient – we did not treat any giants and we tried to exclude obviously cachectic patients. So I would think it corresponds to something like 30 mg/kg of body weight.

TABLE VII

Adverse effects with challenge

Type of adverse effect	Onset PR_x	After challenge	2	3
Nausea	4th day	5th day		
Diarrhea	14th day	7th day	6th day	
Severe stomach pain	2nd day	2nd day		
Nausea	60th day	Diarrhea 28th day	6th day	6th day
Diarrhea	85th day	10th day		
Diarrhea, nausea	6th day	0		

Total	Male	Female	Mean age	Concomitant diseases
6	5	1	62.5 (52–71)	Diabetes 2

TABLE VIII

Discontinuation of R_x

Reason for discontinuation	No.	Onset
Non-drug-related death	1	4th month
Personal physician objected	1	5th month
Personal physician objected	1	2nd month
Left country	1	5th month
Personal problems	1	2nd month
Refused to continue	1	2nd month
Failure to return after first examination	2	2nd month

Total	Male	Female	Mean age	Concomitant diseases
8	2	6	58.6 (43–68)	Diabetes 3 Hepatitis 1

The discontinuation group is shown in Table VIII which gives the reasons for discontinuation of treatment in a total of 8 patients. There were 2 males and 6 females of a mean age of 58.6 years, ranging from 43 to 68 years. This group includes 3 diabetics. One death occurred during the 4th month of treatment without any direct relationship to drug administration. Two patients left the study as their personal physicians objected to their continuing it. One left the country, one had personal problems that prevented the continuation of the study. One patient refused to continue. Two patients failed to return after the first examination, having received their initial supply of drugs.

The results of all tests have at all times been within normal limits in all patients except in patient No.31 who died consequently due to hepatitis contracted independently of this study. Abnormalities in patterns of laboratory results concur with the cause of her death.

For discussion, see p. 300

A STUDY OF THE EFFICACY AND SAFETY OF PYRIDINOLCARBAMATE IN PATIENTS WITH DEMONSTRABLE OCCLUSIVE ARTERIAL DISEASE (DISCUSSION)

E. N. TERRY, W. REDISCH, R. ROUEN and R. H. CLAUSS
Research Clinic, Department of Surgery, New York Medical College, New York, N.Y., U.S.A.

This presentation can be regarded as an interim report of a work still ongoing, with the code still unbroken, without which it cannot be related to administration of active drug or placebo, respectively. Thus it remains ambiguous in the context of this study to determine: (1) the effects of pyridinolcarbamate on the existing atherosclerotic lesion in the arterial tree in the lower extremities; (2) the effect of pyridinolcarbamate on the atherosclerotic lesion in this vascular bed; and (3) the effects of pyridinolcarbamate on clinical manifestations of the disease. Breaking the code and identifying the medication administered is not thought to solve the problem encountered, however tempting such a solution may have seemed.

The inherent problem in any clinical or pharmacological study is to distinguish between 2 or more kinds of treatment or procedure in a given condition or disease. If both treatments measured against each other are 'active' and quantitatively distinguishable, the only impediment to finding an answer to the question posed is in the selection of methods of measurement (including statistics) with inadequate discrimination. In the present study, we were forced, however, to measure the activity of the new drug, pyridinolcarbamate, against a placebo as no other treatment is known for the condition under study. The use of a pharmacologically inert placebo can help to eliminate bias on the part of the physician and psychological effects in the patient. The results of the treatment, though, have to be evaluated against the natural history of the condition under study.

Atherosclerosis is a systemic condition with relentless progression presenting with a wide variety of signs and symptoms. We were, and are, particularly interested in occlusive arterial disease – a manifestation, in the overwhelming majority of cases, of atherosclerosis. Ideally, treatment of a condition or disease should result in restoration of 'normal' (or predisease) physiological conditions. Thus far, no treatment has been found that will re-establish patency and flow in chronically occluded arteries. It has been our experience, as has also been reported by others, that about 40% of reconstructed vessels will restenose and reocclude within about 2 years from the time of surgery. Progress of the existing lesions may also take the same length of time to reach measurable proportions. Thus a finding of 'unchanged' may present a desirable and beneficial result of treatment in atherosclerotic occlusive arterial disease. The results in this study have to be viewed in this light.

However, we will only be able to come up with a definite answer concerning the effectiveness of pyridinolcarbamate administration in atherosclerotic occlusive arterial disease after an adequate length of time has passed to allow for a comparison between the effects of the active drug and of placebo on development and progress of the condition.

We grouped together 3 patients in whom amputation had become necessary. In all 3 treatment was discontinued when surgery became necessary. We felt that, with the stress of surgery, prolonged convalescence and severe limitations on walking subsequent to surgery, these patients were not suited any more for the purposes of this study. Not having broken the code, we do not know yet whether they received the active drug or placebo. Whichever case, it would not have had any influence on the fate of their limb.

Apart from the exogenous factors involved, namely infection, gangrene in diabetics (and 2 of these amputees had severe and partly out of control diabetes) is related to the skin vascular bed of the extremity. We have been able to show that perfusion of skin and muscle vascular beds in reaction to a vasomotor stimulus is in contrary directions, i.e. an increase in skin perfusion is accompanied by a decrease in muscle perfusion. We have referred, in that context, to the interdependence of the vascular beds, which, it should also be noted, are subject to a different regulatory control mechanism.

In our studies, the side-effects most frequently encountered with pyridinolcarbamate administration were related to the gastrointestinal tract: a particularly unpleasant and intractable type of diarrhea led to discontinuation of treatment. The interesting phenomenon was that in the majority of patients diarrhea developed around days 5–6 of treatment.

Thanks to the understanding and willing cooperation of the individuals participating in the study we were able to challenge a number of them after having discontinued medication. Those in whom the first bout of diarrhea had occurred much later in the study reacted to the challenge with onset of diarrhea about day 6 of the medication, too. Bearing in mind a possible dose-response relationship, we had reduced the dose administered during the challenge on some patients, never knowing, however, whether they were receiving active medication or placebo. The recurrence of diarrhea with lower dose challenge would suggest, however, that this effect is not dose-related and has a delayed onset.

The code in this study, as I said, has not been broken yet, so that a formal comparison has to be postponed. Other than for reasons of adverse effects, where the decision to discontinue active participation in the study came from the physician, a number of patients decided against further continuation in the study. Their number is small. In no case was this decision related to the medication. Some of the patients who had suffered from adverse effects as well as some of those who are not continuing in the study are still being seen in the Research Clinic. The follow-up remains identical to that of the active participants in the study. It is hoped that such 'open controls' will provide some additional data on the natural course of atherosclerotic occlusive arterial disease, against which the effects of pyridinolcarbamate have to be matched.

See also p. 300

A STUDY OF THE EFFICACY AND SAFETY OF PYRIDINOLCARBAMATE IN PATIENTS WITH DEMONSTRABLE OCCLUSIVE ARTERIAL DISEASE (DISCUSSION)

R. H. CLAUSS
Research Clinic, Department of Surgery, New York Medical College, New York, N.Y., U.S.A.

Both clinical and laboratory scientists use measurements as the data base from which interpretations emerge. So it is with angiography – interpretations emerge.

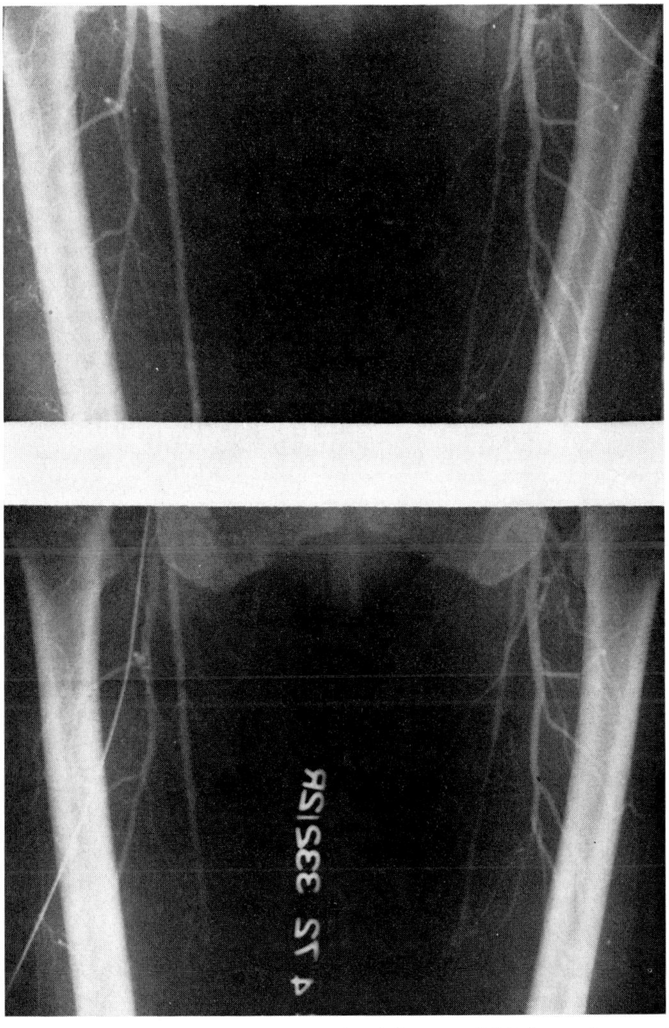

Fig. 1. A new lesion – occlusion – is present in the right superficial femoral artery (at the level of '72' in the identification label). Top, pretreatment, initiated for lesion of left leg arteries.

Angiography *does* have its constants – patients, personnel, equipment, tube-film distance, exposure and processing factors, contrast substances and the rate and volume of injection.

The variables of angiography – interpretations of progression of disease, evidence of change in collateral circulation – are a principal focus of this clinical study with pyridinol-

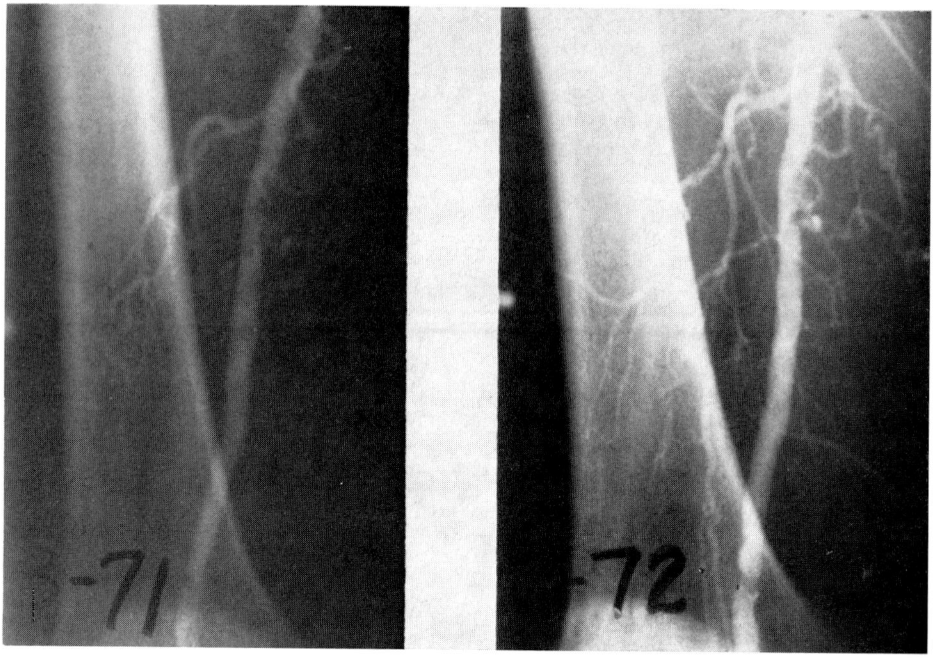

Fig. 2. An increased amount of collateral circulation is present in the thigh despite the absence of a new lesion in the superficial femoral artery.

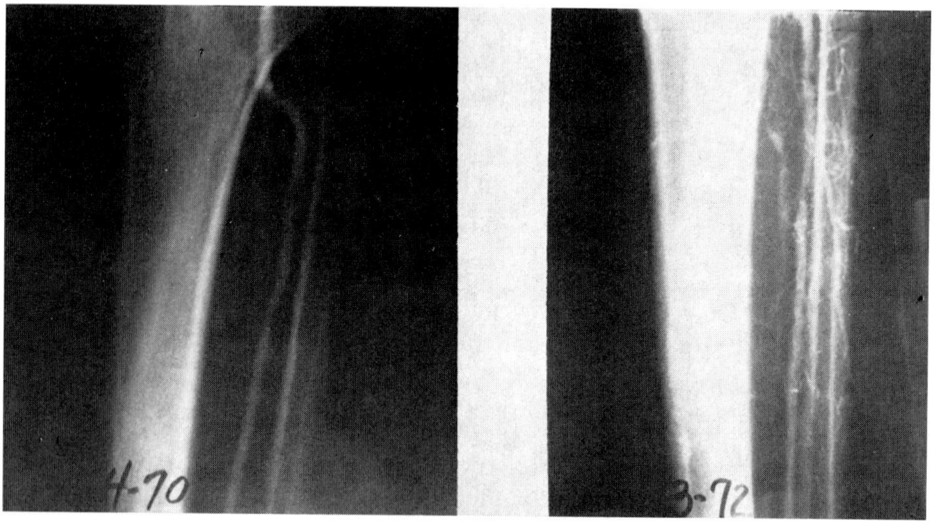

Fig. 3. A markedly increased amount of collateral circulation is present in the distribution of the anterior tibial artery.

carbamate. To attempt to achieve objectivity, our serial angiograms (2 films per sec per field) are interpreted independently by 3 physicians. Each records findings, compares current films with the previous series, and indicates his value judgments – unchanged or new lesion, and collateral the same, less, or more. A conference of the 3 readers discusses any lack of agreement, but the radiologist's interpretation becomes the final record, accepted over the internist's and the surgeon's views.

Examples of angiograms and interpretations follow. The angiograms were made before placebo or pyridinolcarbamate trial was begun, and again 8–12 months after the onset of the double-blind study (see Redisch et al., *This Volume*, pp. 287–294).

Figure 1 shows a new lesion – occlusion – present in the right superficial femoral artery (at the level of '72' in the identification label). Figure 2 shows an increased amount of collateral circulation present in the thigh despite the absence of a new lesion in the superficial femoral artery. Figure 3 shows a markedly increased amount of collateral circulation present in the distribution of the anterior tibial artery.

Examples of no change or of questionable change are not depicted. Numerous examples similar to Figures 1, 2, and 3 were observed.

Our angiograms routinely include the ankle level, and, upon indication, the entire foot and toes.

Angiograms allow us (Drs. Redisch, Terry, Clauss) to make correlations between: (*a*) new lesions and change of symptoms; (*b*) increased collateral circulation and change of symptoms; (*c*) absence of wall lesions *and* alterations in collateral circulation; and, finally, correlations between (*d*) changes in major arteries, flow data, blood, plasma, and formed elements.

See also p. 300

DISCUSSION

Dr. RUTH PICK: Dr. Redisch and Dr. Terry, did you perform any lipid determinations? Did you put your patients on any kind of diet?

Dr. REDISCH: No and yes. We did not perform lipid determinations directly related to the study. We have some lipid determinations running which may, in due time, also contribute to this study, and our work has been generally based on a low saturated-fat diet.

Dr. PRATESI: Dr. Redisch, have you seen any difference between female and male patients? In Italy, female patients with atherosclerosis are diabetic. Have you seen any difference in evolution between male and female patients, because in Italy the atherosclerosis difference is greater and less severe in the female? Is it the same in the United States?

Dr. REDISCH: Yes, Dr. Pratesi. Your question is a very important one. We have really good data to show that the difference in the incidence of atherosclerosis in males and females disappears in the diabetic. Diabetics show no essential difference. This is what you, I am sure, have found.

The second question, whether the form of atherosclerosis or occlusive atherosclerosis is different in males and females, I cannot answer. I do not think I have paid sufficient attention to it, but there is a difference in diabetics and non-diabetics. There is no doubt about that.

A DOUBLE-BLIND CROSS-OVER CLINICAL TRIAL OF PYRIDINOLCARBAMATE IN PERIPHERAL ARTERIAL DISEASE (ARTERIOSCLEROSIS OBLITERANS)*

K. W. WALTON, GILLIAN M. CRAIG,** PATRICIA PRIOR,
J. A. H. WATERHOUSE and J. SKILTON

Department of Experimental Pathology, Social Medicine and Surgery, University of Birmingham, Birmingham, United Kingdom

INTRODUCTION

This paper gives, in outline, the results of a trial of pyridinolcarbamate (PC) that was carried out in Birmingham, England. Several points emerged which are relevant to the design of future trials of PC. Methodology is discussed in some detail at the request of Dr. Numano.

DESIGN OF TRIAL

Thirty-three men with peripheral vascular disease and intermittent claudication took part. No drugs known to affect peripheral blood vessels or clotting mechanisms were given, but any hypotensive or lipid-lowering regimes were continued. The trial was conducted on an out-patient basis and was of double-blind cross-over design. It was carried out between March and October of 1970.

Patients, stratified in respect of blood pressure, smoking habits and disease severity, were divided by random number tables into 3 treatment groups (Table I). Patients with hyperlipid-aemia, including 6 taking clofibrate, were distributed randomly. The criteria used in stratification of patients were: a daily cigarette consumption of less than 10, or more than 10; a mean BP (i.e. systolic + diastolic ÷ 2) of less than 125 or more than 125 mm Hg, as recorded at the initial examination with a mercury sphygmomanometer; and the ability to do more than 50 kg of work, or less than 50 kg of work in a step test during the control period.

After a preliminary control period of 2–3 months, all patients received placebo for 4 weeks. The placebo control period was followed by 3 consecutive 8-week treatment periods, during which patients received placebo, or 1 g or 2 g of PC daily. Patients attended fortnightly for 28 weeks.

TABLE I

Design of double-blind clinical trial (dosage schedules)

Period	Control	Placebo control	Treatment 1	Treatment 2	Treatment 3
Duration (weeks)	8–12	4	8	8	8
Group 1	Nil	Placebo	Placebo	1 g PC	2 g PC
Group 2	Nil	Placebo	1 g PC	2 g PC	Placebo
Group 3	Nil	Placebo	2 g PC	Placebo	1 g PC

* This study was supported by Banyu Pharmaceutical Co., Tokyo and Imperial Chemical Industries.
** Recipient of a British Heart Foundation Research Fellowship.

TABLE II

Frequency and timing of observations

	Week	Blood tests	Pulses	Blood flow	Step test
	0	Profile, Hb, Drug, Lipids		X	
Placebo	2		X		
	4			X	
	6	Profile, Hb	X		X
Period 1	8	Profile, Hb, Drug			
	10		X		X
	12	Profile, Hb, Drug		X	

Period 2: as Period 1 omitting intermediate profile at week 8.
Period 3: as Period 2 plus lipids at week 26.
Urine level of PC and metabolites measured at each visit.

Biochemical profile, Hb, WBC and serum and urine levels of PC were measured at intervals. Table II shows the frequency and timing of observations.

METHODS USED TO ASSESS PERIPHERAL CIRCULATION

Four objective criteria were used, namely digital palpation of leg pulses, work done prior to claudication in a step test, claudication point, and measurement of calf blood flow before and after exercise. No smoking was allowed for 1 hour before appointments. Leg pulses were palpated when both patient and observer had been in a warm room (26–28 °C) for 15 min.

The step test

The step test is a simple method of measuring the total work undertaken before the onset of claudication. The patient rested for 20 min at 28 °C and then stood under a height-measuring gauge with the horizontal bar set 1 inch above his head. He then raised himself up and down until his head just touched the bar 36 times a minute in time with a metronome until claudication began. The number of movements and the duration were noted. After a 20-min rest, the test was repeated and the mean of the 2 tests taken. The total work in kilogram-metres causing claudication was calculated as:

Body weight (kg) × distance lifted (m) × times lifted.

Calf blood flow

It seemed essential to measure calf blood flow, since lack of it was the source of symptoms. We decided against measuring post-ischaemic hyperaemia because of the risk of causing damage by compression of atheromatous arteries. Since resting flow may be normal in obstructive arterial disease, we measured flow after exercise by the method of *venous occlusion plethysmography* as described by Whitney (1953).

A 2-strand Hg in a rubber strain gauge was used, with a Devices pressure transducer and pen recorder. A venous occlusion cuff was placed below the knee, and inflated rapidly to 60 mm Hg during blood flow recordings. A cuff pressure of 40 mm Hg might have been preferable to 60 mm Hg, since the higher pressure may have caused slight underestimation of post-exercise hyperaemia in the patients with low blood pressure (Lorentsen et al., 1970). However, there was no significant difference in results in the 2 blood pressure groups. The strain gauge was placed at mid-calf level at the same distance below the tibial tuberosity on each occasion. It was mounted at a tension of 20 g, with the strands 1 cm apart, and was calibrated on the limb. It remained in position during exercise.

Rhythmic calf muscle exercise was used, since published work by Blair et al. (1959) and Lind and McNicol (1967) suggests that changes produced by arterial occlusion are greater following rhythmic than sustained muscle contraction. A foot exerciser similar to that described by Shepherd (1950) was used. By depressing a foot lever, the patient lifted a 10 lb weight vertically a standard distance 27 times per minute in time to a metronome. Exercise was performed with knee and hip extended, movement being confined to flexion and dorsi-flexion of the foot.

Blood flows were measured with the patient lying supine in an environment box at air temperature between 25 and 26 °C. Four basal blood flows were recorded when the patient had been supine for 20 min. Exercise was then commenced. The number of movements causing claudication (claudication point) were recorded and exercise was terminated 20 movements beyond this. Post-exercise hyperaemia was measured 15 and 45 sec after cessation of exercise, and at frequent intervals for 20 min after exercise. The blood flows at 19 and 20 min were specified 'resting flows'. A standard exercise of 20 movements was then performed, and flows were measured 15 and 45 sec after this (Fig. 1). The following blood flows were used in analysis: (*a*) mean basal flow, (*b*) peak flow after prolonged exercise minus basal flow, (*c*) mean resting flow, and (*d*) peak flow after standard exercise minus basal flow.

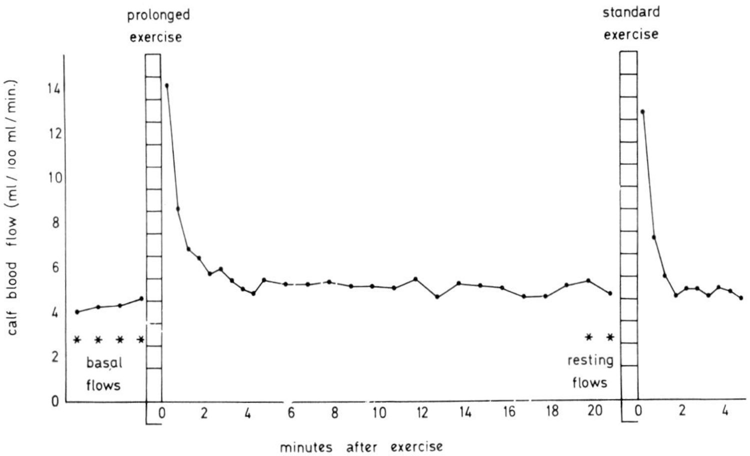

Fig. 1. Typical control calf blood flow result, from one patient (K.W.).

The increase in blood flow following exercise in a limb with occlusive vascular disease has a smaller maximum and a greater duration than normal (Shepherd, 1950). We anticipated that improvement would result in an increase in post-exercise hyperaemia, and a shortening of recovery time. Twenty movements beyond claudication was considered the maximum tolerable exercise.

It was considered justifiable to test the response to a bradykinin antagonist on the basis of changes in post-exercise hyperaemia, since, although bradykinin may contribute to this (Burch and De Pasquale, 1963; Hilton, 1962), more recently the role of osmolarity changes (Arvill et al., 1969; Johansson and Jonsson, 1968; Mellander et al., 1967) and of K ions (Kjellmer, 1965) have been stressed.

RESULTS

Results from 25 of the original 33 participants were analysed. Five sets of results were discarded because of unsatisfactory blood and urine levels of PC. One patient was withdrawn because of a cardiac arrhythmia, one because of diarrhoea and one defaulted.

Results for the step test, claudication point and blood flow were analysed. Digital palpation of leg pulses proved an unreliable method of assessing progress and the results were not used.

Control values

The mean values during the placebo control period were less than those of the control period for all tests, and the variance ratios (control:placebo control) were significantly high ($P < 0.05$). Therefore, in subsequent analyses, treatment period values were tested against both the control period value and a combined control value, this being the mean of control and placebo control values.

Analysis of results in relation to treatment (Fig. 2)

A significant improvement in performance in the step test was apparent when treatment values were compared with the combined control. However, no dose effect could be shown, and the placebo treatment mean exceeded that for 2 g of PC. Claudication point improved during the treatment periods, but not significantly.

Calf blood flow

Calf blood flow did not increase beyond control values with the exception of the mean peak flow after prolonged exercise on 2 g of PC, but this was not significant when compared with

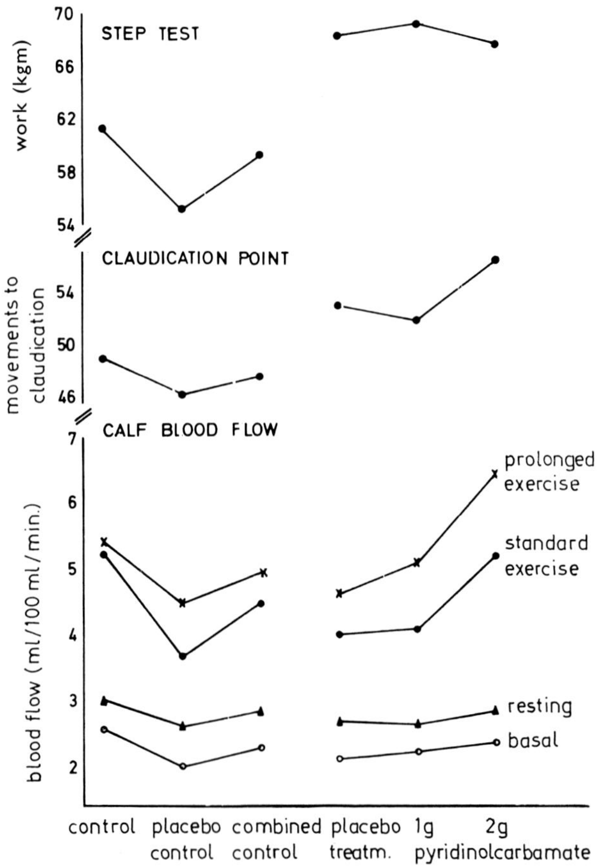

Fig. 2. Mean response over treatment.

the combined control. There was no change in basal blood flow or in 'resting' flow. The mean resting flow exceeded the mean basal flow throughout the trial, and the difference did not diminish with treatment.

The results of a statistically more efficient method of evaluation, using for each patient the deviation from his own control or combined control mean value, showed that performance in the step test decreased significantly in the placebo control period and increased significantly during each treatment period (Table III).

In this analysis, peak flow after standard exercise decreased significantly from control

TABLE III

Mean change in response in relation to treatment. Step test results (kgm work) expressed as mean deviation from control (C) or combined control (CC)

	– C	– CC
Placebo control	– 6.4*	–
Placebo treatment	8.3*	10.6*
1 g PC	7.5*	9.8**
2 g PC	6.2*	8.5**

Significance levels: *P < 0.05; **P < 0.01.

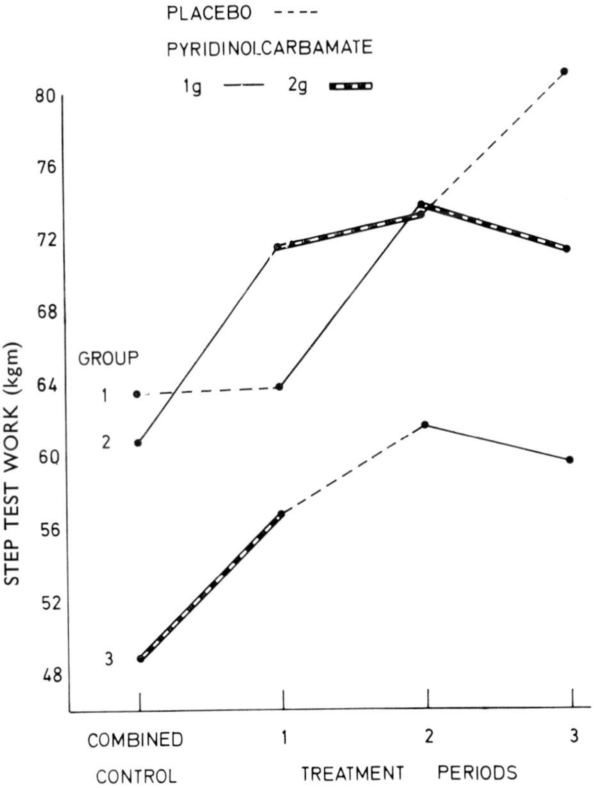

Fig. 3. Step test. Mean results analysed by treatment-schedule groups.

values during the placebo control and placebo treatment period (by 1.80 and 1.33 ml/min/100 ml respectively; $P < 0.01$).

A comparison of results for each test within the 3 treatment groups suggested that randomization within the groups had been satisfactory and the treatment sequence had not significantly affected the response. However, Figure 3 shows that, in Group 1, there was no difference in step test performance between the combined control and placebo treatment, whereas in Groups 2 and 3, in which placebo treatment followed high dosage (2 g) of PC, improvement was maintained on placebo.

Because of the possibility of some 'carry-over' effect during placebo treatment (Shimamoto et al., 1970), a further analysis was undertaken, omitting the placebo treatment results. For each patient, the combined control was subtracted from the combined 1 g and 2 g PC treatment values. Only the step test showed a significant mean difference in response (of +9.33 kgm; $P < 0.001$) during PC treatment.

Analysis of results in relation to time

Since no definite dose-related effect of PC was demonstrable, the data were rearranged and analysed by chronological sequence, irrespective of dose.

Analysis in terms of mean deviation (Tables IV and V) showed a significant increase in the step test over both control and combined control values in treatment Periods 2 and 3. Claudication point and peak calf flow blood after prolonged exercise increased significantly from the combined control value in Periods 2 and 3 respectively. Basal blood flow did not change.

TABLE IV

Change in response over time expressed as mean deviation from control (C) or combined control (CC) values. Step test and claudication point results

Period	Step test (kgm work)		Claudication (movements)	
	−C	−CC	−C	−CC
Placebo control	−6.4 *	−	−1.8	−
Period 1	2.3	4.6	−1.0	−0.08
Period 2	8.5**	10.8***	11.5	12.4*
Period 3	11.2**	13.5**	5.6	8.5

* = $P < 0.05$, ** = $P < 0.01$, *** = $P < 0.001$.

TABLE V

Change in response over time expressed as mean deviation from control (C) or combined control (CC) values. Blood flow results

Period	Peak calf blood flow (ml /100 ml/min) ***		
	Prolonged exercise	Standard exercise	
	−CC	−C	−CC
Placebo control	−	−1.80**	−
Period 1	−0.86	−1.85**	−0.76*
Period 2	0.43	−0.98	0.05
Period 3	1.71*	0.21	1.23

* = $P < 0.05$, ** = $P < 0.01$
*** = Peak post-exercise hyperaemia minus basal flow

Within broad limits, all tests showed the same basic pattern over time, a decrease from control values during the first part of the trial, followed by a rise in the latter half.

Evaluation of seasonal variation effect

The decrease in performance during the placebo control period needed explanation, particularly since, for all tests, the significance of the change in response was due mainly to low values during this period. Ambient temperature was considered as a possible complicating variable.

Step test results were available for subgroups of patients during each calendar week, and these weekly means were plotted above the mean ambient temperature for the corresponding week. Mean monthly step test results for all patients were also compared with mean temperature over the same 4-week periods.

The overall picture (Fig. 4) was of performance following temperature. When a correlation analysis was carried out on mean weekly values over the trial period (both variables in logarithms), a lag period of 1 week gave a correlation coefficient ($r = 0.587$; $P < 0.01$) which was marginally higher than the values for periods of 2–8 weeks.

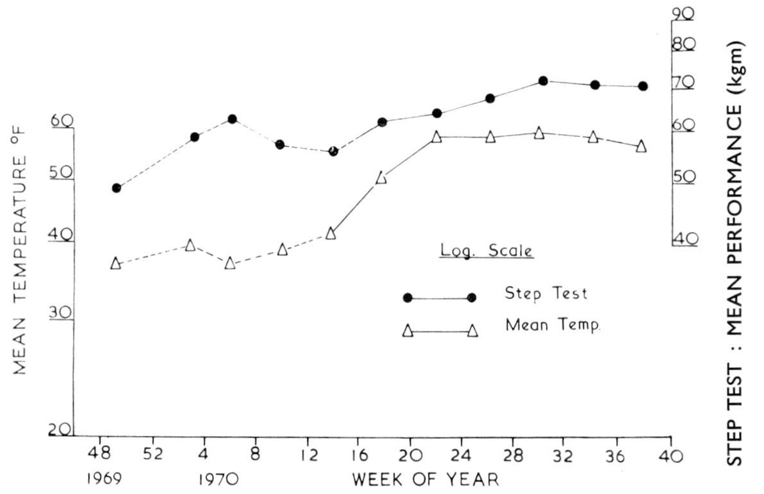

Fig. 4. Mean monthly step test performance with mean temperature for corresponding months. Control period indicated by dotted line. Step test results, mean of 22, 15, 24 and 15 patients for first 4 points in control period, and 25 patients throughout treatment period.

It was possible that a major temperature effect was masking a subordinate drug effect. To isolate a residual element which might correlate with drug dosage, the mean weekly performance value was subtracted from each patient's result for that specific week. The resultant values were then analysed in relation to treatment, but no residual drug effect could be demonstrated. Repeating the procedure with 4-point moving averages of the weekly performance values (to allow for variation between the 4 subgroups on which they were based) gave a similar negative result. The residual values for each patient remained remarkably constant over the trial.

Factors influencing response

The effect of smoking habits, blood pressure and serum cholesterol level on response were examined. Results were analysed in terms of the deviation of each patient from his own control for each factor in the step test, claudication point and peak calf blood flow after prolonged exercise.

For all 3 tests the light smokers improved more than the heavy smokers, but the mean deviations did not achieve the 5% level of significance, and were not clearly related to PC treatment. Neither cholesterol nor blood pressure levels had any consistent or significant effect on tests.

Assessment of subjective changes

Of the 25 final participants, 16 felt better, 8 were unchanged, and one felt worse during treatment. When told that 3 doses of drug had been tested, all expressed surprise.

Side-effects

Four patients developed diarrhoea on the 2 g dose and one of these had to be withdrawn from the trial. In 2 cases, the diarrhoea was accompanied by mild depression and in a third by early waking. One patient became suicidal during treatment with 2 g daily and was withdrawn.

Biochemical and haematological results

The haemoglobin, total and differential white count remained within normal limits during treatment, as did the serum albumin, globulin, sodium, potassium, calcium and SGOT. No consistent changes in total cholesterol were observed between 2 laboratories.

Blood and urine drug levels

The mean blood level of PC on 1 g daily was 9.4 μg/ml, and on 2 g daily was 17.3 μg/ml. The mean urine level of PC and its metabolites was 46.7 μg/ml on 1 g daily and 61.4 μg/ml on 2 g daily.

DISCUSSION

Assessment of the effect of medical treatment of arteriosclerosis is difficult, because patients vary in the nature of spontaneous progression of their signs and symptoms.

Reduction in serum cholesterol improves calf blood flow in cases of Type III hyperlipidaemia with peripheral vascular disease (Zelis et al., 1970). Serum cholesterol did not change significantly in our patients.

Rodbard and Pragay (1968) have postulated that, during a muscle contraction, a metabolite is produced which diffuses out of the muscle cell into the extracellular space, where a specific concentration of the metabolite in contact with a pain receptor causes ischaemic pain. Applying this concept, an improvement in the step test, or in claudication point in the present trial, could be due to decreased production or release of metabolite (perhaps by some hypothetical effect of PC on membrane permeability), more rapid elimination due to improved blood flow, or antagonism of the effect of the metabolite on pain receptors.

The disparity between calf blood flow results and the improvement demonstrated by the step test and, to some extent, claudication point might be explicable if PC acted as an analgesic. Piper and Vane (1969) have shown that the analgesic effect of aspirin may be due to an action whereby it blocks the release of an intermediary vasoactive substance (RCS) produced in response to bradykinin. A study of the effect of PC on ischaemic muscle pain would be valuable.

Performance in the step test improved, but no direct relationship to PC treatment could be shown. The differences were more significant when analysed over time, and improvement correlated with a rise in external temperature during the summer, although physiological tests were all undertaken in a temperature-controlled environment.

Sternieri et al. (1969) have reported seasonal changes in bradykinin sensitivity in the rabbit and rat. If a seasonal variation in bradykinin sensitivity occurs in man, it could influence the response both to endogenous bradykinin and to a bradykinin antagonist such as PC. The effect this may have had on our results is a matter for conjecture, since it is uncertain whether bradykinin has a significant role in peripheral circulatory physiology or in the pathogenesis of atheroma, or whether it contributes to ischaemic muscle pain. However, if bradykinin contributes to ischaemic pain, it is of considerable interest that the painful effect of intra-arterial bradykinin in rabbits is least between April and July (Sternieri et al., 1969), the time when step test performance improved in the present study.

The objective of the Birmingham trial was to confirm the results of Shimamoto et al. (1970), who ascribed the improvement in claudication in 80% of their patients to PC. Although there may be differences in the severity or natural history of the condition between the populations tested, this cannot entirely explain the disparity in results. In our series, although a significant improvement occurred in the step test, no dose-related drug effect could be demonstrated. The results do not decisively exclude a cumulative drug effect, but the fact that claudication point and step test values were decreasing during the latter weeks of the trial throws doubt on the possibility. The proposed seasonal variation effect is supported by the correlation and residual drug effect results and, in the absence of a cumulative drug effect, could account for all the variation found in the step test.

ACKNOWLEDGEMENTS

Thanks are due to Professor Slaney and Mr. F. Ashton for allowing us to study their patients, and to Dr. G. Malone, Staff Nurse R. Arnold and Mrs. M. Cochrane for their assistance. The Staff of the Pharmacy and Departments of Biochemistry and Haematology, Queen Elizabeth Hospital, Birmingham, played a valuable part. Anginin levels were measured by Mrs. D. Dunkerley. Dr. J. Nelms helped with the design and loan of physiological equipment. Finally, we thank the patients for their co-operation and enthusiasm, which enabled the work to be completed.

REFERENCES

ARVILL, A., JOHANSSON, B. and JONSSON, O. (1969): Effects of hyperosmolarity on the volume of vascular smooth muscle cells and the relationship between cell volume and muscle activity. *Acta physiol. scand.*, *75*, 484.

BLAIR, D. A., GLOVER, W. E. and RODDIE, I. C. (1959): The abolition of reactive and post-exercise hyperaemia in the forearm by temporary restriction of arterial inflow. *J. Physiol. (Lond.)*, *148*, 648.

BURCH, G. E. and DE PASQUALE, N. P. (1963): Bradykinin. *Amer. Heart J.*, *65*, 116.

HILTON, S. J. (1962): Local mechanisms regulating peripheral blood flow. *Physiol. Rev.*, *42*, *Suppl. 5*, 265.

JOHANSSON, B. and JONSSON, O. (1968): Cell volume as a factor influencing electrical and mechanical activity of vascular smooth muscle. *Acta physiol. scand.*, *72*, 456.

KJELLMER, I. (1965): The potassium ion as a vasodilator during muscular exercise. *Acta physiol. scand.*, *72*, 456.

LIND, A. R. and MCNICOL, G. W. (1967): Local and central circulatory response to sustained contractions and the effect of free or restricted arterial inflow on post-exercise hyperaemia. *J. Physiol. (Lond.)*, *192*, 575.

LORENTSEN, E., HANSTEEN, V. and SIVERTSSEN, E. (1970): The influence of venous collecting pressure on measurements of calf blood flow by venous occlusion plethysmography. *Angiology*, *21*, 661.

MELLANDER, S., JOHANSSON, B., GRAY, S., JONSSON, O., LUNDVALL, J. and LJUNG, B. (1967): The effects of hyperosmolarity on intact and isolated vascular smooth muscle. Possible role in exercise hyperaemia. *Angiologica*, *4*, 310.

PIPER, P. J. and VANE, V. R. (1969): Release of additional factors in anaphylaxis, and its antagonism by anti-inflammatory drugs. *Nature (Lond.)*, *223*, 29.

RODBARD, S. and PRAGAY, E. B. (1968): Contraction frequency, blood supply and muscle pain. *J. appl. Physiol.*, *24*, 142.

SHEPHERD, J. T. (1950): The blood flow through the calf after exercise in subjects with arteriosclerosis and claudication. *Clin. Sci.*, *9*, 49.
SHIMAMOTO, T., ATSUMI, T., YAMASHITA, S., MOTOMIYA, T., ISOKANE, N., ISHIOKA, T. and SAKUMA, A. (1970): Clinical pharmacologic evaluation of the antiatherosclerotic agent pyridinolcarbamate. A double blind cross-over trial in the treatment of atherosclerosis obliterans. *Amer. Heart J.*, *79*, 5.
STERNIERI, E., MUCCI, P., BERTOLINI, A. and CASTELLI, M. (1969): Variazioni stagionalli nella sensibilità alla bradichinina del coniglio e del ratto. *Bull. Soc. ital. Biol. sper.*, *45*, 421.
WHITNEY, R. J. (1953): Measurement of volume changes in human limbs. *J. Physiol. (Lond.)*, *121*, 1.
ZELIS, R., MASON, D. T., BRAUNWALD, E. and LEVY, R. I. (1970): Effects of hyperlipoproteinaemias and their treatment on the peripheral circulation. *J. clin. Invest.*, *49*, 1007.

DISCUSSION

Dr. REDISCH: Dr. Craig, first my compliments on an excellent study and second, I have a question and a comment. Did you, in addition to the types of exercise you did, also measure post-strangulation hyperaemia (strangulation is the American term for reactive hyperaemia)?

Dr. CRAIG: No, we did not. We tried this during preliminary runs before the trial and decided against it because, although it can be more easily standardized than post-exercise hyperaemia, we thought the risk of causing further arterial damage was too great.

Dr. REDISCH: Yes, your way of doing it is extremely interesting. It showed beautifully that the basal blood flow may be normal in peripheral vascular disease, and it is the response to exercise which is the decisive test of severity. I think we can distinguish between responses in the skin microcirculation and muscle microcirculation. Reactive hyperaemia, as discussed earlier by Professor Pratesi, is really going on primarily in the skin microcirculation, whereas post-exercise hyperaemia, as in your study, takes place predominantly in the muscle and very little in the skin. Do you agree with me there?

Dr. CRAIG: Yes, I think so.

Dr. TERRY: It is a purely technical question. Did you use a constant temperature laboratory for your plethysmography?

Dr. CRAIG: We did not have a constant temperature room. We used an environment box at constant temperature.

Dr. TERRY: You used a temperature of 28 °C, I believe.

Dr. CRAIG: Yes, 26–28 °C.

Dr. TERRY: How long did you allow for patients to adapt to this temperature prior to plethysmography?

Dr. CRAIG: They rested at that temperature for 20 min before the first basal blood flow.

CLINICAL TRIAL OF PYRIDINOLCARBAMATE

Z. JANUSHKEVICHIUS and J. BLOOZHAS
Kaunas Medical Institute, Kaunas, Lithuanian S.S.R., U.S.S.R.

Pyridinolcarbamate, as many experimental and clinical studies have proved, exerts a significant effect not only on the initial stages in the development of atherosclerosis, but upon already damaged vascular wall as well. At present, there is an impression of an unequivocal Anginin effect in a definite number of cases, particularly in those with peripheral vascular involvement. The supposed mechanisms have been described in detail elsewhere (Atsumi et al., 1969; Constantinides, 1969; Miyao, 1969; Shimamoto, 1967, 1968, 1969*a*, *b*; Shimamoto et al., 1966; Yamazaki et al., 1970).

In the Kaunas Medical Institute a clinical and biochemical study was performed, the patients being divided into 3 groups (Table I): Group I, those with predominant coronary atherosclerosis (16 were treated with Anginin and 8 were given placebo); Group II, patients with atherosclerotic peripheral arterial involvement (Anginin 7, placebo 5); and Group III, those with cerebral atherosclerosis (Anginin 5, placebo 0).

TABLE I

Distribution of patients on Anginin and placebo according to location of disorder, sex, and age

	Anginin					Placebo				
	No.	Sex		Average age	Age range	No.	Sex		Average age	Age range
		M	F				M	F		
Coronary vessels	16	13	3	58.8	39–75	8	6	2	63.4	39–74
Peripheral vessels	7	6	1	45.4	25–67	5	4	1	52.8	35–67
Cerebral vessels	5	3	2	53.6	44–66	–	–	–	–	–
Total	28	22	6	54.5	25–75	13	10	3	59.2	35–74

In the group with coronary atherosclerosis (Table II) there were 11 patients (Anginin 4, placebo 7) with acute myocardial infarction, 7 patients (all on Anginin) with previous myocardial infarction, and 6 patients (Anginin 5, placebo 1) with no myocardial infarction.

In addition to routine and special tests, all patients underwent ophthalmological (biomicroscopy, rheo-ophthalmography, blood pressure measurement of conjunctival vessels) and biochemical (complete spectrum of lipids and lipoproteins, blood coagulation factors, metabolic and electrolyte balance) tests. Anginin treatment showed a favourable effect in most of the patients. However, the small number and heterogeneity of the patients did not allow us to make a categorical conclusion, the more so as in 20–30% of cases a therapeutic effect was attained, according to current medical literature and our data, by the use of placebo alone.

1500 mg of Anginin and placebo were given daily for 4–6 months (2 tablets, each containing 250 mg of Anginin and placebo t.i.d.). All patients, with the exception of those suffering from acute myocardial infarction, were on an out-patient regime. A number of patients were even able to continue their routine work. Three patients with coronary atherosclerosis, all

TABLE II

Distribution of patients with coronary atherosclerosis on Anginin and placebo

	Anginin					Placebo				
	No.	Angina pectoris		Heart failure		No.	Angina pectoris		Heart failure	
		I	II	0	I		I	II	0	I
Acute myocardial infarction	4	1	3	3	1	7	5	2	5	2
Previous myocardial infarction	7	4	3	4	3	–	–	–	–	–
No myocardial infarction	5	3	2	5	–	1	–	1	1	–
Total	16	8	8	12	4	8	5	3	6	2

suffering from chronic occlusive vascular disease of the extremities, received no vasodilators; the others were given symptomatic treatment. All patients had undergone an examination and laboratory and other tests were carried out prior to the treatment and then every month during the trial. General improvement of the patients and favourable changes in their laboratory and other tests served as criteria for the assessment of the effectiveness of the treatment.

Anginin treatment was followed by favourable subjective and clinical response in 62.5% of patients with coronary atherosclerosis (in 10 of 16 patients), in 71.4% of the patients with peripheral arterial involvement (5 of 7), and in 3 out of 5 patients suffering from cerebral atherosclerosis (Table III). 37.5% (3 of 8) of patients with coronary atherosclerosis noted some improvement with placebo treatment. There was no improvement after administration of placebo in cases with peripheral arterial involvement.

TABLE III

Results of Anginin and placebo treatment (%)

	Anginin		Placebo	
	Effective	Ineffective	Effective	Ineffective
Coronary vessels	62.5	37.5	37.5	62.5
Peripheral vessels	71.5	29.5	0	100.0
Cerebral vessels	60.0	40.0	–	–

In patients with coronary atherosclerosis there was both subjective and objective improvement, although there was only an insignificant difference in biochemical findings in patients with and without any improvement. The Anginin treatment resulted in disappearance or decrease in ectopic sites of excitation in the myocardium (in 3 patients of 4), decrease in ischaemic signs in the ECG (in 2 patients), and improvement in atrioventricular conduction (in 2 patients) as reported by other authors (Mizuno, 1969; Yamazaki, 1969*a*, *b*; Yamazaki et al., 1970*b*).

The ECG is described of a 42-year-old patient who was given Anginin during the first week following myocardial infarction. The onset of infarction was very dramatic – there was severe pain of long duration and marked weakness. The treatment was begun with the ECG showing a negative T wave in the standard and left chest leads. During Anginin treatment there was no development of necrosis, and the ischaemic signs disappeared after 4 months (Fig. 1).

The ECG of a 60-year-old patient who 3 years ago underwent an anteroseptal transmural myocardial infarction is shown in Figure 2. Until treatment with Anginin the patient suffered frequently from disturbed atrioventricular conduction (in the ECG there is a first-degree A-V block and sometimes a second-degree A-V block occurred). Treatment with atropine or vagolytic drugs resulted only in a temporary effect. During treatment with Anginin A-V conduction became normal and has remained normal to this time.

One 64-year-old patient had a posterior wall myocardial infarction (Fig. 3). During treatment with Anginin frequent premature ventricular beats disappeared over the course of the 2 months' treatment.

The parallel ophthalmological tests were used to make an assessment of the microcirculation. In spite of the fact that ocular vessels have a definite autonomy, our findings established the possibility of estimating to some degree the state of the whole vascular system on the basis of the ocular vessels.

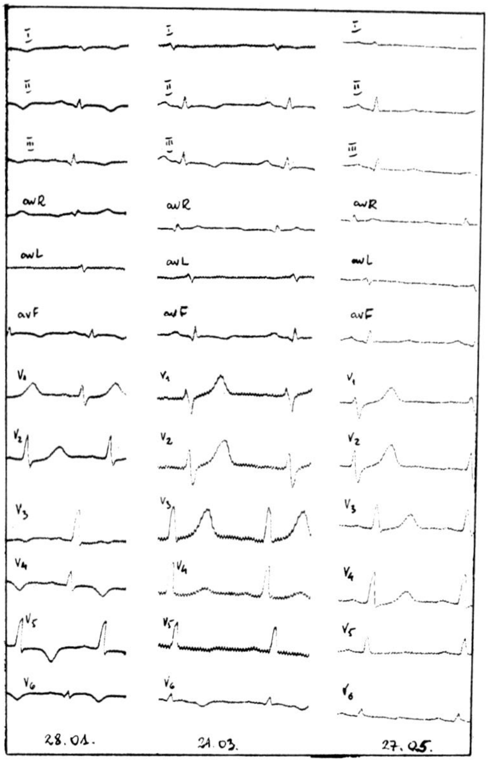

Fig. 1

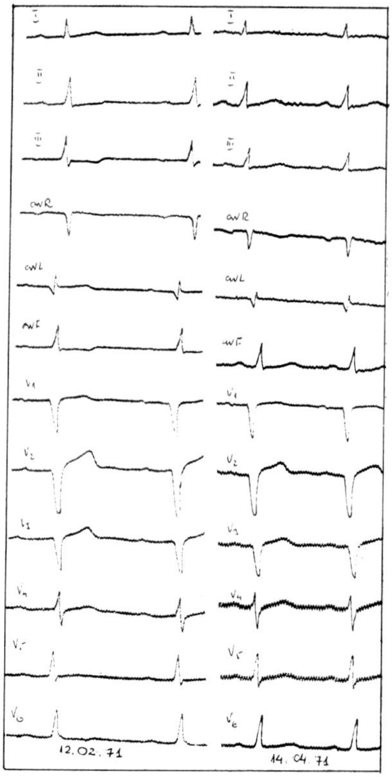

Fig. 2

In patients with peripheral arterial disorders the effect of Anginin was more appreciable. Only one patient denied general improvement. The effect of Anginin in these patients was more controllable as no vasodilators were used and other means of therapy were limited. All patients noted an extension of walking distance and decrease or complete disappearance of leg pains. There was healing of trophic ulceration (2 patients), an increase in the temperature of the extremities and the oscillometric index and peripheral pulsation also showed favourable changes. Ophthalmological investigations (Figs. 4 and 5)* showed that even although the gross changes in the morphology of the vascular wall remained, there were signs of more regular blood flow and of a decrease in erythrocyte aggregation.

Our modest experience in the treatment of cerebral patients permitted us to think that Anginin had a favourable effect on them too. However, the lack of the placebo group did not allow us to correlate our findings.

Interpretation and assessment of the biochemical findings was a more complex task. It has been revealed that biochemical changes were not always linked with the clinical response. The causes of this non-correlation are apparently very intricate and this fact is reflected in the medical literature (De Soldati et al., 1969; Yamazaki, 1969*b*; Yamazaki et al., 1970*b*) and still undefined, though Anginin dosage and duration of its administration could have been implicated.

It has been reported that Anginin had an inhibitory effect on lipid mobilization and stimulated the esterification of free fatty acids (Goto and Nakamura, 1969). In experiments on animals fed on an atherogenic diet Anginin lowered the blood cholesterol level (Goto and

* See p. 316*a*

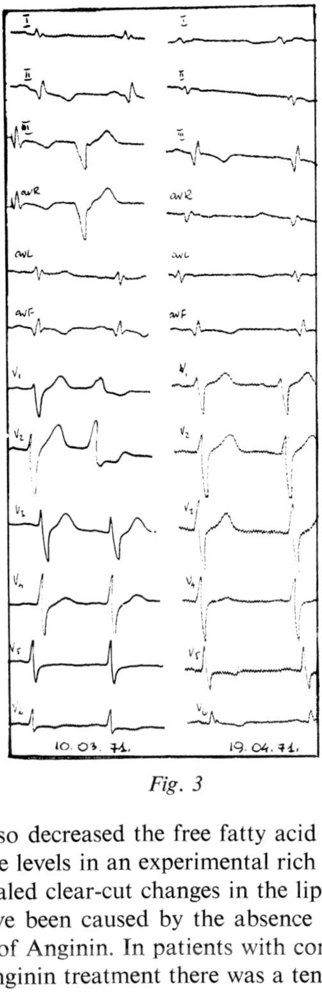

Fig. 3

Nakamura, 1969). Anginin also decreased the free fatty acid level without affecting cholesterol, triglycerides and glucose levels in an experimental rich butter diet in humans.

Our findings have not revealed clear-cut changes in the lipid-lipoprotein spectrum in the patients treated. It might have been caused by the absence of marked hyperlipidaemia in our patients prior to the use of Anginin. In patients with coronary atherosclerosis showing general improvement after Anginin treatment there was a tendency towards lowering of the lipid level (Fig. 6). However, the difference in some indices was insignificant even in comparison with the placebo group. More often than not, most indices returned to the initial level at the end of treatment. One cannot exclude the influence of the psychological factor in accounting for the changes in the placebo group.

Changes in cholesterol level were small and are within the limits of statistically insignificant values (Fig. 6). In two groups of patients (one with the improvement in general state and the other without) changes in cholesterol level are insignificant.

A general tendency to change in the triglyceride (Fig. 6) level is observed after a month of treatment with Anginin. It returns to the initial level.

The changes in the phospholipid level (Fig. 6) are similar to those described above with the exception of a statistically insignificant increase in patients with coronary atherosclerosis who felt improvement in their general state after treatment with Anginin.

Total lipoproteins, as well as their fractions (Fig. 6) (α- and β-lipoproteins), changed independently of the treatment with Anginin or placebo. However, a tendency to a decrease in level is noticed in coronary patients with improvement of state compared to those who received the placebo treatment, although in patients with lesions of the peripheral arteries placebo resulted in the opposite response.

The changes in the blood coagulation system under the influence of Anginin were shown more distinctly in the thrombelastogram (TEG). We have registered prolongation of the TEG reaction time (*r*). The changes in the *r* and *k* indices were more distinct after a month of treatment. At the end of the course of treatment these indices did not differ significantly from the initial one (Fig. 6). Placebo had the same, although less marked, effect. After treatment with Anginin a considerable decrease in blood clot density was observed as shown by the *ma* index of the TEG. The placebo treatment did not give such a response (Fig. 6). The decrease in the *ma* index of the TEG in the placebo group of coronary patients can be explained by the improvement in the clinical state after previous myocardial infarction and treatment with anticoagulants. The changes in thrombin time are small and there was no statistically significant difference between the indices mentioned above (Fig. 6). The fibrinolytic activity, which had different levels at the beginning of the investigation, became equal after the course of treatment (Fig. 6). The greatest difference was obtained in the heparin level (Fig. 6). These changes are similar to those reported by other investigators (De Soldati et al., 1969). A striking feature is the increase in the plasma fibrinogen level in patients of all groups with the exception of those suffering from peripheral atherosclerosis (Fig. 6). We were interested in this observation and have made an attempt to determine its cause: Was there an increase in fibrinogen production or was it released from the conjugated state? The Niewiarowski test with protamine sulphate showed that during Anginin treatment there was an increase in both the free and conjugated fibrinogen level.

Of theoretical and practical interest were the cases of 2 patients on Anginin and anticoagulant (phenyllin) who developed signs of haematuria, and retinal and conjunctival haemorrhage after one month of Anginin treatment, although there was no change in anticoagulant dosage, mode of life or eating habits.

Some patients, particularly those with coronary atherosclerosis, showed resistance to Anginin. Little is known of its cause, but the most important effect is that the Anginin treatment produced no deterioration, the drug itself being well tolerated by the patients and causing no significant complications.

Our findings do not contradict the view that Anginin improves vascular wall metabolism, normalizes its permeability and helps to eliminate products of tissue metabolism. In the patients on Anginin there was a decrease in the lactic acid level.

In our post-infarction centre the 10-year follow-up of patients following myocardial infarction showed that the anticoagulant therapy (phenyllin) exerted a favourable effect. In a group of patients on phenyllin followed for 2 years after myocardial infarction the rate of mortality was 3.2%, re-infarction rate 1.6% and disablement rate 9.7%; in the control group mortality, re-infarction and disablement rate were 14.3%, 11.9% and 22.1%, respectively. It would be very interesting to perform a similar follow-up study with Anginin as well.

At present, the surgical correction of the coronary circulation, particularly reconstructive by-pass surgery, is becoming increasingly more popular. However, the interpretation of the long-term outcome gives rise to much controversy. It would be very useful to study the effect of Anginin on the stability of the reconstructed coronary circulation. At the same time selective coronary arteriography would be helpful in studying the effect of Anginin on the regional main artery stenosis and on generalized stenosis of the 3 main coronary arteries. It would help to explain the effect of Anginin on the two main causes of ischaemic myocardial damage. Finally, it would be useful to study the effect of Anginin on patients with angina pectoris in order to learn about its preventive properties concerning myocardial infarction.

Summing up, our experience in the clinical trial of Anginin showed that a sufficiently effective remedy for the treatment of atherosclerosis has been produced. Anginin is indicated in cases of coronary atherosclerosis and in other atherosclerotic disorders as well, although its effectiveness depends on the site of disease.

Fig. 4. Before Anginin treatment.

Fig. 5. After 4 months of Anginin treatment.

→

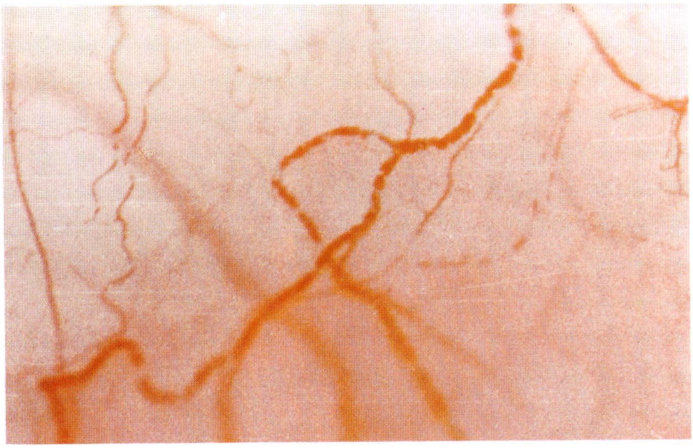

Fig. 4

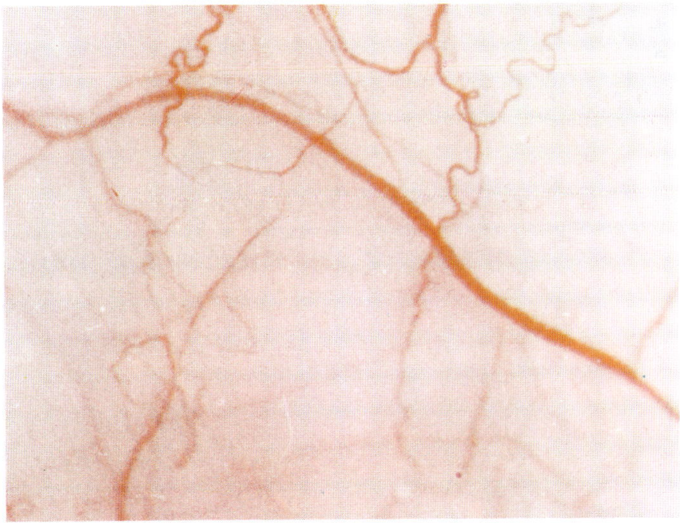

Fig. 5

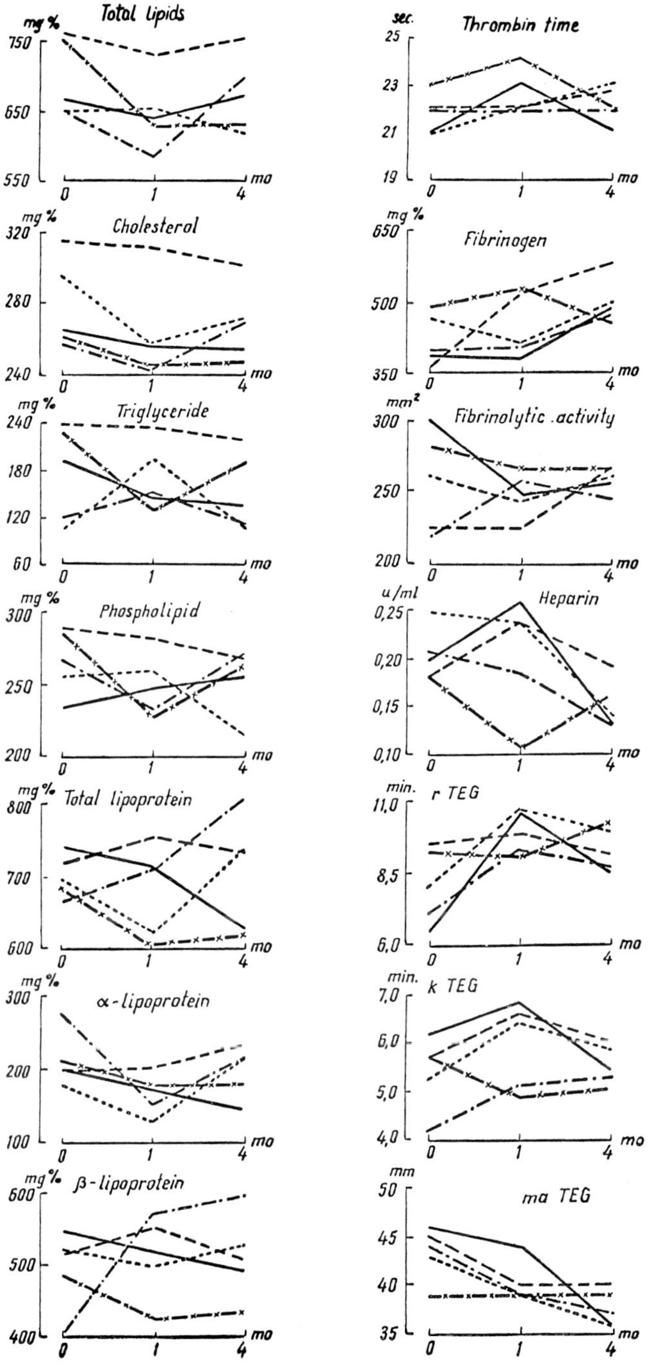
Total lipids
mg %
750
650
550
0 1 4 mo
Thrombin time
sec.
25
23
21
19
0 1 4 mo
Cholesterol
mg %
320
280
240
0 1 4 mo
Fibrinogen
mg %
650
500
350
0 1 4 mo
Triglyceride
mg %
240
180
120
60
0 1 4 mo
Fibrinolytic activity
mm²
300
250
200
0 1 4 mo
Phospholipid
mg %
300
250
200
0 1 4 mo
Heparin
u/ml
0,25
0,20
0,15
0,10
0 1 4 mo
Total lipoprotein
mg %
800
700
600
0 1 4 mo
r TEG
min.
11,0
8,5
6,0
0 1 4 mo
α-lipoprotein
mg %
300
200
100
0 1 4 mo
k TEG
min.
7,0
6,0
5,0
4,0
0 1 4 mo
β-lipoprotein
mg %
600
500
400
0 1 4 mo
ma TEG
mm
50
45
40
35
0 1 4 mo

Fig. 6

REFERENCES

ATSUMI, T., YAMASHITA, S., MOTOMIYA, T., SANO, T., ISOKANE, N., KUARI, A., ISHIOKA, T. and SHIMAMOTO, T. (1969): The pyridinolcarbamate treatment of atherosclerosis obliterans. In: *Atherogenesis. Proceedings, I International Symposium on Atherogenesis, Thrombogenesis and Pyridinolcarbamate Treatment, Tokyo 1967*, pp. 163–170. Editors: T. Shimamoto and F. Numano. ICS 201, Excerpta Medica, Amsterdam.

CONSTANTINIDES, P. (1969): The role of the endothelial barrier in atherosclerosis. In: *Atherogenesis. Proceedings, I International Symposium on Atherogenesis, Thrombogenesis and Pyridinolcarbamate Treatment, Tokyo 1969*, pp. 99–100. Editors: T. Shimamoto and F. Numano. ICS 201, Excerpta Medica, Amsterdam.

DE SOLDATI, L., CASTRO, C., GRILLI, H. and REUSSI, J. (1969): Clinical trials with pyridinolcarbamate on arterial circulation and blood coagulation in patients with atherosclerosis obliterans. In: *Atherogenesis. Proceedings, I International Symposium on Atherogenesis, Thrombogenesis and Pyridinolcarbamate Treatment, Tokyo 1969*, pp. 153–162. Editors: T. Shimamoto and F. Numano. ICS 201, Excerpta Medica, Amsterdam.

GOTO, Y. and NAKAMURA, H. (1969): Effect of pyridinolcarbamate on the plasma lipids and glucose in vivo. In: *Atherogenesis. Proceedings, I International Symposium on Atherogenesis, Thrombogenesis and Pyridinolcarbamate Treatment, Tokyo 1969*, pp. 119–120. Editors: T. Shimamoto and F. Numano. ICS 201, Excerpta Medica, Amsterdam.

MIYAO, S. (1969): The effectiveness of pyridinolcarbamate (Anginin) on cerebral circulation in patients with cerebrovascular disease. In: *Atherogenesis. Proceedings, I International Symposium on Atherogenesis, Thrombogenesis and Pyridinolcarbamate Treatment, Tokyo 1969*, pp. 225–227. Editors: T. Shimamoto and F. Numano. ICS 201, Excerpta Medica, Amsterdam.

MIZUNO, Y. (1969): Effects of pyridinolcarbamate treatment of coronary heart disease. In: *Atherogenesis. Proceedings, I International Symposium on Atherogenesis, Thrombogenesis and Pyridinolcarbamate Treatment, Tokyo 1969*, pp. 261–266. Editors: T. Shimamoto and F. Numano. ICS 201, Excerpta Medica, Amsterdam.

SHIMAMOTO, T. (1967): An antiatherosclerotic, pyridinolcarbamate. Microcirculatory aspects of atherogenesis and thrombogenesis. *Asian med. J. 10/6*,425.

SHIMAMOTO, T. (1968): Microcirculatory aspects of atherogenesis, thrombogenesis, and antiatherosclerotics. *Amer. Heart J., 76/1*, 105.

SHIMAMOTO, T. (1969*a*): An introduction to the investigation of atherogenesis, thrombogenesis and pyridinolcarbamate treatment. Vizualization of the transendothelial passage through intercellular junctions and discovery of endothelial folds and intercellular bridges of vascular endothelium. In: *Atherogenesis. Proceedings, I International Symposium on Atherogenesis, Thrombogenesis and Pyridinolcarbamate Treatment, Tokyo 1969*, pp. 5–27. Editors: T. Shimamoto and F. Numano. ICS 201, Excerpta Medica, Amsterdam.

SHIMAMOTO, T. (1969*b*): Experimental study on atherosclerosis – an attempt at its prevention and treatment. *Acta path. jap., 19/1*, 15.

SHIMAMOTO, T., NUMANO, F. and FUJITA, T. (1966): Atherosclerosis inhibiting effect of an antibradykinin agent, pyridinolcarbamate. *Amer. Heart J., 71/2*, 216.

YAMAZAKI, H. (1969*a*): The effect of pyridinolcarbamate on ischemic ECG changes. In: *Atherogenesis. Proceedings, I International Symposium on Atherogenesis, Thrombogenesis, and Pyridinolcarbamate Treatment, Tokyo 1969*, pp. 285–287. Editors: T. Shimamoto and F. Numano. ICS 201, Excerpta Medica, Amsterdam.

YAMAZAKI, H. (1969*b*): Changes in blood coagulation, platelet count and platelet aggregation induced by endotoxin or exercise and the prevention of these changes by pyridinolcarbamate. In: *Atherogenesis. Proceedings, I International Symposium on Atherogenesis, Thrombogenesis and Pyridinolcarbamate Treatment, Tokyo 1969*, pp. 93–96. Editors: T. Shimamoto and F. Numano. ICS 201, Excerpta Medica, Amsterdam.

YAMAZAKI, H., KOBAYASHI, I. and SHIMAMOTO, T. (1970*a*): Enhancement of ADP-induced platelet aggregation by exercise test in coronary patients and its prevention by pyridinolcarbamate. *Thrombos. Diathes. haemorrh. (Stuttg.), 24/3*, 438.

YAMAZAKI, H. et al. (1970*b*): Electrocardiographic and hematological changes by exercise test in coronary patients and pyridinolcarbamate pretreatment. A double-blind crossover trial. *Amer. Heart J. 79/5*, 640.

THE MEASUREMENT OF BLOOD FLOW THROUGH THE ANTERIOR TIBIAL MUSCLE USING THE ^{133}Xe CLEARANCE METHOD AND ITS CLINICAL EVALUATION

TOSHIYUKI ATSUMI
Department of Medicine, Tokyo Ika-Shika National University,
Tokyo, Japan

In the previous Symposium we reported the results of a double-blind cross-over trial with pyridinolcarbamate and placebo in patients with atherosclerosis obliterans and the summary of our experience in 201 patients treated with this drug for 3 years. This time, I would like to present the results of blood flow measurement through the anterior tibial muscle using the ^{133}Xe clearance method in 129 legs with atherosclerosis obliterans and the results of the augmentation of the blood flow in patients treated with pyridinolcarbamate.

The blood flow through the anterior tibial muscle was measured in 65 patients using the radioactive xenon clearance method originally reported by Lassen in 1964. Blood flow was also measured in 16 individuals who had no arterial obstruction. Resting blood flow was first measured after the bilateral injection of 100-200 μCi of radioactive xenon into the anterior tibial muscle, and then reactive blood flow was measured after releasing a cuff which compressed the upper part of the leg to a pressure above the level of systolic blood pressure for 3 min.

Resting blood flow was 1.57 ± 0.18 ml/100 g/min in the 32 healthy control limbs, 1.83 ± 0.27 ml/100 g/min in 18 unaffected limbs of patients treated with pyridinolcarbamate, and 1.54 ± 0.15 ml/100 g/min in the 54 affected limbs which had been treated with pyridinolcarbamate (Fig. 1). There were no statistically significant differences among these 3 groups. However, the blood flow was significantly decreased in 14 affected limbs which had not been treated with pyridinolcarbamate compared with 54 affected legs which had been treated with pyridinolcarbamate. Muscle blood flow was significantly decreased to 1.0 ± 0.16 ml/100 g/min in the severely affected limbs which had cyanosis or ulcers, although these patients had been treated with pyridinolcarbamate for a long period.

From the above results it can be seen that the measurement of resting blood flow did not succeed in separating the affected limbs from the non-affected limbs, except for severely affected limbs. Moreover, the blood flow varies from time to time, although patients were measured under almost the same conditions. Figure 2 shows the difference in muscle blood flow between the 1st measurement and a 2nd which was obtained 1 week after the 1st measurement. There are apparent differences between the data of the 2 measurements. For example, in my legs, muscle blood flow was calculated as 0.67 ml/100 g/min in the 1st measurement and 1.6 ml/100 g/min in the 2nd in the right leg; and in the left leg, they were calculated as 0.53 and 1.5 ml/100 g/min. Therefore, it was concluded that the measurement of resting blood flow was not suitable to evaluate the severity of circulatory disturbance in patients with occlusive arterial disease and also was not beneficial to evaluate the improvement in the peripheral circulation by the medical treatment.

On the other hand, the data obtained from the measurement of postischemic reactive blood flow is satisfactory in evaluating the effectiveness of the drug treatment, because its repeat variability was in a narrow range (Table I) and it succeeded in separating the affected leg from the non-affected leg as shown in the following 2 figures. Figure 3 shows reactive blood flow obtained in a 66-year-old healthy man and in a 74-year-old man with hypertension.

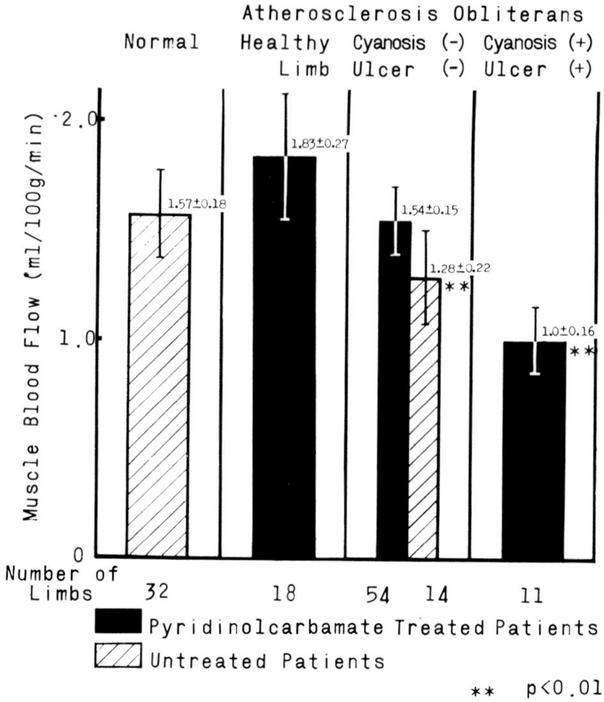

Fig. 1. Blood flow through tibialis anterior muscle measured by ^{133}Xe.

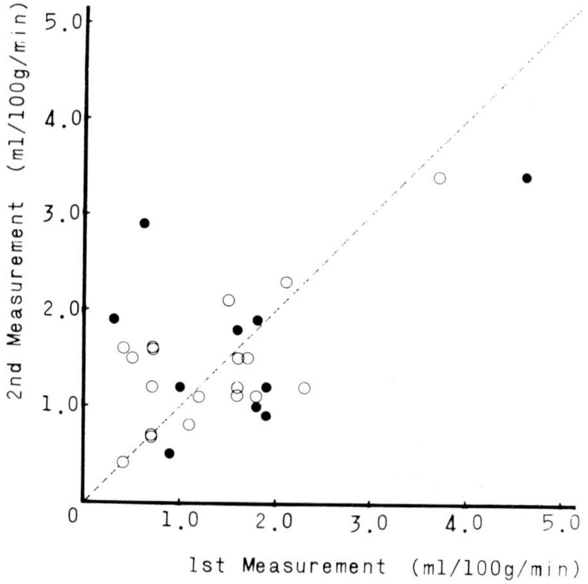

Fig. 2. Difference between 1st and 2nd measurements of muscle blood flow.
• Affected limbs. ○ Healthy limbs.

TABLE I

Repeat variability of reactive blood flow through anterior tibial muscle measured by ^{133}Xe

	1	2	3	4	Mean	SD
M.M. 31 yr male	11.5	10.5	10.1	12.0	11.0	±0.44
H.K. 70 yr male	13.5	11.4	12.8	9.5	11.8	±0.88

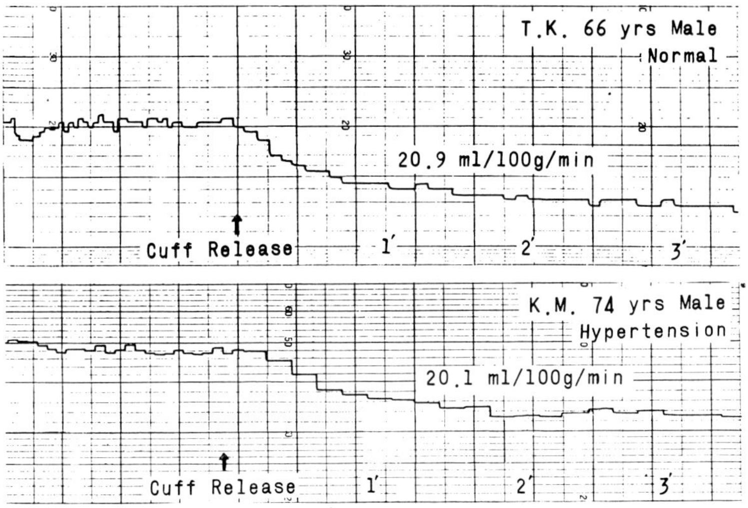

Fig. 3. Reactive blood flow through anterior tibial muscle in a healthy male and in a hypertensive patient.

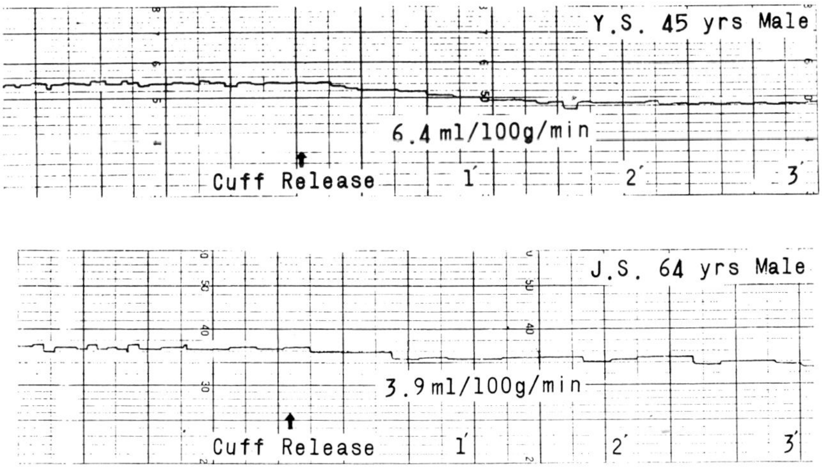

Fig. 4. Reactive blood flow through anterior tibial muscle in 2 patients with atherosclerosis obliterans.

Mean muscle blood flow was calculated during the first 30 sec after restoring rapid blood flow. Reactive muscle blood flow was 20.9 and 20.1 ml/100 g/min in these individuals. On the other hand, postischemic reactive muscle blood flow decreased to 6.4 and 3.9 ml in 2 patients with atherosclerosis obliterans (Fig 4).

Postischemic reactive blood flow was 19.6±1.2 ml/100 g/min in normal limbs, 13.0±2.56 ml/100 g/min in 6 limbs of hypertensive patients, 9.3±1.52 ml/100 g/min in 11 patients with atherosclerosis obliterans who had not been treated with pyridinolcarbamate and 11.7±1.26 ml/100 g/min in 45 patients treated with pyridinolcarbamate. Reactive blood flows in the latter 3 groups were significantly decreased from those in the normal subjects, although resting blood flow did not show any statistically significant difference between these 4 groups (Fig. 5).

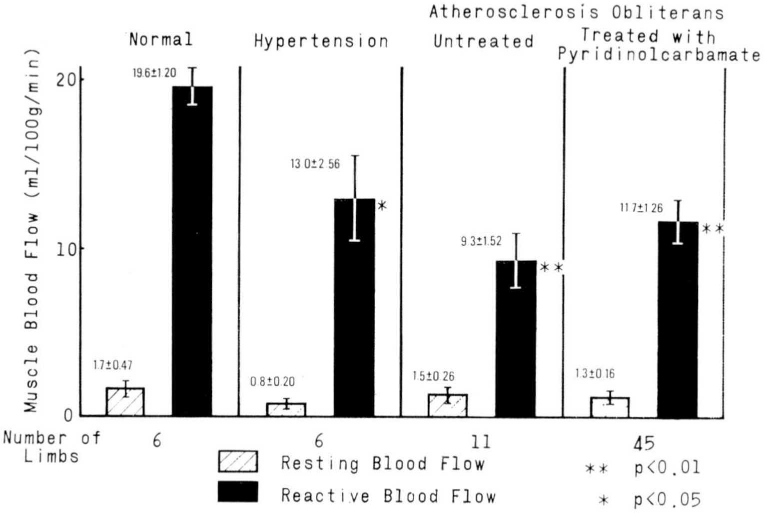

Fig. 5. Resting and postischemic reactive blood flow through anterior tibial muscle measured by ^{133}Xe.

As already known, the crest time on a toe plethysmogram is prolonged in patients with occlusive arterial disease, and the plethysmogram is not recorded as a wave in severely affected legs. In the upper diagram of Figure 6, mean resting blood flow is classified into 5 groups according to the length of crest time. As you can see, there are no statistically significant differences in the resting blood flow among these 5 groups. However, reactive blood flow tended to decrease as the crest time was prolonged as shown in the lower diagram. The mean reactive blood flow was 15.4±1.9 ml/100 g/min in the unaffected limbs whose crest time was under 0.2 sec. However, it was 7.7±0.94, 7.9±1.65 and 7.7±2.10 ml/100 g/min in the affected limbs whose crest time was 0.3–0.4 sec, 0.4–0.5 sec, and in the severely affected limbs whose plethysmograms were not recorded as a wave. There were statistically significant differences between these latter 3 groups and the normal group.

Serial measurement of reactive blood flow was performed in 7 patients with atherosclerosis obliterans for 2–50 weeks of continuous treatment with pyridinolcarbamate (Fig. 7). Reactive blood flow was increased after pyridinolcarbamate in 6 out of the 7 patients. In one patient, reactive blood flow decreased after the initial temporary increase. This patient showed a slight improvement in claudication within the first 5 weeks of treatment. However, intermittent claudication deteriorated thereafter, although he was continuously treated with pyridinolcarbamate.

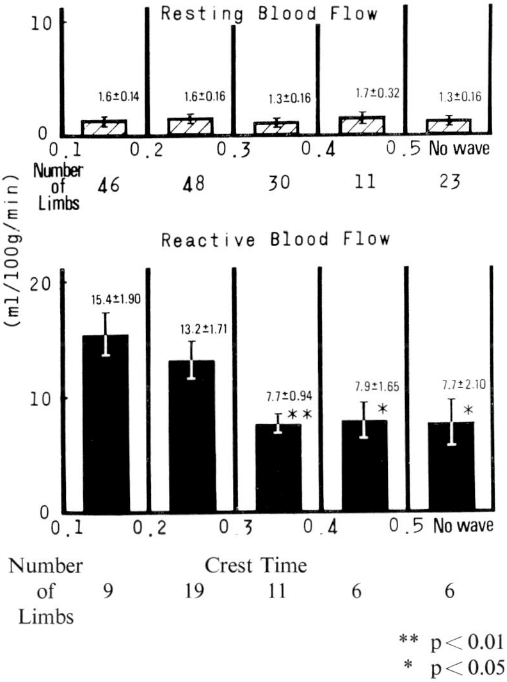

Fig. 6. Correlation between crest time in the plethysmogram and blood flow through anterior tibial muscle measured by ^{133}Xe.

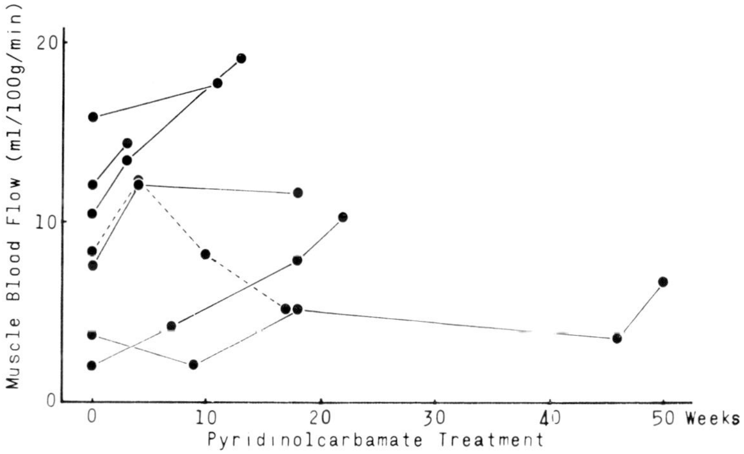

Fig. 7. Reactive blood flow through anterior tibial muscle in patients with atherosclerosis obliterans treated with pyridinolcarbamate.

Finally, I will describe one case whose reactive blood flow through anterior tibial muscle was serially measured before and after pyridinolcarbamate treatment. This patient had complained of intermittent claudication and had to stop twice when walking about 200 meters. Reactive blood flow was 2.0 ml/100 g/min before treatment. Blood flow increased to 4.0 ml/100 g/min after 7 weeks of treatment. At this stage, intermittent claudication was so improved that he stopped only once when walking the same distance. Thereafter, blood flow

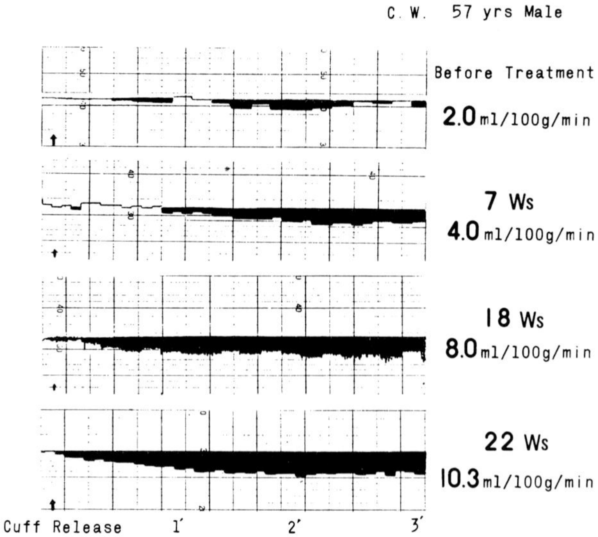

Fig. 8. Serial recordings of reactive blood flow through anterior tibial muscle in a patient with atherosclerosis obliterans treated with pyridinolcarbamate.

increased to 8.0 and 10.3 ml/100 g/min after 18 and 22 weeks of treatment, respectively (Fig. 8). Ultimately, his symptoms improved and he was able to walk the above-mentioned distance without stopping.

In conclusion, the measurement of reactive blood flow using the ^{133}Xe clearance method seems to be useful in evaluating objectively the effectiveness of pyridinolcarbamate treatment in patients with atherosclerosis obliterans.

PERIPHERAL ARTERITIS – INFECTIOUS AETIOLOGY

J. G. BERNARD and E. MOREL
108, Boulevard Raspail, Paris 6e, France

In hypersensitivity reactions of whatever kind the vascular system plays an important role. It carries antigens, antibodies, soluble complexes and complement, immunocompetent cells, mastocytes, eosinophils, neutrophils, and polynuclear cells.

The fixation of antigens on the vascular endothelium is possible including bacteria, rickettsiae, and viruses.

According to the circumstances it induces:

1. An instant hypersensitivity reaction by acquired anaphylactic antibodies (IgM, IgA) and spontaneous anaphylactic antibodies (IgE) (Fig. 1).

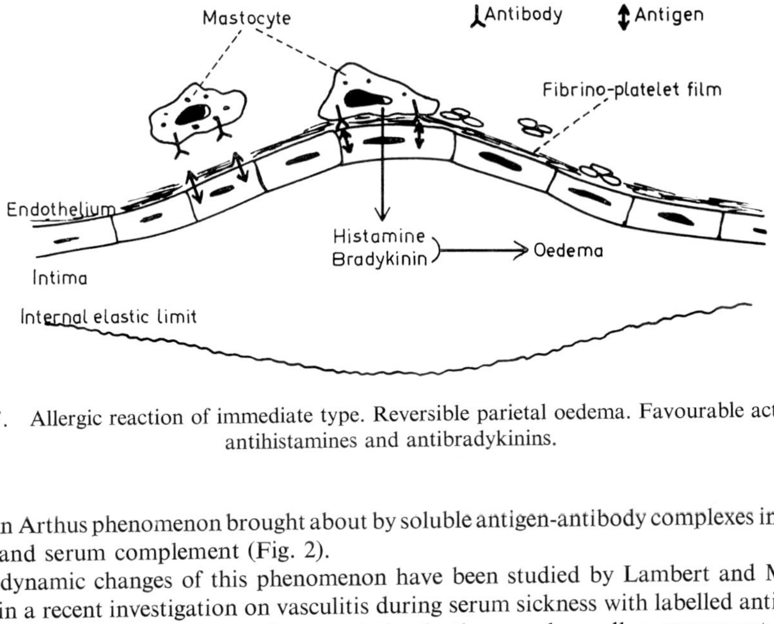

Fig. 1. Allergic reaction of immediate type. Reversible parietal oedema. Favourable action of antihistamines and antibradykinins.

2. An Arthus phenomenon brought about by soluble antigen-antibody complexes in antigen excess and serum complement (Fig. 2).

The dynamic changes of this phenomenon have been studied by Lambert and Miescher (1971) in a recent investigation on vasculitis during serum sickness with labelled antigen and antibodies. They observed an antigen persisting in the vascular wall, a permanent reaction with the circulating antibodies which turned the soluble antigen-antibody complex into large insoluble complement-fixing complexes, and continual replacement of the antibodies fixed on the vascular walls.

3. A phenomenon of late hypersensitivity, with emigration of immunocompetent or normal round cells out of the capillary and the constitution of a perivascular lymphocytic cuff which is typical of the inflammatory granuloma and able to damage the vasa vasorum of the large arteries.

4. A Sanarelli-Shwartzman phenomenon (Fig. 3) in which two different proteins act: one leads to polynuclear margination, the other to rupture of the leukocytic lysosomes and

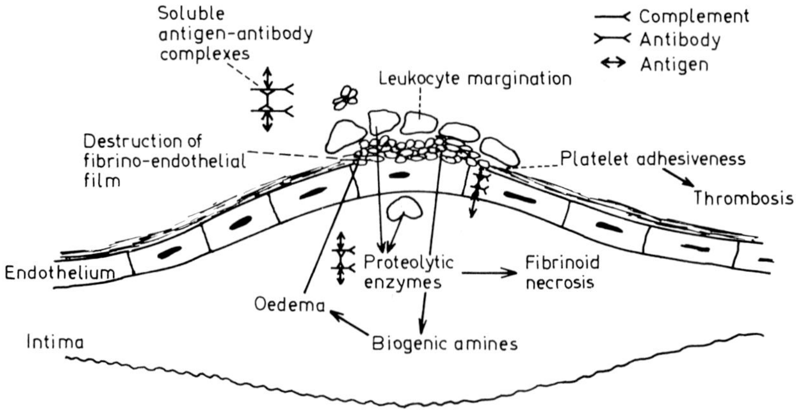

Fig. 2. Arthus phenomenon – soluble antigen-antibody complexes. Intimal necrosis due to lesion. Protective effect of heparin.

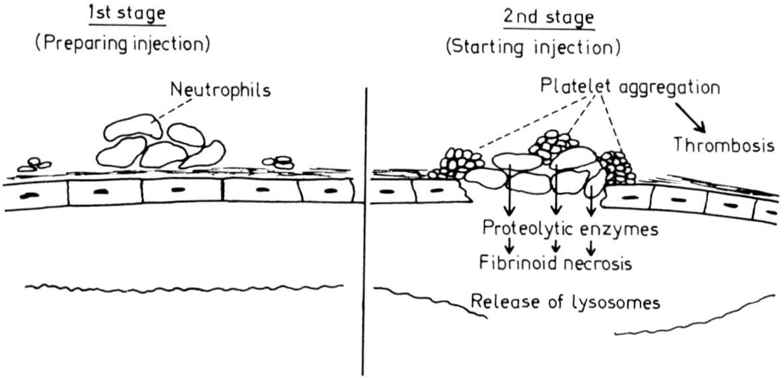

Fig. 3. Sanarelli-Shwartzman phenomenon. Protective effect of heparin.

destruction of the fibrin-platelet clot and vascular endothelium, liberating proteolytic enzymes.

This short introduction indicates how much the vascular wall is subject to numerous kinds of attack, which all cause a more or less reversible vascular intimal injury, particularly reproducible as long as the antigen remains.

The early, rapid vascular complications of infectious diseases are less known nowadays than in the past because of the rapid action of antibiotics. The rickettsiae show a particular affinity for the arteriolar capillary system (Fraenkel nodule) or the vascular system as is shown by the frequency of arteritis of the viscera and limbs in rickettsial diseases. However, everybody agrees on the presence of more slowly progressing forms with incomplete regression (Dawidowskie, 1924). In 1943, at autopsy of Russian prisoners killed by typhus, Schopper noticed many cases of clinically undiagnosed thrombotic endarteritis. In 1914, having described thromboangiitis obliterans in the same population in which Brill in New York had noticed recurrent typhus, Buerger suspected a rickettsial aetiology. This idea was followed by many authors (Goodman, 1917, 1941) between the two World Wars, but the suspected infectious aetiology was never proved. It became forgotten among the many clinical details which were linked to the clear anatomical description of Buerger. It was hidden by all the metabolic, neuroendocrinological aetiology which we regard as a consequence and not as a cause of the initial rupture of the arterial intima, progressive changes that follow the specific injury and replace by degrees the initial inflammatory features.

In 1958, with P. Giroud and our research fellows (Bernard et al., 1959), we proved not only its clinical and histological reality, but also its serological and microbiological reality (strain isolation). Since that time, these observations have been confirmed by other authors (Rollier, 1959; Nicolau, 1964). Brill's and Buerger's first hypothesis, as well as their students' and successors' work, has been confirmed, thanks especially to the contribution of serological techniques.

Rickettsial infection manifests itself after an incubation period of 2 or 3 weeks through a sharp clinical attack which conforms with the classical description of endemic typhus by Prowaczeki. Its spread affects the vascular system where it becomes clinical (vascular gangrene, acute arteritis, etc.) or latent (strain isolation from vascular fragments, Fraenkel nodules, etc.). The clinical improvement is not connected with the disappearance of the rickettsiae from the organism. The rickettsiae remain present as is proven by the frequent occurrence of relapses.

The idea of latent infection, proved by Nicolle as far back as 1909 (Nicolle and Conseil, 1952), explains either the long incubation or clinical relapses occurring after an initial phase of unapparent infection. It depends on a precarious immunological balance between the host and the infectious agent which was called 'premunition immunity' by Sergent et al. (1949) and is indicated by the persistence of specific antibodies. This immunological state and its possible variations due to specific, para-specific or non-specific external influences can bring about at any time one of the intimal injury mechanisms from each of the pathogenic routes shown in Figure 4. Rickettsiae have a particular affinity for the lymph nodes (Price, 1955) and the vascular endothelium.

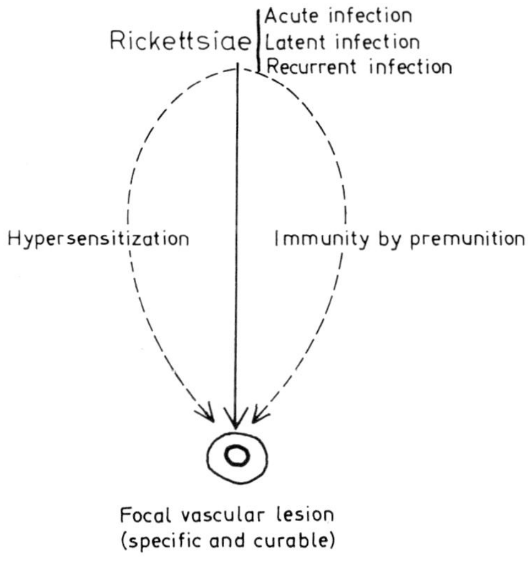

Fig. 4. Pathogenic routes of intimal injury.

This effect is not specific to the rickettsiae. Let us mention the bacterial endotoxins, particularly salmonella, which we studied in 1964. The intimal injury releases chemical intermediaries, disturbs neurohormonal regulator systems, and induces proteolytic enzyme activation and blood coagulation variations. Some other noxious agents can interfere with this.

When irreversible intimal injury occurs (Fig. 5) as a consequence of the hypersensitivity

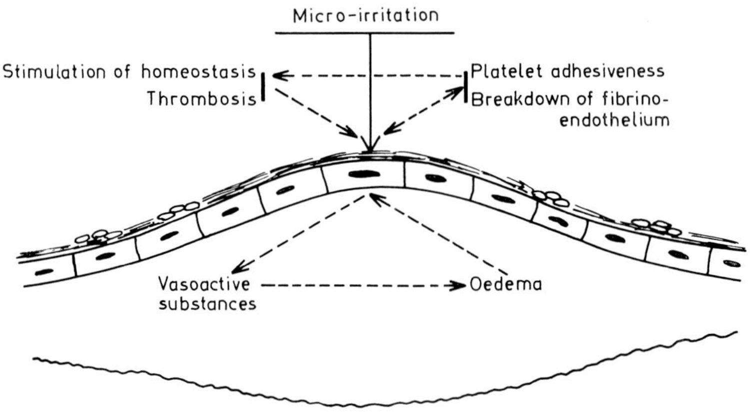

Fig. 5. Non-specific lesion stage of allergic and para-allergic stress.

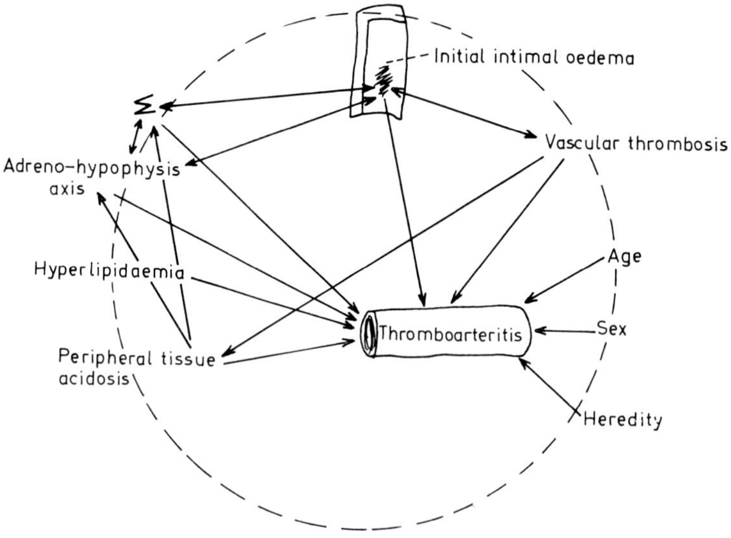

Fig. 6. Pathogenetic vicious circle leading to the clinical lesion.

conditions mentioned under Sections 1, 2 and 3, a pathogenic vicious circle is set up (Fig. 6) depending partly upon the lesion itself, which constitutes an irritating vagosympathetic and endocrine centre, and partly upon the patient (heredity, age, metabolic habits, etc.). At this stage of endarteritis obliterans the initial specific lesions loose their specificity and have the appearance of a common arteriosclerotic lesion.

According to this hypothesis, Anginin in the initial or postspecific period exerts 2 main effects of its own: (*a*) on the vasoactive tissue substances set free by the infectious injury (in particular due to its antibradykinin effect); and (*b*) on haemostasis due to its antagonistic effect on platelet adhesiveness and thromboplastin stimulation.

Thus we return, on the one hand, to Shimamoto's initial hypothesis about Anginin's preventive action – in which it acts directly on the vascular endothelium but not on the vasa vasorum (or secondarily at that level) – and, on the other hand, to our clinical observations on the more efficient action of the drug during periods of inflammatory aggravation of the arterial disease.

SUMMARY

Certain infections, in particular with rickettsiae, have a known affinity for the vascular walls. Their persistence in this location, once the frequently subclinical invasive phase is over, leads to local reactions (oedema, microthromboses, etc.) in connection with variations in Arthus-type or delayed hypersensitivity, or in the patient's immunological condition. With the occurrence of non-specific reactions, a positive vicious circle, in which the chief part is played by irritation of the autonomic nervous system and imbalance of the pituitary-adrenal axis, is set up. Its final result is thrombogenic endarteritis in which the infections and immunological factors, even if they persist, have lost their pathogenic character but with resultant sclerosis of the walls and thrombosis of the vascular lumen.

REFERENCES

BERNARD, J. G. (1964): Endotoxines bactériennes et lésions du système vasculaire. *Rev. Immunol. (Paris)*, *28*, 251.

BERNARD, J. G., GIROUD, P., PFISTER, R. and HUGONOT, R. (1959): Le problème étiologique des thromboartérites oblitérantes du jeune adulte. *Sem. Hôp. Paris*, *35*, 326.

BUERGER, L. (1914): Is thromboangiitis obliterans an infectious disease? *J. Surg. Gynec. Obstet.*, *19*, 582.

DAWIDOWSKIE, J. W. (1924): Die pathologische Anatomie und Pathologie des Fleckfiebers. *Ergebn. allg. Path. path. Anat.*, *20*, 571.

GOODMAN, C. (1917): Thromboangiitis obliterans. Further confirmation of its relation to typhus fever. *Med. Rec.*, *92*, 275.

GOODMAN, C. (1941): Thromboangiitis obliterans and typhus. *J. Mt Sinai Hosp.*, *7*, 391.

LAMBERT, P. and MIESCHER, P. A. (1971): Aspect dynamique de la pathogénie des vascularites d'origine allergique. *Schweiz. med. Wschr.*, *101*, 1797.

NICOLAU, S. S. (1964): Recherches sur l'étiologie rickettsienne et pararickettsienne de certaines angiopathies - Rapport. In: *Proceedings, V International Congress of Angiology, Paris, 1964.*

NICOLLE, C. and CONSEIL, E. (1952): *Typhus Exanthématique – Nouveau Traité de Médecine, Vol. II.* Masson et Cie, Paris.

PRICE, W. H. (1955): Survivance interépidémique du virus du typhus épidémique. *J. Bact.*, *69*, 106.

ROLLIER, R. (1959): Artériolites, thrombophlébites, gangrènes insulaires bénignes – acropathies mutilantes, rickettsioses et néo-rickettsioses. *Bull. Soc. franç. Derm.*, *3*, 333.

SERGENT, E., PARROT, L., HORRENBEGER, R. (1949): De la prévention des épidémies de typhus exanthématique en Afrique du Nord. *Bull. Acad. nat. Méd. (Paris)*, *133*, 62.

SCHOPPER, W. (1943): Zur Pathologie des Fleckfiebers. *Virchows Arch. path. Anat.*, *310*, 70.

CLINICAL USE OF PYRIDINOLCARBAMATE IN PATIENTS WITH AORTITIS SYNDROME

T. KOKUBU

Department of Medicine, Osaka University Hospital, Osaka, Japan

At the First International Symposium, I presented our experience with pyridinolcarbamate administered to patients with aortitis syndrome, especially pulseless disease or so-called Takayasu's disease. Since then, the number of patients treated with pyridinolcarbamate has increased to 11 and the administration period ranges from 3 months to 5 years. Improvement was judged on the basis of the following findings as seen in Table I. For clinical evaluation of pyridinolcarbamate treatment in pulseless disease, our attention was mainly focussed upon objective findings, especially the sonogram from upper-limb arterial blood flow which was repeatedly estimated by means of the ultrasonic Doppler technique. In 6 out of 11 cases successful results were obtained, 4 cases showed no change, and in 1 case the severe aortitis syndrome was worsened.

I would like to describe one case (Fig. 1) of a 21-year-old man admitted to our clinic in April, 1965, with inflammatory signs and symptoms. Angiography revealed that the left

TABLE I

Clinical evaluation of pyridinolcarbamate in pulseless disease

1. Subjective complaints
   - Attacks of dizziness and syncope
   - Coldness, paresthesia or fatigue in the arms
   - Cerebral symptoms on postural change
   - Shoulder pain, headache, etc.
2. Objective and laboratory findings
   - Status of pulsation in radial artery
   - Blood pressure (R, L)
   - ESR
   - Leukocyte count
   - CRP reaction, RA, ASLO, Rose-Waaler
3. Estimation of blood flow in upper-limb arteries by means of ultrasonic Doppler technique (Kaneko, Shiraishi)

TABLE II

Liver function tests in the course of pyridinolcarbamate treatment

Case	Months treated	Icterus index	Kunkel(U)	GPT(U)	GOT(U)	Al-pase(U)
1	51	5	5	41	32	7.5
2	3	10	7	42	26	5.0
6	15	5	7	6	14	6.5
7	23	5	5	34	27	
9	3	5	7	22	22	11.5
11	8	5	7	32	22	5.0

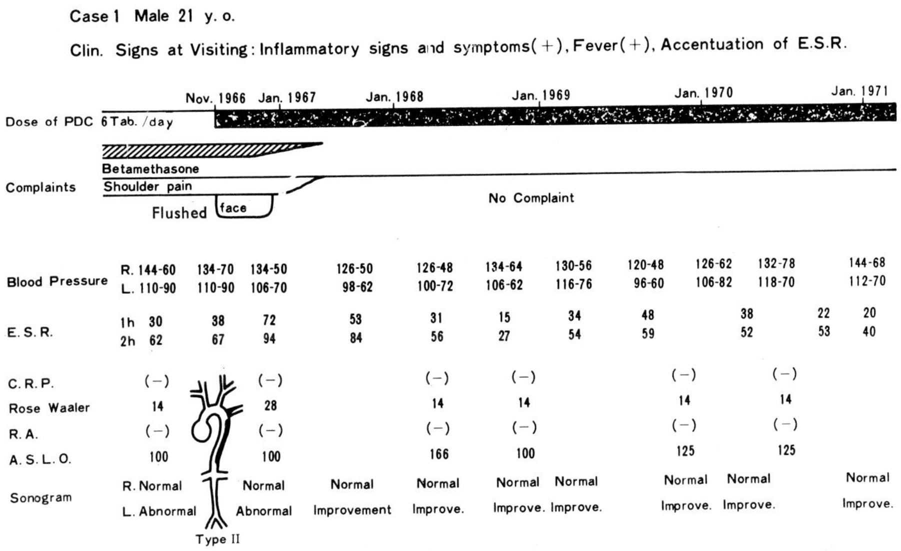

Fig. 1. Male patient, 21 years of age. Clinical signs at examination: inflammatory signs and symptoms (+), fever (+), accentuation of ESR.

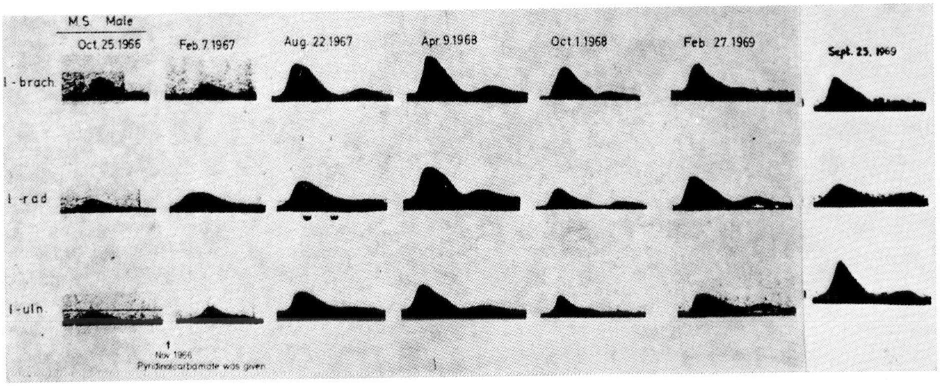

Fig. 2. Abnormal sonographic patterns from left-side upper-limb arteries of patient seen in Fig. 1.

subclavian artery was markedly narrowed. He was immediately given corticosteroid therapy until April, 1967. After disappearance of the inflammatory signs and symptoms, he received only pyridinolcarbamate treatment over a period of 5 years. The patient had normal sonograms from the right brachial, radial and ulnar arteries.

Figure 2 shows abnormal sonographic patterns from the left-side upper-limb arteries of the patient. These sonograms indicate the decrease of blood flow from the upper-limb arteries. It can be seen that improvements in patterns are obtained at about 5 months after the beginning of pyridinolcarbamate administration.

As side-effects, in a few patients gastrointestinal disturbances, such as nausea, epigastric pain and anorexia, were observed in the early stages of treatment. However, no liver damage was observed in liver function tests (Table II).

In summary, after disappearance of the inflammatory process, the long-term use of pyridinolcarbamate might be effective for the improvement of blood flow of peripheral arteries in Takayasu's disease.

CLINICAL EXPERIENCE WITH PYRIDINOLCARBAMATE IN VENOUS DISEASES

CL. ELBAZ
7, Rue de Passy, Paris 16e, France

I would like to discuss my experience with pyridinolcarbamate in certain types of venous pathology. Pyridinolcarbamate was given in the treatment of complications of varicose veins and for sequelae of the postthrombotic syndrome.

1. Varicosities and edema (6 cases)

Edema regressed rapidly in 5 out of 6 cases.

2. Varicose ulcers (22 cases)

This is the most important part of our clinical experience. We made a selection of severe ulcers, treated for months by classical methods without any improvement and complicated by indurated cellulitis and eczema.

The results of our experience are as follows:
a. Action on the ulcer: Complete healing, 16 cases; improvement, 7 cases; no change, 4 cases.
b. Action on pain: Excellent results in 15 out of 21 cases. Most of the time it goes together with healing of the ulcer but sometimes appears alone, long before healing, 2 or 3 days after the treatment starts. One can ask whether pyridinolcarbamate has an analgesic action by itself.
c. Action on indurated cellulitis: The action is less evident but it is known that it takes a long time to heal: Complete healing, 5 cases; improvement, 11 cases.
d. Action on eczema is quite good with improvement and healing in 8 out of 9 cases.
e. Action on edema: We observed excellent results especially in very severe chronic edema involving the whole leg in spite of compression and classical treatment.

3. Postthrombotic syndrome (11 cases)

In 9 out of 11 cases, we noticed improvement of all the symptoms, especially of edema, but also the healing of painful ulcers and a decrease in inflammatory cellulitis. But the treatment has to be extended over 2 or 3 months.

4. Inflammatory cellulitis (22 cases)

Indurated cellulitis is one of the most severe complications of varicose veins and its treatment is very difficult and disappointing because of the interaction of venous insufficiency with lymphatic stasis and arteriolar spasm. In 14 out of 22 cases we noticed a good improvement as a result of treatment with pyridinolcarbamate. Redness decreased and the tissue became less swollen.

In conclusion, the results of our experience with pyridinolcarbamate in the treatment of severe venous diseases are quite good.

DYNAMIC FLUORESCEIN ANGIOGRAPHY

A New Method for Assessment of Skin Circulation of the Limbs in Peripheral Arterial Disease*

F. LUND and S. LUND
Stureby Sjukhus Geriatric Unit, Enskede, Stockholm, Sweden

INTRODUCTION

In peripheral obliterative arterial disease the danger to the limb and possibly to the life of the patient arises not from a deficiency of blood flow through exercising muscles as in claudication, but from interference with blood flow through the skin of the distal parts.

Many of the methods for investigation of peripheral circulation concern muscular blood flow but there are also some which assess skin circulation. In fact, digital plethysmography, whether the venous occlusion procedure or pulse volume recording with analysis of the pulse contour and amplitude (Lund, 1955; Lund and Hellström, 1969; Strandness, 1969; Hallböök, 1971) are used, measures mainly circulatory conditions of the skin. Recording of digital pulsations by means of a strain gauge is also used in measurement of blood pressure in the digits (Gundersen, 1972; Lassen et al., 1972). Other techniques which primarily measure skin blood flow are thermometry and thermovision-thermography (with recording of long-wave infrared radiation) as well as clearance studies by use of radioisotopes (Kövamees, 1968; Larsen, 1972).

During recent years, interest in our laboratory has been focussed upon 2 other methods, viz. vital capillary microscopy (Fagrell and Lund, 1969; Fagrell, 1972) and the elevation-dependency tests (Lund et al., 1969, *This Volume*, pp. 281–286). Recording by standardized color photography in cases of ischemic skin lesions should not be forgotten as a simple, indirect, and very illustrative way of following changes in nutritional blood flow of the skin (Lund, *This Volume*, pp. 269–280).

Still, there is a need for additional new techniques to aid diagnosis and prognosis. This is desirable not least for evaluation of new non-surgical and surgical measures in acute as well as in chronic arterial occlusion. Furthermore, methods are required to study the degree of impaired blood flow and to delineate the lowest level of skin viability, making it easier to decide on the indications for amputation and its proper level. Recently we have developed a method for dynamic fluorescein angiography of limbs by rapid-sequence still photography. This is a new technique for assessment both of the arterial circulation time in the limbs, which is affected by macrovascular changes, and of the adequacy of skin microcirculation as revealed by the pattern of fluorescence. One major advantage of the method is that it will give an over-all view of the skin circulation in the limb by 'one single series of shots'.

This procedure is preferable to cinerecording with 8 or 16 mm film, although the latter method will give a continuous record of the natural course of the progression of fluorescence to distal parts of the limbs. The use of sequential still photography with 24 × 36 mm film permits much greater accuracy in the study of detail because of the larger size of frames, a finer-grained film emulsion, smaller aperture on exposure due to the intense flashlight and consequently a greater depth of field.

* This investigation was supported in part by a grant from the Albert and Gerda Svensson Foundation for Medical Research especially in the fields of Peripheral Circulation and Microcirculation.

In X-ray arteriography large and middle sized arteries, their main branches and also to some extent the larger collaterals are visualized. Therefore, this method is of great value in arterial reconstructive surgery and also for exact interpretation of results obtained with new indirect methods during their phase of development. However, X-ray arteriography provides little or no information on the smaller vessels and the circulatory function at the arteriolar-capillary level in the skin. Information of that type can be obtained by sequential fluorescein angiography, preferably after intra-arterial administration of the dye which gives higher regional concentrations than the intravenous route. The usefulness of intra-arterial fluorescein in peripheral arterial disease was shown by Moore and Campbell (1947) who improved wheal-fluorescence (Neller, 1945) by injecting the dye intra-arterially, and also by Guagliano (1958), Lowry et al. (1964), Schwartz (1965), and Harner et al. (1969).

However, it should be recognized that the influence of time after fluorescein injection is of the greatest importance in the evaluation of these rapidly developing and changing phenomena. Estimation of the circulation time exclusively by visual observation of the appearance of fluorescence at different levels of the limbs during illumination with a Wood's ultraviolet mercury vapor lamp and subsequent isolated photography of the fluorescence pattern, even if repeated at longer intervals (Pearson, 1968), cannot be accepted as an adequate standard of research technique. Demonstration of the inherent advantages of fluorescein angiography requires recording of the dynamic sequence of events by serial photographic exposures at short intervals starting from the very moment of fluorescein injection. Modern electronic phototechniques including fast repetitive high-power flashes and electrically driven cameras with automatic-timed exposures at very short intervals (down to 1–2 sec) render this possible.

The principle of this serial technique has been used in ophthalmology, usually after intravenous injection of fluorescein, for fluorescence photography of the retinal vessels (cf. the monograph by Rosen, 1969) and in neurosurgery for angiography of the epicerebral vessels (Feindel et al., 1967; Järpe, 1968, 1969). The method has, however, not previously been adopted for use in the field of peripheral arterial disease or otherwise for visualizing blood circulation of the skin.

In the present study the equipment for sequential fluorescein angiography of the limbs is described. A technique for bilateral injection of fluorescein into the femoral arteries is used rendering simultaneous serial fluorescein angiography of both legs possible.

EQUIPMENT

Equipment for intra-arterial injection of fluorescein (cf. Plate I, Fig. 1b) *

Cannula The 'Infart Tefnyl Cannula' (No. 35007-145 Stille-Werner AB, Stockholm) was used. It consists of an inner stylet of flexible steel wire and an outer Teflon cannula provided with a Luer lock and a stopcock (length 7 cm, outer diameter 1.45 mm and lumen 1.00 mm). In bilateral angiography both femoral arteries are cannulated.

Other parts of the injection system Teflon communication tubes (No. 33-7302 or 33-7305 Stille-Werner AB, Stockholm), also with Luer locks and stopcocks (length 20 or 50 cm, outer diameter 1.75 mm and lumen 1.3 mm) are connected to the cannulae. These parts of the injection system are joined by a Y-shaped metal tube of stainless steel (No. 25971 Kifa AB, Stockholm), to which the syringe containing the fluorescein solution is attached. This metal piece is the same as that used for bilateral contrast injection in X-ray arteriography. The syringe during and after injection should be handled at a distance from the patient in order not to disturb the photography, and the use of 50 cm extension tubes may be advisable.

Fluorescein solution An isotonic, i.e. 3.3%, solution of sodium fluorescein is prepared by dilution of a 20% base solution (Militär-Apoteket, Karolinska Sjukhuset, Stockholm) in 6 volumes of sterile distilled water. For simultaneous injection of 10 ml of the 3.3% solution of sodium fluorescein into the femoral artery of each leg a syringe of 25 or 30 ml is recommended since the 'dead space' of the

* See p. 340*a*

injection system (Y-shaped metal tube, Teflon communication tubes and cannulae) has a capacity of about 4 ml.

Photographic equipment

Camera A Nikon F electrically driven camera with cassettes for 250 exposures (24 × 36 mm) with a Micro Nikkor Auto 55 mm/3,5 lens was used. In the preliminary studies a zoom lens (Nikkor Auto Zoom 43-86 mm/3,5) was tried for rapid transition from an over-all view of the legs to close-up photography of special skin areas, e.g. the feet. However, because of the rapid spread of fluorescence from proximal to distal parts of the leg which may vary from case to case, it has been found preferable in continued studies to use 2 electrically driven cameras working simultaneously. In one of them the standard lens (Mikro Nikkor Auto 55 mm/3,5) is used for an over-all view of the whole legs and in the other a telephoto lens (Nikkor Auto 135 mm/3,5) for close-up pictures of the feet or other areas of special interest.

Illumination Two flashes of type Pro-1 fed by a generator (Profoto AB, Scheffersgatan 6-8, Stockholm) are used. The generator supplies 600 Wsec to each of the flashes with a repetitive frequency of down to 1 flash every 2 sec.

Filters An excitation filter, Schott glass filter BG 3*, is mounted in front of the flashes. A barrier filter, Schott glas filter GG 495*, is fitted to the camera lens**. The fluorescence exciting ultraviolet and blue wavelengths transmitted through the excitation filter of the flashes are unable to pass through the barrier filter of the camera, while the yellow-green fluorescence wavelengths pass freely and are recorded on the film.

Accessories for camera operation and for automatically timed exposures A 220 V rectifier and transformer, supplying 12 V to the electric motors. Relay boxes. Impulse-giving intervallometer (Pelling and Cross), for use as 'pacemaker' for flashes and cameras at a speed between 1 and 30 sec.

Film 35 mm Agfachrome 50 S Professional; 30 m = about 750 exposures.

Time marking of the pictures is achieved by means of a chronometer (a large stopwatch) with phosphorescent figures and hands, which emit an intense fluorescence when illuminated by ultraviolet light.

TECHNICAL PROCEDURE

General experimental conditions

The patient should be kept warm during examination to avoid the error associated with vasoconstriction. This is of particular importance for out-patients, who are not in bed prior to examination. Skin temperature measurements of fingers and toes (thermocouple) are used to ensure that the patient is at least moderately vasodilated. During the cold seasons of the year induction of vasodilatation may be required for out-patients and sometimes also for in-patients. Oral intake of alcohol and moderate warming of the body in a heating box are used. During investigation the legs of the patients are uncovered and the temperature of the examination room should be high, at least 25 °C, to prevent the return of vasoconstriction. A standardized technique for induction of moderate vasodilatation, with subsequent skin temperature measurements, before fluorescein examination is preferable in obliterative arterial disease to exclude false influences of vasoconstriction (cf. Lund, 1955; Lund and Hellström, 1969).

On the other hand, if in future studies the fluorescein angiography is used in vasospastic disease, vasoconstriction should not be inhibited before fluorescein injection (preferably by the intravenous route of administration). The influence of induced vasodilatation could later on be evaluated by comparison of the fluorescence pattern with the recordings during vasoconstriction.

Before fluorescein angiography, the skin of the legs should be thoroughly examined for

* Jenaer Glaswerk Schott & Gen., D-65 Mainz 1, Federal Republic of Germany.

** These filters are identical to those described by Järpe (1968) for use in fluorescein angiography of the epicerebral circulation.

ischemic or other lesions as well as for the presence and location of skin pigmentation, and edema. Pigmentation as seen in venous insufficiency may be the reason for erroneous interpretation, as fluorescence in the areas of skin pigmentation will remain fainter and spotted: or at least a normal pattern of fluorescence will be retarded. If such skin changes are observed, a preceding ordinary color photograph would seem to be advisable for later comparison with the fluorescence pictures.

Arterial cannulation and fluorescein injection (Plate I, Fig. 1b)

The areas over the femoral arteries to be catheterized were anesthetized with 1 % lignocaine (Xylocaine, Astra AB, Södertälje, Sweden). Prior to introduction of the catheter into the artery the skin should be punctured by a larger needle to avoid damage to the Teflon catheter tip as it passes through tough skin. After the artery has been punctured, the outer catheter is advanced over the stylet and pushed into the blood vessel for a distance of 2 or 3 cm while the stylet is successively withdrawn.

Neither during catheter introduction into the artery nor afterwards may the stylet be reinserted as the catheter could be perforated and part of it cut off to form an embolus. After complete withdrawal of the stylet the handle of the catheter with the stopcock is attached to the skin by adhesive plaster to ensure that the cannula will not slip out during the investigation. A Teflon communication tube is also used. The principle of the technique corresponds to that described by Westberg (1970) for cannulation of the carotid artery in cerebral X-ray arteriography by a similar but longer and somewhat softer polythene catheter.

While a similar procedure is repeated for puncture of the other femoral artery, the injection system of the side injected first is intermittently flushed with saline and checked for free flow. Finally the cannula systems of both sides are joined by the 'upper' branches of the Y-shaped metal piece. A syringe with saline is coupled to the 'lower' branch and the function of the whole system is checked by flushing and aspiration.

As soon as the photographic equipment is ready for action, the saline syringe is substituted by the syringe containing 24 ml of the 3.3 % solution of sodium fluorescein. The total contents of the syringe are now rapidly injected by hand, the injection being completed in a few seconds. Thus 10 ml of the fluorescein solution are injected into the femoral artery of each leg, as 4 ml of the solution are retained in the cannulation system.

Photographic procedure

The camera (or cameras, if another camera with a telephoto lens is used for simultaneous close-up photography of the feet) was fixed to a specially made metal support attached to the ceiling. Use of a separate free-standing camera stand was thus unnecessary. The vertical distance between camera (or cameras) and the legs of the recumbent subject was about 1.6 m.

For uniform bilateral illumination of both legs the 2 stands supporting the flashes were placed on each side of the patient in such a way that the legs were illuminated obliquely from above. A distance of 1.3 m was chosen and a lighting angle (between lamp-subject axis and lens-subject axis) of at least 55°, i.e. a total angle between both flashes and the subject of at least 110°. Shadowing of the feet during photography may easily occur if they are kept in a semivertical as well as a vertical position. This can be avoided by directing both or at least one of the flashes to some degree towards the feet. An illumination arrangement including 4 flashes might be preferable but has, however, not yet been used in our study.

The phosphorescent chronometer placed closely to the legs of the patient and the intervallometer for rapid-sequence photography are started at the moment of fluorescein injection. Exposures at intervals of 2 sec seem to be suitable during the first minute and at 4 sec during the 2nd minute. Thereafter still longer intervals (8 or 15 sec) may be used for another 2 or 3 min. Time-setting of the intervallometer can easily be adjusted gradually during the investigation.

In advanced arterial insufficiency with impending or manifest ischemic lesions of the feet the examination should properly be supplemented and concluded by separate photographs of the soles of the feet, or other areas which are not included in ordinary sequential photography. If skin circulation of, e.g., the soles is of greater interest than that of other parts of the legs, the whole study can of course be concentrated on this area and sequential photography can be focussed on the soles from the start.

By use of these exposure rates about 60 time-marked frames will be obtained. The whole of the series is at first analysed as a consecutive reproduction of the appearance and propagation of fluorescence, representing blood flow to the skin of the limbs. Later, selected illustrative exposures may be picked out for future demonstration of circulation time and fluorescence pattern.

PRELIMINARY RESULTS OBTAINED BY INTRA-ARTERIAL FLUORESCEIN ADMINISTRATION

Without sequential photography

Before the equipment for serial photography was ready for use, assessment of the fluorescence pattern after intra-arterial injection of fluorescein, using a Wood's lamp, was attempted by inspection only in 5 patients. Areas of different intensity in fluorescence were marked with color pencils and the marks were later recorded by ordinary color photography. Undoubtedly some valuable information could be obtained, particularly as regards delineation of non-viable tissues. As the fluorescence pattern is changing gradually within a few minutes following the injection, observation and recording by drawing and/or separate fluorescence photographs have to be performed at regular intervals, at least every minute. Recordings taken after 2 or 3 min proved to be more suitable for evaluation of circulatory conditions than those obtained after 1 min. However, it was difficult to follow the propagation of the fluorescence and change of its intensity by this means. The very rapid sequence of events immediately after injection, i.e. the arterial circulation time to different levels of the leg, was particularly difficult, if not impossible, to study with any acceptable accuracy. As soon as the equipment for sequential photography was set up, the former more simple procedure was abandoned. However, the experience gained during these preliminary attempts have in some technical details benefited the development of dynamic fluorescein angiography.

Sequential photography

So far, sequential fluorescein angiography has been performed in 5 cases. More extensive experience with the method has to be acquired than provided by this limited material before the method can be evaluated conclusively and before more definite instructions can be given.

The efficacy of the method will be illustrated by description of a case of acute arterial occlusion in whom fluorescein angiography was performed before and after thrombolysis of the superficial femoral artery by brinase. Further details of this case, particularly referring to laboratory examinations during the thrombolytic procedure, will be included in a separate report to be published later (Frisch and Lund, 1973). From a methodological point of view, this case is of particular interest as subsequent examinations revealed improvement of the arterial pathway in the thigh. However, foot circulation deteriorated at the same time, resulting in progressive gangrene, and this proved to be due mainly to extensive venous thrombosis of the lower leg.

The thrombolytic effect of brinase* (Protease I from the mould of *Aspergillus oryzae*) has been established clinically in acute arterial occlusion by means of repeated X-ray arteriography performed before, between and after intra-arterial infusions of the enzyme (Lund et al., 1968*a*, *b*). However, at the same time local side-effects indicating increased vascular permeability were observed (Lund et al., 1968*b*). Subsequent experimental studies in dogs demonstrated that these side-effects were mainly caused by an interaction between the X-ray contrast medium used (Urographin 60%) and degrada-

* Astra AB, Södertälje, Sweden.

tion products formed during thrombolysis (Frisch et al., 1970, 1971). By omission of the X-ray contrast, or by occlusion of the artery by means of ligature instead of thrombosis, a significant increase in vascular permeability could be avoided in these experiments. For further clinical investigations of this thrombolytic procedure another control method had to be found which was more suitable than X-ray arteriography and which could be used in addition to available clinico-physiological techniques. In fact, this need was the incitement for development of dynamic fluorescein angiography.

Case report

The patient was a 90-year-old woman, non-diabetic, with acute arterial occlusion of the right superficial femoral artery for approximately 24 hours, in all probability of thrombotic and not of embolic origin, and incipient gangrene of the foot. Examination of pulsations by palpation and by the Doppler ultrasound technique showed an arterial block beginning 3–4 cm below the inguinal ligament. The skin temperature gradient of the leg showed an upper moderate temperature demarcation line a hand's breadth below the knee joint with another colder temperature demarcation line on the distal part of the foot proximal to the toes. Oscillometry indicated arterial block located at the most proximal part of the thigh with minimal deflections up to the proximal part of the thigh. The left leg had normal findings with pulsations palpable as distal as the foot level. Reconstructive arterial surgery of the right leg could not be considered, in the opinion of the surgeons.

After the initial examination including also fluorescein angiography, brinase treatment was started. Two intravenous brinase infusions (75 and 90 mg respectively within about 1 hour) were given at 2 days' interval. After these 2 treatments the temperature difference between the 2 legs at the level of the lower leg was less than before therapy. Moreover, progression of gangrene was possibly less rapid than expected. Two days after the second intravenous infusion, an intra-arterial brinase infusion (50 mg in 1 hour) was given. Before, during and after all infusions blood samples were obtained for laboratory analysis of coagulation, fibrinolysis and protease inhibitors.

Palpation 2 days after the intra-arterial infusion revealed the surprising finding of marked arterial pulsations in the right thigh. By palpation and Doppler examination arterial pulsations could be shown as far down as 10 cm above the patella, thus even distally to the entrance of the artery into Hunter's canal. Oscillometry showed an obvious increase in deflections from proximal parts of the thigh, but from its most distal level still only minimal deflections. The temperature difference between the 2 legs at the level of the lower leg showed a further decrease.

However, the ischemia of the foot exhibited further deterioration with progression of the gangrenous changes in spite of signs apparently indicating considerable reopening of the right superficial femoral artery. This discrepancy was still more accentuated during the following days and an amputation proved unavoidable. The patient had a low thigh amputation as she would be mainly bedridden in the future because of her other diseases and as a prosthesis was not considered suitable.

The concurrently observed signs of improvement in arterial circulation of the leg and clinical deterioration of the foot gangrene stood out as confusing findings. Examination of the amputated limb provided the explanation. On the arterial side only limited thrombotic deposits of recent type were found, besides atheromatosis, e.g. a stenosis at the femoro-popliteal junction. Thus there was relatively little thrombosis of the arterial system as evidenced both by X-ray arteriography of the amputated limb and by dissection. However, extensive venous thrombosis was found in the whole of the lower leg, affecting all large veins as well as many muscular veins. Clinically, the patient had shown edema of the foot which increased during treatment. The gangrene of the foot showing progression in spite of considerable reconstruction of the arterial pathway was thus rather of venous origin than an arterial gangrene.

Fluorescein angiography A comparison between recordings before and after recanalization of the right superficial artery is illustrated in Plate I, Figures 1*a* and 1*b*. In Figure 1*a* selected exposures from the prethrombolytic fluorescein angiography have been arranged in the following vertical order (top to bottom): at the start of intra-arterial fluorescein injection, and about 20, 30, 45, 60 and 120 sec after injection. The topmost frame shows the background color of the leg itself before any fluorescence is visible. Figure 1*b* shows the corresponding arrangement of exposures selected from the postthrombolytic angiography. However, the first frame at the top illustrates the technical procedure used in bilateral intra-arterial administration of fluorescein.

After 20 sec (2nd frame from top) the comparison between Figures 1*a* and 1*b* shows a common feature, viz. fluorescence has advanced farther down the diseased right leg than the healthy left leg. This difference might seem paradoxical at first. However, in occlusion or marked stenosis of the superficial femoral artery and particularly of its proximal part, more blood is forced to the periphery through the deep femoral artery and its branches, e.g. the medial and the lateral circumflex femoral arteries, which also supply the skin of the upper thigh. It is obvious that this difference between the legs is more marked before (Fig. 1*a*) than after recanalization of the upper and middle part of the right superficial artery (Fig. 1*b*). In Figure 1*a* fluorescence extends as a luminous tongue, while the border is more distinct in Figure 1*b*.

Furthermore, in Figure 1*a* the anterior area of the right knee exhibits an early fluorescence in contrast to the darker distal part of the thigh, especially its medial aspect which shows no fluorescence at all. These colored spots at the knee correspond to a descending branch from the lateral circumflex femoral artery which also originates from the deep femoral arterial system. Fluorescence of the right knee can also be observed in Figure 1*b*, possibly a little less luminous. In the left leg there is no knee fluorescence, neither in Figure 1*a* nor in Figure 1*b*.

After 30 sec (3rd frame from top) a darker triangular field, the contours of which were already being drawn after 20 sec, is observed in the medial lower region of the right thigh in Figure 1*a*. This fluorescence defect is interpreted as a sign of occlusion of the superficial femoral artery blocking the origin of branches which supply that skin area with blood. In Figure 1*b* this region shows fluorescence, indicating blood flow through corresponding branches of the superficial femoral artery which have been reopened by the thrombolytic procedure.

After 45 sec (4th frame from top) the darker triangular field in the lower medial region of the right thigh is still visible in Figure 1*a*. In this phase fluorescence descends down to the upper part of the lower legs in the left as well as in the right thigh. In the right leg there is also a fluorescent area at the ankle while on the left, healthy side serving as a control the plantar side of the foot and the toes are luminous because of blood conveyed directly to these areas via deep arteries of the lower leg. After thrombolysis (Fig. 1*b*) the fluorescence of the right side also includes parts of the distal lower leg due possibly to reopening of the saphenous branch of the descending genicular artery from the superficial femoral artery. On the left control side fluorescence has in fact been retarded as compared to the same phase of the initial examination (Fig. 1*a*). This occurs both in the proximal lower leg and in the soles and toes. The delay may be secondary to general circulation factors, or possibly also to some difference between the 2 sequences in respect of synchronization of fluorescein injection and start of chronometry. Whatever the cause of this delay on the left side may be, the simultaneously occurring increased spread on the right side to the distal lower leg should be interpreted as a sign of improved blood flow through the skin-supplying branches and collaterals of the main arteries.

After 60 sec (2nd frame from bottom) most of the right foot in Figure 1*a* is still dark and a border of fluorescence is seen rather high up on the foot. The left control leg now demonstrates a more or less intense over-all fluorescence involving also the distal parts of the lower leg and the dorsum of the foot, with the exception of some black spots. These patches, which cause a certain irregularity of the pattern, are due to skin pigmentation.

In the right leg of Figure 1*b* the border of fluorescence is located a little higher up as compared to the same phase in Figure 1*a*. Now a smaller part of the heel is fluorescent than in Figure 1*a*. From the clinical and patho-anatomical point of view this finding is in accordance with the progressive nutritional deficiency of the foot due to extensive venous thrombosis of the lower leg, with subsequent circulatory arrest of the foot caused by obstruction of venous outflow. In Figure 1*b* the retardation of the spread of fluorescence in the left control leg as noticed in this series after 45 sec is again seen. In fact the actual fluorescence distribution of the left leg after 60 sec is just similar to that after 45 sec in Figure 1*a*.

After 120 sec (bottom frame): In the right leg of Figure 1*a* recorded at a time when foot ischemia was less marked, an obvious distal displacement of the border of fluorescence has occurred during the minute between the exposures at 60 sec and 120 sec. A larger part of the foot is now fluorescent, including the whole of the heel except a small dark area in which a black skin necrosis had developed. As mentioned above, the recording in Figure 1*b* was made when ischemia of the right foot was more advanced due to venous obstruction. The border of fluorescence has moved distally since the 60 sec recording, but still only to a demarcation line located rather high up on the dorsum of the foot and including solely the back part of the heel.

There is now an over-all fluorescence of the left control not only in Figure 1*a* but also in Figure 1*b*. The patchy pattern caused by pigmentations is less marked. Two black areas in Figure 1*b* located on the anterior surface of the lower leg correspond to an adhesive plaster covering a traumatic skin lesion and to a limited hemorrhage around it.

In this case unfortunately no recordings were obtained during the 3rd and 4th minute after fluorescein injection, but only after 12–15 min. Clinically progressive signs of pre-necrosis and necrosis developed as characterized by increased edema, marked discoloration, blisters and even black skin necrosis within the non-fluorescent areas of the right foot.

DISCUSSION AND CONCLUSIONS

Comments on some observations and results in the case described and others not reported here

Apparently arterial occlusion and marked stenosis of the superficial femoral artery do not in themselves prolong circulation time to the skin of the thigh as evidenced by the spread of fluorescence. On the contrary, such obliterations may in fact shorten the circulation time and speed up the spread of fluorescence, at least to the proximal and lateral part of the thigh, as a comparatively larger amount of blood is forced out to the periphery through branches of the deep femoral artery supplying the skin. Also, for the same reason assessment of the inguinal

→

Fig. 1a, b. 90-year-old woman with acute arterial occlusion of right superficial femoral artery, in all probability of thrombotic and not of embolic origin. Left leg, normal findings.
Considerable thrombolysis of right femoral occlusion by brinase treatment. Nevertheless, deterioration of foot ischemia because of concomitant extensive venous thrombosis in the lower leg.
Selected fluorescein angiograms (about 20, 30, 45, 60 and 120 sec after injection of the dye) have been chosen from 2 rapid-sequence series: before and after arterial thrombolysis; 1 week between examinations.
Fig. 1a. Before thrombolysis of right superficial femoral artery.
Fig. 1b. After thrombolysis. This Figure also includes at the top an illustration of the procedure used in bilateral intra-arterial injection of fluorescein. The stage shown is the moment of aspiration of blood just before the syringe with saline is substituted for another containing 24 ml of 3.3 % sodium fluorescein solution. In injection 4 ml of the solution will be retained in the cannulation system.
For detailed description of the changes in skin fluorescence observed in recordings at different phases after injection of fluorescein, see text, pp. 339–340.
Note that the position of the chronometer is upside down in Fig. 1*a*!

0 sec.

20 sec.

30 sec.

45 sec.

60 sec.

120 sec.

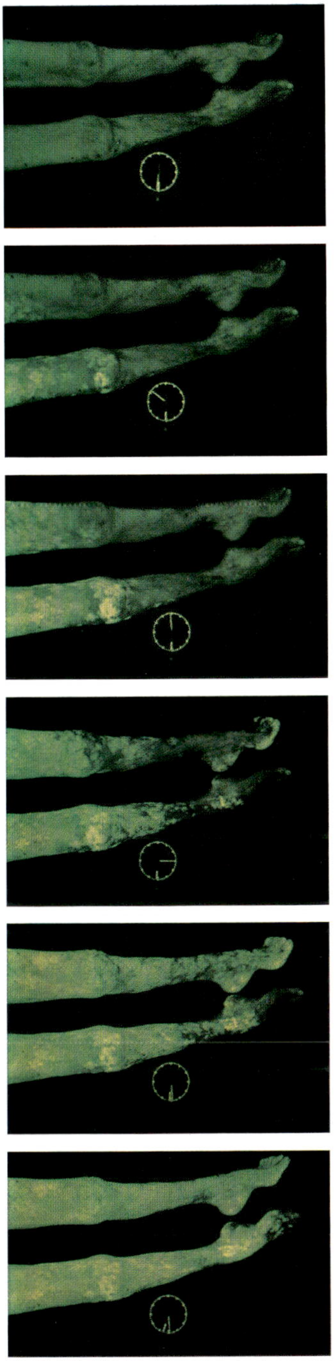

Fig. 1a

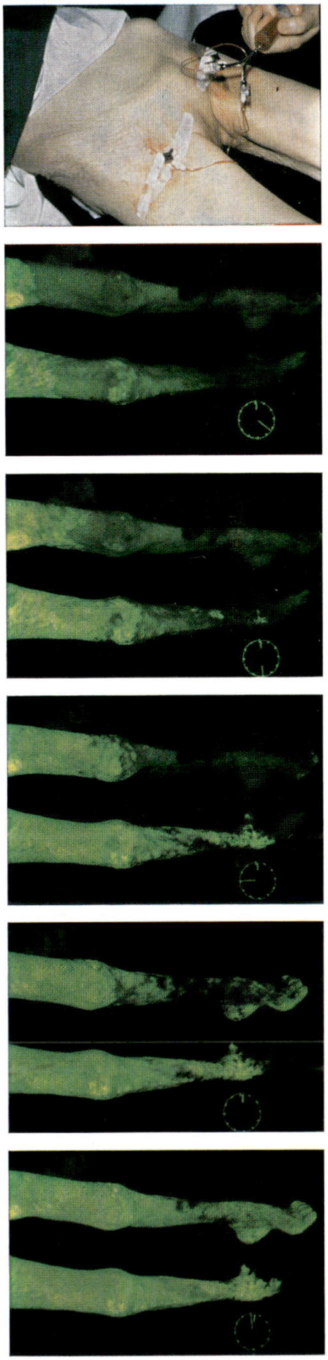

Fig. 1b

ligament–knee circulation time seems to be a very unreliable indicator, at least if a short circulation time over this distance is taken as a sign of non-obstructed arteries. The anterior side of the knee is supplied by a directly descending branch forming part of the deep femoral arterial system. If the normal pathway through the superficial femoral artery is obstructed, blood will be transferred straight down to the knee which actually will show fluorescence before the distal part of the thigh.

So far, we have not had an opportunity to demonstrate whether the same mechanism also applies to blood supply of the skin in the lower leg, e.g. in occlusion of the lower popliteal artery. However, we found in the leg without obstruction, as evidenced by extensive clinico-physiological investigation, that fluorescence as an indicator of blood supply did not gradually propagate downwards from the knee to the distal lower leg, the ankles and finally the foot. Instead, blood passed directly down to the foot, in particular to the sole and the toes, through the deep main arteries of the lower leg arriving in the foot before it reached the small of the leg.

These observations differ in fundamental points from the data on average circulation times to different levels of the legs in normals and various disease groups as given by Lowry et al. (1964). Their data were based on ocular inspection of fluorescence spread during illumination with a Wood's lamp in a total of 30 cases. Our own preliminary study by means of a similar simple set-up showed the difficulties in following the rapid propagation of fluorescence, and changes in its intensity without rapid-sequence angiography.

Furthermore, we have demonstrated that a triangular dark field may for some time be observed in the lower medial region of the thigh if the upper superficial femoral artery is occluded. This implies retarded blood supply to that area due to obstruction of blood flow through the ordinary direct branches from the superficial femoral artery. In principle, this would seem to be the same phenomenon which Widmer and Hürliman (1966) used to localize the position of the needle in intra-arterial therapy by means of initial fluorescein injection and ultraviolet illumination.

It seems very reasonable to assume that obstruction of blood flow in other branches of the arterial system in the legs will become visible in sequential fluorescein angiography as a similar retardation of the appearance of fluorescence in the corresponding skin areas. Because of good collateral blood flow this delay does not need to be associated with any marked impairment in nutritional blood flow and danger of subsequent tissue damage. It is just a delay, possibly combined with some reduction in total blood flow.

Thus an obstruction of a main artery may have 2 consequences: (1) increased flow through branches and collaterals originating above the block, which can be recorded by fluorescein angiography if these vessels also include skin branches; (2) a reduced, or at least delayed, blood flow to skin areas which are mainly supplied by branches originating from the main artery below the beginning of the block. By using fluorescein angiography such phenomena can be recorded in moderate circulatory disturbances at more proximal levels of the limbs, e.g. in the thigh.

At the borderline of areas with severe impairment in nutritional blood flow as usually occurs in distal parts of the legs, the spread of fluorescence will be greatly retarded (impending or pre-necrosis) or definitely stopped (necrosis). A proximal transitional zone of very retarded progression of fluorescence with lower intensity seems to precede the absolute demarcation line characterized by completely blocked spread.

Our experience is limited and the whole of the problem, in particular the degree of delayed spread in severe circulatory impairment, has to be thoroughly studied in future work. Therefore recordings should be done not only at short intervals during the first 2 min after injection when things happen more rapidly but also at successively prolonged intervals during at least the next 2 or 3 min, in order to follow a possible slow spread of fluorescence. For such purposes, the combined photographic set-up will be very useful, including another camera with a telephoto lens for close-up recording of the feet.

Severely impaired circulation not only causes delayed appearance of fluorescence, but also delayed disappearance when the dye finally has entered incompletely devitalized tissues. Thus, additional information on blood flow can be obtained by subsequent follow-up. We would suggest intervals of 1-2 hours to follow the disappearance of the dye, i.e. the removal of tissue fluid. This clearance function, which also represents the degree of impaired microcirculation, is of course influenced by the presence of edema. Some interesting experimental observations on the appearance as well as on the disappearance rate of fluorescence in ischemic pregangrenous tissues were included in a study on peripheral gangrene in the rat tail (Lund, 1951).

Prognostic value of fluorescein angiography Other authors (e.g. Schwartz, 1965) have previously demonstrated the value of intra-arterial fluorescein as a prognostic test method for assessment of the healing tendency in distal circulatory disturbances and in ulcerations of the lower leg or the foot. However, they did not use serial photography. Our own preliminary studies with their more simple procedure confirmed this to some degree. The introduction of sequential fluorescein angiography means a more quantitative and exact approach in prognostic predictions, as indicated by our findings. Use of the method in a more extended patient series including normal legs and various disease groups is required.

Other comparative methods to be used in future evaluation of dynamic fluorescein angiography

There was striking agreement between the changes assessed by fluorescein angiography and those found by pulse recording methods and by measurement of skin temperature of the legs in the described case. Of particular interest was the similarity of findings obtained by skin temperature measurement. Agreement was not only found in the distal part of the leg showing severely disturbed circulation, but also the paradoxically increased spread of fluorescence on the right thigh and knee corresponded to a higher skin temperature as compared to the left thigh. Unfortunately the triangular area in the lower medial region of the right thigh showing a delay in spread of fluorescence was not subjected to a special temperature study. It will be most interesting to compare results obtained by fluorescence angiography with those assessed by the other skin circulation methods mentioned in the introduction, particularly with an over-all assessment of the surface temperature as recorded by thermography.

For better assessment of the relationship between obstructions in the major circulation and the resultant changes in skin blood flow as revealed by fluorescein angiography, ordinary clinical and indirect clinicophysiological methods alone are not sufficient. A series of cases studied also by X-ray arteriography is desirable, to be collected preferably among patients in whom reconstructive arterial surgery is considered. It would be worth attempting to combine both methods subsequently during the same investigation in order to avoid 2 separate arterial punctures. It might be expected that on the basis of such a comparative study fluorescein angiography may in future clinical work be a substitute for X-ray arteriography in many non-surgical cases where the indications for the latter method are only relative. In the actual case described in this paper X-ray arteriography, which would have been very useful for interpretation, was not performed since reconstructive arterial surgery was out of the question.

Other applications of the method

So far, we have mainly focussed our interest on the intra-arterial route of administration in peripheral arterial disease, not only in acute arterial occlusion but also in chronic cases, which are a much more common disease group. This procedure makes it possible to determine the circulation time in the legs more exactly as the dye is introduced directly into the artery itself. This results in a higher concentration of dye in the blood and thus in pictures which are more accessible for interpretation. In addition to the reported findings, isolated trials with sequential photography following intravenous administration have been made. Moreover, in the intra-arterial studies some interesting observations on the fluorescence of skin areas other than the legs after recirculation of the dye with subsequent systemic distribution were carried out.

It is therefore intended to adapt the dosage of fluorescein and the photographic technique in order to make discrimination between different intensities in skin fluorescence possible also after intravenous injection. This route of administration may be expected to extend considerably the scope of dynamic fluorescence and may be preferable, e.g. in evaluation of vasoactive drugs and other therapeutic procedures in both acute and particularly in chronic cases. It will also facilitate examination of cases with high obstructions to the aorta or the iliac arteries. Intravenous fluorescein is in itself to some degree a practical procedure in peripheral vascular disease, as already demonstrated by Lange and Boyd (1942, 1943) before the wheal fluorescence modification was introduced by Neller (1945) and later adapted by Ejrup (1953) as an exercise test.

By use of sequential photography of the skin after intravenous fluorescein challenging opportunities would present themselves for clinical research and diagnosis in such fields as heart failure, shock, burns, skin grafting and superficial tumors. This technique, preferably by the intra-arterial route, might be applied furthermore during surgery to visualize disturbed circulation in various organs, e.g. the liver, intestines, kidneys, and possibly also the heart in surgical treatment of ischemic heart disease, i.e. fields of research in some of which fluorescein examination without sequential angiography has previously been used to advantage (cf. also Schaefer and Baldwin, 1970).

For such purposes the period of development of the film, anyhow of color film, will generally constitute a great limitation and disadvantage, especially if the results are to be used as a guidance to the surgeon. Therefore, the passage of dye through the organ under study may be observed by the supplementation of photo equipment with a television camera and videotape recording. An immediate playback of the tape provides informative data without delay, although the quality of the reproduction will not be comparable to photography with ordinary film. In intra-arterial injection a smaller amount of fluorescein can be used which permits repeated angiography during operation. The television and videotape pictures may be obtained by cinephotography or possibly by rapid-sequence still photo recording. A simultaneous, permanent, high-quality record on ordinary film can be obtained by a separate camera.

Rapid-sequence infrared absorption angiography after injection of indocyanine green (Choromokos et al., 1969) represents another interesting approach to similar problems applicable particularly in experimental work but possibly also for some clinical purposes. The rapid clearance of indocyanine green by the liver almost completely within its first passage makes recirculation negligible and allows repeated recordings without background interference from residual dye in the plasma.

Comments on clinical toxicity and untoward effects of fluorescein injections

A very low toxicity of fluorescein has been a prerequisite for the extensive use of fluorescein injections, e.g. in ophthalmology and other clinical fields. This question might, however, be brought up for reconsideration as fluorescein injections are now used in patients with peripheral vascular disease who are often in a poor general condition because of old age and/or concomitant diseases. As a matter of fact, the new possibilities for the use of sequential fluorescein angiography suggested above, which are outside the fields of ophthalmology, neurosurgery and peripheral vascular disease, concern patients who probably are more easily affected by possible toxic influences. Some data on the incidence of unwanted systemic side-effects of fluorescein would therefore seem to be desirable.

In Goodman and Gilman (1966) it is quite briefly stated that practically no unwanted effects accompany the *intravenous administration of fluorescein* and that only an occasional patient may experience nausea and vomiting. It is added that injections may be repeated at intervals of several days without ill-effects. The dye is said to be non-toxic in animals.

According to Rosen (1969) transient nausea starting approximately half a minute after intravenous injection (3 ml of 25% sodium fluorescein) is reported by about 5% of patients.

Few patients actually vomit, probably depending on the gastric contents at the time of injection. Two cases of acute shock reaction to the dye have been reported in the literature, both patients having a history of asthma and hay fever. Rosen gives a small test dose of fluorescein prior to the large volume injection necessary for fluorescence photography of the eye if there are any signs in the history suggesting an allergic type of illness or previous reaction to the substance. If there is a negative history, he proceeds immediately with injection of the full fluorescein dose. Apparently a concentrated hyperosmotic solution of sodium fluorescein can be injected intravenously without local side-effects from the tissues or the recipient vessels. Correct intravascular injection is of course a condition.

In *intra-arterial injection* the danger of nausea as a systemic side-effect is less probable than in intravenous injection. On the other hand, the intra-arterial procedure may to a greater extent be accompanied by local and regional effects. The studies by Lowry et al. (1964) and by Schwartz (1965) comprised a series of more than 30 cases each receiving an intra-arterial injection of a moderately hyperosmotic fluorescein solution (5%) without any general or local complications being observed.

However, 2 points must be recalled:

1. Arterial puncture is not a harmless procedure to the vessel. It should always be performed with as gentle a technique as possible, whether a metal cannula or a Teflon catheter is used. We found a thin Teflon catheter with an outer diameter of 1.45 mm sufficient for rapid injection of the solution. The catheter need not be pushed into the artery for a distance of more than 2 or 3 cm and it is withdrawn about 5 minutes after the injection, as soon as the 'sequential phase' of photography has ended. This procedure will markedly reduce the danger of cellular aggregation and thrombosis on the catheter. After withdrawal of the catheter, compressive massage at the puncture site is essential to avoid hemorrhage.

2. The possibility cannot be excluded that a hyperosmotic fluorescein solution may have some unfavorable effects on blood cells and vessel walls when it passes directly from a larger vessel to a vascular region with a slow, possibly an extremely slow, circulation. We therefore prefer to use an isotonic solution (3.3%). This factor would not play the same role in intravenous administration where even a very hyperosmotic solution, e.g. 20 or 25%, will soon be diluted as it passes rapidly from smaller to larger vessels, at any rate before finally reaching the terminal vascular bed.

Compared with the strongly hyperosmotic contrast medium necessary in X-ray angiography, the possibility of using an isotonic solution in intra-arterial fluorescein angiography of the limbs represents an advantage which can be assumed to eliminate the danger of possible local side-effects on blood cells and the vessel wall.

SUMMARY

For dynamic fluorescein angiography of the limbs by rapid-sequence still photographic recording, fast repetitive high-power flashes and electrically driven cameras were used with automatically timed exposures at very short intervals down to 1–2 sec. This procedure is preferable to cine-recording with 8 or 16 mm film, although that method will give a continuous reproduction of the natural course of fluorescence progression to the distal parts of the limbs. The use of sequential still photographic recording with 24 × 36 mm film permits much greater accuracy in study of details because of the larger size of frames, a more fine-grained film emulsion, and more intense illumination by the flashlight.

The procedure makes possible a record of the rapidly developing and changing phenomena after injection of fluorescein corresponding to the circulation time in the limb and the microflow pattern of the skin. The principle of the serial technique has been used in ophthalmology and neurosurgery. However, it has not previously been adopted for use in the field of peripheral vascular disease or otherwise for studies of skin circulation.

Intrafemoral arterial injection of the fluorescein solution gives a higher regional concentration, a more intense fluorescence of the skin and better possibilities to discriminate between different degrees of intensity in the fluorescence pattern. A technique of bilateral injection of fluorescein into the femoral arteries is used giving simultaneous serial fluorescein angiography of both legs. The intravenous procedure is more simple and practicable. On the other hand, good photographic recording of variations in the induced fluorescence of the skin will be more complicated as the fluorescence is fainter. For some purposes this approach may prove preferable.

Clinical application of dynamic fluorescein angiography showed promising results. It may provide important diagnostic possibilities as regards the localization and extent of gross arterial obstructions, the lowest level of skin viability in acute or advanced chronic arterial obstructions, the healing probability of ischemic ulcers etc. An interesting finding in a patient suffering from acute occlusion of the superficial femoral artery was the paradoxically faster progression downwards of skin fluorescence in the thigh of the diseased leg compared to the other leg without obstruction. This phenomenon is due to increased blood flow through skin branches from the deep femoral artery originating above the block. At the same time, skin areas supplied by the superficial femoral artery showed a retarded appearance of fluorescence.

The method is useful for evaluation of therapeutic measures in acute arterial occlusion as evidenced in this case by the change in the fluorescence pattern of the skin after considerable thrombolysis of the occluded superficial artery by a thrombolytic enzyme, brinase.

Of greater importance is the possibility that dynamic fluorescein angiography may be used to advantage in the more common disease group of chronic obliterative arterial disease for the evaluation of the effect of vasoactive drugs and other treatment regimes on the long-term course of the disease.

REFERENCES

CHOROMOKOS, E., KOGURE, K. and DAVID, N. J. (1969): Infrared absorption angiography. *J. biol. photogr. Ass.*, *37*, 100.

EJRUP, B. (1953): Fluorescein after exercise: a method of investigation in peripheral arterial diseases. *Angiology*, *4*, 253.

FAGRELL, B. (1972): Vital capillaroscopy. A clinical method for studying changes in skin microcirculation in patients suffering from vascular disorders of the leg. *Angiology*, *23*, 284.

FAGRELL, B. and LUND, F. (1969): Vital capillary microscopy as a test method for therapeutic procedures in peripheral vascular diseases. In: *Proceedings, International Congress on Clinical Evaluation of Testing Methods of Vasoactive Drug Effects, Rome 1968*, p. 329. Edizione CEPI, Rome.

FEINDEL, W., YAMAMOTO, Y. L. and HODGE, CH. P. (1967): Intracarotid fluorescein angiography: A new method for examination of the epicerebral circulation in man. *Canad. med. Ass. J.*, *96*, 1.

FRISCH, P., HEDIN, L., LUND, F. and MAGNUSSON, G. (1970): Regionale intraarterielle Thrombolyse mit Protease. I. Tierexperimentelle Untersuchung über Interferenz mit Röntgenkontrastmittel. In: *Thrombose und Embolie. XII Hamburger Symposium über Blutgerinnung, 1969*, Teil B. 'Neue Möglichkeiten', p. 321. Editors: R. Marx and H. A. Thies. F. K. Schattauer Verlag, Stuttgart.

FRISCH, P. and LUND, F. (1973): Laboratory tests in arterial thrombolysis with brinase. To be published.

FRISCH, P., LUND, F., MOLLER, G., HEDIN, L. and MAGNUSSON, G. (1971): Permeability changes in the dog by repeated arteriography during regional intra-arterial thrombolysis with brinase. In: *Proceedings, VI European Conference on Microcirculation, Aalborg 1970*, p. 399. S. Karger, Basel.

GOODMAN, L. S. and GILMAN, A. (1966): *The Pharmacological Basis of Therapeutics. A Textbook of Pharmacology, Toxicology and Therapeutics for Physicians and Medical Students, 3rd ed.*, p. 1045. The Macmillan Press Ltd., New York-London-Toronto.

GUAGLIANO, G. (1958): La fluorescinografia nelle arteriopatie obliteranti chroniche periferiche. *Minerva cardioangiol.*, *6/2.*

GUNDERSEN, J. (1972): Segmental measurements of systolic blood pressure in the extremities including the thumb and the great toe. *Acta chir. scand., Suppl. 426.*

HALLBÖÖK, T. (1971): Blood flow measurements with strain gauge plethysmography in the early post-operative course after reconstructive arterial surgery of lower limb. *Acta chir. scand.*, *137*, 233.

HARNER, R. C., RHAME, D. W. and THOROUGHMAN, J. C. (1969): Intra-arterial fluorescein in the evaluation of a vasodilator drug. *Sth. med. J., 62,* 424.

JÄRPE, S. (1968): Cortical fluorescein angiography in neurosurgery. *Acta neurol. scand., 44,* 177.

JÄRPE, S. (1969): Pre-operative fluorescein angiography of the cerebral cortex. In: *Fluorescence Photography of the Eye*, Chapter 'Photography with fluorescein - further applications', p. 299. Editor: E. S. Rosen. Butterworth, London.

KÖVAMEES, A. (1968): Skin blood flow in obliterative arterial disease of the leg. *Acta chir. scand., Suppl. 397.*

LANGE, K. and BOYD, L. J. (1942): The use of fluorescein to determine the adequacy of circulation. *Med. Clin. N. Amer., 26,* 943.

LANGE, K. and BOYD, L. J. (1943): The technique of the fluorescein test to determine the adequacy of circulation in peripheral vascular diseases, the circulation time and capillary permeability. *Bull. N. Y. Med. Coll., 6,* 78.

LARSEN, O. A. (1972): Xenon-133 methods for determining peripheral blood flow and blood pressure in patients with occlusive arterial disease. *Angiology, 23,* 153.

LASSEN, N. A., TVEDEGAARD, E., JEPPESEN, F. I., NIELSEN, P. E., BELL, G. and GUNDERSEN, J. (1972): Distal blood pressure measurement in occlusive arterial disease: Strain gauge compared to Xenon-133. *Angiology, 23,* 211.

LOWRY, K., KIRKPATRICK, J. F. and THOROUGHMAN, J. C. (1964): Evaluation of peripheral vascular disease using intra-arterial fluorescein. *Amer. Surg., 30,* 35.

LUND, F. (1951): Vasodilator drugs against experimental peripheral gangrene. A method of testing the effect of vasodilator drugs on constricted peripheral vessels. *Acta physiol. scand., 23, Suppl. 82,* 43, 58.

LUND, F. (1955): Morphological analysis of the digital volume pulse as a diagnostic method. In: *Comptes Rendus, II Congrès Internationale d'Angéiologie, Fribourg (Suisse) 1955,* p. 233. Editors: L. Laszt, R. Meier and A. Müller. Editions Universitaires, Fribourg.

LUND, F. (1973): Pyridinolcarbamate treatment in peripheral obliterative atherosclerosis with ischemic skin lesions and its evaluation. *This Volume*, pp. 281–286.

LUND, F., ALGOTSSON, A. and LUND, S. (1973): Elevation and dependency tests in peripheral vascular disease. Standardization and increased accuracy by use of modern electronic photo-techniques. *This Volume*, pp. 287–294.

LUND, F. and HELLSTRÖM, L. (1969): Evaluation of oscillography and digital volume pulse recording as compared to arteriography in follow-up studies of occlusive arterial disease. With application to long-term nicotinic acid treatment. In: *Proceedings, International Congress on Clinical Evaluation of Testing Methods of Vasoactive Drug Effects, Rome 1968*, p. 199. Edizione CEPI, Rome.

LUND, F., HELLSTRÖM, L. and FRISCH, P. (1968*a*): Combined arteriography and regional thrombolytic therapy. *Opusc. med. (Stockh.), 13,* 281.

LUND, F., HELLSTRÖM, L. and FRISCH, P. (1968*b*): Side effects observed in combined arteriography and regional thrombolytic therapy with Protease I. *Opusc. med. (Stockh.), 13,* 396.

LUND, F., HELLSTRÖM, L. and FRISCH, P. (1969): Pulse recording and arteriography in a long-term study with pyridinolcarbamate. In: *Atherogenesis. Proceedings, I Symposium on Atherogenesis, Thrombogenesis and Pyridinolcarbamate Treatment, Tokyo 1969*, pp. 181–190. Editors: T. Shimamoto and F. Numano. ICS 201, Excerpta Medica, Amsterdam.

MOORE, G. E. and CAMPBELL, G. S. (1947): Intra-arterial fluorescein for evaluation of peripheral vascular disease. *Proc. Soc. exp. Biol. (N.Y.), 65,* 297.

NELLER, J. L. (1945): The use of fluorescent wheals in determining extent and degree of peripheral vascular insufficiency. *Ann. Surg., 122,* 898.

PEARSON, B. (1968): Unpublished study. Cited by Rosen (1969), pp. 300, 306.

ROSEN, E. S. (1969): *Fluorescence Photography of The Eye.* Butterworth, London.

SCHAEFER, D. T. and BALDWIN, E. L. (1970): The photography of fluorescein-dye fluorescence in surgery. *J. biol. photogr. Ass., 38,* 70.

SCHWARTZ, W. W. (1965): Intra-arterial fluorescein in the diagnosis of arterial disease in the lower extremity. *J. Amer. osteopath. Ass, 65,* 1300.

STRANDNESS JR, D. E. (1969): *Peripheral Arterial Disease*, p. 92. J. and A. Churchill Ltd, London.

WESTBERG, G. (1970): Cannula for injection of contrast medium in cerebral angiography. *Acta radiol. Diagn., 10,* 553.

WIDMER L. and HÜRLIMANN, F. (1966): Erhöht die intraarterielle Zufuhr eines Pharmakons dessen Konzentration in den Akren? *Z. Kreisl.-forsch., 55,* 410.

ANGININ IN THE TREATMENT OF PATIENTS WITH CHRONIC CORONARY INSUFFICIENCY

I. K. SHKHVATSABAYA
Miasnikov Institute of Cardiology, Academy of Medical Sciences, Moscow, U.S.S.R.

I wish to present some preliminary data of the study which is going on in the Institute of Cardiology in Moscow on the treatment of patients with coronary heart disease with Anginin. I should say that this is an ordinary trial of Anginin so I am not going to discuss scientific approaches and the scientific sides of the problem. Just some clinical experience will be presented.

Everybody knows that the problem of treatment of patients with coronary heart disease is quite difficult. It is difficult to evaluate the real effect of the drug and the effectiveness of treatment. Up to now we have experience on about 1,400 patients who have been treated with different kinds of drugs and almost all of the patients who were treated with these drugs had an approximately similar response to the drugs (about 67–80% of the patients had a positive response). It should be stressed that evaluation of treatment of such patients is very difficult because objective signs of coronary insufficiency are not very expressive. In our trial Anginin was studied under clinical conditions in a double-blind trial in 66 patients with chronic coronary insufficiency including 11 cases with the combination of atherosclerosis obliterans with the symptoms of intermittent claudication and an additional 6 patients with atherosclerosis obliterans but without symptoms of coronary heart disease. Treatment was started within 7–10 days of the control period. During this period, the patients did not receive any medicine, which gave us an opportunity to assess the clinical course of the disease and to follow the patients and their reactions to any environmental influences.

During this period we were able to make a more exact diagnosis and to assess the disease pattern (angina of effort, angina at rest or cardialgia of non-coronary origin). Correct diagnosis was very important to assess the real effect of treatment. At that time we tried to perform a physical examination of the patients including ECG, rheography, in some cases coronary angiography etc. One of the criteria of treatment which we used in this type of study was measuring of tolerance to physical strain by means of bicycle ergonometry or by measuring the walking distance. The results of our study are described below.

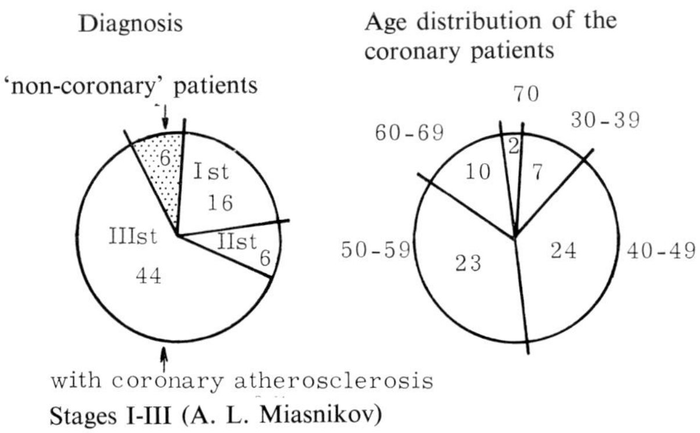

Fig. 1. Diagnosis and age distribution of patients studied.

Figure 1 shows the diagnosis in the group of patients who have been studied. They are divided into 4 groups: (1) 16 patients, with the primary stage of the disease, i.e. those patients with coronary insufficiency who have not had previous myocardial infarction; (2) 6 patients with coronary insufficiency who had recent myocardial infarction; (3) patients who had previous myocardial infarction in the past (44 patients); and (4) 6 patients who had no symptoms of coronary heart disease but had only arteriosclerosis obliterans (we called these 'non-coronary patients'). There were 72 patients in total. The age distribution was between 30 and 70, and there were 70 males and 2 females. We would prefer to have males because it would be easier to operate on them and, as you know, the clinical picture is more significant and more typical in males.

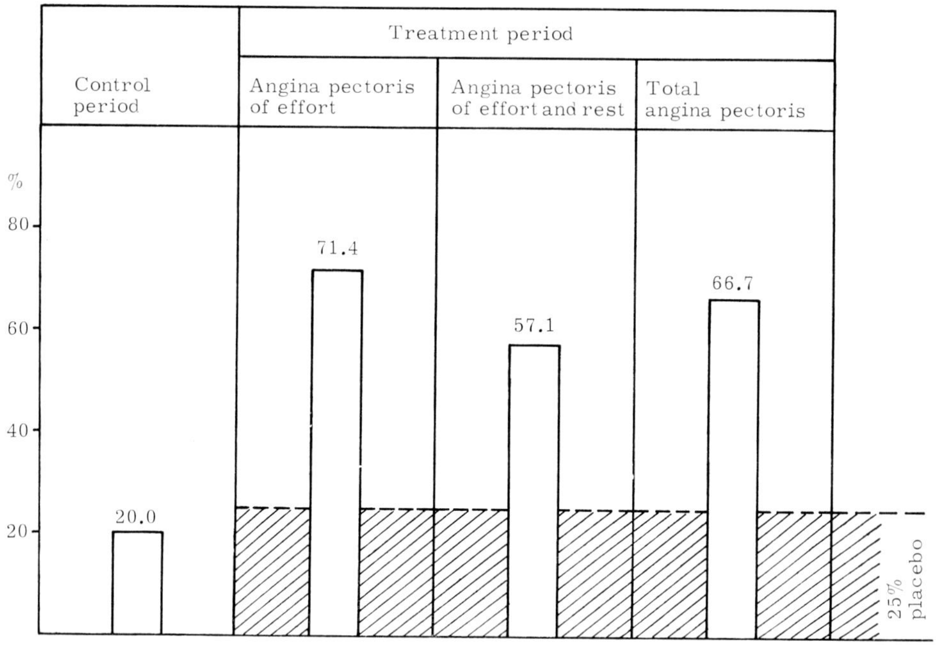

Fig. 2. Effect of Anginin treatment of chronic coronary insufficiency (double-blind trial).

Figure 2 shows the effect of Anginin treatment in patients with chronic coronary insufficiency. At the control period, positive results were observed in 20% of the patients. This is important in assessing the results of treatment. In the placebo group, which comprised 20 patients, 25% positive results were observed (5 out of 20 patients). Completely positive results (i.e. improvement in the clinical state) were observed in 66.7% of patients. However, I should like to stress the following:

We divided all patients with chronic insufficiency into two groups: one group with angina pectoris of effort and another group with angina pectoris of effort and at rest. The results were in accordance with those groups. In the first group we got positive results in 71.4%, in the second group in only 51.1%. Thus, when you treat patients with angina pectoris, it is probably reasonable to divide them into two or several groups. It depends on the interest and type of study. Figure 3 shows that the best results were obtained in patients with atherosclerosis obliterans (82.4%). Improvement of the symptoms of disease was found to be within 2–3 weeks of the treatment. In Figure 4 you can see a case with improvement in the rheograms observed 8 weeks after Anginin treatment. Figure 5 shows patients who, during

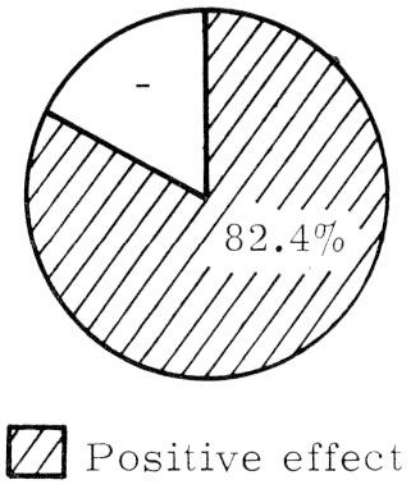

Fig. 3. Effect of Anginin treatment on atherosclerosis obliterans.

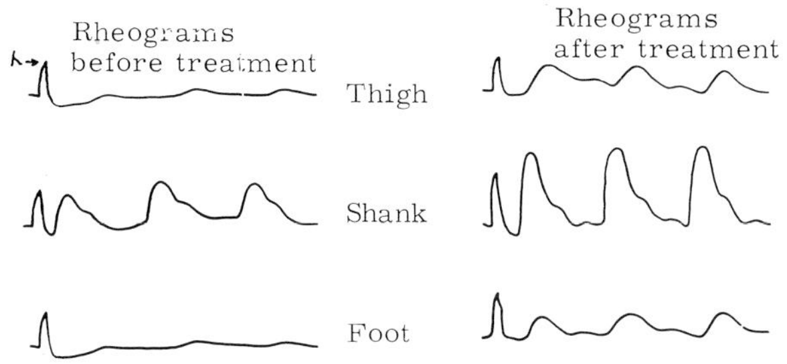

Fig. 4. Results of Anginin treatment (8 weeks) in patient S. H. with atherosclerosis obliterans.

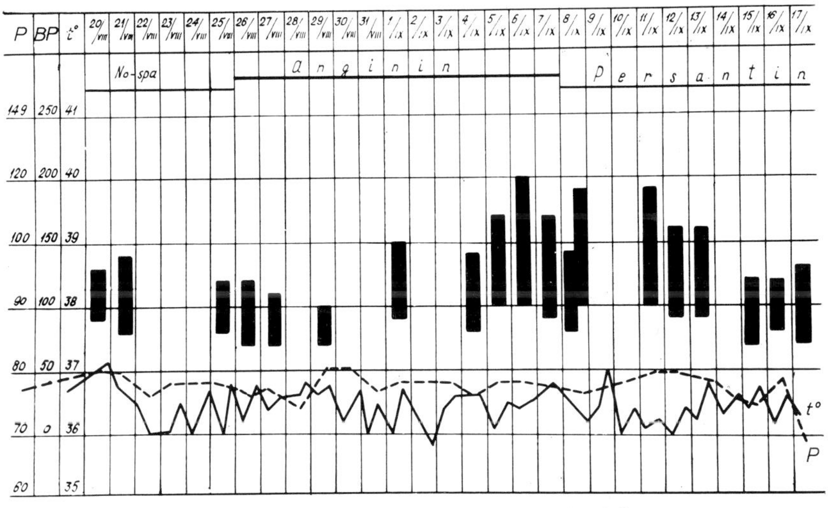

Fig. 5. Hypertensive reactions in patients during Anginin treatment.
Patient B., age 52. P = pulse; BP = blood pressure; t° = temperature.

Anginin treatment, demonstrated hypertensive reactions. Out of 72 patients there were 2 patients who demonstrated such a reaction. This reaction could be called a hypertensive crisis because it presented a typical clinical picture with hypertensive encephalopathy, tachycardia etc. After the Anginin was stopped, the hypertensive reactions disappeared, so I think the data presented by Dr. Spector are very different as regards the explanation of this type of reaction in these patients. Apart from this, the side-effects observed were that some patients developed allergic reactions on the skin but these disappeared very quickly after stopping Anginin treatment.

Unfortunately, we have not studied the mechanism of Anginin in coronary heart disease, but we have now started to do so in experimental laboratories, and I think in a year we will be able to present some details. However, I think that the most important factor which could be related to positive effects of Anginin in coronary heart disease is its effect on the microcirculation. Such a mechanism has been shown by participants in relation to the peripheral circulation. It is well known that the microcirculation is related very closely to autoregulation of coronary flow. It could be possible to understand the positive effect of Anginin in coronary patients by means of this kind of action of Anginin. But this is a speculation and should be studied in detail.

In summary, Anginin was effective in the treatment of patients with angina pectoris of effort (71.4%) and less effective in patients with angina pectoris of effort and at rest (57.1%). Anginin seems to be most suitable in the treatment of angina pectoris of effort in combination with intermittent claudication induced by atherosclerosis obliterans. In hypertensive patients the use of Anginin should be studied more carefully.

DISCUSSION

Dr. AUSTIN: I would like to ask some questions in relation to the two patients who had an hypertensive effect. Firstly, were these patients hypertensive or mildly hypertensive to begin with? Secondly, did they show changes in pulse rate? Thirdly, did they show any evidence of central nervous system excitation?

Dr. SHKHVATSABAYA: These patients were hypertensive and showed a labile transitory hypertension. When we started to treat them, their blood pressure was normal, but some time before treatment they experienced elevation of blood pressure. Secondly, they had very rapid pulse rates during the administration of Anginin, but not before.

Dr. AUSTIN: How rapid?

Dr. SHKHVATSABAYA: About 100. But I cannot tell you exactly. I remember that these two patients had symptoms of sympathetic overactivity. They experienced headache and different kinds of reactions, typical of hypertension.

Dr. AUSTIN: My question relates to their level of nervous system hyperreactivity. Were they excitable?

Dr. SHKHVATSABAYA: Oh yes, they were very excitable. Many patients with coronary heart disease and hypertension are excitable.

Dr. NUMANO: Thank you, Dr. Shkhvatsabaya, for your very interesting data. I should like to ask one question. Did you discover some relationship between the effectiveness of this drug and the age of the patients? Was age a factor?

Dr. SHKHVATSABAYA: I cannot say, because we did not study this particularly. But the material could be analysed from this point of view.

CHANGES IN MYOCARDIAL CONTRACTILE STRENGTH BEFORE AND AFTER ADMINISTRATION OF PYRIDINOLCARBAMATE IN PATIENTS WITH ISCHEMIC HEART DISEASE

M. YOSHIMURA
2nd Department of Internal Medicine, Japan Medical School, Tokyo, Japan

I should like to present some data concerning myocardial contractility which we measured before and after the administration of pyridinolcarbamate.

The myocardial contractile strength was estimated as a function of pressure elevation in the left ventricle during the isometric contraction phase. In the isometric left ventricular contraction period (t^i), left ventricular myocardial strength (F) produces the pressure elevation in the left ventricle up to end-diastolic aortic pressure ($Pd \fallingdotseq$ diastolic blood pressure) from almost zero ($\fallingdotseq$ left atrial pressure). A force f (dynes) can be represented as in the following formula:

$$f = m \frac{d^2 l}{dt^2},$$

where m is mass (g), dl indicates distance of displacement (cm), dt is time needed for displacement (sec), and d^2l/dt^2 represents acceleration of displacement (cm/sec^2). The isometric myocardial contractile strength to raise a column of mercury to height h (cm) in the U-tube of a mercury manometer against gravity indicates the level of diastolic pressure. This U-tube of the manometer has an area of 1 cm^2 in cross-section. Therefore the index of isometric left ventricular contractile strength F (dynes) can be represented as follows:

$$F = 13.6 \times 1 \times h \times \left\{ \frac{h}{(t^i)^2} + 980 \right\},$$

where *13.6* is density of mercury, h indicates height of the mercury column (cm) which represents the diastolic blood pressure (mm Hg), and t^i indicates duration of isometric left ventricular contraction (sec). $h/(t^i)^2$ indicates acceleration of displacement of the mercury column in height, and *980* is acceleration due to gravity. We determined t^i by mechanocardiography by a polygraphic recording technique (phonocardiogram, apex cardiogram and external sphygmogram) (Oreshkov, 1965). Thus we measured the index of myocardial contractile strength F in 11 patients with coronary sclerotic heart disease before and after administration of pyridinolcarbamate as shown in Figure 1.

There were 3 patients who showed no improvement in myocardial contractility F (Fig. 1). In these patients there was gradual reduction in myocardial contractility in 19 weeks after administration of pyridinolcarbamate, and one patient finally showed apparent signs of heart failure. However, in 8 other patients, a significant increase in myocardial contractility was observed. The broken line in Figure 1 indicates the lower limit of normal values of myocardial contractility. Two patients showed an apparent increase in myocardial contractility but one showed signs of side-effects, e.g. nausea and vomiting. We therefore stopped pyridinolcarbamate treatment, after which her myocardial contractility again showed a significant reduction. There was another patient who showed a slight increase in myocardial contractility after administration of pyridinolcarbamate, but he died due to severe myo-

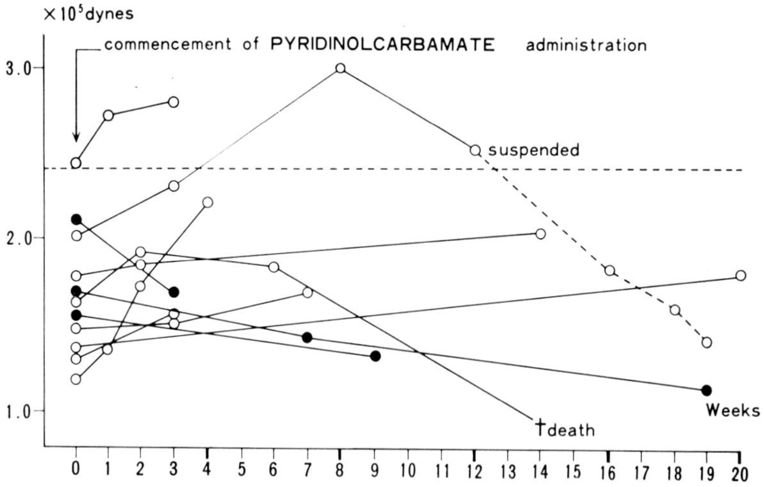

Fig. 1. Changes in index of myocardial contractile strength before and after administration of pyridinolcarbamate in patients with ischemic heart disease.

cardial infarction. We had a control group whose myocardial contractility did not show any significant change after administration of pyridinolcarbamate. I assume that these effects of pyridinolcarbamate in the patients with ischemic heart disease are probably due to the disappearance of edematous changes in the aortic wall and, in consequence, there will be a successful increase in coronary blood flow.

REFERENCE

OreshKov, V. (1965): Indirect measurement of isovolumetric contraction time on the basis of polygraphic tracing (apexcardiogram, carotid tracing and phonocardiogram). *Cardiologia (Basel)*, *47*, 315.

DISCUSSION

Dr. Kipshidze: What dose of pyridinolcarbamate did you give the 2 patients for 9 weeks who exhibited increased contractility? Can you tell me something about the mechanism of increased contractility, because 9 weeks is too short to expect twice as much increased contractility.

Dr. Yoshimura: These patients had signs of weakness, and they showed a significant reduction in contractility. Reduced contractility is hardly increased without digitalis. I think many patients showed a significant increase in contractility after administration of pyridinolcarbamate. However, a very rapid increase in contractility is observed in some patients. I consider it to be the result of the disappearance of the edema in the aorta, which is probably due to the antibradykinin action of pyridinolcarbamate. If the edematous change in the aorta disappears, the entrance of the coronary artery will expand, thus causing an increase in coronary blood flow and myocardial contractility.

Dr. Kipshidze: What age were these 2 patients?

Dr. Yoshimura: Over 40 years old.

Dr. Janushkevichius: Did you measure left ventricular pressure and what was the diastolic pressure?

Dr. YOSHIMURO: No, it was an indirect measurement; we did not use the cardiac catheter. We determined the left ventricular isovolumetric contraction time by polygraphic external tracings and also determined the blood pressure indirectly.

Dr. SHKHVATSABAYA: Could you tell me what was the clinical state of the patients who got the depression of contractility? How do you explain the depression of contractility in some patients?

Dr. YOSHIMURA: In answer to the first question, I would like to say that these patients showed signs of heart failure during or after exercise, e.g. palpitation, breath-shortening and fatigue in the lower extremities during exercise, but they showed no signs of angina pectoris or signs suggesting myocardial infarction, i.e. silent ischemic heart disease. One patient died due to an attack of myocardial infarction. At autopsy, we found the myocardial infarcts.

In answer to the second question, there were one or two patients who showed a gradual decline in myocardial contractility. It is difficult to explain, but I think these patients did not show a lower initial myocardial contractility than others. Moreover, these patients showed a significant fall in diastolic blood pressure after administration of pyridinolcarbamate. It might be possible to decrease the coronary blood flow in a condition with lower diastolic blood pressure.

EVALUATION OF ANGININ IN THE TREATMENT OF PATIENTS WITH ANGINA PECTORIS

H. I. RUSSEK
St. Barnabas Hospital, Staten Island, N.Y., U.S.A.

Determination of the efficacy of any drug for the treatment of angina pectoris cannot be made from a study of such factors as cellular anatomy or physiology, hemodynamic alterations, changes in metabolism, or modifications in myocardial mechanics or energetics. This is because potent agents frequently have multiple actions, some favorable for the myocardium, some unfavorable and some even unknown. For example, the beneficial influence of nitroglycerin, which has been in use for 100 years, still evades our complete understanding. The drug appears to have a favorable effect by dilating the coronary arteries and in particular the coronary collaterals. It would also seem to have desirable actions in diminishing the venous return to the heart and in reducing blood pressure, responses contributing to a decrease in heart work and oxygen consumption. But nitroglycerin also exerts adverse effects by producing tachycardia and an increase in contractility, factors augmenting the oxygen requirements for myocardial contraction. Thus, in some patients, these adverse effects may cancel out the favorable actions of the drug. Indeed, we have reported some years ago that there are patients in whom the use of nitroglycerin actually produces a paradoxical response. In these, the exercise-electrocardiographic patterns were actually made worse by the administration of nitroglycerin. So, obviously, in evaluating the response to any antianginal agent, it is the sum total of all the actions of the drug, those positive and those negative, favorable and unfavorable, which determines whether or not that drug has value in the treatment of angina pectoris. In the last analysis, the efficacy of any drug for angina pectoris will depend

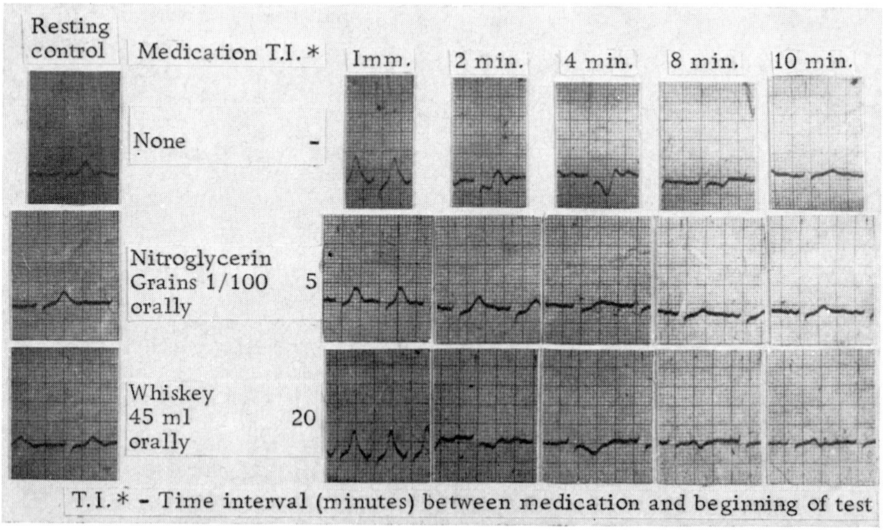

Fig. 1. Comparative electrocardiographic responses to exercise following either nitroglycerin or whiskey.

on whether it can favorably influence, in the ischemic area of the myocardium, the ratio between oxygen delivery and myocardial oxygen demands. Even today there is no method comparable to the long-used exercise-electrocardiographic test which provides a kind of mirror that reflects what is going on in the myocardium with respect to ischemic changes. The illustrations that follow are examples of the value of this method of study.

Twenty-five years ago, alcohol was considered only second to nitroglycerin for the treatment of angina pectoris. All the textbooks and all authorities recommended the use of whiskey for patients with angina. Figure 1, which was made about 25 years ago, shows the results in one of about a dozen patients who responded to exercise in a very predictable way under controlled circumstances after placebo. They were then given either nitroglycerin or whiskey under identical conditions and the measured exercise was repeated. It was found that, while whiskey prevented the pain induced by exercise just as nitroglycerin had done, whiskey failed in all of the patients studied to alter favorably the ischemic electrocardiographic patterns induced by exercise.

Our efforts, therefore, have been directed toward selecting patients whose responses from day to day under controlled circumstances are predictable in terms of ischemic electrocardiographic patterns. In the study shown in Figure 2, a placebo was given to the patient and he

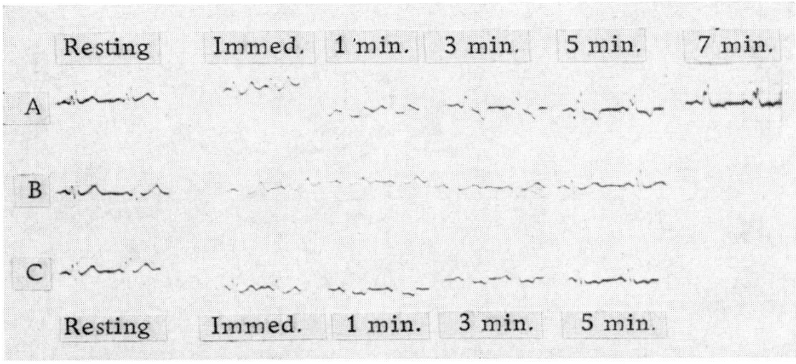

Fig. 2. Comparative electrocardiographic responses to exercise following placebo and Isordil sublingual (5 mg) in patient B.C. A: Exercise (28 steps) to the point of pain following placebo. B: Same exercise (28 steps) 1 hour after Isordil sublingual (5 mg). No pain. C: Exercise (46 steps) to the point of pain 1 hour after Isordil sublingual (5 mg).

was then exercised to the point of pain; this was 28 trips on the Master 2-step staircase. You see the markedly ischemic pattern which he developed. When the patient performed the same exercise, but this time after 5 mg of isosorbide dinitrate sublingually, you can see that the previously observed ischemic electrocardiographic pattern did not appear and the patient experienced no discomfort. On the third occasion, we administered isosorbide dinitrate again, but this time permitted the patient to exercise to the point of pain and it was found that he could then traverse the 2-step staircase 46 times (instead of 28) before he developed angina and the typical ECG findings.

This then represents a technique for evaluating the modifying influence of a drug upon the exercise-electrocardiographic response and upon the patient's capacity to exercise without pain.

A demonstration of the multiple effects produced by drugs can be appreciated from a study of propranolol and isosorbide dinitrate. Propranolol is commonly recognized today as a valuable drug for the treatment of angina pectoris. Yet, in many patients this agent does not materially influence the exercise-electrocardiographic test or the frequency and severity of angina. As I shall show later, this is because of the multiple actions of propranolol. In some cases, the favorable effects are cancelled out by the unfavorable ones. In the case shown in

Figure 3, a 65-year-old male, propranolol given in a 40 mg dose, 2 hours before the test, had little effect on the electrocardiographic response or the development of angina. On another occasion, when the same patient was given isosorbide dinitrate, 5 mg sublingually, there was again little or no favorable response. But strangely enough, when both drugs were administered concomitantly, propranolol 2 hours before the test and isosorbide dinitrate 1 hour before the test, we observed this rather remarkable response in terms of normalization of the exercise-electrocardiogram and absence of pain.

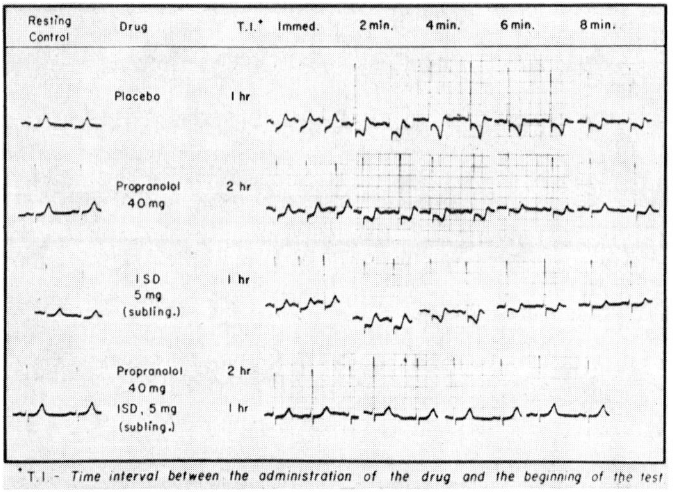

Fig. 3. Comparative electrocardiographic responses (lead V_5) to standard exercise (26 trips) following propranolol and/or isosorbide dinitrate (ISD) in a 65-year-old male patient (R.D.).

So, as a result of this observation, we began to study patients with refractory angina pectoris to determine whether we could, by combining both of these drugs, improve the electrocardiographic response and also the capacity to exercise without pain. Figure 4 shows another case in which we uncovered the same phenomenon, namely a synergistic response to propranolol and isosorbide dinitrate.

Figure 5 also shows studies in a patient with refractory angina pectoris; he was unresponsive to Isordil alone, poorly responsive to propranolol alone, but with the combination of drugs he has shown a remarkable response.

Despite the very easily demonstrable effect from the use of these drugs in angina pectoris, it is unfortunate that the agents are currently being used rather improperly in the treatment of this syndrome. The dose employed for propranolol is frequently not optimal. It is often not given in proper chronological sequence with regard to isosorbide dinitrate. Moreover, the only agent we have found truly effective synergistically in the nitrate series, besides isosorbide dinitrate (Isordil) by the sublingual route, is nitroglycerin. All oral preparations, even of Isordil or nitroglycerin and such oral formulations as PETN (pentaerythritol tetranitrate) and ETN (erythrityl tetranitrate), showed unpredictable or unsatisfactory response.

Now the point I am trying to make is that when one is going to administer these drugs for their synergistic interaction one has to know the time of onset of action and the duration of activity of each agent. Since isosorbide dinitrate sublingually begins to work within 5 min but has a duration of effect of approximately $1\frac{1}{2}$ hours, while propranolol has an onset of action in about 1 hour and a duration of activity of some 4 hours, to obtain the best response from these agents one must administer the propranolol before the meal and isosorbide dinitrate sublingually after the meal. With such a regimen both agents will be working concomitantly

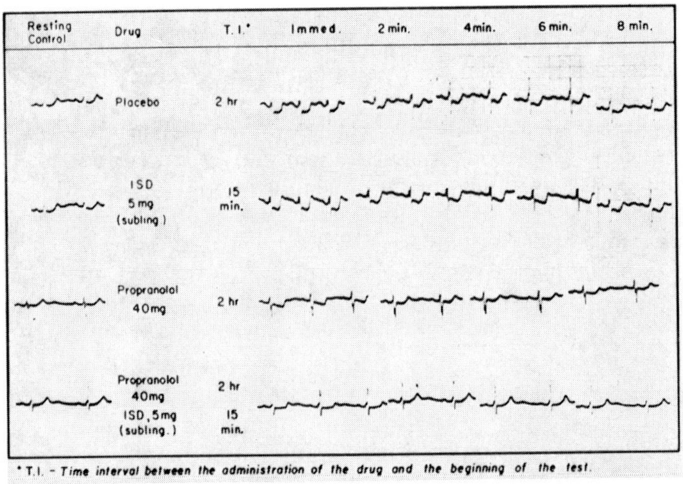

Fig. 4. Comparative electrocardiographic responses (lead V_5) to standard exercise (8 trips) following propranolol and/or isosorbide dinitrate (ISD) in a 77-year-old female patient (H.F.).

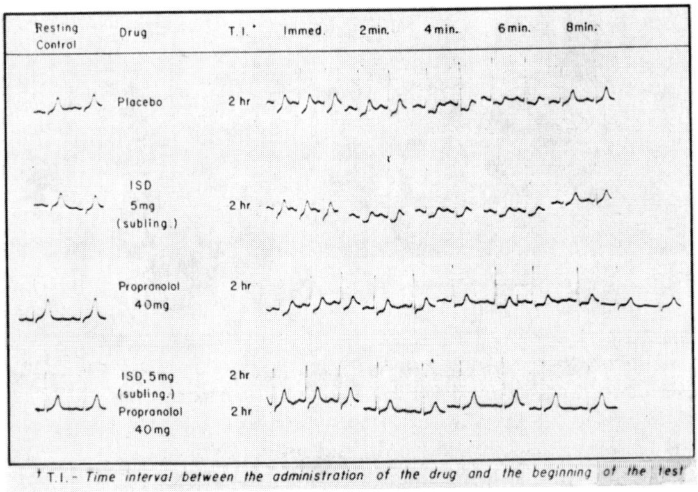

Fig. 5. Comparative electrocardiographic responses (lead V_5) to standard exercise (30 trips) following propranolol and/or isosorbide dinitrate (ISD) in a 60-year-old male patient (A.S.).

when the patient resumes his postprandial activity. Unless this is done, the synergistic effect is not obtained as long as possible and when it is most needed.

Now this leads us to a consideration of the multiple actions of potent drugs. If we consider the nitrates, it is known that these agents have a favorable effect in decreasing intramyocardial tension and in increasing regional coronary blood flow to ischemic myocardium. But they also have adverse effects in increasing heart rate and augmenting cardiac contractility. Propranolol, on the other hand, decreases the myocardial oxygen requirements by influencing factors responsible for myocardial oxygen consumption. But it is believed that propranolol, like all β-blockers, tends to decrease the coronary blood flow. This is therefore an unfavorable effect which may negate the desirable actions of the drug. Consider, however, what happens when these drugs (propranolol and a potent nitrate) are combined. One observes a cancelling out of the adverse effects of the nitrate and propranolol, respectively. The final result is a decrease in myocardial oxygen requirement with an increase in coronary flow, a response which seems to explain what appears to be a 1 + 1 = 4 phenomenon when we administer both these drugs together. Thus, there is frequently an increase in exercise tolerance in these patients by almost 100% with the combination, as compared to about 25% with Isordil or propranolol alone.

I have only recently begun to study Anginin in the treatment of angina pectoris and I was only able to do this through the kind cooperation of Professor Redisch who made the drug available to me about 3 months ago. So what I have to offer are very preliminary observations. In the case shown in Figure 6, a 56-year-old male patient who was studied with cine-angio-

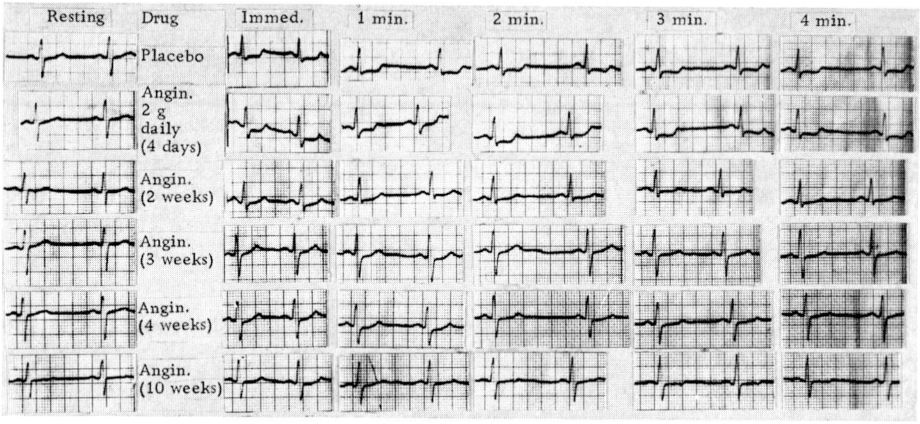

Fig. 6. Exercise-electrocardiographic tests (30 trips) showing lead V_4 in a 56-year-old male patient (R.M.) with angina pectoris receiving placebo or Anginin.

graphy and found to have triple coronary artery disease with diffuse involvement of the entire coronary tree, surgery was considered inadvisable because of the diffuse nature of the disease. He was treated with propranolol and Isordil and despite significant symptomatic improvement remained markedly disabled. This patient had not slept in his bed for more than 1 year; just assuming the supine position produced the repetitive attacks of angina pectoris. I was unable to discontinue Isordil and propranolol in this patient because of the severity of symptoms. In all of his tests therefore, Isordil was administered sublingually 10 min before exercise and propranolol 1 hour before testing. In addition, he was given either Anginin placebo or Anginin itself. After recording the response to Anginin placebo, Anginin was administered in a 2 g daily dose for 4 days when the tests were again repeated. We saw very little change as compared with the placebo control. We kept the patient on Anginin for 2 weeks on the dosage of 2 g per day and then began to observe a rather improved response compared with the control. In 3 weeks this favorable response had been maintained; in 4 weeks it was similarly present but from 4 to 10 weeks there seemed to be a slow deterioration.

This patient while on therapy volunteered the information that for the first time in a year he had been able to sleep in his bed without the need for sitting up in a chair all night. You can take that for what it may be worth.

The second patient whom I had an opportunity to study was a 53-year-old male who received placebo and after exercising to the point of pain developed the usual ischemic ST and T wave changes in the post-exercise electrocardiogram (Fig. 7). He was then given 1 g of Anginin and he was retested in the manner reported by Dr. Yamazaki and Professor Shimamoto and his group. After a one-shot dose of Anginin with repeat exercise 3 hours thereafter, we found a rather striking response which tends to confirm the observations of this group.

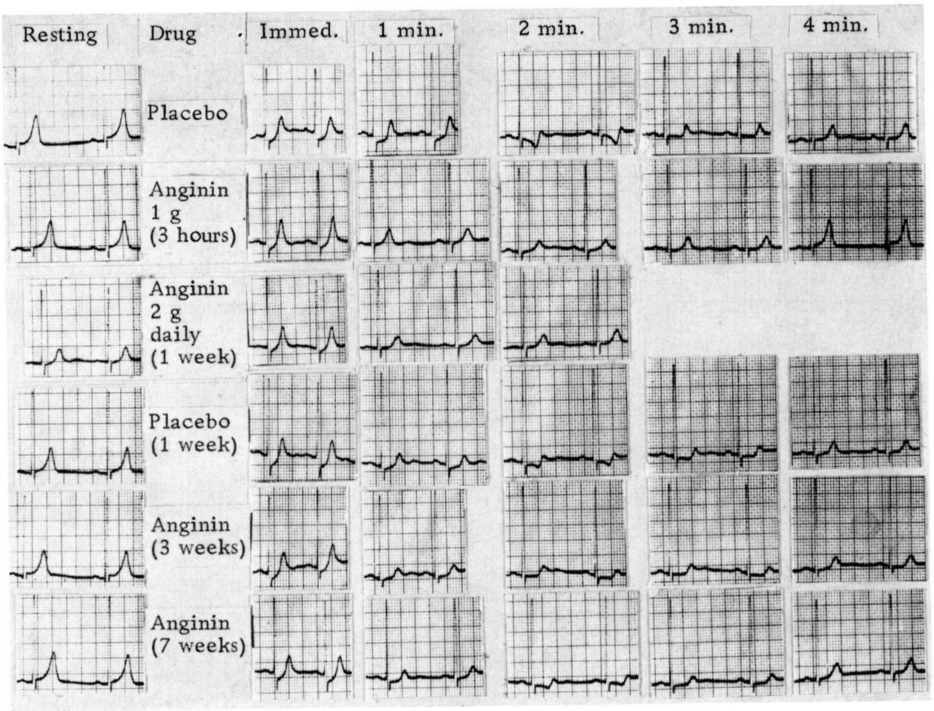

Fig. 7. Exercise-electrocardiographic tests (40 trips) showing lead V_4 in a 53-year-old patient (A.K.) with angina pectoris receiving placebo or Anginin.

When Anginin was given to this patient in a 2 g daily dose for 1 week the response continued to be favorably maintained. We then substituted placebo and you can see the deterioration in the electrocardiographic response when this was done. Upon restarting Anginin therapy again, after 1 week on placebo, the tests were repeated after 3 weeks but the exercise-electrocardiographic responses have not appeared as good as when the drug was administered during the initial period of 1 week.

Figure 8 shows another case, that of a 61-year-old male, whose response on placebo was characterized by marked ischemic changes. Anginin was given in a 1 g dose and the patient was tested 3 hours later. There was some improvement in the response but it was not a normal pattern. Anginin was then given in a dose of 2 g daily for 1 week and here you see a completely normal response after 1 week of therapy. At 2 weeks, this response was still maintained. We then gave him placebo; this was done shortly before I set out for Japan and after 1 week on placebo therapy you can see definite deterioration in the electrocardiographic response to standard exercise.

The fourth patient whom we had an opportunity to study showed no significant change from the administration of Anginin as compared with the findings during placebo control

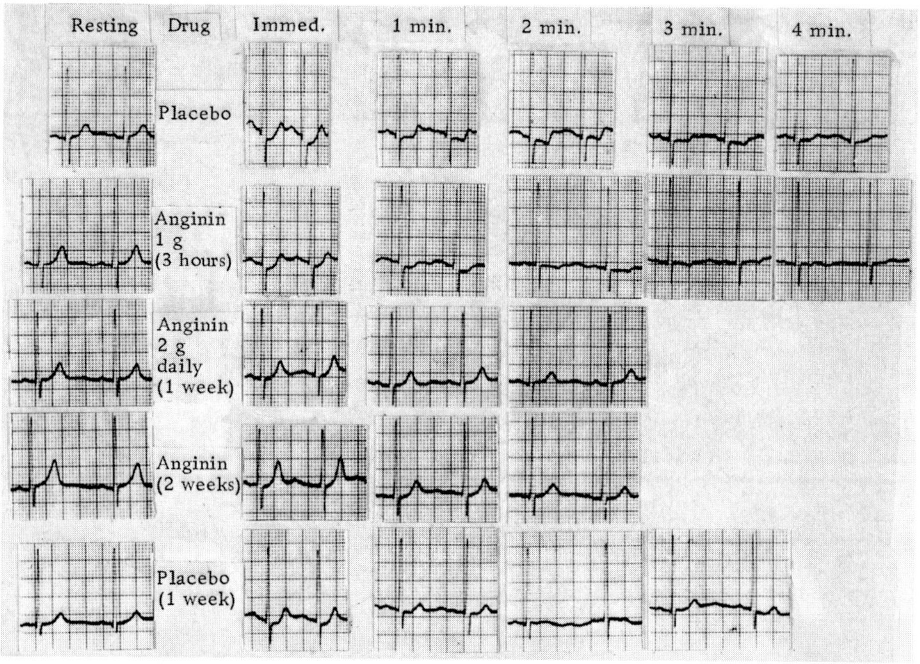

Fig. 8. Exercise-electrocardiographic tests (26 trips) showing lead V_4 in a 61-year-old male patient (R.S.) with angina pectoris receiving placebo or Anginin.

(Figs. 9 and 10). If anyone doubts that one can study drugs by means of repetitive studies with the same patient acting as his own control, this is a pretty good example of the almost finger-print type of response that one gets with careful selection of patients having a stable form of coronary insufficiency. These are the kinds of patients whom we use for drug testing, not

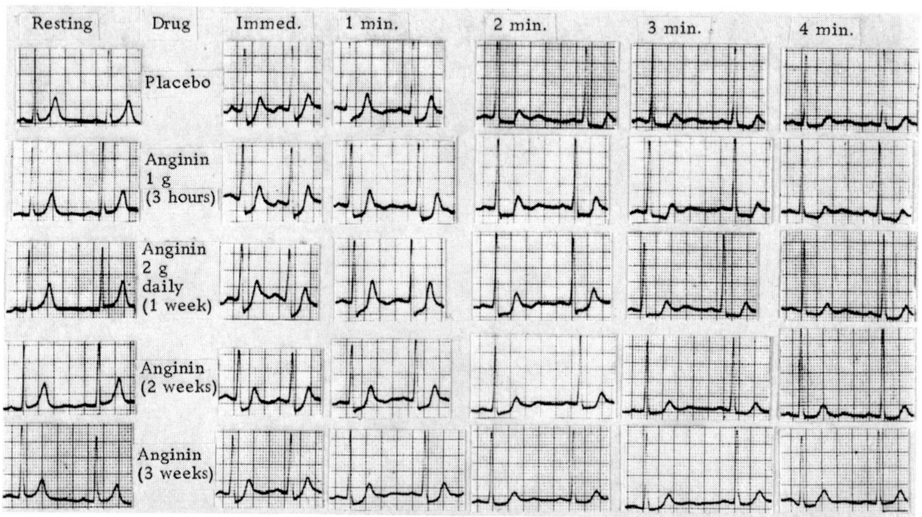

Fig. 9

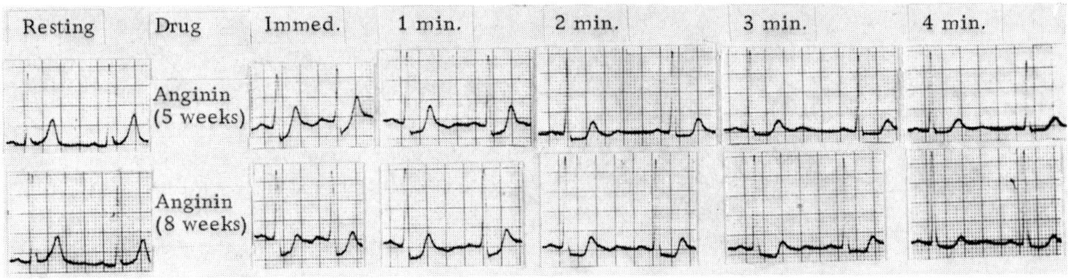

Figs. 9 and 10. Exercise-electrocardiographic tests (30 trips) showing lead V_4 in a patient (A.S.) with angina pectoris receiving placebo or Anginin.

the kind of patient who will show one type of response one day and an entirely different response on the following day. Now, that is all I have to report because this is a very preliminary study; but from the vantage point of one who has studied patients with all kinds of drugs over the past 25 years, I am encouraged by these preliminary observations. Just how this drug is acting in the cases that have shown favorable response remains to be elucidated.

DISCUSSION

Dr. Kipshidze: I would like to ask if you use a combination of Anginin or propranolol or liquorice together.

Dr. Russek: I have not used a combination of drugs except in the very first case in which propranolol and Isordil were employed in order to protect the patient from the risk of exercise. As a matter of fact I would not have been able to exercise the patient very much if he had not had these drugs. In the other patients I have not combined a nitrate or propranolol with Anginin as yet. This is something which hopefully we will do in the future.

Dr. Kipshidze: How long a time does the effect of Anginin last? Suppose you gave Anginin and discontinued it. After 1 week, do you have the same effect?

Dr. Russek: I think I showed that, if you give the patient Anginin 1 week and then substitute a placebo and have him come back a week later, the effect seems to be gone. At least, it seemed so with these very few. So within 1 week the effect is lost. I do not know whether it is lost sooner than that, but it may well be.

Unidentified speaker: Dr. Russek, do you not think large-scale studies involving controlled observations in many patients are essential for valid results?

Dr. Russek: I think in the area of coronary disease, for all practical purposes, it is an extremely difficult thing to match control patients with treated patients. It is an ideal which has never been achieved in the past and I doubt whether it will be achieved in the future because there are so many variables from patient to patient. Unless patients are chosen at random and literally thousands of patients are included, you cannot expect a cancelling out of these variables. Certainly if you take such numbers as 50 or 100 or 200 patients, I do not think you will get comparable series. I do think that having the patient serve as his own control in relatively short-term studies, before the natural course of the disease influences his symptomatology, is perhaps the best, presently available technique. For example, to demonstrate that whisky was not a favorable drug in angina pectoris was not a difficult thing to do. You did not need a hundred patients. If you took a dozen patients carefully selected and tested them in this manner, I think you would be able to convince everyone of your results.

Dr. Pratesi: Do you not think the proper use of drugs could prevent sudden death?

Dr. Russek: I agree with you and I think this is a subject for a new symposium. I would like to say this with regard to sudden death. The great emphasis has been on the use of antiarrhythmic agents, but we know that just as there are silent myocardial infarctions, there is the equivalent in 'silent' angina pectoris. If we exercise our patients and find ST segment changes but no pain, those patients probably should be treated just as though they had symptoms, because if we are to make any inroads against the problem of sudden death, these ischemic changes should be prevented since they may well trigger fatal ventricular fibrillation. Such patients may therefore require not only antiarrhythmic agents but also effective anti-ischemic drugs.

EVALUATION OF AN ANTIANGINAL DRUG

LEON DE SOLDATI

Servicio de Cardiología, Hospital Alvear, Buenos Aires, Argentina

I think that the evaluation of an antianginal drug is always difficult. Dr. Russek has given a beautiful presentation of acute clinical trials using the ECG and effort test.

But I consider it necessary to establish the most useful criteria to: (*a*) diagnose the anginal syndrome, (*b*) confirm the presence of ischemic heart disease, and (*c*) evaluate the efficacy of an antianginal drug.

In order to diagnose the anginal syndrome the following must be taken into consideration:

1. Main symptoms

a. Chest pain (or other known localization of the pain) produced by 'stress' situations
b. Duration: 1–5 min
c. Relief by rest or nitroglycerine

2. Associated symptoms

a. Sense of choking or inability to breathe
b. Anxiety
c. Sweating, belching, flatulence

The objective confirmation of ischemic heart disease can be made as follows:

1. ECG: rest and graded exercise test
2. Ballistocardiogram
3. Apex cardiogram: 'a' wave
4. Coronary arteriography: asynergic ventricular contraction
5. Radioactive rubidium
6. Evidence of myocardial glycolysis (myocardial lactate A-V difference)

Referring to points 4 and 5, I want to emphasize that ischemic heart disease has been frequently demonstrated with patent coronary arteries. Thus, lack of abnormalities in coronary arteries or coronary blood flow does not rule out ischemic heart disease.

Furthermore, according to the *Nomenclature and Criteria for Diagnosis of Diseases of the Heart and Blood Vessels* (New York Heart Association, 1964) the anginal syndrome 'is a physiological diagnosis and is not synonymous with coronary atherosclerosis. The underlying mechanism is ischemia of the heart muscle: thus any factor which invokes this mechanism can initiate the anginal syndrome'.

Taking into consideration different aspects of coronary insufficiency, the evaluation of antianginal drugs can be made from the following:

1. Anginal syndrome (using a double-blind test): pain – frequency, severity, duration and grade of stress inducing pain

2. Coronary circulation: coronary arteriography, radioisotope techniques

3. Myocardial contractility: apex cardiogram, ballistocardiogram, left ventricular end-diastolic pressure, ventriculography

4. Myocardial metabolism: electrocardiogram, lactate extraction, arterial-coronary sinus difference of potassium.

Some of these methods cannot be used as a routine, but ECG (rest and exercise tests), radio-isotopes, apex cardiogram, ballistocardiogram, etc. combined with a double-blind test, should prove useful.

REFERENCE

NEW YORK HEART ASSOCIATION (1964): *Nomenclature and Criteria for Diagnosis of Diseases of the Heart and Blood Vessels, 6th ed.* Criteria Committee, New York Heart Association.

ETIOLOGY OF ACUTE AND CHRONIC A–V BLOCK IN RELATION TO ATHEROSCLEROSIS

ALFRED PICK
Heart Station, Cardiovascular Institute, Michael Reese Hospital and Medical Center, Chicago, Ill., U.S.A.

Although, in the context of this Symposium, I have no data to present concerning pyridinolcarbamate, Prof. Shimamoto and Dr. Numano kindly permitted me to raise an important question referring to the relationship of atrioventricular (A-V) block to atherosclerotic heart disease. In the past the two, when occurring in older people, were thought to be closely associated. Today it is recognized that in the adult there is an important difference in the pathogenesis of acute and chronic block. Up to about age 50, A–V block develops suddenly, mostly in the early stage of myocardial infarction as a consequence of coronary artery disease. In elderly patients, on the other hand, A–V block sets in gradually, in several stages, and ischemic heart disease is found at autopsy in only 15% of the cases. This was evident in a series of 100

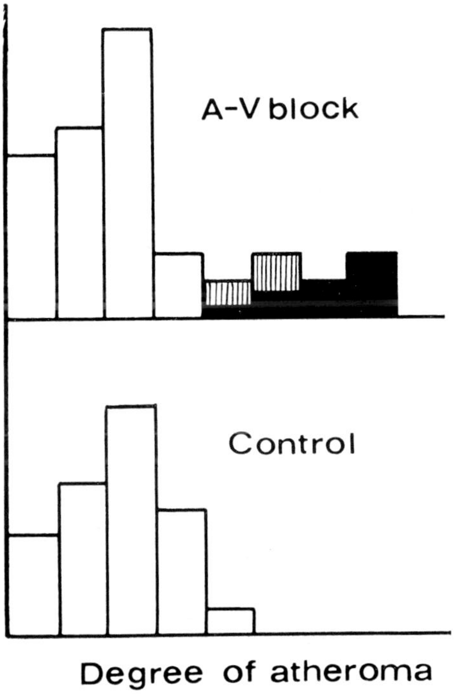

Fig. 1. The degree of coronary artery stenosis in hearts from patients with chronic A–V block is compared with that in hearts from control subjects. The A–V block group contains a number of patients with significant coronary artery stenosis which may be responsible for conduction system damage (solid squares) or coincidental (hatched squares). However, the majority of patients with A–V block (open squares) have no more arterial stenosis than control cases.

TABLE I

Causes of chronic A-V block (100 cases coming to autopsy) *

Idiopathic bilateral bundle branch fibrosis		46
Ischemic coronary artery disease		
Destruction of both bundle branches	14	
Destruction of A-V node	1	
Cardiomyopathy		13
Calcific valve disease		8
Myocarditis		4
Connective tissue disorder		3
Amyloidosis		3
Transfusion siderosis (only A-V node affected)		2
Congenital heart block (only main bundle affected)		3
Gumma of I-V septum		3
	Total	100

* Davies (1971)

such cases studied in London by Davies (1971). Table I shows some of the data from his recent monograph on the subject. Coronary artery disease, together with other known etiologic factors, accounted for only 54% of the cases. Figure 1 shows that significant coronary disease was about the same in hearts with chronic A–V block as in control hearts without block. Although this fact had been pointed out in 1912 by Bachmann in Germany and again in 1931 by Mahaim in Switzerland, it was not appreciated fully until the late Dr. Lenègre in

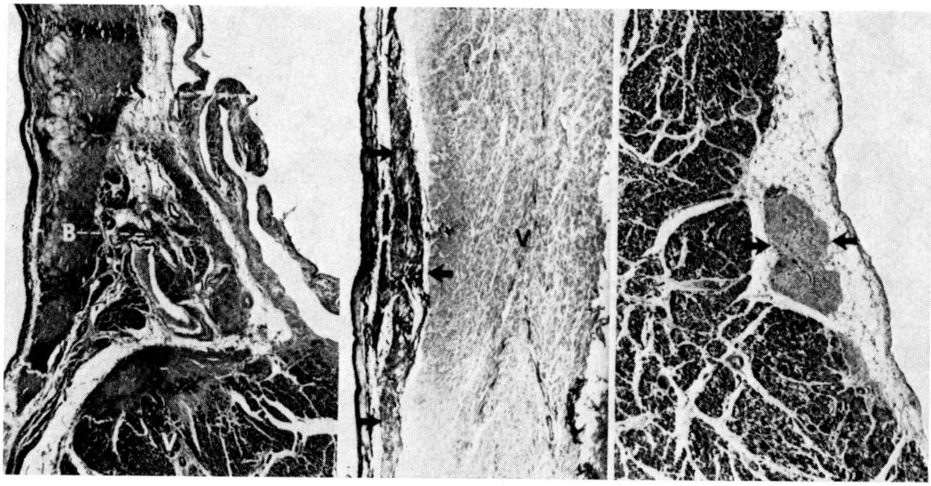

Fig. 2. 71-year-old man with Stokes-Adams attacks. ECG: Complete A–V dissociation due to advanced A–V block. *Left panel:* branching portion of A–V bundle showing fibrosis of right side with arteriolosclerosis. Hematoxylin-eosin stain; reduced from × 45. B = A–V bundle; V = ventricular septum. *Middle panel:* Left bundle branch showing fibrosis. Weigert-Van Gieson stain; reduced from × 45. *Right panel:* Right bundle branch at junction of first and second portions showing replacement by connective tissue. Hematoxylin-eosin stain; reduced from × 45. In middle and right panels, arrows point to left and right bundle branch in various views.

Reproduced from Lev et al. (1970) by permission of The American Heart Association, Inc.

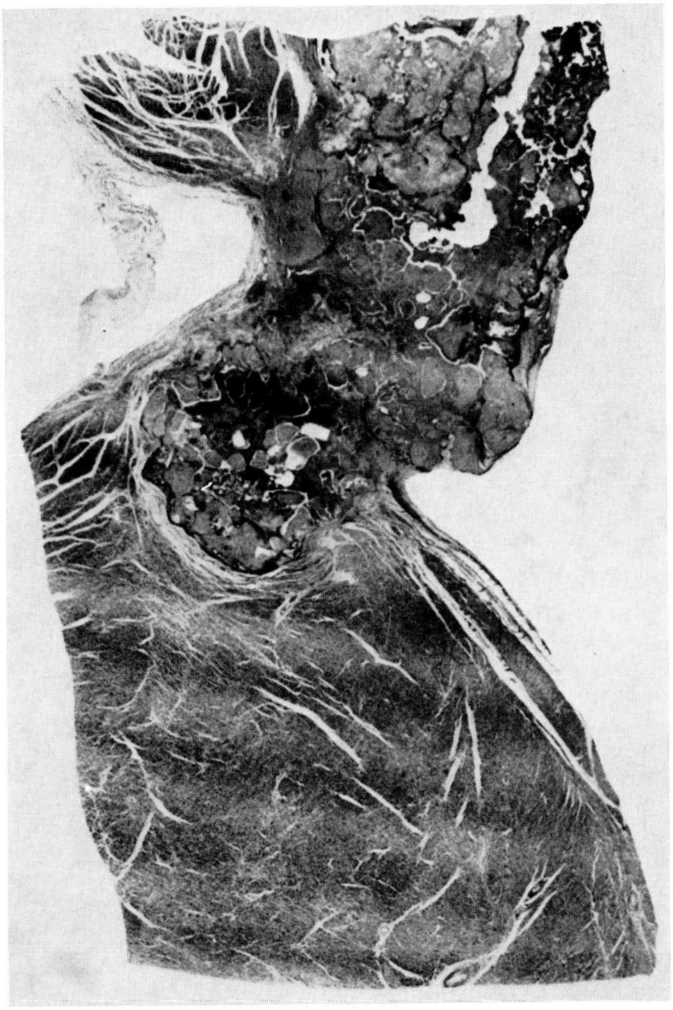

Fig. 3. 56-year-old man with Stokes-Adams attacks. ECG: Intermittent complete A–V block due to bilateral bundle branch block. A calcific destructive lesion of the bicuspid aortic valve penetrates into the summit of the ventricular septum and interrupts the A–V conduction system at the bifurcation and in the initial parts of both bundle branches.

Paris started his brilliant clinicopathologic correlations (Lenègre, 1958; Lenègre and Moreau, 1963), which have been confirmed and amplified by Dr. Lev in Chicago (Lev, 1964; Lev et al., 1970). At about the same time Dr. Rosenbaum in Buenos Aires (Rosenbaum et al., 1970) introduced his concept of a trifascicular intraventricular conduction system which allowed multiple pathologic lesions to be readily recognized in the electrocardiogram.

What then is the etiologic factor that accounts for the production of A–V block in the 50% of patients in whom the cause was not obvious? Lenègre described a primary sclerodegenerative process of unknown nature restricted to one or more fascicles of the specific ventricular conduction system. Lev, on the other hand, described, under the name of 'sclerosis of the left side of the cardiac skeleton', fibrocalcareous lesions involving the summit of the ventricular septum or extending into the branching part of the conduction system from a calcified mitral annulus or aortic valve. Figure 2, from our studies, shows an example of Lenègre's disease, and Figure 3 an example of Lev's disease, in patients who died during Stokes-Adams attacks and who, at autopsy, displayed no, or only minimal, coronary arterial disease.

In the state of our present knowledge we can, thanks to Rosenbaum's work, recognize certain electrocardiographic patterns that sooner or later, but invariably, will lead to complete A–V block and the Stokes-Adams syndrome. We know how to treat and keep a patient alive, after he has survived his first attack of cardiac syncope, by chronic electrical pacing of the heart. But, lacking knowledge of the pathogenesis of Lev's and Lenègre's diseases, what can we do to prevent or at least arrest them?

This is the question I pose to this distinguished audience: Is perhaps (and hopefully) Anginin able to influence the course of these diseases, to prevent Stokes-Adams attacks, or at least postpone for years the time when the life of a patient will have to depend on the correct function of an electronic instrument?

I believe that some of the slides shown by Dr. Janushkevichius may show us a way in this direction.

REFERENCES

DAVIES, M. J. (1971): *Pathology of Conducting Tissue of the Heart.* Butterworth and Co., London.

BACHMANN, G. (1912): A physiologico-pathological study of a case of heart block occurring in a dog as a result of natural causes. *J. exp. Med., 16*, 25.

LENÈGRE, J. (1958): *Contribution à l'Etude des Blocs de Branch.* J. B. Ballière et Fils, Paris.

LENÈGRE, J. and MOREAU, P. (1963): Le bloc auriculo-ventriculaire chronique: Etude anatomique, clinique et histologique. *Arch. Mal. Cœur, 56*, 867.

LEV, M. (1964): The pathology of complete atrioventricular block. *Progr. cardiovasc. Dis., 6*, 317.

LEV, M., KINARE, S. G. and PICK, A. (1970): The pathogenesis of atrioventricular block in coronary disease. *Circulation, 42*, 409.

MAHAIM, I. (1931): *Maladies Organiques du Faisceau de His-Tawara.* Masson et Cie., Paris.

ROSENBAUM, M. B., ELIZARI, M. V. and LAZZARI, J. O. (1970): *The Hemiblocks.* Tampa Tracings, Oldsmar, Fla.

MECHANISMS OF CARDIAC ARRHYTHMIAS: FROM HYPOTHESIS TO PHYSIOLOGIC FACT

ALFRED PICK

Cardiovascular Institute, Michael Reese Hospital and Medical Center, Chicago, Ill., U.S.A.

Recent years have witnessed a revival of interest in mechanisms of cardiac arrhythmias as refined recording techniques developed in the animal laboratory became applicable to the human heart. Today, controlled electrical pacing of the atria and/or the ventricles, direct recordings of the activity of the human conduction system and especially a combination of the 2 methods permits (*a*) reproduction at will of a great number of disorders of cardiac rhythm known to occur spontaneously (Langendorf and Pick, 1971) and thus (*b*) testing of the validity of interpretations arrived at by deductive speculation. In this presentation I intend to demonstrate this on some selected examples, leaning on our own experience as well as on work by others found in the literature.

CONCEALED A–V CONDUCTION

In Figure 1 is shown an exact replica in man of an experiment performed in the dog heart in 1925 by Lewis and Master. Rapid pacing of the atria resulted in a 2:1 ventricular response at a P–R of 0.28 sec. When the pacing rate was reduced to one-half, 1:1 response resulted with

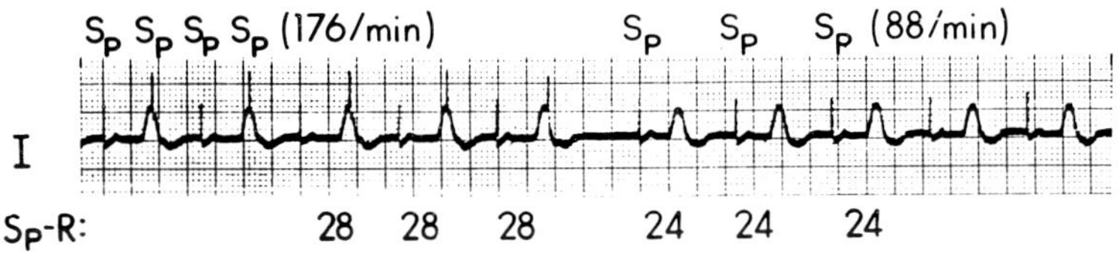

Fig. 1. Concealed A–V conduction in rapid atrial pacing. S_p = atrial response to pacer stimulus.

P–R interval shortened to 0.24 sec. The assumption is that the longer P–R is the after-effect of concealed conduction into the A–V node of the apparently blocked stimulus. This we could verify (Fig. 2) by repeating such an experiment with His bundle recording. In panel B, during rapid pacing of the atria, alternate impulses (S) are not followed by a His deflection while the A–H interval of conducted impulses measures 170 sec. Thus there is A–V nodal block at a 2:1 conduction ratio. At half the stimulation rate in panel C, there is ventricular response to each stimulus, with A–H reduced to 110 msec, corresponding to that of the control panel A, at a sinus rate of 70.

Perhaps the most convincing documentation of the concealment of an impulse within the A–V junction was recently provided for the case of so-called pseudo A–V block. Figure 3 shows in Lead II sudden prolongation, followed by failure of conduction in a regular sinus rhythm. As indicated in the diagram, this is attributed to after-effects of 2 premature A–V junctional discharges blocked in both directions. Documentation of such an event was provided by Rosen et al. (1970), who proved the concealed junctional discharge in man by recording

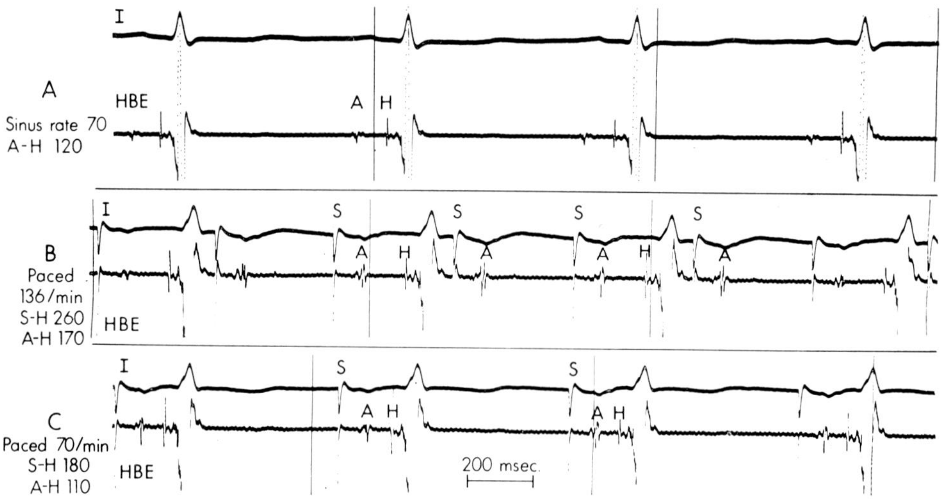

Fig. 2. Concealed A–V conduction demonstrated by His bundle recording during rapid atrial pacing. Panel A: Control before pacing. S = stimulus artifact in His bundle electrogram (HBE). A = atrial potential; H = His potential; A–H = transnodal conduction time (approximate).

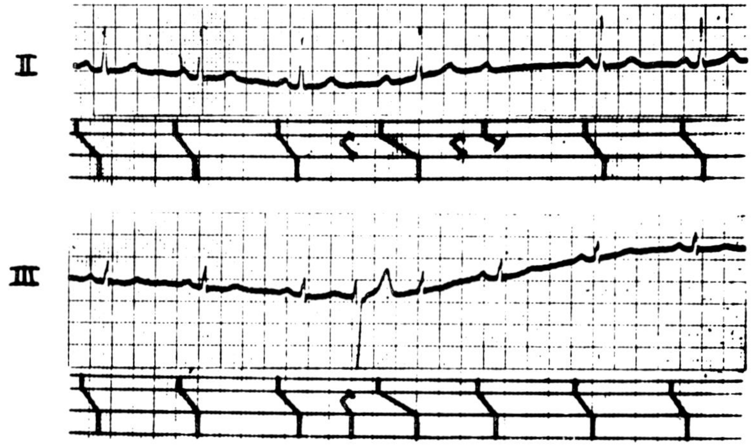

Fig. 3. First-degree, and Type I second-degree, A–V block imitated by blocked A–V junctional premature beats.

His bundle potentials in a corresponding case. Moore et al. (1971) reproduced it experimentally in the rabbit heart through a microelectrode impaled into the A–V junction.

MECHANISMS OF SUPRAVENTRICULAR (A–V JUNCTIONAL) TACHYCARDIAS

Continued reciprocal beating of atria and ventricles can today be presumed as the cause of many, although not all, supraventricular paroxysmal tachycardias. Leaning on convincing experimental data found in the animal (Janse et al., 1971; Mendez and Moe, 1966; Moe and Mendez, 1966) and in man (Coumel et al., 1967; Wellens, 1971) spontaneous initiation and termination of paroxysms can now be understood in physiologic terms. One such instance is

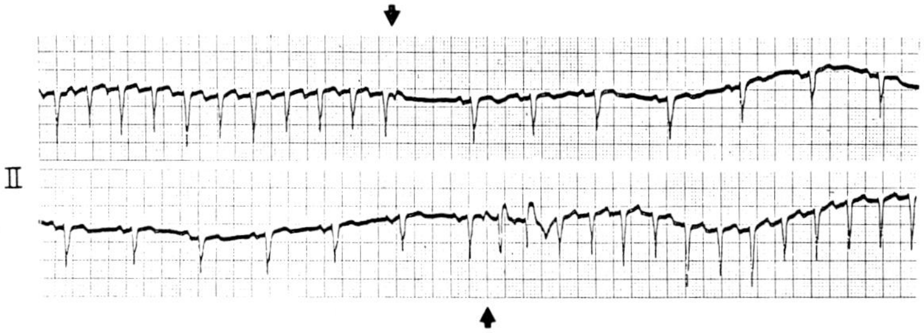

Fig. 4. Termination (↓) and resumption (↑) of reciprocating supraventricular paroxysmal tachycardia by atrial premature beats. The right bundle branch block contour of the first and second beat of the recurrent tachycardia is due to aberrant ventricular conduction.

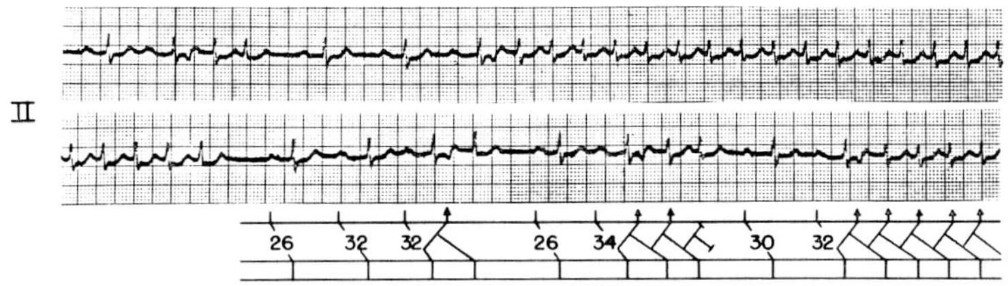

Fig. 5. Repetitive reciprocating supraventricular tachycardia initiated by critical (0.32–0.34 sec) P–R prolongation in Type I second-degree A–V block (caused by digitalis).

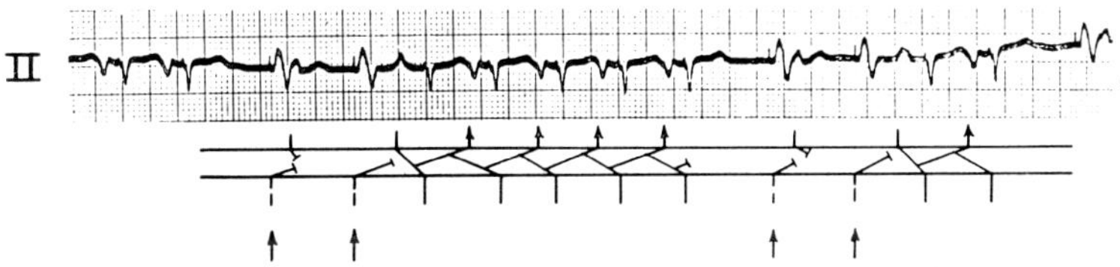

Fig. 6. Intermittent reciprocating supraventricular tachycardia initiated by prolonged A–V conduction time of ventricular captures during A–V dissociation resulting from ventricular pacing.

illustrated in Figure 4. In the upper strip, a junctional circus movement can be postulated to be interrupted when a spontaneous premature atrial discharge at the upper arrow invades and blocks the circus path; it is resumed in the lower strip when a similar spontaneous atrial ectopic impulse, at the lower arrow, conducted with delay to the ventricles, initiates repetitive alternating echoes of atria and ventricles. We also can now understand why in Type I A–V block, as illustrated in Figure 5, paroxysms of reciprocating tachycardia prevent the completion of a Wenckebach period, once a critically prolonged P–R is reached: it sets the stage for the first as well as consecutive re-entry processes in the A–V junction. Another more rare example of the crucial role of slowed A–V conduction in the initiation and perpetuation of atrial and ventricular echoes is shown in Figure 6. During demand pacing of the ventricles, indicated by the pairs of upright arrows, A–V dissociation is transiently replaced by atrioventricular reciprocation subsequent to the prolonged P–R interval of a ventricular capture by a sinus impulse.

However, not all known varieties of junctional tachycardia have their experimental counterpart. Continued reciprocation remains to be proved in cases with a bidirectional exit block. In Figure 7 is shown an example with 2 diagrams which may or may not require amendment. In a junctional tachycardia there is repetitive group beating of the ventricles and

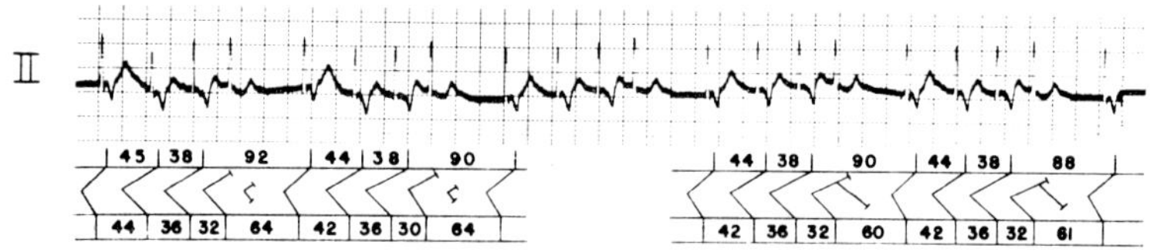

Fig. 7. A–V junctional tachycardia with Wenckebach periods of forward and retrograde conduction. For explanation of the 2 diagrams, see text.

atria, corresponding to a 5:4 antegrade and a 5:3 retrograde Type I block. In the left diagram, a continuous regular junctional discharge is assumed; at the right, concealed subatrial antegrade re-entry is assumed, resetting the cycle of the junctional focus.

DUAL A–V PATHWAYS vs SUPERNORMAL A–V CONDUCTION

Reciprocal beating is one of the manifestations in the human heart of the experimentally proved existence of at least 2 A–V transmission systems having different functional properties (Mendez and Moe, 1966). These potential re-entry pathways may not be utilized to their entire length and the sweep may be incomplete. Thus, in 1950, we explained a curious case (Fig. 8) of slow junctional rhythm, in which R–P intervals and junctional cycles alternated concomitantly, by concealed antegrade re-entry, postponing the next junctional discharge. This is evident in the lower panel where each R–P of 0.20 sec is followed by an R–R of 1.08 sec, while R–P intervals of 0.28 sec lead to R–R prolongation to 1.36 sec. The clue to an interpretation was found in the upper record of another day. Here it could be seen that the prolongation of the ventricular interval to 1.24 sec was the result of junctional re-entry, actually completed in the middle, but concealed at both ends of the record. By the same token, we explained in another case (Fig. 9) of incomplete A–V dissociation failure of a

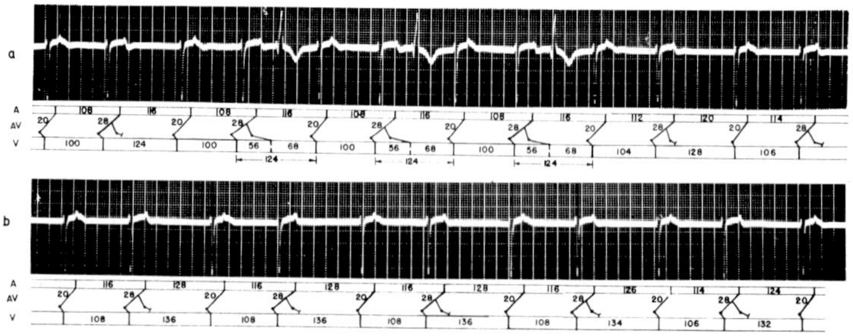

Fig. 8. Concealed (blocked) reciprocal beating in A–V junctional rhythm with delayed retrograde conduction. Note that in (b) the longer R–P interval of 0.28 is always followed by prolongation of the manifest junctional cycle from 1.08 to 1.36 sec.

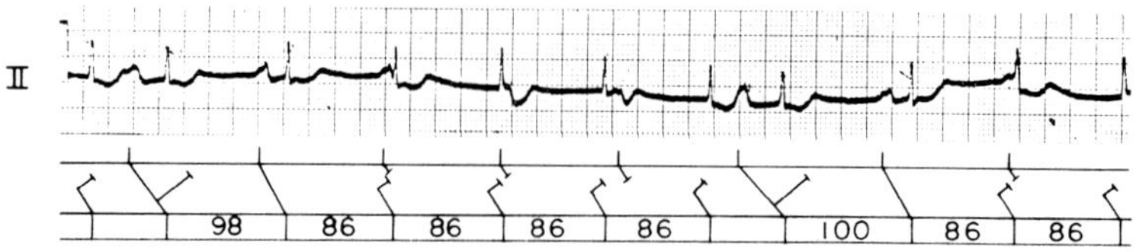

Fig. 9. Concealed retrograde re-entry (attempt at atrial echo) in incomplete A–V dissociation which developed after acceleration of A–V junctional impulse formation by digitalis.

junctional escape to occur at the expected time of 0.86 sec by a concealed retrograde re-entry attempt induced by prolonged antegrade conduction of early ventricular captures.

Leaning on experimental data available in the literature, we can now interpret with confidence other variants of such mechanisms, e.g. some atypical features of atrioventricular Wenckebach periods. Figure 10 is an unusual electrocardiogram in which 4 different events have been labelled *a* to *d* for presentation. Part *d* shows a simple 3:2 Wenckebach period. In *a* to *c* the sequence of regular sinus impulses is disturbed by atrial echoes induced by greater delay in antegrade conduction. These echoes occur regardless of whether the initiating sinus impulse reaches the ventricles as in *c* or fails to do so as in *a* and *b*. However, when it fails, the unused portion of the antegrade path provides a potential avenue for a ventricular echo, a sweep which is actually completed in portion *b*.

In the Wenckebach periods shown in Figure 11, the arrow indicates that, against the rule, the increment in P–R is largest before the dropped beat. Previously we tried to explain this by assuming a critical state of A–V conductivity before its total failure (Pick et al., 1962). Today we can attribute it to the after-effect of an attempted re-entry via a retrograde path that has opened up after sufficient delay of antegrade conduction. In Figure 12 an opposite event is seen. In the middle of a Wenckebach period, at the arrow, P–R unexpectedly shortens

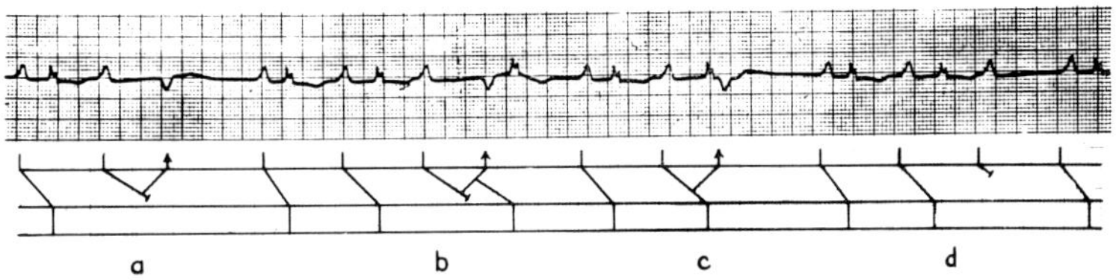

Fig. 10. Second-degree A–V block (Type I) with concealed A–V conduction with 3 atrial echoes and 1 ventricular echo.

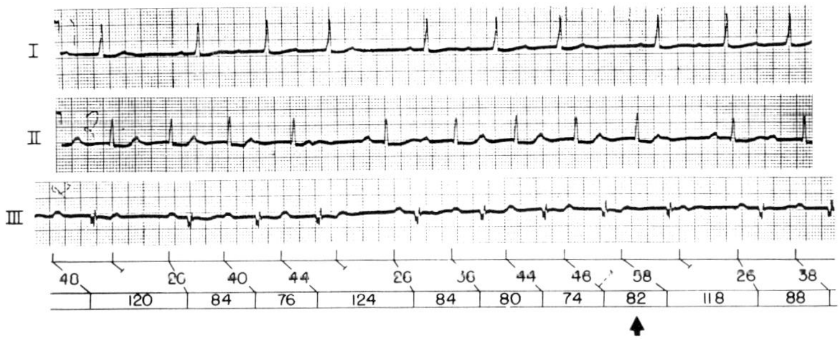

Fig. 11. Concealed re-entry in the A–V junction (attempt at atrial echo) causing an 'atypical' Wenckebach period.

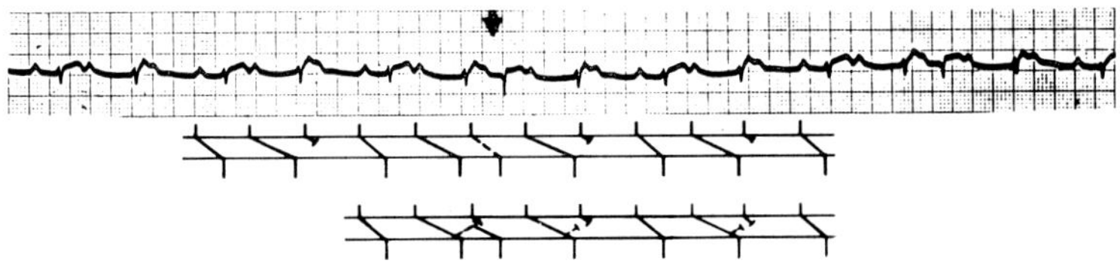

Fig. 12. Atypical Wenckebach periods due to a double A–V path (upper diagram) or concealed retrograde, followed by manifest antegrade, re-entry (lower diagram) in the A–V junction.

before the period is resumed and completed. Previously (Pick et al., 1962) we thought that this might be due to supernormal conduction through depressed A–V junctional tissues. In the light of advanced knowledge other interpretations appear more likely. In the upper diagram, 2 longitudinally dissociated conduction pathways with different conduction speeds are considered. In the lower diagram, the premature QRS is unrelated to the P wave preceding it. Rather it is a ventricular echo reflected from an abortive attempt at an atrial echo.

The concept of supernormal A–V conduction is hypothetical and indeed was severely criticized by Moe et al. (1968). It is unlikely in the case of unexpected shortening of conduction time of successive impulses traveling in the *same* direction. However, we still consider the mechanism of supernormal conduction in cases of advanced A–V block (Fig. 13) when captures occur exclusively and predictably in a narrow limited early period of the ventricular cycle. In the example shown, the range for A–V conduction, expressed in R–P intervals, is 0.16–0.22 sec. We attribute this to backward penetration of ventricular impulses, transiently converting a region of unidirectional conduction into one of supernormal conduction. We also have no other explanation for cases of Type II A–V block such as that shown in Figure 14, in which resumption of A–V conduction is clearly dependent on the

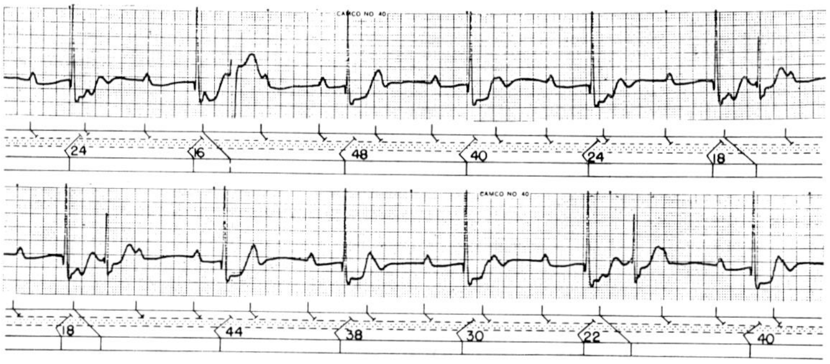

Fig. 13. Incomplete A–V dissociation due to advanced unidirectional A–V block. Concealed retrograde conduction of idioventricular impulses permits ventricular capture by sinus impulses (with aberrant ventricular conduction) only during a supernormal phase of A–V conduction.

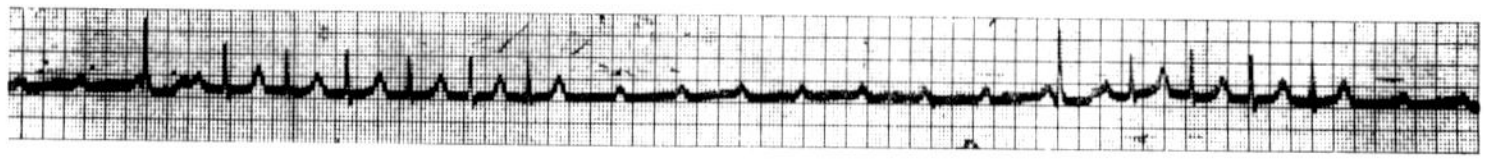

Fig. 14. Sudden protracted ventricular arrest in Type II second-degree A–V block. A–V conduction is resumed following spontaneous escape of a subsidiary ectopic pacemaker.

appearance of a junctional or ventricular escape beat. Perhaps a clue may be the experimental demonstration of summation effects of subthreshold action potentials in Purkinje fibers (Cranefield and Hoffman, 1971).

Figure 15 shows a case of 2:1 A–V block with 2 different P–R intervals published in 1938 by Katz's associates (Gertz et al., 1938). This is probably the first *clinical* instance in which operation of 2 pathways in a single A–V junction was taken into consideration. Watanabe (1967) reproduced this in an alternating form in the rabbit heart and showed by microelectrodes that the cause was alternating depth of penetration of the N region of the A–V junction by blocked atrial impulses. This explanation, however, cannot readily apply to a random variation of P–R intervals nor to alternation of P–R intervals in 1:1 conduction, as illustrated in Figure 16. This is a record which we, probably erroneously, published as an example of supernormal A–V conduction, because the less prolonged P–R followed against the rule

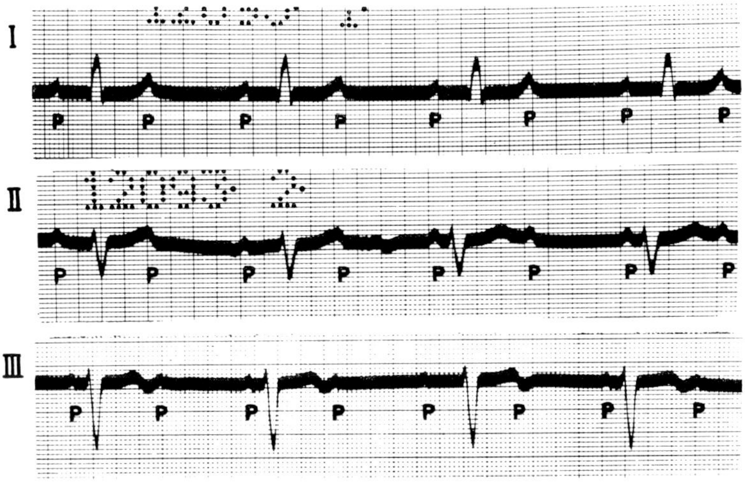

Fig. 15. 2:1 A–V block in bilateral (right and left anterior fascicular) bundle branch system block. Note 2 fixed ranges (0.16 and 0.34 sec) of P–R intervals in the conducted beats.

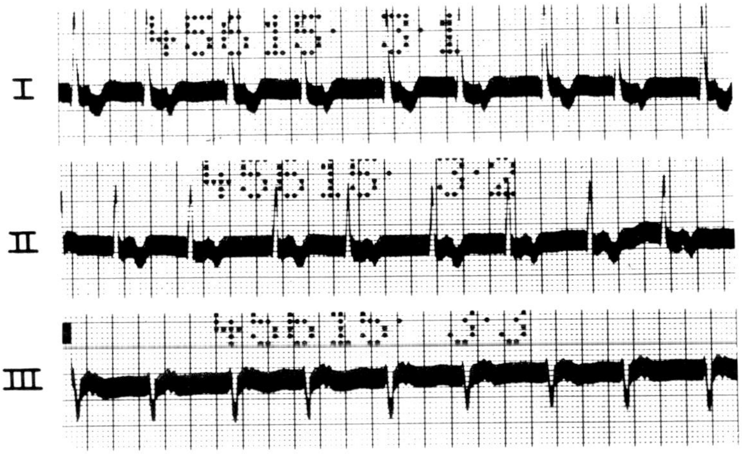

Fig. 16. First-degree A–V block with alternation of P–R intervals (causing ventricular bigeminy). For interpretation, see text and Fig. 17.

the shorter R–P distance. Moe et al. (1968) have provided diagrams of alternative explanations for such observations based on dissociation of the upper junction into 2 pathways α and β, having different refractoriness and conduction speeds. An attempt at reinterpretation of our case on this basis is presented in Figure 17. A is the diagram of the originally proposed and discarded explanation by supernormal A–V conduction. In B and C longitudinally dissociated pathways α and β are assumed, each of which can be entered only by alternate atrial impulses due to a 2:1 block. Diagram A postulates shorter refractoriness and faster conduction in pathway α. In B the α path also has a shorter refractory period but slower conduction with partial retrograde penetration of pathway β. Added to this is diagram D of an entirely different but possible explanation: a 2:1 block in a single path, in which conducted beats alternate with junctional escapes.

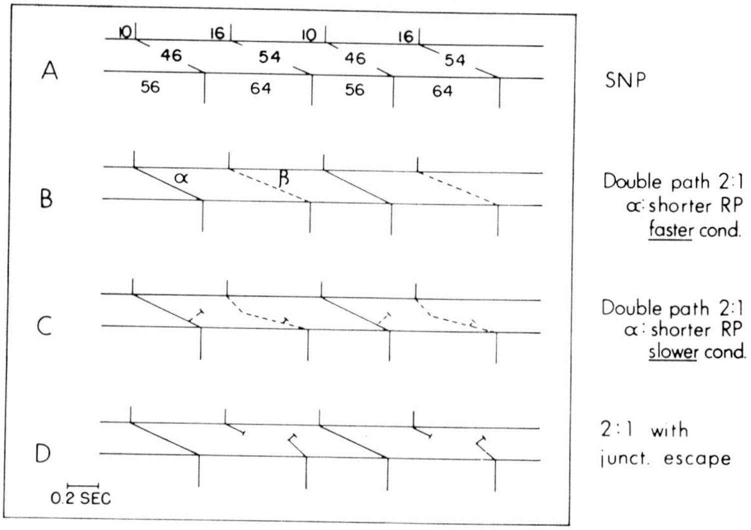

Fig. 17. Diagrammatic interpretation of Fig. 16. The numbers in diagram A represent (in sec/100) R–P intervals in the upper level, P–R intervals in the middle level and R–R intervals in the lowest level. SNP = supernormal phase of A–V conduction. Two A–V pathways (α and β) are indicated in diagrams B and C by solid and broken diagonal lines.

THE PRE-EXCITATION (WPW) SYNDROME

A discussion of a dual A–V conduction system would be incomplete without consideration of the pre-excitation syndrome. In the context of my topic I should like to make only some historical remarks and present some puzzling clinical observations with tentative but as yet unproved interpretations. In a diagram (Fig. 18) devised in 1955, we postulated (Pick and Katz, 1955) that the A–V bypass may not be total as in path #1, but take off as, in path #3, in a lower part of the A–V node instead in the atria. This assumption appeared necessary to account for cases of pre-excitation associated with A–V block. For instance (Fig. 19), in a case of first-degree A–V block it was found that intermittent pre-excitation shortened the P–R from 0.30 sec to not less than 0.24 sec. Or, in the case shown in Figure 20, the question had to be answered why pre-excitation present in 1962 did not prevent a 2:1 block recorded 2 years earlier. Today, this speculation can be considered justified thanks to detailed anatomical studies (James, 1961; Lev, 1966) and physiologic experiments (Coumel et al., 1971; Wellens, 1971). Our simple basic diagram of partial bypass fibers has been amplified by inclusion of James and Mahaim fibers in a diagram by Durrer et al. (1970). In a series of other diagrams presented by Coumel et al. (1971) in France a correlation was made of the function of the various known partial and total bypasses with their electrocardiographic manifestations, including His bundle recording. In one of these, it is postulated that James fibers bypass the A–V node to enter the His bundle, and the delta wave is caused by independent Mahaim fibers which bypass the ventricular conduction system. That had been previously predicted from standard electrocardiograms in one of our own cases and was then confirmed post mortem by Lev et al. (1966) in a meticulous study of serial sections of the A–V junction.

However, these diagrams cover only the relation of bypasses to the normal A–V junction. What about varieties of their terminal insertion? In a case of pre-excitation Type A in combination with a right bundle branch block (Fig. 21) we attributed persistence of the latter

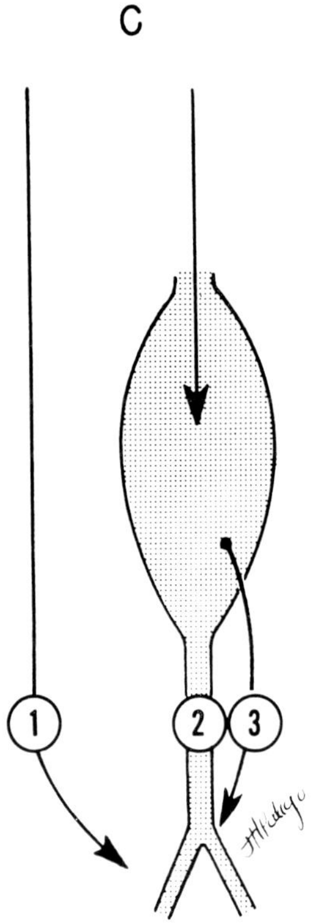

Fig. 18. Schematic representation of pathways for A–V conduction in ventricular pre-excitation. (2) normal path through A–V node and bundle of His; (1) total A–V bypass; (3) partial A–V bypass.

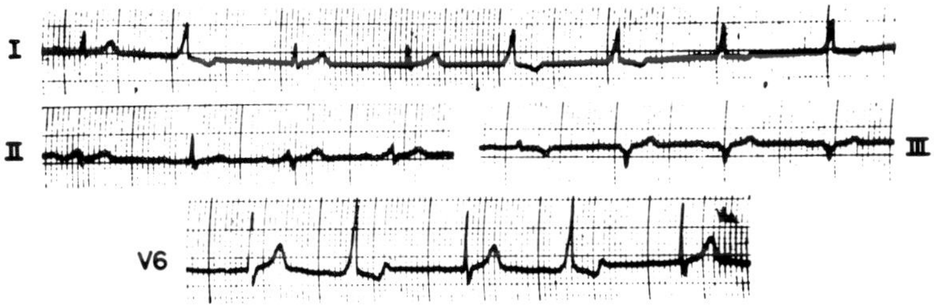

Fig. 19. Intermittent ventricular pre-excitation with first-degree A–V block.

to a bypass pre-exciting the contralateral left ventricle (Pick and Fisch, 1958). But this assumption was untenable in another case of intermittent right bundle branch block associated with pre-excitation of Type B (Fig. 22). Note that in the framed Lead V_1 a deep negative delta wave is followed by a large late R wave. Here right-sided pre-excitation did not preclude the bundle branch block in the ipsilateral ventricle. Pending a better explanation, based on anatomical and physiologic study of such cases, we propose that a complete right-sided A–V bypass could insert proximal to the region of block in the right ventricular conduction system.

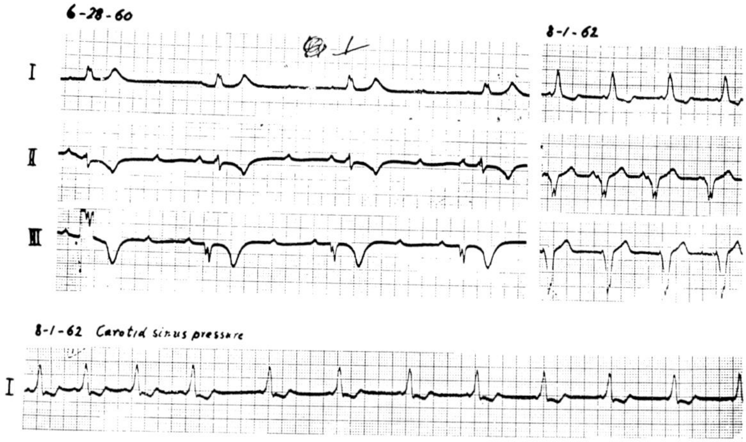

Fig. 20. In 1960: 3:1 A–V block during recent ischemia of the inferior wall. 1962: 1:1 conduction with ventricular pre-excitation.

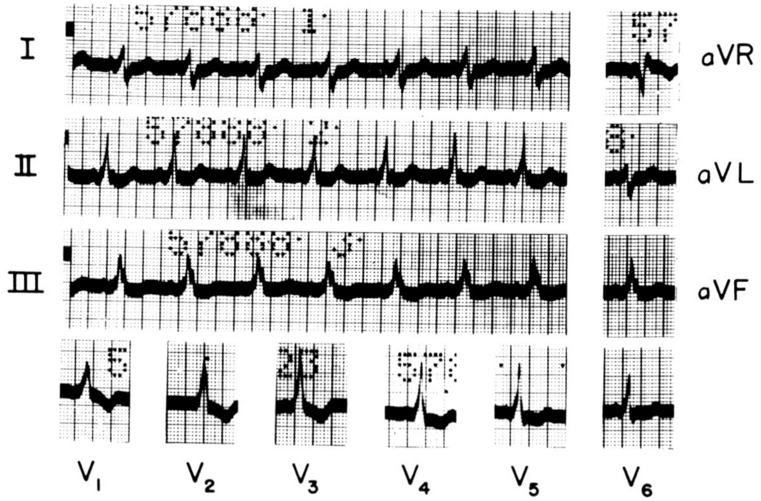

Fig. 21. Ventricular pre-excitation Type A in the presence of a right bundle branch block.

JUNCTIONAL ESCAPE WITH ABERRANT VENTRICULAR CONDUCTION

In the electrocardiogram shown in Figure 23, obtained from a digitalized case of atrial fibrillation, regular escape beats, the smaller QRS complexes in each lead, show a higher degree of right bundle branch block than the faster conducted ones. The following 5 explanations have been offered for this apparent paradox: origin of the escapes in or close to Mahaim fibers (Pick, 1956); Phase 4 depolarization (Singer and Ten Eick, 1971); origin in one of the fascicles of the ventricular conduction system (Rosenbaum, 1969); functional dissociation within a bundle branch (Wellens, 1969); and supernormality of intraventricular conduction (Friedberg, 1971). The first and the last are purely hypothetical and may apply only exceptionally. For the effects of Phase 4 depolarization Singer and Ten Eick (1971) have provided experimental evidence in microelectrode studies of automatic Purkinje cells. Aberration of

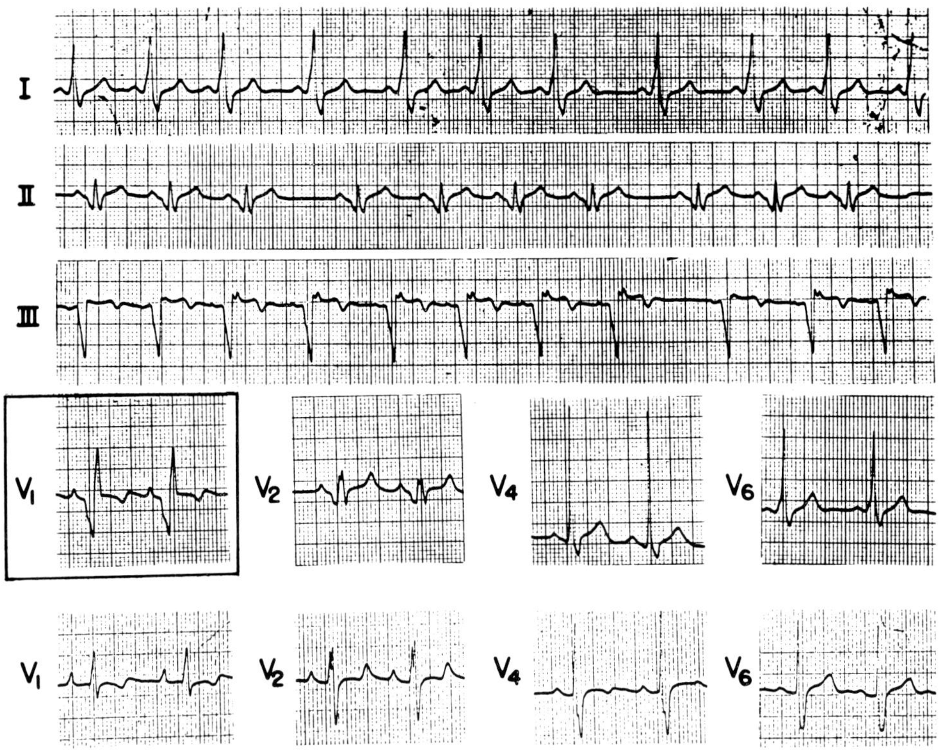

Fig. 22. Intermittent ventricular pre-excitation Type B in the presence of right bundle branch block. Pre-excitation is seen in the limb leads and upper series of chest leads, and has disappeared in the lower series, V_1 to V_6.

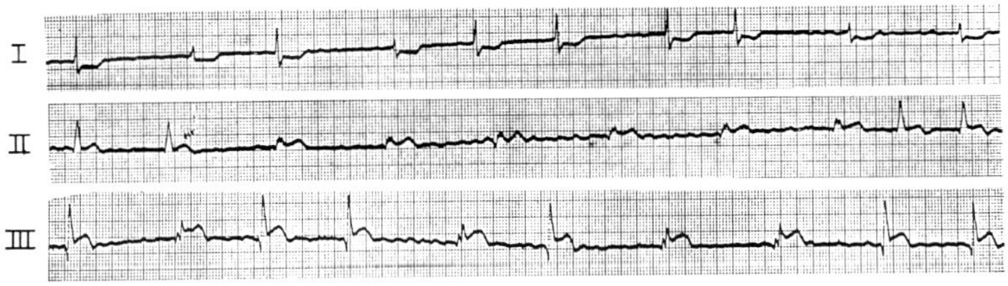

Fig. 23. Atrial fibrillation with slow ventricular response and A–V junctional escape with aberrant ventricular conduction (smaller QRS complexes in each lead) causing temporary A–V dissociation in the middle of Lead II.

R–S–T depends on the magnitude of the transmembrane potential at the time of an ectopic impulse. This take-off potential may be reduced due to (*a*) incomplete repolarization in the case of a premature impulse or (*b*) diastolic Phase 4 depolarization with a late impulse. The latter mechanism is most likely in cases like the one illustrated in Figure 24. Normal intraventricular conduction is maintained up to a cycle length of 112; it is slightly aberrant with a cycle of 116 and totally aberrant with cycles equal to or longer than 120. In other cases Rosenbaum's (1969) concept of fascicular origin can be more readily applied (Fig. 25). In this case of atrial fibrillation, escape beats can be identified in the routine electrocardiogram on top by their constant long cycle, as well as by the pattern of a posterior fascicular block.

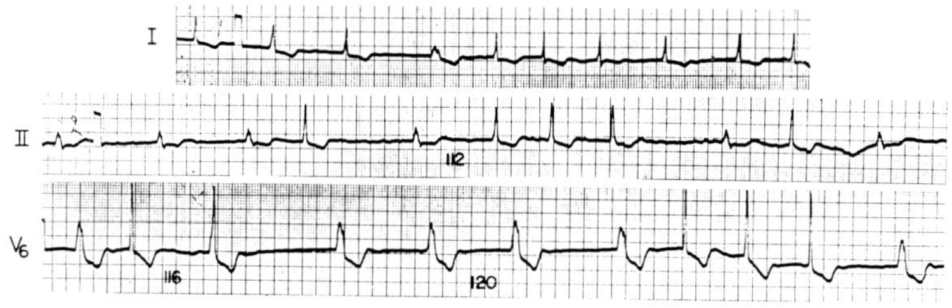

Fig. 24. Intermittent (bradycardia dependent) left bundle branch block in atrial fibrillation and left ventricular hypertrophy. The degree of the intraventricular conduction disturbance is determined by the cycle length.

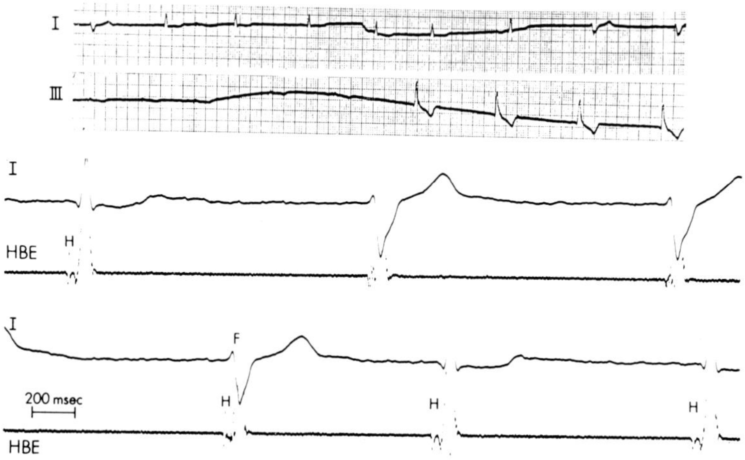

Fig. 25. Atrial fibrillation with a slow ventricular response and repetitive escape of a subsidiary pacemaker, probably located in the anterior fascicle of the left bundle branch. His bundle recordings (HBE) reveal that H potentials precede only conducted beats and a fusion beat (F).

Their ventricular origin, presumably in the left anterior fascicle, could be documented in the His electrogram. They lack an H deflection which precedes at a normal H–V interval the conducted beats and the fusion beat (F) in the lowest panel.

However, the possibility of supernormal conduction in depressed bundle branches cannot be entirely dismissed and I should like to present one pertinent example (Fig. 26). In a case of left bundle branch block, premature beats show a typical contour of a bifascicular, right and left anterior, conduction defect. Conceivably, the ectopic beats could arise in the posterior fascicle of the left bundle branch system, distal to a region of high predivisional block. However, it could also be postulated that supernormal conduction through the left bundle unmasks a latent block in the right bundle branch system.

TYPE I (WENCKEBACH) BLOCK IN THE PERIPHERAL CONDUCTION SYSTEM

I will conclude my discussion with one more aspect of abnormal intraventricular conduction, highlighting how new techniques have borne out hypotheses. Figure 27 is a case of intermittent ventricular bigeminy with dropping out of a ventricular premature beat after progressive lengthening of the coupling interval from 54 to 70. Here we speculated on an intraventricular Wenckebach mechanism located either in a re-entry path or at the Purkinje-

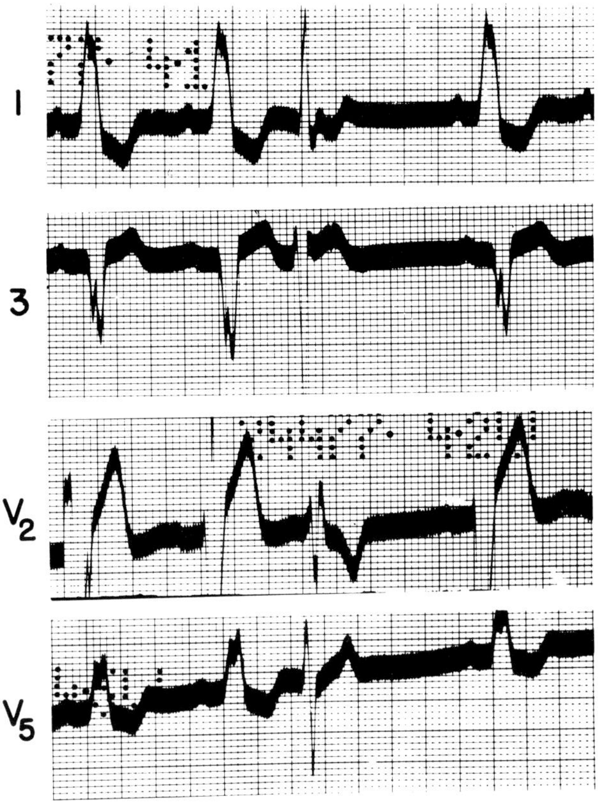

Fig. 26. Left bundle branch block (QRS 0.16 sec) with premature beats of bilateral (right and left anterior fascicular) bundle branch block configuration having less QRS prolongation (0.14 sec).

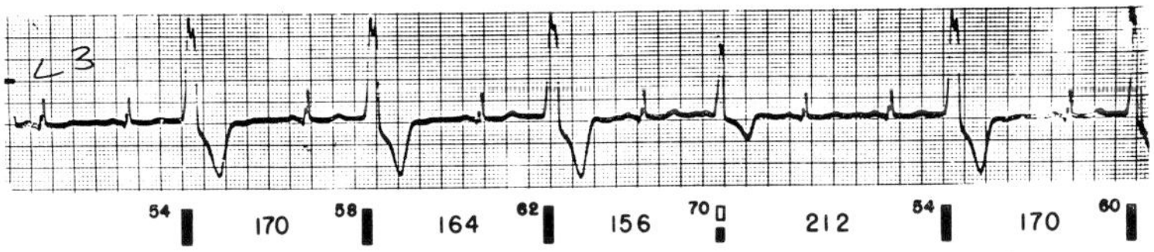

Fig. 27. Intermittent ventricular bigeminy. Progressive prolongation of coupling interval (upper small numbers) of ventricular premature beats. The longest coupling (0.70 sec) before intermission approaches the length of the sinus cycle, resulting in a ventricular fusion beat (interrupted white-black bar in the diagram). Note that the irregular interectopic intervals (lower larger numbers) have the structure of a Wenckebach period.

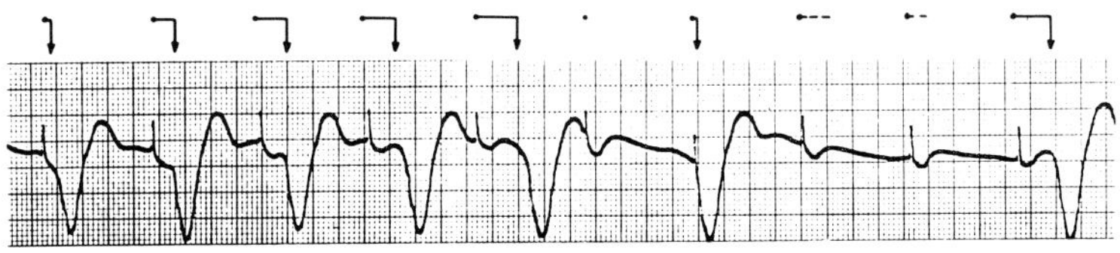

Fig. 28. Type I exit block of impulses of a failing artificial ventricular pacemaker. In the diagram the dots indicate pacer discharge, horizontal lines the duration of latency of ventricular responses (↓), interrupted horizontal lines decremental (concealed) conduction from point of stimulation into surrounding myocardium.

myocardial junction. Support for this assumption we found in a patient with pacemaker dysfunction (Fig. 28). Progressively longer stimulus to response intervals preceded a nonresponse. The prolonged latency after 2 successive failures, as seen at the end of the record, we attributed to decremental propagation of the pacer stimulus. That a Wenckebach type of block can indeed occur between contractile myocardium and Purkinje fibers was shown in 1961 by Alanis et al. in Mexico in the rapidly driven dog heart. Recently Greenspan et al. (1971) documented this in hypoxic canine Purkinje fibers as well as in excised human ventricular tissue perfused by potassium in high concentration.

REFERENCES

ALANIS, J., BENITEZ, D. and PILAR, G. (1961): A functional discontinuity between the Purkinje and ventricular muscle cells. *Acta physiol. lat.-amer.*, *11*, 171.

CASTILLO, C. A. and CASTELLANOS JR., A. (1970): The mechanism of ventricular preexcitation as studied by His bundle electrogram. In: *Proceedings, Symposium on Cardiac Arrhythmias, 1970*, p. 329. AB Astra, Denmark.

COUMEL, P., CABROL, C., FABIATO, A., GOURGON, R. and SLAMA, S. (1967): Tachycardie permanente par rhythme réciproque. I. Preuves de diagnostic par stimulation auriculaire et ventriculaire. II. Traitement par l'implantation intracorporelle d'une stimulateur cardiaque avec entraînement simultané de l'oreillette et du ventricule. *Arch. Mal. Cœur*, *60*, 1830, 1850.

COUMEL, P., WAYNEBERGER, M., SLAMA, R. and BOUVRAIN, Y. (1971): Intérêt de l'enregistrement de potentiels Hisiens au cours du syndrome de Wolff-Parkinson-White; à propos de six observations. *Acta cardiol. (Brux.)*, *26*, 188.

CRANEFIELD, P. F. and HOFFMAN, B. F. (1971): Conduction of the cardiac impulse. II. Summation and inhibition. *Circulat. Res.*, *28*, 220.

DURRER, D., SCHUILENBURG, R. M. and WELLENS, H. J. J. (1970): Preexcitation revisited. *Amer. J. Cardiol.*, *25*, 690.

FRIEDBERG, H. D. (1971): Mechanism of the Wedensky phenomenon in the left bundle branch. *Amer. J. Cardiol.*, *27*, 698.

GERTZ, G., KAPLAN, H. A., KAPLAN, L. G. and WEINSTEIN, W. (1938): Cardiac syncope due to paroxysms of ventricular flutter, fibrillation and asystole in a patient with varying degrees of A–V block and intraventricular block. *Amer. Heart J.*, *16*, 225.

GREENSPAN, K., ANDERSON, G. J. and FISCH, C. (1971): Electrophysiologic correlate of exit block. *Amer. J. Cardiol.*, *28*, 197.

JAMES, T. N. (1961): Morphology of the human atrio-ventricular node with remarks pertinent to its electrophysiology. *Amer. Heart J.*, *62*, 756.

JANSE, M. J., VAN CAPELL, F. J. L., FREUD, G. E. and DURRER, D. (1971): Circus movement within the AV node as a basis for supraventricular tachycardia as shown by multiple microelectrode recording in the isolated rabbit heart. *Circulat. Res.*, *28*, 403.

KATZ, L. N. and PICK, A. (1956): *Clinical Electrocardiography. Part I. The Arrhythmias.* Lea and Febiger, Philadelphia, Pa.

LANGENDORF, R. and PICK, A. (1971): Artificial pacing of the human heart. Its contribution to the understanding of arrhythmias. *Amer. J. Cardiol.*, *28*, 516.

LEV, M. (1966): Anatomic considerations of anomalous A–V pathways. In: *Mechanisms and Therapy of Cardiac Arrhythmias*, p. 665. Editors: L. S. Dreifus and W. Likoff. Grune and Stratton, Inc., New York, N.Y.

LEV, M., LEFFLER, W. B., LANGENDORF, R. and PICK, A. (1966): Anatomic findings in a case of ventricular preexcitation (WPW) terminating in complete atrioventricular block. *Circulation*, *34*, 718.

LEWIS, T. and MASTER, A. M. (1925): Observations upon conduction in the mammalian heart. *Heart*, *12*, 209.

MENDEZ, C. and MOE, G. K. (1966): Demonstration of a dual A–V nodal conduction system in the isolated rabbit heart. *Circulat. Res.*, *19*, 378.

MOE, G. K., CHILDERS, R. W. and MERIDETH, J. (1968): An appraisal of 'supernormal' A–V conduction. *Circulation*, *38*, 5.

Moe, G. K. and Mendez, C. (1966): The physiologic basis of reciprocal rhythm. *Progr. cardiovasc. Dis.*, *8*, 461.

Moore, E. N., Knoebel, S. B. and Spear, J. F. (1971): Concealed conduction. *Amer. J. Cardiol.*, *28*, 406.

Pick, A. (1956): Aberrant ventricular conduction of escaped beats: Preferential and accessory pathways in the A–V junction. *Circulation*, *13*, 702.

Pick, A. (1966): Electrocardiographic features of exit block. In: *Mechanisms and Therapy of Cardiac Arrhythmias*, p. 469. Editors: L. S. Dreifus and W. Likoff. Grune and Stratton, Inc., New York, N.Y.

Pick, A. and Fisch, C. (1958): Ventricular pre-excitation (WPW) in the presence of bundle branch block. *Amer. Heart J.*, *55*, 504.

Pick, A. and Katz, L. N. (1955): Disturbances of impulse formation and conduction in the pre-excitation (WPW) syndrome – their bearing on its mechanism. *Amer. J. Med.*, *19*, 422.

Pick, A., Langendorf, R. and Katz, L. N. (1962): The supernormal phase of atrioventricular conduction. I. Fundamental mechanisms. *Circulation*, *24*, 388.

Rosen, K. M., Rahimtoola, S. H. and Gunnar, R. M. (1970): Pseudo A–V block secondary to premature nonpropagated His bundle depolarizations. Documentation by His bundle electrocardiography. *Circulation*, *42*, 367.

Rosenbaum, M. B. (1969): Classification of ventricular extrasystoles according to form. *J. Electrocardiol.*, *2*, 289.

Singer, D. H. and Ten Eick, R. E. (1971): Aberrancy: Electrophysiologic aspects. *Amer. J. Cardiol.*, *28*, 381.

Watanabe, Y. (1967): A–V conduction disturbances and electrophysiology. *Igaku no Ayumi*, *69*, 339.

Wellens, H. (1969): Unusual occurrence of nonaberrant conduction in patients with atrial fibrillation and aberrant conduction. *Amer. Heart J.*, *77*, 158.

Wellens, H. J. J. (1971): *Electrical Stimulation of the Heart in the Study and Treatment of Tachycardias.* University Park Press, Baltimore, Md.

THE EFFECT OF PYRIDINOLCARBAMATE ON THE PLATELET RESPONSE TO ADP IN PATIENTS WITH INTERMITTENT CLAUDICATION

R. C. COTTON, K. BLOOR and G. ARCHIBALD

University Department of Surgery, Manchester Royal Infirmary and Research Department, I.C.I. Pharmaceuticals Division, Alderley Park, Macclesfield, Cheshire, United Kingdom

Virchow (1856, 1871) regarded atheromatous lesions as inflammatory in origin. He considered that the initial arterial change was intimal oedema and the fibrous thickening and fatty degeneration were interpreted as resulting from long-continued irritation. Shimamoto (1963) has revived this hypothesis. He considers that even in patients with advanced atherosclerotic lesions oedematous areas are present in the vessel wall which could contribute to the narrowing of the lumen of the artery (Shimamoto, 1969). He has produced oedematous swelling of the subendothelial and muscular layers of large arteries in monkeys and rabbits using single doses of adrenalin or cholesterol (Shimamoto, 1963). Adhesion of platelets and leucocytes to the endothelial surface was seen to occur as part of the reaction. Compounds which inhibit this so-called oedematous arterial reaction were also found to interfere with the deposition of cholesterol in the arteries of cholesterol-fed rabbits. The most effective compound, of those investigated, was pyridinolcarbamate.

During the investigation of patients with intermittent claudication who were receiving pyridinolcarbamate we measured the effect of the compound on platelet function. We considered that change in platelet function might reflect events occurring in the arterial wall. The sensitivity of the platelets to ADP was measured in a group of patients with peripheral atherosclerosis and the results compared with those obtained in apparently healthy subjects. Further measurements were then made in a number of these patients while they were receiving pyridinolcarbamate.

Twenty-one patients with peripheral atherosclerosis and 25 normal subjects were investigated. The latter were apparently healthy male subjects on the staff of I.C.I. These were selected so that there were 2 groups of widely different ages. One group consisted of subjects of age range 20–30 years; the other group consisted of subjects in the 40–60 age range. The mean age of the latter group did not differ significantly from the patient group (Table I).

On each blood sample the platelet response to 4 concentrations of ADP was measured. Plasma fibrinogen, erythrocyte sedimentation rate (ESR), white cell count, platelet count

TABLE I

Age range in patients with peripheral atherosclerosis and apparently healthy subjects investigated

Group	Number	Age (years) (mean $\pm$ SEM)
Patients with atherosclerosis	21	56.9 ± 1.7
Normal males	14	52.9 ± 1.9
Normal males	11	24.2 ± 0.9

and blood level of pyridinolcarbamate and its metabolites were also measured. The apparatus used for the measurement of platelet aggregation was constructed from details given by Swank et al. (1964) and the method was similar to that described by Dhall and Matheson (1969). Two ml of the citrated blood-ADP mixture was forced at a constant rate through a screen containing 20 × 20 μ perforations. The changes in pressure which occurred proximal to the screen were transmitted to a strain gauge transducer and recorded. The maximal pressure which develops has been shown to correlate with the degree of platelet aggregation (Dhall et al., 1969).

The results (Fig. 1) indicated that in the group of patients with peripheral atherosclerosis

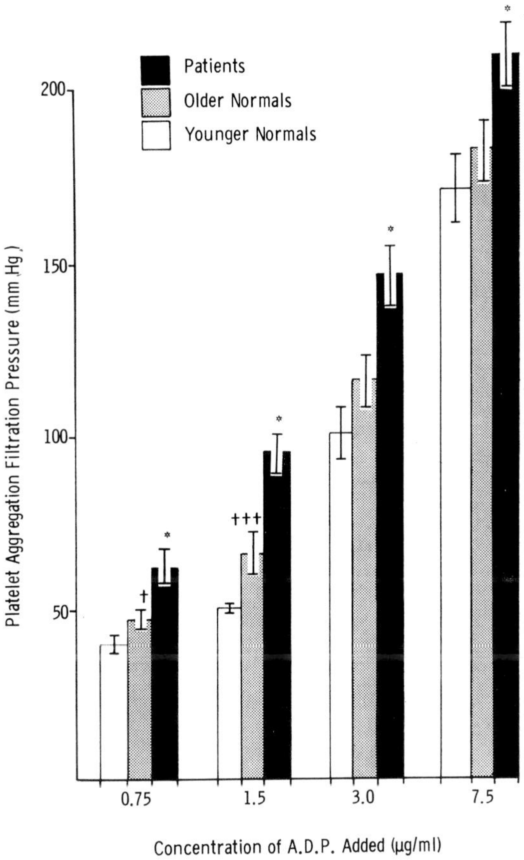

Fig. 1. Platelet response to ADP in a group of patients with peripheral atherosclerosis and in apparently healthy normal subjects. * = $p < 0.02$ – significance of difference from older normal subjects; + = $p < 0.02$, + + + = $p < 0.001$ – significance of difference from younger normal subjects.

there was a statistically significant increase in the platelet response to ADP compared with values obtained in normal subjects of similar age. This effect was significant at each of the concentrations of ADP tested. In the younger normal subjects the mean value for platelet aggregation filtration pressure (PAFP), at each concentration of ADP, was lower than that of the older subjects. This difference was statistically significant using the 0.75 μg/ml and 1.5 μg/ml strengths of ADP. Plasma fibrinogen levels and ESR values followed the same trend (Table II). There was no significant correlation between PAFP and platelet count,

TABLE II

Comparisons between platelet count, haematocrit, white cell count, fibrinogen and ESR in patients with peripheral atherosclerosis and normal subjects

Group	Platelet count (thousands per mm^3)	Haematocrit (%)	White cell count/mm^3	Plasma fibrinogen (mg %)	ESR (mm in 1st hr)
Peripheral atherosclerosis (21)	238.2 ± 18.0	41.3 ± 1.09*	$8,657 \pm 420$	486.8 ± 50.6*	27.3 ± 6.4**
Normal subjects age 40–60 yr (14)	190.9 ± 18.2	44.5 ± 0.53	$7,521 \pm 445$	$349.1 \pm 19.6^{+}$	$5.5 \pm 0.9^{+}$
Normal subjects age 20–30 yr (11)	177.9 ± 7.9	44.7 ± 0.75	$7,118 \pm 422$	281.8 ± 13.4	2.8 ± 0.3

* $= p < 0.02$, ** $= p < 0.01$ – significance of difference from 40–60 age group.
\+ $= p < 0.01$ – significance of difference from 20–30 age group.

white cell count, ESR, plasma fibrinogen or haematocrit in either the normal or the atherosclerotic groups of patients.

Thirteen of the patients were then treated with pyridinolcarbamate, 250 mg 3 times daily for the first week and then 500 mg 3 times daily for the rest of the period of study. Further blood samples were then taken, initially at weekly intervals and then every 2–4 weeks. No change in PAFP was apparent during the first 4 weeks of treatment. However, after 5 weeks there was a significant reduction in the platelet response to ADP and a further reduction occurred by the 11th to 16th week of therapy (Fig. 2). At this time there was also a significant reduction in the plasma fibrinogen level. This was reduced from a mean value ($\pm$SEM) of 470.0 ± 29.4 mg% to 397.0 ± 17.1 mg% ($p < 0.05$).

We have no knowledge of the mechanism producing an increase in sensitivity of the platelets to ADP in these patients with peripheral atherosclerosis. The fact that platelet sensitivity to ADP increases with age and that there is a further increase in patients with clinical evidence of atherosclerosis suggests that this phenomenon may correlate with the degree of atherosclerosis. Pilgeram (1961) has made similar comments regarding changes in plasma fibrinogen concentration with increasing age.

The mechanism by which pyridinolcarbamate reduces the platelet response to ADP in these patients is also speculative. We have not been able to demonstrate any activity on platelet aggregation in vitro using final concentrations of pyridinolcarbamate of up to 4 times that obtained in vivo. We found that the blood level of the compound remained more or less constant at about 30 μg/ml from the second week of treatment onwards, whereas the platelet response to ADP was diminishing from the 5th to the 16th week of treatment. It is possible therefore that the effect on platelet function is an indirect one. Samama (1971) found that

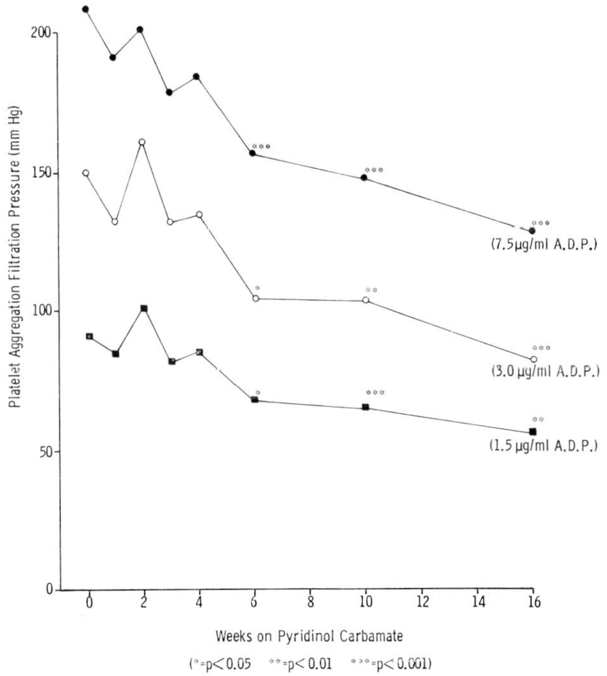

Fig. 2. Effect of pyridinolcarbamate treatment on platelet response to ADP in patients with peripheral atherosclerosis. Each point represents the mean values obtained for each concentration of ADP in 13 patients.

pyridinolcarbamate reduced the platelet aggregation response to adrenaline as well as to ADP in patients with atherosclerosis. He considered that this was an indirect effect.

We have gained some further insight into the pharmacological activity of pyridinolcarbamate following the use of the compound in diabetic rats and in rats with adjuvant arthritis. In one of these experiments the effect of pyridinolcarbamate on blood changes in rats with streptozotocin-induced diabetes was investigated. Two groups of diabetic rats were used. One group received the compound in the diet at a dose required to give blood levels similar to that obtained in patients receiving 1,500 mg daily (20–40 μg/ml). The other group received a normal diet. After 9 weeks of this regime blood samples were taken and the animals were killed. It was apparent (Fig. 3) that in the pyridinolcarbamate group of animals there was a reversal of the abnormal trend found in the haematological results in the untreated diabetic rats. The total serum protein, which was reduced in the control diabetic rats, was significantly

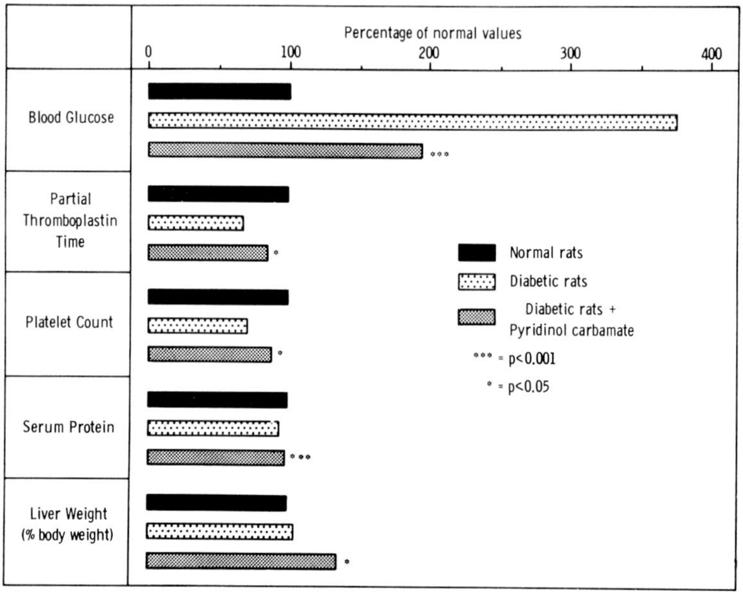

Fig. 3. Effect of pyridinolcarbamate on blood changes in streptozotocin-induced diabetes in the rat.

increased in the treated group. Blood glucose levels were significantly reduced towards normal values; there was significant lengthening of partial thromboplastin clotting times and a rise in platelet count towards normal values in the group receiving pyridinolcarbamate. There was also an increase in liver weight relative to body weight in this group. At no stage of the experiment was there any significant difference in the body weights between the control diabetic rats and the diabetic rats treated with pyridinolcarbamate.

The mechanism producing the shortened clotting times and reduction in platelet counts in the diabetic rats is not known. These changes could conceivably be due to the release of circulating procoagulant factors from the tissues or blood vessels into the circulation and that pyridinolcarbamate is able to interfere with the release of these factors.

In a further experiment the effect of pyridinolcarbamate on adjuvant arthritic rats was investigated. Rats with arthritic lesions of 3 weeks' duration were used. These were divided into 3 groups. One group received pyridinolcarbamate at the same dose as in the previous experiment, another group received β-hydroxyethylrutoside (Paroven) in a similar dose and the third group received a normal diet without added treatment. At the end of the 4 weeks it was noted (Fig. 4) that the spleen weight, which is increased in the untreated arthritic rats, was of normal size in the pyridinolcarbamate-treated group and in the group receiving the rutosides. In contrast to the diabetic rats no increase in liver weight was produced in the arthritic rats receiving pyridinolcarbamate. A significant reduction in the raised plasma fibrinogen levels was produced in the arthritic rats receiving pyridinolcarbamate or rutosides.

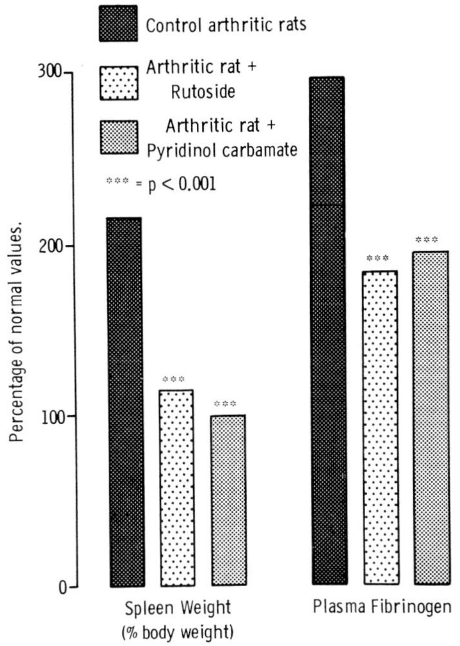

Fig. 4. Effect of pyridinolcarbamate and β-hydroxyethylrutoside on spleen weight and plasma fibrinogen in adjuvant arthritic rats.

As a result of these animal experiments it is tempting to postulate that in the human disease situation the compound is preventing the release into the circulation of substances causing aggregation of platelets and stimulation of fibrinogen synthesis. The increase in sensitivity of the platelets to ADP in the patients studied here, before treatment, could be an indication that they have been affected by some agent which is being released into the circulation. Pyridinolcarbamate may inhibit the release or neutralize the effects of such an agent. Platelet turnover in the presence of the compound, in the early treatment period, may therefore result in platelet populations containing an increasing proportion of platelets which have not been exposed to the type of environment which was present before therapy. Thus by the 5th week of treatment the numbers of relatively normal platelets (according to their response to ADP) may be such that they are detectable in the test system.

In a number of trials of pyridinolcarbamate in patients with peripheral atherosclerosis it was claimed that the compound produced an improvement in blood flow in the affected limbs after a few months of treatment (De Soldati et al., 1969; Bronstein et al., 1969; Shimamoto et al., 1970). The compound has no vasodilator activity and it is suggested that the drug produced its effect through a direct or indirect action on the atheromatous areas in the affected arteries resulting in some degree of resolution of the arterial lesions (Shimamoto et al., 1970). The Framingham study indicated that the rate of remission of symptoms of intermittent claudication is high. Among those who were followed for 4 or more years from the onset of their symptoms 45% had disappearance of their symptoms for at least 4 years (Kannel and Shurtleff, 1971). This factor must be taken into account in evaluating the efficacy of therapy and in the planning of clinical trials involving patients with arteriosclerosis obliterans. We would therefore be interested to see results of controlled trials involving large numbers of patients who have received pyridinolcarbamate over several years.

REFERENCES

BRONSTEIN, J., GALEANO, J. C. and SOUTRIC, J. L. (1969): Results obtained with pyridinolcarbamate in the treatment of atherosclerosis in different sectors of the organism. In: *Atherogenesis. Proceedings, I International Symposium on Atherogenesis, Thrombogenesis and Pyridinolcarbamate Treatment, Tokyo 1969*, pp. 251–259. Editors: T. Shimamoto and F. Numano. ICS 201, Excerpta Medica, Amsterdam.

DE SOLDATI, L., CASTRO, C. M., GRILLI, H. and REUSSI, J. (1969): Clinical trials with pyridinolcarbamate on arterial circulation and blood coagulation in patients with atherosclerosis obliterans. In: *Atherogenesis. Proceedings, I International Symposium on Atherogenesis, Thrombogenesis and Pyridinolcarbamate Treatment, Tokyo 1969*, pp. 153–162. Editors: T. Shimamoto and F. Numano. ICS 201, Excerpta Medica, Amsterdam.

DHALL, D. P., ENGESET, J., MCKENZIE, F. N. and MATHESON, N. A. (1969): Screen filtration pressure of blood – An evaluation. *Cardiovasc. Res.*, *3*, 147.

DHALL, D. P. and MATHESON, N. A. (1969): Platelet aggregation filtration pressure – A method of measuring platelet aggregation in whole blood. *Cardiovasc. Res.*, *3*, 155.

KANNEL, W. B. and SHURTLEFF, D. (1971): The natural history of arteriosclerosis obliterans. *Cardiovasc. Clin.*, *3*, 37.

PILGERAM, L. O. (1961): Relation of plasma fibrinogen concentration changes to human arteriosclerosis. *J. appl. Physiol.*, *16*, 660.

SAMAMA, M. (1971): Personal communication.

SHIMAMOTO, T. (1963): The relationship of edematous reaction in arteries to atherosclerosis and thrombosis. *J. Atheroscler. Res.*, *3*, 87.

SHIMAMOTO, T. (1969): Visualization of the transendothelial passage through intercellular junctions and discovery of endothelial folds and intercellular bridges of vascular endothelium. In: *Atherogenesis. Proceedings, I International Symposium on Atherogenesis, Thrombogenesis and Pyridinolcarbamate Treatment, Tokyo 1969*, pp. 5–27. Editors: T. Shimamoto and F. Numano. ICS 201, Excerpta Medica, Amsterdam.

SHIMAMOTO, T., ATSUMI, T., YAMASHITA, S., MOTOMIYA, T., ISOKANE, N., ISHIOKA, T. and SAKUMA, A. (1970): Clinical pharmacologic evaluation of the antiatherosclerotic agent, pyridinol carbamate. A double-blind cross over trial in the treatment of atherosclerosis obliterans. *Amer. Heart J.*, *79*, 5.

SWANK, R. L., ROTH, J. G. and JANSEN, J. (1964): Screen filtration pressure method and adhesiveness and aggregation of blood cells. *J. appl. Physiol.*, *19*, 340.

VIRCHOW, R. (1856): *Gesammelte Abhandlungen zur wissenschaftlichen Medizin.* Staatsdruckerei, Frankfurt.

VIRCHOW, R. (1871): *Die celluläre Pathologie, in ihrer Begrundung auf physiologische und pathologische Gewebelehre.* Berlin.

DISCUSSION

Dr. HENRY: How long did you wait after the addition of ADP to make the pressure measurements?

Dr. COTTON: 60 sec. In preliminary investigations we measured the pressure response after various periods of time and found that the maximum response to ADP was around 60 sec after the addition of this agent. This is in accord with the observations of Dhall and Matheson (1969).

Dr. SPECTOR: Could you indicate a little bit more about the clinical state of the patients studied? Are you especially interested in whether any of them has aberrations in cholesterol or triglycerides?

Dr. Cotton: We measured the levels of cholesterol and the Sf 0–20 and Sf 20–400 lipoproteins in all of these patients. The serum cholesterol and lipoproteins were not significantly raised in these patients as compared with the older normal subjects. Your question is also of interest because we have noted that with progression of the disease the serum cholesterol level actually falls. Six of the 21 patients we investigated required amputation 1 or 2 months later. The mean serum cholesterol level in these 6 patients was significantly lower than the mean value for cholesterol in the rest of the group.

Dr. Camerini-Davalos: I wonder if you would like to suggest some explanation for the effect of pyridinolcarbamate on the blood glucose levels in your streptozotocin animals because in our KK mice with almost normal amounts of insulin the compound had no effect on blood glucose. In our animals we gave the compound by a stomach tube. Would you like to suggest the mechanism?

Dr. Cotton: I find the interpretation of this result difficult because this is not my field. In our experiment pyridinolcarbamate was incorporated in the diet. The blood level of pyridinolcarbamate would therefore fluctuate during the day according to their feeding habits. Over the 24 hour period we obtained blood values up to 90 μg/ml and as low as 5–10 μg/ml and the mean value was close to 40 μg/ml (which is the level obtained in patients on treatment). The animals were therefore under the influence of the compound for most of the 24 hours and one wonders whether our results differ from yours because of this. I would also hesitate to compare the changes found in streptozotocin-induced diabetes in rats with those found in your KK mice. We were also intrigued by the increase in size of the livers of our diabetic rats treated with pyridinolcarbamate. We found no increase in liver size in control rats dosed with equivalent amounts of the compound. We wondered whether there were changes in gluconeogenesis in the diabetic rats on pyridinolcarbamate which might affect the blood sugar levels. These results are preliminary ones and obviously further work is required on the mechanism of action of pyridinolcarbamate in this situation.

Dr. W. Oppermann: The blood sugar levels in your streptozotocin-induced diabetic rats is much higher than ours. You are therefore more prone to find an effect on blood sugar levels because you are dealing with much higher levels to begin with.

Dr. Cotton: Yes, this is possible.

EFFECT OF PYRIDINOLCARBAMATE TREATMENT ON ADP-INDUCED PLATELET ADHESIVENESS*

S. BYGDEMAN and F. LUND

Department of Clinical Physiology, Karolinska Institutet at the Serafimerhospital and Stureby Sjukhus Geriatric Unit, Enskede, Stockholm, Sweden

The effect of pyridinolcarbamate treatment on ADP-induced platelet adhesiveness to glass was studied in 20 patients with peripheral occlusive atherosclerosis. The investigation was initiated by a preliminary study in 3 patients which indicated a decrease of platelet adhesiveness induced by pyridinolcarbamate (referred to by Lund et al., 1969).

The patients were given pyridinolcarbamate in a dose of 250 mg 3 times daily for the first week and thereafter the dose was increased to 500 mg 3 times daily.

TABLE I

Effect of pyridinolcarbamate treatment on ADP-induced platelet adhesiveness to glass. ADP concentration 0.10 and 0.15 μg/ml plasma

Patient	Platelet adhesiveness (%)									
	ADP concentration 0.10 μg/ml					ADP concentration 0.15 μg/ml				
	Control	Weeks of treatment				Control	Weeks of treatment			
		2	5	9	18		2	5	9	18
1	39	50	6	50	29	57	69	49	56	56
2	38	46	28	26	24	59	72	44	44	61
3	33	20	–	6	8	58	45	–	12	15
4	61	40	53	–	–	75	60	66	–	–
5	31	32	24	31	–	49	46	35	48	–
6	25	25	30	–	–	37	35	42	46	–
7	60	87	65	–	–	76	89	71	–	–
8	89	90	51	72	–	88	94	70	86	–
9	52	–	54	48	–	63	–	65	66	–
10	24	–	19	–	–	37	–	30	–	–
11	52	59	53	46	–	77	72	71	64	–
12	44	38	14	28	–	68	65	34	44	–
13	30	35	39	40	–	41	59	65	57	–
14	34	18	21	33	–	48	55	45	55	–
15	59	48	52	46	–	70	72	68	64	–
16	39	42	40	62	–	68	77	63	79	–
17	37	61	66	33	–	85	84	86	68	–
18	70	29	34	65	–	69	49	52	79	–
19	32	43	52	25	–	49	65	69	54	–
20	56	38	38	33	–	69	52	54	52	–
Mean	45	45	39	40	(20)	62	64	57	57	(44)

* This investigation was supported in part by a research grant from the Swedish Medical Research Council No. 14X-1019-08B.

ADP-induced platelet adhesiveness was determined by the method of Hellem et al. (1963). Blood samples were taken in the morning from the antecubital vein with the patient fasting. The blood was collected in glass tubes containing 1/10 Vol 3.13 % trisodium citrate dihydrate. Platelet-rich plasma was prepared by centrifuging the blood at $290 \times g$ at room temperature for 15 min. Platelet counts were determined with an electronic particle counter (Celloscope 202, Ljungberg Ltd, Stockholm) at an accuracy of $\pm 2\%$. The citrated platelet-rich plasma was passed through a glass bead column under standardized conditions immediately after the addition of ADP. The number of adhesive platelets was taken as the difference between the platelet count before and after the passage and expressed in percent of the original number.

Platelet adhesiveness was determined prior to the start of pyridinolcarbamate treatment (control value) and following 2, 5 and 9 and, in 3 patients, 18 weeks of treatment. The ADP concentrations used were 0.10 and 0.15 μg/ml plasma. The results are summarized in Table I. Although pyridinolcarbamate treatment induced a substantial decrease in platelet adhesiveness in some of the patients, the overall change in adhesiveness was small and was not statistically significant. The results therefore do not support the assumption that a therapeutic effect of pyridinolcarbamate in peripheral atherosclerotic disease in man is secondary to an inhibition of ADP-induced platelet adhesiveness as evaluated by Hellem's method.

In a few preliminary experiments the effect of pyridinolcarbamate on ADP-induced platelet aggregation in vitro was studied by the turbidometric method of Born. The results indicated that no inhibitory effect could be observed unless very high concentrations (500 μg/ml plasma) of pyridinolcarbamate were used.

REFERENCES

HELLEM, A. J., ÖDEGAARD, A. E. and SKÅLHEGG, B. A. (1963): Investigations on adenosinediphosphate (ADP) induced platelet adhesiveness in vitro. I. The ADP-platelet reactions in various experimental conditions. *Thrombos. Diathes. haemorrh. (Stuttg.)*, *10*, 61.

LUND, F., HELLSTRÖM, L. and FRISCH, P. (1969): Pulse recording and arteriography in a long-term study with pyridinolcarbamate. In: *Atherogenesis. Proceedings, I International Symposium on Atherogenesis, Thrombogenesis and Pyridinolcarbamate Treatment, Tokyo 1969*, pp. 181–193. Editors: T. Shimamoto and F. Numano. ICS 201, Excerpta Medica, Amsterdam.

THE STUDY OF PYRIDINOLCARBAMATE IN HEALTHY SUBJECTS*

R. MALLEIN, J. RONDELET, M. BOUCHERAT and Mlle H. AVENUE
Hôpital de l'Antiquaille, Lyon, France

STUDY OF PYRIDINOLCARBAMATE IN THE BLOOD-STREAM

The authors have studied blood levels obtained following the administration of a unit dose of 1 g pyridinolcarbamate. For this purpose they have used spectrophotometric analysis at 264 nm, after chloroform extraction. All analyses were carried out after subtraction of a reference value (chloroform extraction of serum from the subject studied, this being done immediately prior to administration of the drug.)

Figure 1 shows blood concentration curves obtained in 10 subjects during a period of 8 hours. Following administration of the drug, maximum concentration appeared between the 2nd and 9th hours, with an average maximum level at the 5th hour (26 μg).

Figure 2 shows blood concentration curves obtained in 4 subjects over 24 hours. Concentration appeared close to 10 μg at the 24th hour.

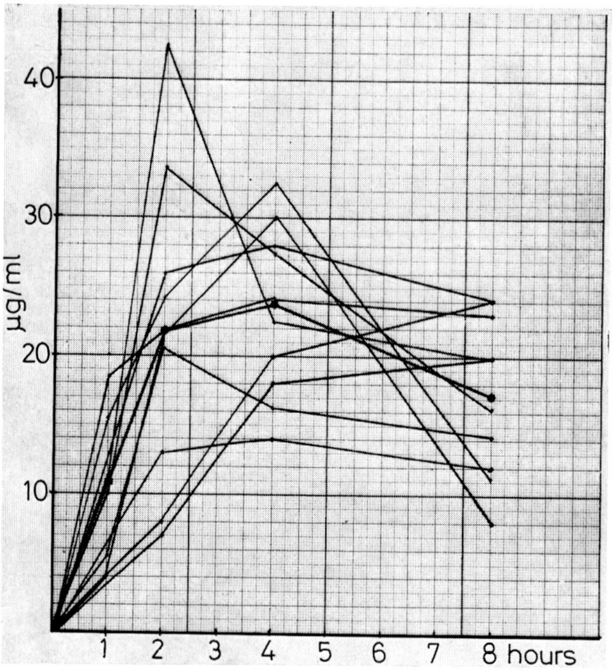

Fig. 1. Pyridinolcarbamate 1 g. Blood concentration curves obtained in 10 subjects during a period of 8 hours.

* Presented by Dr. A. Perrin, Hôpital Cardiovasculaire et Pneumologique, Bron, France.

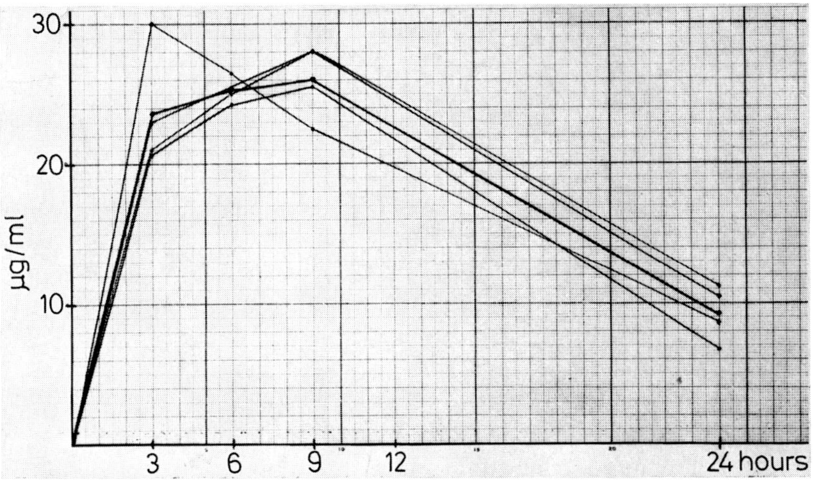

Fig. 2. Pyridinolcarbamate 1 g. Blood concentration curves obtained in 4 subjects over 24 hours.

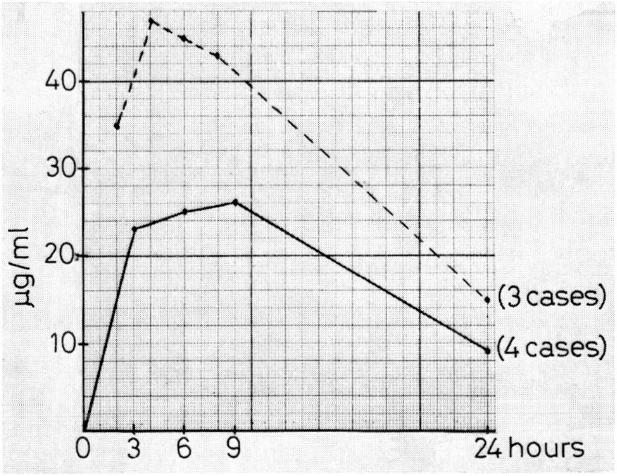

Fig. 3. Pyridinolcarbamate 1 g. Blood concentration curves obtained over 24 hours.
---- Japanese study; ——— our results.

Figure 3 shows blood concentrations over 24 hours in a Japanese study (upper curve, average for 3 subjects) and a curve based on our results (lower curve, average for 4 subjects). (It is possible that the Japanese authors (Maezawa et al., 1965) have not discounted the optical density obtained with the reference serum, hence the inflated results.)

The half-life of pyridinolcarbamate calculated on the basis of the blood concentration curves varies between 5 and 12 hours, and the shape of the curves is in favour of prolonged elimination of the pyridinolcarbamate.

URINARY EXCRETION OF PYRIDINOLCARBAMATE. EVIDENCE OF 2 METABOLITES

The authors have perfected a technique of chromatographic isolation followed by spectrophotometric analysis, which has enabled them to demonstrate the presence in the urine of

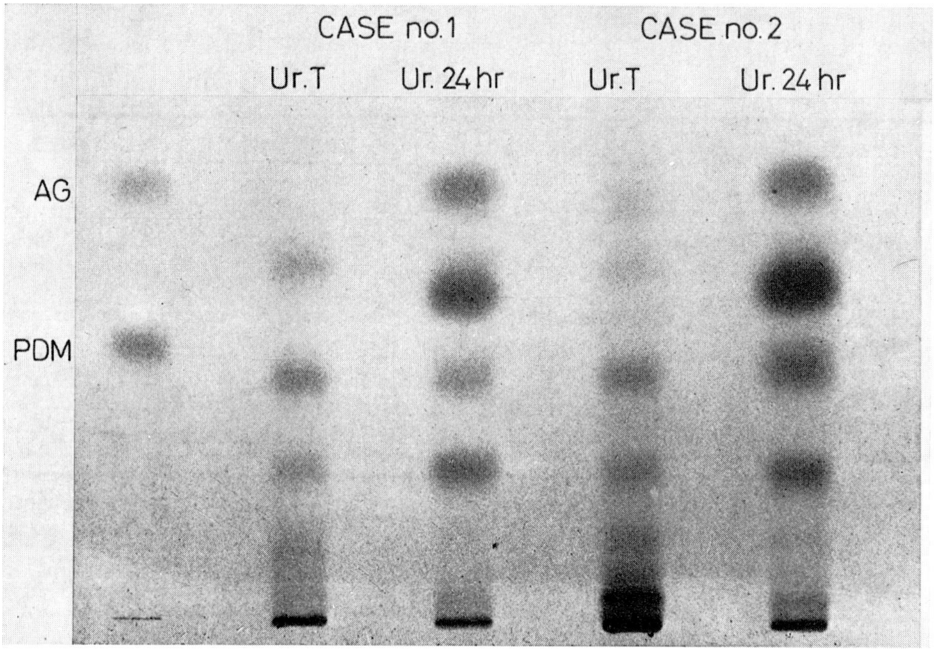

Fig. 4. Ultraviolet photo of a chromatographic plate. Far left, standard sample. 1st and 3rd columns, control urine; 2nd and 4th columns, urine from subjects treated with pyridinolcarbamate. AG = Anginin, PDM = 2,6-pyridinedimethanol. For further explanation, see text.

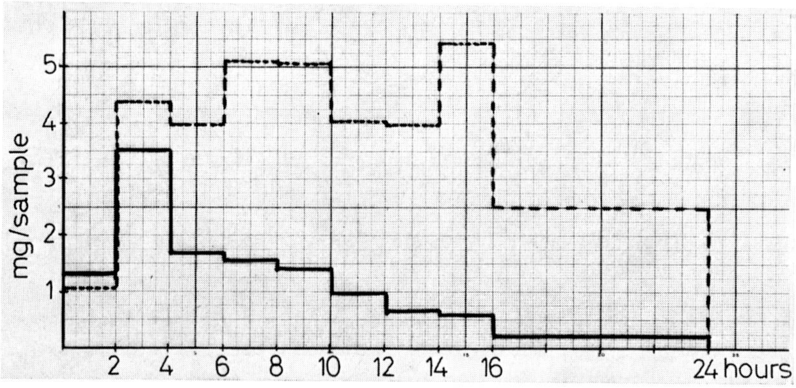

Fig. 5. Elimination of urinary metabolites over 24 hours.
——— pyridinolcarbamate; ----- second metabolite.

subjects treated with pyridinolcarbamate, of 2 metabolites of different Rf, which are excreted in varying proportions: (1) Rf 0.52 which is unmodified pyridinolcarbamate; (2) Rf 0.39 which has an identified structure.

Figure 4 is an ultraviolet photo of a chromatographic plate. Different chromatographic spots in dark blue on a light-blue base can be clearly observed (1st and 3rd columns, control urine; 2nd and 4th columns, urine from subjects treated with the drug). In the urine from subjects treated with the drug, there are 2 additional spots: (1) Rf 0.52 which corresponds to the pyridinolcarbamate and (2) Rf 0.39 which corresponds to the second metabolite. The variation of these metabolites with time is of interest.

Figure 5 shows elimination of the 2 urinary metabolites over a 24-hour consecutive period. Pyridinolcarbamate, the first metabolite, predominates only during the first 2 hours. From the 3rd hour onwards there is a progressive increase in the second metabolite. At the 6th hour, the level of the second metabolite is 4 times greater than that of the pyridinolcarbamate.

Figure 6 shows elimination of a unit dose of 1 g pyridinolcarbamate over a period of 5 days. The first metabolite is found only during the first 24 hours; the second is found in decreasing quantities over the following 3 days.

Figure 7 shows urinary elimination of the metabolites during a 4-day course of treatment (1 g pyridinolcarbamate per day). During the 4 days of treatment, the 2 metabolites are

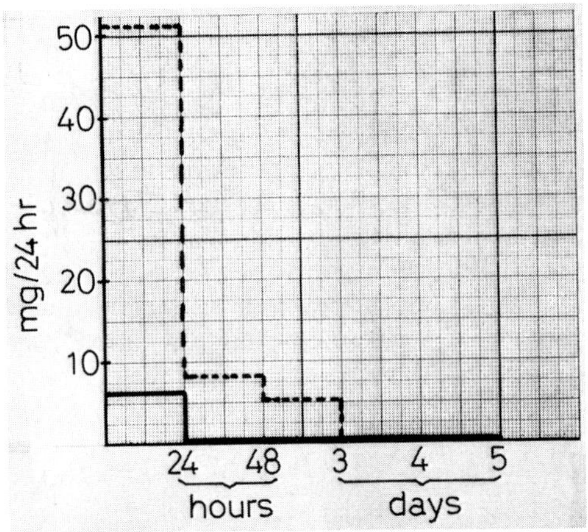

Fig. 6. Subject O.R. Urinary metabolites of a unit dose of pyridinolcarbamate over a period of 5 days. ——— pyridinolcarbamate; ---- second metabolite.

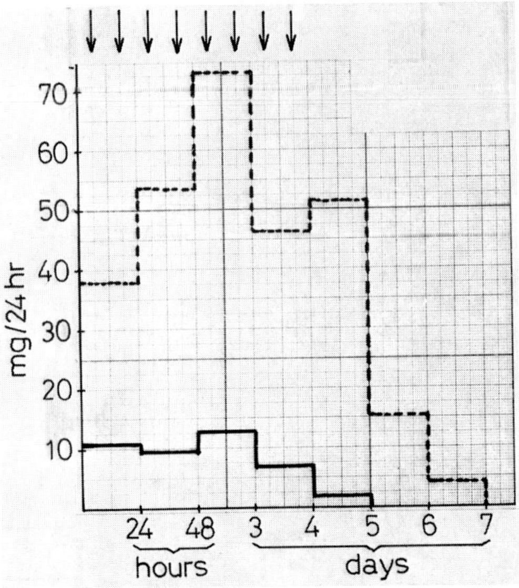

Fig. 7. Urinary elimination of metabolites during a 4-day course of pyridinolcarbamate treatment (1 g/day). Each arrow corresponds to 500 mg. ——— pyridinolcarbamate; ---- second metabolite.

present, the second predominating between 4 and 5 times. After termination of treatment, the first metabolite persists for no more than 24 hours, then disappears completely in favour of the second, the latter being found for a further 3 consecutive days after termination of treatment.

CONCLUSION

This study shows that the first urinary metabolite, pyridinolcarbamate, predominates for no more than the first 2 hours, then disappears progressively in favour of the second metabolite, this being the only one of the two still found after 24 hours. This shows that the transformation of pyridinolcarbamate into the second metabolite, in a healthy subject, is complete within a period of 24 hours after administration.

SUMMARY

The authors have studied the kinetics of pyridinolcarbamate in the blood and urine of healthy, adult male subjects, who received a unit dose of 1 g pyridinolcarbamate.

The blood levels of pyridinolcarbamate were measured in serum samples, after chloroform extraction and spectrophotometric reading at 264 nm. For a unit dose of 1 g pyridinolcarbamate, maximum blood levels varied from 14 to 42 μg/ml with an average maximum of 26 μg. The half-life of pyridinolcarbamate varies between 5 and 12 hours.

The authors have made a particular study of the urinary metabolites of pyridinolcarbamate. They have perfected a technique for chromatographic isolation, followed by spectrophotometric analysis, which has enabled them to demonstrate the presence in the urine of subjects treated with pyridinolcarbamate of 2 metabolites of different Rf, which are eliminated in varying proportions.

The percentage urinary elimination of the total metabolites of pyridinolcarbamate over 24 hours varies from 6.67 to 11.7% with an average of 8.22%.

The authors have shown that the first metabolite (pyridinolcarbamate) predominates only during the first 2 hours after treatment, then disappears progressively in favour of the second metabolite (monodemethylpyridinolcarbamate), which is the only one of the two still found after 24 hours.

It therefore appears that transformation of pyridinolcarbamate into the second metabolite in a healthy subject is complete within 24 hours.

REFERENCE

MAEZAWA, H., ATSUMI, T., SAGAWA, N., SANO, T. and ODAKURA, T. (1965): *Ochanomizu med. J.*, *13/3*.

SUBJECT INDEX

A

INDEX OF AUTHORS